FAILED INTUBATION

| Can't intubate | *Reposition pillows* |

⇓

| Try a gum elastic bougie STOP trying if unsuccessful × 2 attempts | *Use a McCoy blade* |

⇓

| CALL FOR HELP | *Senior anaesthetist* |

⇓

| Maintain cricoid pressure |

⇓

| WAKE UP & POSTPONE SURGERY | ⇐ | IN THE PATIENT'S BEST INTERESTS SHOULD YOU... | ⇒ | CONTINUE ANAESTHESIA & SURGERY |

⇓

| Can you ventilate and oxygenate? | No⇒ | Progress down this list until you can oxygenate...
• Insert Guedel airway
• Two hands to mask
• Nasal airway
• LMA/COPA/Combitube
• Release cricoid
• Needle cricothyroidotomy | ⇐No | Can you ventilate and oxygenate? |

⇓YES (left) ⇓YES (right)

| • Wake up the patient
• Regional technique?
• Awake fibreoptic? | | | | • Continue on a mask
• Consider an LMA
• Allow spontaneous ventilation
• Deepen volatile agent |

D1322978

Oxford Handbook of Anaesthesia

Keith G. Allman
Consultant Anaesthetist

and

Iain H. Wilson
Consultant Anaesthetist
both at the Royal Devon and Exeter Hospital, UK

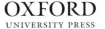

OXFORD
UNIVERSITY PRESS

OXFORD

UNIVERSITY PRESS

Great Clarendon Street, Oxford OX2 6DP

Oxford University Press is a department of the University of Oxford.
It furthers the University's objective of excellence in research, scholarship,
and education by publishing worldwide in

Oxford New York

Auckland Bangkok Buenos Aires Cape Town Chennai Dar es Salaam
Delhi Hong Kong Istanbul Karachi Kolkata Kuala Lumpur Madrid
Melbourne Mexico City Mumbai Nairobi São Paulo Shanghai
Taipei Tokyo Toronto

Oxford is a registered trade mark of Oxford University Press
in the UK and in certain other countries

Published in the United States
by Oxford University Press Inc., New York

A catalogue record for this title is available from the British Library

Library of Congress Cataloguing in Publication Data

Oxford handbook of anaesthesia/[edited by] Keith Allman and Iain Wilson.
(Oxford medical publications)
Includes index.
1. Anesthesia – Handbooks, manuals, etc.   I. Title: Handbook of anaesthesia
II. Allman, Keith   III. Wilson, Iain, Dr.   IV. Series.
[DNLM: 1. Anesthesia – methods – Handbooks   2. Anesthetics – Handbooks.
3. Surgical Procedures, Operative – Handbooks. WO 231 098 2001]
RD82.2.096 2001   617.9'6 – dc21   2001036909
ISBN 0 19 263273 6 (alk. paper)
10 9 8 7 6 5 4 3 2

Typeset in Minion
by EXPO Holdings, Malaysia
Printed in Italy
on acid-free paper by
LegoPrint S.p.A.

Preface

This handbook is aimed at anaesthetists who have received at least basic training in anaesthesia. It does not tell the reader how to give an anaesthetic, but aims to help decide the best anaesthetic for different situations. We have tried to be selective about the contents of the book and have omitted some of the more traditional, but less relevant, topics for our target audience. The text is split into sections:

Section I (Chapters 1–12) gives standard information on pre-operative considerations such as consent and preoperative investigations and details the implications of pre-existing medical conditions. We have provided information about further reading for many of the varied conditions that are met in clinical practice, and have tried to give practical advice whenever possible, though in many situations the evidence base for choosing one technique over another is not available.

Section II (Chapters 13–33) gives practical, comprehensive advice for different surgical specialities. When compiling this section we asked colleagues with specific areas of expertise to describe their standard approach for their most common operations. The techniques and practical considerations described are not meant to be exclusive, but do represent a standard approach to many of the more common procedures. We hope these clinical descriptions will help anaesthetists working outside their immediate areas of expertise. In no way can guidelines substitute for supervized training but it is a fact of life that although anaesthetists are specialized by day, out of hours many of us have to be prepared to deal with a considerably wider range of surgery. We have included some details on more specialized areas of surgery such as cardiac surgery, neurosurgery and liver transplantation to give a basic grounding to trainees rotating through these fields.

Section III (Chapter 34) covers obstetric anaesthetic practice and Section IV (Chapter 35) covers paediatric and neonatal anaesthesia. Section V (Chapter 36) covers anaesthetic emergencies. Section VI (Chapters 37–48) discusses a range of practical issues such as airway assessment. Section VII deals with acute pain issues and Section VIII is concerned with regional anaesthesia.

Also included are appendices containing a drug formulary, infusion regimes, and normal values.

We hope that this handbook will be useful to a variety of anaesthetists. The exam candidate should find many basic principles listed and trainees should find the information concerning different areas of anaesthesia useful when moving between specialities. We hope that more senior colleagues will also find much of the information useful, both in theatre and when preparing a teaching session.

The book represents many hours of work by many people, and we owe thanks to the numerous persons who helped with the project. In particular we acknowledge the support given by our wives and families.

We are keen to receive comments about the book; its imperfections and deficiencies are as important as any positive feedback. Also, if you know of any better approaches to the problems or operations listed, or would like to add material not covered, please e-mail us. Try also to suggest which sections should be deleted.

Despite exhaustive efforts to check for drug dose errors, it is possible that some exist, please check carefully.

Keith Allman and Iain Wilson
2001
oxford.handbook.anaesthesia@ukgateway.net

Contents

Section IV
Paediatric and neonatal anaesthesia

Section VII
Acute pain

Section VIII
Regional anaesthesia

List of abbreviations

A&E	Accident and emergency
AAA	Abdominal aortic aneurysm
ABC	airway, breathing, circulation
ABG	Arterial blood gas
ACT	Activated clotting time
ADH	Antidiuretic hormone
AF	Atrial fibrillation
ALS	advanced life support
ALT	alanine aminotransferase
AMD	airway management device
AP	Anteroposterior
APTR	activated partial thromboplastin ratio
APTT	Activated partial thromboplastin time
ARDS	Acute respiratory distress syndrome
ASA	American Society of Anesthesiologists
ASD	Atrio-septal defect
AV	Atrioventricular
bd	twice daily
BIPAP	Biphasic positive airways pressure
BMI	Body mass index
BNF	British National Formulary
BP	Blood pressure
C&S	Culture and sensitivity
CABG	Coronary arterial bypass grafting
CBF	Cerebral blood flow
CCU	Coronary care unit
CEA	Caudal extradural analgesia
Ch	Charrière (French) gauge (also FG or Fr)
CK-MB	creatine kinase - myocardial isoenzyme
CMV	Cytomegalovirus
CNS	Central nervous system

COAD	Chronic obstructive airways disease
COETT	Cuffed oral endotracheal tube
COHb	carboxyhaemoglobin
COPA	cuffed oropharyngeal airway
COPD	Chronic obstructive pulmonary disease
CPAP	Continuous positive airway pressure
CPB	Cardiopulmonary bypass
CPK	creatine (phospho)kinase
CPP	Cerebral perfusion pressure
CPR	Cardio-pulmonary resuscitation
CSE	Combined spinal/epidural
CSF	Cerebrospinal fluid
CT	Computed tomography
CVA	Cerebrovascular accident
CVE	Cerebrovascular episode/event
CVP	Central venous pressure
CVS	Cardiovascular system
DDAVP	Desmopressin
DHCA	Deep hypothermic circulatory arrest
DIC	Disseminated intravascular coagulation
DLT	Double lumen [endobronchial] tube
DVT	Deep vein thrombosis
ECF	Extracellular fluid
ECG	Electrocardiogram
EEG	Electroencephalogram
EMD	electromechanical dissociation
EMG	Electromyograph
EMLA	Eutectic mixture of local anaesthetic
ENT	Ear, nose, and throat
ERPC	Evacuation of retained products of conception
$ETCO_2$	End tidal CO_2
ETT/ET	Endotracheal tube
EUA	Examination under anaesthetic
FBC	Full blood count
FEV_1	Forced expiration in 1 s
FG	French gauge (also Fr or Ch)
FGF	Fresh gas flow

FiO$_2$	Fractional inspired oxygen content
FM	Face mask
FFP	Fresh frozen plasma
Fr	French gauge (also FG or Ch)
FRC	Functional residual capacity
FVC	Forced vital capacity
G	Gauge (standard wire gauge)
G-6-PD	glucose 6-phosphate dehydrogenase
GA	General anaesthetic
G&S	Group and save
GCS	Glasgow coma score
GI(T)	Gastrointestinal (tract)
GTN	Glyceryl trinitrate
HAS	human albumin solution
Hct	Haematocrit
HDU	High-dependency unit
HELLP	Haemolysis, elevated liver enzymes, low platelets
HME	heat and moisture exchanger
HOCM	Hypertrophic obstructive cardiomyopathy
HPA	Hypothalamic–pituitary–adrenal
HRT	Hormone replacement therapy
IABP	Intra-aortic balloon pump
IBP	invasive blood pressure
ICP	Intracranial pressure
ICU	Intensive care unit
ID	Internal diameter
IDDM	Insulin-dependent diabetes mellitus
I:E ratio	Inspired: expired ratio
IHD	Ischaemic heart disease
ILMA	Intubating laryngeal mask airway
IM	intra-muscular
INR	International normalized ratio
IO	intra-osseous
IOP	Intraocular pressure
IPPV	Intermittent positive pressure ventilation
ITP	Idiopathic thrombocytopenic purpura
ITU	Intensive therapy unit

IV	Intravenous
IVC	Inferior vena cava
IVI	Intravenous infusion
IVRA	Intravenous regional anaesthesia
JVP	Jugular venous pressure
LA	Local anaesthetic
LFT	Liver function test
LMA	Laryngeal mask airway
LMWH	Low-molecular-weight heparin
LV	Left ventricle/ventricular
LSCS	lower segment caesarean section
LVEDP	left ventricular end diastolic pressure
LVF	Left ventricular failure
LVH	Left ventricular hypertrophy
MAC	Minimal alveolar concentration
MAOI	Monoamine oxidase inhibitor
MAP	Mean arterial pressure
MCV	Mean corpuscular volume
MH	Malignant hyperthermia
MI	Myocardial infarction
MIBG	*Meta*-iodobenzylguanidine
MRI	Magnetic resonance imaging
MRSA	Methicillin-resistant *Staphylococcus aureus*
MST	morphine sulphate
MUA	Manipulation under anaesthesia
NCA	Nurse-controlled analgesia
NIBP	Non-invasive blood pressure
NIDDM	Non-insulin-dependent diabetes mellitus
NIPPV	Non-invasive positive pressure ventilation
NMDA	N-methyl-D-aspartate
nocte	at night
NR	not recommended
NSAID	Non-steroidal anti-inflammatory drug
OCP	Oral contraceptive pill
od	once daily
OLV	One-lung ventilation
ORIF	Open reduction internal fixation

PA	Pulmonary artery/arterial
PA	postero-anterior
$PaCO_2$	Arterial partial pressure of CO_2
PAFC	pulmonary artery flotation catheter
PaO_2	Arterial partial pressure of O_2
P_AO_2	alveolar partial pressure of oxygen
PAOP	Pulmonary artery occlusion pressure
PAP	pulmonary artery pressure
PAWP	pulmonary artery wedge pressure
PCA	Patient-controlled analgesia
PCEA	Patient-controlled epidural analgesia
PCWP	Pulmonary capillary wedge pressure
PDA	Patent ductus arteriosus
PE	Pulmonary embolism
PEFR	peak expiratory flow rate
PEEP	Positive end expiratory pressure
PND	Paroxysmal nocturnal dyspnoea
PO	per os (oral)
PONV	Postoperative nausea and vomiting
POP	plaster of paris
$P\bar{v}CO_2$	Mixed venous partial pressure of CO_2
PR	per rectum
prn/PRN	'as required'
PT	prothrombin time
PVC	Polyvinyl chloride
PVR	Pulmonary vascular resistance
qds	four times daily
RAE	Ring, Adair, and Elwyn [tube]
RS	respiratory system
RSI	Rapid sequence induction
RV	right ventricle/ventricular
SA	Sinoatrial
SaO_2	Arterial oxygen saturation
SBE	subacute bacterial endocarditis
SpO_2	Arterial oxygen saturation
SC	Subcutaneous
SCBU	Special care baby unit

SIRS	Systemic inflammatory response syndrome
SL	sublingual
SLT	Single lumen tube
SjO_2	jugular mixed venous oxygen saturation
SNP	sodium nitroprusside
SSRI	Selective serotonin reuptake inhibitor
(S)TOP	(suction) termination of pregnancy
SV	Spontaneous ventilation
SVC	Superior vena cava
$S\bar{v}O_2$	Mixed venous oxygen saturation
SVR	Systemic vascular resistance
SVT	Supraventricular tachycardia
TCD	transcranial Doppler
TCI	Target-controlled infusion
tds	three times daily
TEDS	Thromboembolism stockings
TENS	Transcutaneous electrical nerve stimulation
THR	total hip replacement
TIA	Transient ischaemic attack
TIVA	Total intravenous anaesthesia
TKR	total knee replacement
TPN	Total parenteral nutrition
TURP	Transurethral resection of the prostate
U&E	Urea + electrolytes
URTI	Upper respiratory tract infection
VATS	Video-assisted thoracoscopic surgery
VF	Ventricular fibrillation
VP	Venous pressure
V/Q	ventilation/perfusion
VR	Ventricular rate
VSD	Ventriculo septal defect
V_t or V_T	Tidal volume
VT	Ventricular tachycardia
WBC	White blood cell count
WPW	Wolf Parkinson White
X-match	Cross-match

Major contributors

Anna Batchelor, Consultant Anaesthetist, Newcastle

Mark Bellamy, Consultant in Transplant Anaesthesia and Intensive Care, Leeds

Simon Berg, Consultant Paediatric Anaesthetist, Oxford

Colin Berry, Consultant Anaesthetist, Exeter

Bruce Campbell, Professor of Vascular Surgery, Exeter

Charles Collins, Consultant Anaesthetist, Exeter

David Conn, Consultant in Anaesthesia and Pain Management, Exeter

Peter Davies, Consultant Anaesthetist, Plymouth

Chris Day, Consultant in Anaesthesia and Intensive Care, Exeter

Alasdair Dow, Consultant in Anaesthesia and Intensive Care, Exeter

James Eldridge, Consultant Obstetric Anaesthetist, Portsmouth

Andrew Farmery, Consultant Anaesthetist and Honorary Senior Lecturer, Oxford

Gordon French, Consultant Anaesthetist, Northampton

Jane Halsall, Associate Specialist Malignant Hyperthermia Unit, Leeds

Paul Harvey, Consultant Anaesthetist, Plymouth

Graham Hocking, Specialist Registrar, Royal Air Force

Gavin Kenny, Professor of Anaesthesia, Glasgow

John Lehane, Consultant Anaesthetist, Oxford

Alex Manara, Consultant Neuroanaesthetist, Bristol

Paul Marshall, Consultant in Anaesthesia and Pain Management, Exeter

Peter MacIntyre, Consultant in Anaesthesia and Pain Management, Exeter

Andrew McIndoe, Consultant Anaesthetist and Senior Lecturer, Bristol

Marina Morgan, Consultant Microbiologist, Exeter

Julia Munn, Consultant in Anaesthesia and Intensive Care, Exeter

Julie Murdoch, Clinical Nurse Specialist, Exeter

Peter Murphy, Consultant in Paediatric Anaesthesia and Intensive Care, Bristol

Barry Nicholls, Consultant Anaesthetist, Taunton

Jonathan Purday, Consultant in Anaesthesia and Intensive Care, Exeter

Jerry Nolan, Consultant in Anaesthesia and Intensive Care, Bath

Fred Roberts, Consultant Anaesthetist, Exeter

Mathew Roberts, Consultant Anaesthetist, Royal Army Medical Corps

John Saddler, Consultant Anaesthetist, Exeter

David Sanders, Consultant Anaesthetist, Exeter

Babinder Sandhar, Consultant Anaesthetist, Exeter

Peter Schranz, Consultant Trauma Surgeon, Exeter

Michael Sinclair, Consultant Cardiothoracic Anaesthetist, Oxford

Mark Stoneham, Consultant Anaesthetist, Oxford

Andrew Teasdale, Consultant Anaesthetist, Exeter

Richard Telford, Consultant Anaesthetist, Exeter

Jonathan Warwick, Consultant Anaesthetist, Oxford

David Wilkinson, Medical Artist, Exeter

We would also like to thank the many anaesthetic trainees who have contributed material, Prof Anthony Nicholls and Martin Dresner (Leeds) for expert advice, and the locals of the Manor Inn (Lower Ashton) for support during editorial meetings.

Section I
Preoperative assessment and preparation for anaesthesia

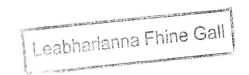

Chapter 1
General considerations

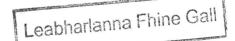

Consent

Background

All competent patients have the right to give or withhold consent for treatment or examination. To obtain consent, the patient must be given sufficient details and information about the procedure to enable a proper decision to be taken. Any procedure undertaken without the patient's consent may be considered an assault in a civil court and may be regarded as serious professional misconduct by the General Medical Council.

Consent may be implied (i.e. the patient willingly cooperates with the procedure), or it may be expressed in written or oral form.

Information

The patient needs sufficient information to allow them to make a considered judgement. This should include:

* A description of the proposed procedure.
* Discussion of alternative options.
* Discussion of the possible complications and their likelihood.
* Discussion of the benefits versus risks.

There is no legal requirement to discuss every possible complication and side-effect but the patient must be warned of any common or serious risks.

Risk

In order to appreciate risk the patient needs to be told of the likelihood of the complication occurring and this should be put into context by using an analogy from everyday life.

* Negligible risk: frequency less than 1:1000 000, i.e. the risk of dying from lightening strike.
* Minimum risk: frequency 1:100 000–1000 000, i.e. the risk of dying on the railways.
* Very low risk: frequency 1:10 000–1:100 000, i.e. the annual risk of dying of an accident at home or at work.
* Low risk: frequency 1:1000 – 10 000, i.e. the annual risk of dying in a road traffic accident.
* Moderate risk: frequency 1:100 to 1:1000, i.e. the risk of death from natural causes for patients over 40 within the next year.
* High risk: frequency greater than 1:100, i.e. the isk of developing diarrhoea after antibiotics.

In addition to the frequency of the risk, the seriousness must be considered. It could be considered negligent to not discuss an infrequent complication, which could result in permanent disability or death. In some patients risk may be increased due to concurrent disease and they should be informed of this. A balance must be achieved between telling the patient enough to enable them to give informed consent, and providing extensive details which result in confusing or needlessly frightening the patient.

Competence

Adult patients who are able to make decisions on their own about their treatment are considered competent. This means that they must be capable of understanding and remembering the information given about the procedure, and be able to weigh up the risks and benefits to arrive at a balanced choice. For competent patients, no other person can consent or refuse treatment on their behalf.

Children and young adults

- Over the age of 16 years, competent young adults can give consent for any treatment without obtaining separate consent from a parent or guardian.
- Children under 16 years who demonstrate the ability to fully appreciate the risks and benefits of the treatment planned may also be considered competent to give consent.
- If a 'competent' child refuses treatment, but the parent has consented, the treatment should only proceed if failure to do so would result in death or permanent injury.
- Parental consent should be sought for any patient under 18 years who is not competent to give consent. If such a child refuses treatment, judgement needs to be exercised by the parent and the doctor as to the level of restraint that is acceptable, depending on the urgency of the case. It may be better to postpone the case until adequate premedication can be given.
- In life-threatening situations, verbal consent by telephone is adequate and essential treatment can be started in the absence of parental authorization.
- Where the child or parent refuse essential treatment, a Ward of Court order can be obtained, but this should not delay the provision of emergency therapy. The Court order enables the doctor to proceed with the treatment lawfully.

Restricted consent

- Some patients may consent to treatment in general, but refuse consent for certain aspects of the treatment, e.g. Jehovah's Witness patients who refuse blood transfusion.
- Restricted consent should be discussed with the patient, in the presence of a witness, so that they are fully aware of the implications of withholding the treatments refused.
- The details of the restriction should be carefully documented on the consent form.
- The patient's wishes must be respected.

Treatment without consent

- In an emergency, consent is not necessary for life-saving procedures.
- Unconscious patients may be given essential treatment without consent. It is good practice to consult with the next of kin, but they cannot give or refuse consent for adult patients.
- Patients who are 'incompetent' may be given treatment provided it is in their best interest.
- Patients detained under the Mental Health Act 1983 may be treated for the mental disorder without consent but not for physical disorder unless they are 'incompetent'. Electroconvulsive therapy requires the patient's consent or the second opinion of an authorized medical practitioner.

Advance statements (directives)

Some patients indicate their preferences regarding treatment in an advance statement (advance directive or living will). The instructions are issued by patients when they are competent, for use when they become unable to express their wishes. Provided the clinical situation falls within the terms of the statement, the wishes of the patient must be respected. The advance statement is usually used to refuse consent for certain treatments, and cannot be used to compel clinicians to perform specific procedures.

Research

- All clinical research requires Research Ethics Committee approval.
- Voluntary consent is required from competent patients, who must be given full information about the purpose of the research, risks involved, and benefits (if any).
- It must be made clear that the patient is not obliged to participate and that they may withdraw from the study at any time. The patient should be reassured that this will not affect their clinical management.
- Patients who are incompetent may only be included in therapeutic research which is in their best interest.
- Competent children are allowed to give consent for therapeutic research associated with minimal risk.
- Parental consent is required for incompetent children.

Teaching

Students must not take part in clinical procedures without the patient's consent. This applies to medical students, student nurses, and trainee paramedical staff.

Documentation

The anaesthetic plan discussed and agreed with the patient should be documented, including a list of the risks which have been explained. Separate written consent is not required for local or regional anaesthesia. The Department of Health recommends that written consent should be obtained for general anaesthesia but the Working Party of the Association of Anaesthetists concluded that this was not necessary.

Further reading

Association of Anaesthetists of Great Britain and Ireland (1999). *Information and consent for anaesthesia.*
General Medical Council (1998). *Seeking patient's consent: the ethical considerations.*
Gilberthorpe J (1997). *Consent to treatment.* The Medical Defence Union, London.
Jones HJS, de Cossart L (1999). Risk scoring in surgical patients. *British Journal of Surgery,* **86**,149–57.

Routine preoperative investigations

A system of routine preoperative investigations for in-patients prior to elective surgery is suggested below. Check local hospital policy. See also p. 272 for day surgery recommendations.

Test	Indications
Urinalysis	All patients: for sugar, blood, and protein
ECG	Age > 50 years
	History of heart disease, hypertension or chronic lung disease
	A normal previous trace within 1 year is acceptable unless there is a recent cardiac history
FBC	Males > 40 years
	All females
	All major surgery
	Whenever anaemia is suspected
Creatinine and electrolytes	Age > 60 years
	All major surgery
	Diuretic drugs
	Suspected renal disease
Blood glucose	Diabetic patients
	Glycosuria
Coagulation screen	History of bleeding tendency (some units measure before major surgery)
Sickle cell test	Black patients with unknown sickle status. If positive then haemoglobin electrophoresis should be performed
Pregnancy test	Whenever there is any chance of pregnancy
Chest radiograph	Not routine
	Acute cardiac or chest disease
	Chronic cardiac or chest disease that has worsened in the last year
	Risk of pulmonary TB (recent arrival from the developing world or immunocompromise)
	Malignant disease

Premedication drugs

See also paediatric premedication (p. 815).

It is well recognized that a clear explanation of anticipated events and a rapport with the anaesthetic team provides more effective anxiolysis than drugs. Premedication is much less commonly prescribed than a few years ago but is still indicated in anxious patients and those in whom there is an increased risk of gastro-oesophageal reflux. Suitable drugs are listed below. Many patients benefit from sedation the night before surgery.

Sedatives: 1 h preoperatively unless otherwise indicated

Benzodiazepines	PO	Lormetazepam	0.5–1.5 mg
		Temazepam	10–30 mg
		Lorazepam (2 h preop.)	1.0–2.5 mg
		Midazolam	0.2–0.5 mg/kg
	IM	Midazolam (20–40 min preop.)	2–10 mg
Non-benzodiazepines	PO	Zopiclone	3.75–7.5 mg

Analgesic drugs

Opioids	Morphine	IM or SC	10–15 mg
	Pethidine	IM	50–100 mg
NSAIDs	Diclofenac	PO or PR	50–100 mg
Other	Paracetamol	PO or PR	1 g

Prokinetic drugs

Metoclopramide	PO, IV, IM	10 mg

Gastric pH increasing drugs

Ranitidine	PO	150–300 mg night before and 2 h preop.
	Slow IV or IM	50 mg 2 h preop.
Omeprazole	PO	40 mg night before and 2–4 h preop.
	IV infusion	40 mg over 30 min
Sodium citrate (0.3 M)	PO	30 ml 10 min preop.

Fasting

Background

Pulmonary aspiration of gastric contents is associated with significant morbidity and mortality. Factors predisposing to regurgitation and pulmonary aspiration include inadequate anaesthesia, pregnancy, obesity, difficult airway, emergency surgery, full stomach, and altered gastrointestinal motility.

Aspiration of 30–40 ml of gastric contents can cause serious pulmonary damage—fasting before anaesthesia aims to reduce the volume of gastric contents.

Gastric physiology

- The preoperative fasting period depends upon the type of food and fluids consumed.
- Clear fluids are emptied from the stomach in an exponential manner with a half-life of 10–20 min, resulting in complete clearance within 2 h of ingestion. Examples of clear fluids include water, fruit juices without pulp, carbonated beverages, clear tea, and black coffee but not alcoholic drinks.
- Gastric emptying of solids is much slower than for fluids and varies depending upon the type of food ingested. Foods with a high fat or meat content require eight or more hours to be emptied from the stomach, whereas a light meal such as toast is usually cleared in 4 h. Milk is considered a solid, because when mixed with gastric juice, it thickens and congeals. However, a small amount of milk (10 ml) added to tea or coffee, does not cause any increase in gastric volume or acidity. Cow's milk takes up to 5 h to empty from the stomach. Human breast milk has a lower fat and protein content and is emptied at a faster rate.

ASA fasting guidelines

In 1999, the American Society of Anesthesiologists (ASA) made the following recommendations on preoperative fasting in elective, healthy patients:

Ingested material	Minimum fast
Clear liquids	2 h
Breast milk	4 h
Infant formula milk	4–6 h
Non-human milk	6 h
Light meal	6 h

Delayed gastric emptying

- Delayed gastric emptying due to metabolic causes (e.g. poorly controlled diabetes mellitus, renal failure), decreased gastric motility (e.g. head injury), or pyloric obstruction (e.g. pyloric stenosis) will primarily affect emptying of solids, particularly high-cellulose foods such as carrots and peas. Gastric emptying of clear fluids is only affected in the advanced stages.
- Gastro-oesophageal reflux may be associated with delayed gastric emptying of solids, but emptying of liquids is not affected.

- Raised intra-abdominal pressure (e.g. pregnancy, obesity) predisposes to passive regurgitation.
- Opioids cause marked delays in gastric emptying.
- Trauma delays gastric emptying. The time interval between the last oral intake and the injury is considered as the fasting period and a rapid sequence induction should be used if this interval is short. The time taken to return to normal gastric emptying after trauma has not been established, and varies depending upon the degree of trauma and the level of pain. The best indicators are probably signs of normal gastric motility such as normal bowel sounds and patient hunger.
- Anxiety has not been shown to have any consistent effect on gastric emptying.
- Oral premedications given 1 h before surgery are without adverse effect on gastric volume on induction of anaesthesia. Studies on oral premedication with midazolam 30 min preoperatively have not reported any link with gastric regurgitation or aspiration.

Chemical control of gastric acidity and volume

- Antacids can be used to neutralize acid in the stomach thereby reducing the risk of damage should aspiration occur. Particulate antacids are not recommended. Sodium citrate solution administered shortly before induction is the is the agent of choice in high-risk cases (e.g. pregnancy) but this results in an increase in gastric volume.
- H_2 blockers/proton pump inhibitors decrease secretion of acid in the stomach and should be used for high-risk patients. Ideally, these agents should be administered on the evening before surgery (or early morning for an afternoon list) and a second dose given 2 h preoperatively. Although these agents are generally very effective, there is a small failure rate and therefore other precautions to prevent aspiration are necessary.
- Gastric motility enhancing agents such as metoclopramide increase gastric emptying in healthy patients, but a clear benefit in trauma patients has not been demonstrated. Metoclopramide is more effective IV than orally.
- Anticholinergic agents do not have a significant effect and are not routinely recommended.
- Pregnant patients should be given ranitidine 150 mg on the evening before elective surgery (or at 0700h for an afternoon list) and again 2 h preoperatively. During labour, high-risk patients should be given oral ranitidine, 150 mg 6-hourly. For emergency cases, ranitidine 50 mg intravenously should be given at the earliest opportunity. In addition, 30 ml of 0.3 M sodium citrate should be given to neutralize any residual gastric acid.

The ASA do not recommend routine use of these agents in healthy, elective patients.

Further reading

Maltby R (1993). New guidelines for preoperative fasting. *Canadian Journal of Anaesthesia*, **40**, R113–R117.
Practice guidelines for preoperative fasting and the use of pharmacological agents for the prevention of pulmonary aspiration: application to healthy patients undergoing elective procedures (1999). *Anesthesiology*, **90**, 896–905.

Prophylaxis of venous thromboembolism

Introduction

- PE is responsible for 10% of all hospital deaths.
- Without prophylaxis 40–80% of high-risk patients develop detectable DVT and up to 10% die from PE.
- Most PEs result from DVTs which start in the venous plexuses of the legs and which then extend up into the common femoral and iliac veins.
- Calf vein DVT is detectable in up to 10% of low-risk patients, but seldom extends into proximal veins.
- DVT can result in chronic leg swelling, skin changes, and ulceration (post phlebitic syndrome).

Reasons for an increased risk of venous thromboembolism at the time of an operation include:

- Hypercoagulability caused by surgery or other factors (cancer, hormone therapy).
- Stasis of blood in the venous plexuses of the leg during anaesthesia.
- Further stasis due to reduced mobility after the operation.
- Damage to veins at the time of surgery.
- Interference with venous return (pregnancy, pelvic surgery, pneumo-peritoneum during laparoscopic surgery).
- Dehydration.
- Conditions causing poor cardiac output.

Remember that any patient confined to bed is at risk of venous thrombo-embolism, even if they have not had an operation, and particularly if other risk factors are present. This applies especially to ill, elderly patients who need prophylaxis from the time of admission.

Risk factors for venous thromboembolism

Patients can be divided into three categories of risk, low, medium, or high, dependent upon the type of operation, patient factors, and associated diseases.

- Duration and type of operation:
  - Operations lasting less than 30 min are considered minor (low risk) and more than 30 min major (higher risk).
  - Particularly high-risk procedures include major joint replacements (hip and knee) and surgery to the abdomen and pelvis.
- Patient factors:
  - previous history of DVT or PE
  - thrombophilia
  - pregnancy, puerperium, oestrogen therapy (contraceptive pill, HRT)
  - age over 40 (risk increases with age)
  - obesity and immobility
  - varicose veins (in abdominal and pelvic surgery, but no evidence of increased risk for varicose vein surgery).

- Associated disease:
  - malignancy (especially metastatic, or in abdomen/pelvis)
  - trauma (especially spinal cord injury and lower limb fractures)
  - heart failure, recent myocardial infarction
  - systemic infection
  - lower limb paralysis (e.g. after stroke)
  - haematological diseases (polycythaemia, leukaemia, paraproteinaemia)
  - other diseases, including nephrotic syndrome and inflammatory bowel disease.

For example, a fit patient over 40 having minor surgery is low risk, whilst a fit patient under 40 having major abdominal surgery is moderate risk; and an elderly patient having pelvic surgery for cancer is high risk for thrombo-embolism.

Methods of prophylaxis

Every hospital should have a policy detailing local practice. General measures which seem logical include:

- avoidance of prolonged immobility (encourage early mobilization)
- avoidance of dehydration.

Subcutaneous heparin

Subcutaneous heparin reduces the incidence of DVT and fatal PE by about two-thirds. Traditionally, unfractionated (ordinary) heparin has been used, but there are advantages to the newer low-molecular-weight heparins.

The small risk of bleeding when using epidural analgesia can be minimized by giving LMWH on the evening before surgery, so that 12 h or more have elapsed before the epidural is inserted (LMWH plasma half-life is 4 h). (See also epidural, p. 998.)

Subcutaneous heparin is usually stopped when patients are fully mobile, or when they leave hospital. However, the incidence of late DVT in orthopaedic practice can be reduced by extended prophylaxis (up to 35 days).

Traditional low-dose unfractionated heparin

Start 2 h before operation in fit patients, and on admission if unfit or immobile

Dose is 5000 units 12-hourly or 8-hourly (8-hourly administration may give greater protection, and should be used for very high risk patients)

Some increase in the risk of bleeding and haematoma formation

---

Low-molecular-weight heparins (LMWHs)

A little more effective than unfractionated heparin in reducing DVT and PE, particularly in trials on hip and knee replacement

Minor bleeding complications, fewer than unfractionated heparin

Daily dosage which is more convenient, but LMWHs more expensive

Daily doses are: certoparin 3000 units, dalteparin 2500 units, enoxaparin 2000 units, tinzaparin 3500 units

Graduated compression stockings (antiembolism stockings)

- These reduce the risk of DVT, but are not proven to reduce PE.
- May give enhanced protection when used in combination with subcutaneous heparin.
- Below-the-knee stockings are probably as effective as above-the-knee stockings.
- Stockings are probably advisable in patients having laparoscopic procedures.
- Fit with care and monitor for pressure damage: they should be avoided in patients with severe arterial disease of the legs (check ankle systolic pressure if in doubt).

Intermittent pneumatic compression devices

- These devices compress the leg (35–40 mmHg) for about 10 s every minute, promoting venous flow.
- These are as effective as heparin in reducing the incidence of DVT.
- Used particularly in orthopaedic practice to avoid the bleeding risks of heparin, or in combination with heparin.
- Foot pumps are similar, and promote blood flow by compressing the venous plexuses of the feet.

Warfarin, dextran, and aspirin.

- Warfarin is used most often in orthopaedic practice, where there is good evidence of its efficacy in relation to hip operations. It may be given either as a fixed low dose (2 mg/day), or as a monitored dose (target INR 2.0–3.0). It is often started the day before operation, but may be given at 2 mg/day for 2 weeks preoperatively, and then as a higher monitored dose after the operation.
- Dextran (Dextran 70 and 40) is as effective as subcutaneous heparin in preventing DVT and PE, but is not often used because it requires intravenous infusion. Fluid overload is a risk, and anaphylaxis can occasionally occur.
- Aspirin provides some protection against venous thromboembolism, but is less effective than other methods.

Choice of anaesthetic

- Local anaesthesia eliminates the lower limb immobility associated with general anaesthesia.
- Regional anaesthesia (spinal/epidural) appears to be protective in certain kinds of surgery, especially hip/knee replacement.

Oral contraceptive pills (OCPs) and venous thromboembolism

- The risk of spontaneous venous thrombosis is increased in women taking combined OCPs, particularly third-generation pills containing desogestrel or gestodene.
- OCPs may increase the risk of perioperative thromboembolism by up to 3 to 4 times but the evidence is not compelling (small studies with varying results).
- The risk may decrease the longer an individual takes a combined OCP.
- Progestogen only OCPs (and injectable progestogen contraceptives) have not been associated with an increased risk of DVT or PE.

Advice on perioperative management is conflicting. Manufacturers and the British National Formulary recommend stopping combined OCPs 4 weeks before major operations, and restarting only after the menstrual period at least 2 weeks following full mobilization. By contrast, specialist groups advise that the OCP should not routinely be stopped, because of insufficient evidence of risk, and the danger of unwanted pregnancy.

A reasonable policy is as follows:

- There is no need to stop progestogen only contraceptives at the time of any operation.
- There is no need to stop combined OCPs for minor operations.
- There is no possibility of stopping any contraceptives for emergency surgery.
- For patients on combined OCPs facing major elective surgery the decision should be made on an individual basis, balancing the risk of thromboembolism, the possibility of unwanted pregnancy, and the preferences of the patient.
- Remember that other factors (e.g. obesity) may increase the risk and influence the decision.
- Patients having intermediate or major surgery when taking the combined OCP should receive subcutaneous LMWH and wear antiembolism stockings.
- In selected cases consider a change to depot progestogen injections.
- Always record decisions about contraceptives in the casenotes, including a record about discussion with the patient.
- If the OCP is stopped, advice must be given about alternative contraceptive measures, and a pregnancy test may be needed before operation if there is a possibility of unprotected intercourse.

Hormone replacement therapy (HRT) and venous thromboembolism

- The incidence of spontaneous venous thromboembolism is increased from 3 to 10 women per 10 000 per annum by HRT, but there are no good data on perioperative risk.
- Stopping HRT may cause recurrence of troublesome menopausal symptoms.
- Despite published recommendations, the advice of specialist groups and common practice suggest that HRT should not be stopped perioperatively as a routine.
- Women having major operations whilst on HRT should receive subcutaneous LMWH, perhaps combined with antiembolism stockings.

Further reading

Clagett GP, Anderson FA, Heit J, Levine MN, Wheeler HB (1995). Prophylaxis of venous thromboembolism. *Chest*, **108**, 31S–34S.

Drugs in the peri-operative period: 3—Hormonal contraceptives and hormone replacement therapy (1999). *Drugs and Therapeutics Bulletin*, **37**, 78–80.

Low molecular weight heparins for venous thromboembolism (1998). *Drugs and Therapeutics Bulletin*, **36**, 25–32.

Thromboembolic Risk Factors (THRIFT) Consensus Group (1992). Risk of and prophylaxis for venous thromboembolism in hospital patients. *British Medical Journal*, **305**, 567–74.

Preoperative optimization

Results of studies into high-risk patients undergoing major surgery[1–3] have shown that critical attention to cardiovascular and respiratory function in the perioperative period improves outcome.

The following criteria have been used to identify high-risk surgical patients:

- severe cardiovascular disease
- severe respiratory disease
- aortic surgery
- major surgery for malignancy (cystectomy, oesophagectomy, etc.)
- surgery for abdominal sepsis
- haemodynamic instability due to an acute abdominal problem.

It has been suggested that haemodynamic monitoring should start in the preoperative period using a pulmonary artery catheter to assess fluid requirement and cardiac output. Patients in these studies were given blood if anaemic and oxygen if hypoxic and subsequently colloid with or without an inotrope until a predetermined level of pulmonary capillary wedge pressure and oxygen delivery was achieved. This approach has been shown to reduce mortality, morbidity, and length of stay in the ICU and hospital.

Unfortunately, most ICUs do not have the capacity to admit all such high-risk patients. However, close monitoring of fluid status and replacing fluids more aggressively in emergency patients perioperatively may also improve outcome. Such measures would not necessarily need to be undertaken in the ICU but could be performed on the ward, in the anaesthetic room, or in the recovery area.

Elective or emergency patients who may benefit from a period of preoperative preparation in the ICU should be discussed with the anaesthetists or the ICU team as early as possible.

1   Boyd O, Grounds RM, Bennett ED (1993). A randomized clinical trial of the effect of deliberate perioperative increase of oxygen delivery on mortality in high-risk surgical patients. *Journal of the American Medical Association*, **270**, 2699–707.

2   Sinclair S, James S, Singer M (1997). Intraoperative intravascular volume optimization and length of hospital stay after repair of proximal femur fracture: randomized control trial. *British Medical Journal*, **315**, 909–12.

3   Wilson J, Woods I, Fawcett J, Whall R, Dibb W, Morris C, McManus E (1999). Reducing the risk of major elective surgery: randomised control trial of preoperative optimization of oxygen delivery. *British Medical Journal*, **318**, 1099–103.

When not to operate

When a patient is critically ill and likely to die from a surgical condition it is very difficult to decide not to operate, but however hard, it is an extremely important decision which will need much thought and discussion with the patient, the family, and senior colleagues in both anaesthesia and surgery. Many factors, such as the patient's medical condition, functional ability, and mental state, need to be considered in addition to the surgical pathology. The functional status of a patient with end-stage respiratory disease or heart failure, for instance, will almost certainly be worse following major surgery and this should be considered in the decision-making process. The patient's GP can often give an invaluable insight into their normal medical condition and their wishes. To decide to operate 'because the patient is going to die anyway' is avoiding the issue and may deprive the patient and family of their final hours or days together.

The problem of surgeons, often trainees, deciding to operate on patients in whom the prognosis is hopeless, has been highlighted a number of times in the CEPOD reports.[4]

---

4 *Confidential Enquiry into Perioperative Deaths* (1987) prepared by N Buck, HB Devlin and JN Lunn.

When and how to book intensive care

Criteria for planned admission to ICU or HDU following *elective* surgery include:

- The nature of the surgery alone, e.g. aortic surgery, some thoracic or upper GI surgery, extensive pelvic or spinal surgery. Cardiac and neurosurgery are usually dealt with in separate units.
- A patient with severe pre-existing medical problems in whom the added insult of surgery and anaesthesia may result in established organ failure unless closely monitored and meticulously managed postoperatively, e.g. a patient with very severe lung disease or left ventricular dysfunction undergoing a routine laparotomy or hip replacement.
- Individual surgical or department policies.

If you are unsure about a patient's need for ICU discuss it with the intensive care and ward staff. Inform the patient that you are intending to admit him to intensive care, explain the reasons and what may be expected in terms of monitoring, alarms, ventilation, drips, etc. Elective cases intended for the ICU/HDU should be booked as far in advance as possible to allow planning of staffing etc. This is most commonly done via the ICU ward clerk or secretary. On the day of surgery it is better to cancel major elective surgery when an ICU bed is not available than attempt a complex case with makeshift arrangements that may not serve the patient effectively.

Perioperative guidelines for body piercing jewellery

The prevalence of body piercing has been increasing in recent years. Patients are often reluctant to remove such jewellery due to difficulties with reinsertion postoperatively. The following are general recommendations for when such items should be removed prior to surgery.

All body piercing should be removed prior to anaesthesia and surgery in the following situations:

- All tongue and lip jewellery should be removed prior to any general anaesthetic. Such items may cause airway obstruction, or enter the tracheobronchial tree if dislodged.
- Any nasal septum, nose, or ear piercing should be removed prior to ENT surgery.
- Body piercing jewellery should also be removed if
  - it is at risk of being caught or ripped out, e.g. by ECG leads, surgical drapes, surgical instruments, or towel clips
  - if there is any risk of pressure damage, e.g. chin or lip piercing (pressure from a face mask), nipple piercing (if patient is to be positioned prone)
  - if the piercing is in close proximity to the surgical site.
- Any piercing with signs of infection around the site should also be removed, due to possible focus of infection. This may also preclude some types of 'clean' surgery.

Body piercing does not always have to be removed for:

- Male catheterization in a patient with penile piercing—the ring can often be pulled to one side.
- Surgery distant from the site of female/male genital piercing.

If body piercing jewellery is to be left *in situ*:

- It should be taped over preoperatively—if possible.
- The site and nature of piercing should be documented on the preoperative checklist.
- A check should be performed to ensure the item is still *in situ* postoperatively.

Further reading

Perioperative guidelines for principles of safe practice with reference to surgical patients with body piercing (1999). *British Journal of Theatre Nursing*, **9**, 469.

Chapter 2
Cardiovascular disease

Chris Day

Ischaemic heart disease

Cardiovascular disease accounts for the majority of perioperative deaths. Preoperative detection, investigation, treatment, and risk assessment helps minimize perioperative morbidity and mortality.

History

- The first presentation of ischaemic heart disease (IHD) is acute myocardial infarction (MI) in 50% of patients.
- Identify previously undiagnosed or misdiagnosed angina, CCF, arrhythmia, or old MI. In established IHD any change in symptoms should be noted.
- Prognostic co-morbidities should be identified (hypertension, diabetes mellitus, renal impairment, peripheral vascular disease, cerebrovascular disease, or pulmonary disease).
- A patient who has had a CABG within 5 years and has no symptoms may be considered a normal preoperative risk.
- The patient's functional capacity should be determined as this has been shown to correlate well with maximal oxygen uptake on a treadmill and is prognostically important. This can be quantified in MET (metabolic equivalents). Mobility problems limit this assessment. Patients who can exercise at 4 MET or greater present a low risk of perioperative morbidity:
  - 1 MET—eating and dressing
  - 3 MET—light housework or walk 100 m at 3.2–4.8 km/h (2–3 mph)
  - 4 MET—climb a flight of stairs
  - 6–7 MET—short run.

Examination

Aim to identify CCF, valvular heart disease, and concurrent pulmonary disease.

Special investigations

- An ECG should be performed on all patients over 50 years scheduled for surgery and in younger patients with risk factors for IHD. Changes from previous traces should be investigated. Bundle branch block may predispose to bradyarrhythmias or AF but 24-h ECG monitoring is only necessary if there is a history of palpitations or blackouts.
- Stress testing: an ECG during treadmill exercise can be used to assess cardiovascular risk. In those unable to exercise a pharmacological (dipyridamole, adenosine, or dobutamine) stress test may be used. It has a high negative predictive value but a low positive predictive value and tests may be equivocal. Testing is useful for assessing patients of intermediate or high risk for elective surgery of at least intermediate risk (see tables). Patients with left bundle branch block or abnormal resting ECGs are often not suitable, as reliable ECG changes may not be seen.
- Coronary arteriography assesses the requirement for revascularization. It is rarely justifiable solely to enable another operation. However, patients with severe, uncontrolled IHD are occasionally discovered during preoperative screening that may require urgent CABG. Preoperative cardiological referral is essential.

Perioperative management

- All patients should be informed about the risks of surgery and alternatives.

- Consider referral to a cardiologist to ensure optimal medical management or evaluation for CABG (see tables). Small, randomized controlled trials have shown survival benefits if patients are treated with a beta-blocker in the perioperative period. This should be considered in patients at risk with no contraindication. (Mangano *et al.*[1] administered 10 mg atenolol in divided doses IV 30 min before surgery, repeated after surgery, and then daily for up to 7 days. 50–100 mg orally was substituted postoperatively when possible.)

- Beta-blockers should be continued and given IV if GI absorption is impaired.

- Nitrates should be given preoperatively. In high-risk patients they can be continued IV or transdermally if GI absorption is impaired. In low-risk patients they can be resumed when stable postoperatively.

- Calcium antagonists should be given preoperatively and resumed as soon as possible postoperatively. The dihydropyridine group (especially short-acting nifedipine) may add to the risk of acute MI. These should be substituted to another class or converted to Adalat LA (NB: nifedipine SR is not long-acting.)

- ACE inhibitors improve survival in patients with left ventricular dysfunction due to IHD. They should be given preoperatively and resumed postoperatively as soon as GI absorption resumes. If they have been stopped for several days restarting at a reduced dose may be prudent as most of these drugs are associated with first-dose hypotension. Administration may be associated with marked hypotension on induction.

- In addition to standard monitoring, invasive arterial BP, CVP, or the use of an oesophageal Doppler should be considered for high/intermediate-risk patients undergoing major surgery. ECG monitoring should be with the CM5 configuration or alternative (p. 930).

- The anaesthetic technique should minimize myocardial ischaemia (increased by tachycardia, diastolic hypotension, and systolic hypertension). Anxiolytic premedication may be helpful. Analgesia is important: regional blocks can be very effective but central neuraxial blocks require care and experience.

- Blood loss needs accurate replacement and haemoglobin should be maintained by regular measurement.

- Myocardial ischaemia occurs often during emergence and extubation. Hypertension and tachycardia should be anticipated and avoided. 'Deep' extubation or the use of a short-acting beta-blocker should be considered.

- Consider admission to HDU postoperatively where careful monitoring and interventions can be continued in high-risk patients.

- Following major surgery, all patients at risk should have supplemental oxygen for 3 to 4 days postoperatively, particularly at night.

- Antiemetics such as cyclizine and hyoscine can cause tachycardia and may exacerbate ischaemia.

1 Mangano DT, Layug EL, Wallace A, Tateo I for the Multicenter Study of Perioperative Ischemia Research Group (1996). Effect of atenolol in mortality and cardiovascular morbidity after non-cardiac surgery. *New England Journal of Medicine*, **335**, 1713–20.

Cardiac risk (% figures relate to combined risk of MI and/or death)

	Major risk (<5%)	Intermediate risk (1–5%)	Minor risk (<1%)
IHD	MI <1 month. Unstable/severe angina	Previous MI. Stable angina	Abnormal ECG
CCF	Decompensated	Compensated (optimal treatment)	Reduced exercise capacity
Arrhythmia	Malignant SVT/VT with rapid ventricular rate. Heart block		Abnormal, e.g. AF
Other	Severe valvular disease	Diabetes	CVE. Uncontrolled hypertension. Age

Surgical risk

High: >5% death/ non-fatal MI	Major emergency surgery (esp. in elderly)
	Aortic/major vascular surgery
	Prolonged surgery with large fluid shifts
Intermediate: <5%	Carotid endarterectomy
	Head and neck
	Orthopaedic
	Prostatic
Low: <1%	Endoscopic
	Cataract extraction
	Superficial surgery (incl. breast)

Cardiological referral

	Exercise tolerance: Any	<4 MET	>4 MET	<4 MET	>4 MET
	Cardiac risk: Major	Intermediate		Minor	
Surgery risk					
High	Refer	Refer	Refer	Refer	Operate
Intermediate	Refer	Refer	Operate	Operate	Operate
Low	Refer	Operate	Operate	Operate	Operate

Perioperative acute myocardial infarction

- Occurs most frequently 3 to 4 days after surgery. Symptoms may be atypical and up to 20% may be silent. The mortality rate is up to 50%. Diagnostic criteria vary but sole reliance on CK-MB assay will over estimate the incidence of MI especially in patients with ischaemic limbs or after aortic surgery.

- Therapeutic options are reduced because thrombolysis is generally contraindicated. Other treatments are possible: aspirin (150 mg od) and beta-blockers (atenolol 5 mg IV followed by 50–100 mg PO daily) should be used as normal. Acute angioplasty for myocardial infarction is probably at least as effective as thrombolysis. Refer immediately to a cardiologist to consider angioplasty or occasionally surgical revascularization.

Further reading

Guidelines for perioperative cardiovascular evaluation for non cardiac surgery (1996). *Circulation*, **93**, 1286–317.

Howell SJ, Sear JW, Foex P (2001). Perioperative β-blockade: a useful treatment that should be greeted with cautious enthusiasm. British Journal of Anaesthesia, **86**, 160–4.

Poldermans D, Boersma E, Bax JJ, *et al.* (1999). The effect of bisoprolol on perioperative mortality and myocardial infarction in high-risk patients undergoing vascular surgery. *New England Journal of Medicine*, **341**, 1789–94.

Turner M, Haywood G (1998). Preoperative assessment of cardiac risk for non-cardiac surgery. *Journal of the Royal College of Physicians of London*, **32**, 545–7.

Heart failure

Heart failure is associated with perioperative morbidity and mortality. Acute heart failure may present as pulmonary oedema (LVF) or hypoperfusion (cardiogenic shock). Chronic or congestive cardiac failure is typically described with peripheral oedema and an elevated JVP.

Aetiology of heart failure

Right heart failure	Left heart failure
Chronic lung disease	Ischaemic heart disease
Chronic pulmonary thromboembolism	Dilated cardiomyopathy (idiopathic, alcohol, myocarditis, familial)
Primary pulmonary hypertension	Hypertension
Right ventricular cardiomyopathy	Drugs (beta-blockers, Ca-channel blockers, antiarrhythmics)
	Sepsis, HOCM*, restrictive cardiomyopathy, hypo- or hyperthyroidism

*Hypertrophic obstructive cardiomyopathy.

Treatment

- Diuretics: reduce peripheral and pulmonary congestion.
- Vasodilators: ACE inhibitors (and angiotensin-II receptor antagonists) and nitrates.
- Anticoagulants: reduce the incidence of thromboembolic events.
- Inotropes: digoxin.
- Antiarrhythmics.
- Beta-blockers: occasionally used by cardiologists if controlling the heart rate outweighs the risks of myocardial depression.

Preoperative assessment

History and examination should identify present or recent episodes of decompensated heart failure (any within 6 months adversely affects risk). Attempts should be made to identify a cause for any decompensation (recent MI, new anaemia, progression of disease, or non-compliance with drugs).

Investigations

- ECG: may suggest aetiology, and comparison with previous traces may explain deterioration.
- Chest radiograph: if symptoms are stable and the last one is less than 12 months old it does not need repeating.
- Echocardiography should be performed in poorly controlled patients and for quantification of degree of cardiac dysfunction (see also p. 343).

Perioperative management

- Perioperative mortality is high and increases with worsening left ventricular dysfunction. Non-essential surgery should be avoided. Where possible perform surgery under a local or regional block.

- Postoperative admission to HDU/ICU should be arranged before starting major surgery. In some centres preoperative admission for optimization is considered.

- Sedative premedication is generally well tolerated except for cor pulmonale when even a slight worsening of hypoxia or acidosis can increase pulmonary vascular resistance and exacerbate heart failure.

- Patients on digoxin and nitrates should receive them preoperatively. Digoxin should be given IV postoperatively if the patient is in AF but can usually be safely omitted until a patient is eating again if they are in sinus rhythm. Nitrates can be given transdermally whilst the patient is not eating.

- ACE inhibitors should generally be given preoperatively, although a degree of hypotension on induction is to be expected. Postoperatively they should be resumed as soon as the patient is absorbing. If they have been omitted for 3 or more days they should be reintroduced at a low dose to minimize the first-dose hypotensive effect.

- Diuretics are often omitted preoperatively as the patient may lose an unknown intravascular volume and is to receive a vasodilating anaesthetic. Postoperative diuretic requirements vary and should be given after consideration of fluid balance and measured cardiovascular variables.

- Following central neuraxial blocks it may be necessary to prescribe a dose of diuretic to compensate for the contraction of the intravascular space that occurs when the block wears off.

- Anaesthetic technique should minimize negative inotropy, tachycardia, diastolic hypotension, and systolic hypertension. No technique is clearly superior but these high-risk anaesthetics should be given by an experienced anaesthetist. Measurement of CVP is valuable and this may be complemented by use of intra-arterial BP, PAOP measurement, or oesophageal Doppler/transoesophageal echo.

- Renal perfusion is easily compromised in these patients—monitor hourly urine volumes. If the urine output falls, hypovolaemia should be excluded and adequate perfusion pressure ensured before diuretics are used even if a preoperative dose has been omitted. NSAIDs are a potent renal insult in these patients and their use requires care.

- All patients should have supplemental oxygen for 3 to 4 days after major surgery.

- Good analgesia is essential to minimize the detrimental effects of catecholamine release in response to pain.

Hypertension

Approximately 15% of patients are hypertensive (diastolic BP > 90 mmHg). Moderate hypertension (100–115 mmHg) and well-controlled hypertension has not been shown to be an independent risk factor for cardiovascular complications although it is a marker of coronary artery disease. Preoperative hypertension is associated with exaggerated intra-operative swings, which can be associated with myocardial ischaemia.

Potential problems

- There is an increased risk of acute MI, CVA, and renal impairment.
- Antihypertensive drugs exaggerate the hypotension caused by hypovolaemia because of attenuation of vasoconstriction or tachycardia in response to hypovolaemia.
- ACE inhibitors may increase the risk of renal failure due to effects on glomerular blood flow.

Perioperative management

- BP on admission is frequently elevated. Repeated measurement, liaison with the GP, or rechecking after an anxiolytic can help differentiate between genuine and anxiety-related hypertension. (NB: 'white coat' hypertension is not necessarily a benign disease.)
- Assessment should focus on end organ damage (retinal, renal, and vascular bruits) and associated diseases (mainly coronary artery disease).
- If severe diastolic hypertension (> 115 mmHg) is present, whenever possible surgery should be cancelled and the patient investigated and treated for at least 4 weeks before returning for surgery.
- If moderate diastolic hypertension (100–115 mmHg) is present and there is evidence of end organ damage then management is as for severe elevation. If there is no end organ damage then control over a few days is usually safe.
- Mild diastolic hypertension (< 100 mmHg) is likely to benefit from beta-blockade providing there is no contraindication, but there is little increased risk.
- Preoperatively all normal antihypertensive drugs should be given. Sedative premeds are well tolerated if desired. If not already on a beta-blocker and one is not contraindicated then perioperative administration may reduce the risk of cardiac complications.
- No anaesthetic technique is superior. Good analgesia is important to minimize hypertensive swings. Although effective, central neuraxial blocks can result in profound hypotension so frequent or continuous measurement of blood pressure is required.
- If hypertension is severe or preoperative control is poor and major or emergency surgery is planned invasive monitoring of BP and CVP and postoperative admission to HDU is advisable.

Cardiomyopathy

There are three subgroups of cardiomyopathy: dilated, constrictive, and restrictive. They are pathophysiologically quite distinct, are associated with different problems and require different approaches.

Dilated cardiomyopathy

* There is systolic impairment of the LV, although in the early stages there may be no discernible dilation. There are many aetiologies (alcohol, vitamin deficiencies, drugs) but the commonest is ischaemic heart disease.
* The commonest problems encountered are heart failure, arrhythmias (AF and VT), and emboli from left-sided cardiac cavities. Thus they are treated with combinations of diuretics, ACE inhibitors, vasodilators, anticoagulants, and antiarrhythmics.
* Perioperative management is the same as for heart failure due to ischaemic heart disease.

Hypertrophic obstructive cardiomyopathy

* An inherited condition in which excessive muscle bulk impinges on the LV outflow tract causing obstruction that increases during systole. There is a spectrum of severity with some patients having a normal exercise tolerance. Others may have exertional dyspnoea, angina, dizziness, or syncope. Some cases present as sudden death.
* Diagnosis is made by echocardiography, but suspicions should be raised by a family history, heaving or double apex, an aortic systolic murmur but without a slow rising pulse of aortic stenosis. The ECG often shows evidence of LVH.
* These patients benefit from negative inotropic agents like beta-blockers or verapamil. Pacemakers are also sometimes used. Hypovolaemia or vasodilatation can precipitate myocardial ischaemia and rapid decompensation.
* Perioperatively all normal drugs should be given. If hypovolaemia is possible (such as patients receiving bowel prep) then an IVI should be started before theatre. Invasive measurement of arterial BP and CVP or oesophageal Doppler will help avoid significant hypotension or hypovolaemia. If there is significant hypotension, this is best treated by correcting hypovolaemia and using an alpha agonist (metaraminol), which will minimize tachycardia. Postoperatively these patients should receive supplemental oxygen and be managed on an HDU with an emphasis on accurate fluid balance.

Restrictive cardiomyopathy

* An exceedingly rare condition. The commonest cause is myocardial infiltration by amyloid. Exercise tolerance is generally impaired but symptoms are often vague. Echocardiography shows predominant diastolic dysfunction and a fixed stroke volume.
* These patients respond poorly to conventional treatments for heart failure but may be sensitive to diuretics.
* The rarity of this condition accounts for the paucity of data on which to base anaesthetic technique. They often have a high resting pulse rate and tolerate pharmacological bradycardia poorly. Increases in systemic vascular resistance may further reduce cardiac output and increased catecholamines (endogenous or exogenous) may further impair diastolic dysfunction.

Arrhythmias

Established atrial fibrillation

- Echocardiography to assess LV function, left atrium size, and the mitral valve should be performed if there is significant exertional dyspnoea or angina. Digoxin level if on more than 375 μg or symptoms of toxicity (nausea is most common)
- Ventricular rate should be 60–90 beats/min (almost always increases on induction of anaesthesia).

Intra-operative atrial fibrillation (p. 831, 934)

- Exclude precipitating causes such as hypovolaemia, hypoxia, hypokalemia, hypomagnesemia, and misplaced CVP lines.
- If the BP is compromised synchronized d.c. cardioversion (200 J then 360 J) is often the quickest way to restore sinus rhythm.
- If drug treatment is preferred consider esmolol, amiodarone, flecainide, or digoxin.

Atrial flutter

The management of this condition is the same as for AF. If the diagnosis is not clear then administration of adenosine will slow the ventricular response and make the flutter waves more obvious.

Paroxysmal junctional tachycardia

- This often occurs in young patients and the heart is structurally normal. Patients should normally be investigated by a cardiologist prior to elective surgery.
- Preoperatively the frequency of episodes and usual treatment should be noted.
- If the ECG shows a short PR and delta wave then the patient has Wolf–Parkinson–White syndrome and digoxin is contraindicated as it may increase conduction through the accessory pathway and progress to VF.
- Treatments include beta-blockers, Ca-channel antagonists, flecainide, propafenone, or amiodarone (p. 933).

Intra-operative junctional tachycardia (SVT)

See p. 933.

Ventricular premature beats (VPB)

- These are common, increase with age, and are generally benign. They can, however, be associated with underlying cardiac disease. They may be asymptomatic or the cause of an 'erratic' heartbeat.
- The presence of VPBs should prompt a search for underlying heart disease but any increase in risk is secondary to the underlying disease and not the VPBs. Attempts to suppress them may increase mortality. Treatment should only be directed at underlying heart disease.

Ventricular tachycardia (VT)

- VT occurs more commonly than previously recognized. It does not necessarily result in cardiac arrest but is almost always associated with significant ventricular disease. Patients with a history of VT will usually be taking an antiarrhythmic agent or have an implantable defibrillator (see p. 33).

* Antiarrhythmic drugs should be given pre- and postoperatively. If a patient is not eating postoperatively then therapy should be continued IV until oral drugs are being absorbed.
* An implantable defibrillator should be turned off just before surgery and turned back on immediately before the patient leaves theatre. This is done by a cardiology technician and prevents diathermy interference being interpreted as VT/VF.

Intraoperative ventricular tachycardia
See pp. 937, 829.

Intraoperative ventricular fibrillation
See pp. 938, 826.

Sick sinus syndrome

* This may be due to idiopathic fibrosis of the sinus node, ischaemic heart disease, cardiomyopathy, or myocarditis.
* It is characterized by sinus bradycardia, sinoatrial block, or sinus arrest but may also occur with paroxysmal atrial fibrillation, flutter or re-entrant tachycardias. However, the ECG may be normal and it is best diagnosed by ambulatory monitoring of the ECG.
* Symptomatic patients should have a pacemaker fitted but may also require antiarrhythmics to prevent the tachyarrhythmias.
* If a patient has no pacemaker then anaesthetic drugs may exacerbate the bradycardia or induce sinus arrest (a long pause may then 'escape' into a tachyarrhythmia).
* Facilities should be available for pacing, and tachyarrhythmias managed appropriately.

Disturbances of conduction (heart block)

The wave of electrical excitation that spreads from the sinoatrial node to the ventricles via the conduction pathways may be delayed or blocked at any point.

First-degree block

There is a delay in conduction from the sinoatrial node to the ventricles, and this appears as a prolongation of the PR interval ie greater than 0.2 s. It is normally benign but may progress to second-degree block, usually of the Mobitz type I. First-degree heart block is not usually a problem during anaesthesia.

Second-degree block—Mobitz type I (Wenkebach)

There is progressive lengthening of the PR interval and then failure of conduction of an atrial beat. This is followed by a conducted beat with a short PR interval and then the cycle repeats itself. This occurs commonly after an inferior myocardial infarction, and tends to be self-limiting. It does not normally require treatment although a 2:1 type block may develop with haemodynamic instability.

Second-degree block—Mobitz type II

If excitation intermittently fails to pass through the AV node or the bundle of His, this is the Mobitz type II phenomenon. Most beats are conducted normally but occasionally there is an atrial contraction without a subsequent ventricular contraction. This often progresses to complete heart block and if recognized preoperatively will need expert assessment and pacing.

Second-degree block—2:1 type

There may be alternate conducted and non-conducted beats, resulting in two P waves for every QRS complex—this is 2:1 block. A 3:1 block may also occur, with one conducted beat and two non-conducted beats. This may also herald complete heart block, and in most situations a temporary transvenous pacing wire is required preoperatively.

Third-degree block/complete heart block

There is complete failure of conduction between the atria and the ventricles. The ventricles are therefore excited by a slow escape mechanism from a focus within them. There is no relationship between the P wave and the QRS complex, which is abnormally shaped. It may occur occasionally as a transient phenomenon in theatre due to severe vagal stimulation, in which case it often responds to stopping surgery and intravenous atropine. When it occurs in association with acute inferior myocardial infarction, it is due to AV nodal ischaemia and is often transient. Very rarely it may be congenital. However, if it occurs with anterior myocardial infarction it indicates more extensive damage including the His–Purkinje system. It may also occur as a chronic state usually due to fibrosis around the bundle of His.

Bundle branch block

If there is a delay in depolarization of the right or left bundle branches, this will cause a delay in depolarization of part of the ventricular muscle with subsequent QRS widening. Diagnosis of which bundle is blocked can only be achieved by analysing a full 12–lead ECG.

Right bundle branch block

The characteristic pattern here is of wide complexes with an 'RSR' in lead V1 (so that it may appear 'M' shaped) and in V6 a small initial negative downward deflection followed by a larger upwards positive wave and then a second downward wave. In addition there are also often secondary changes in ventricular repolarization with ST segment depression in the right precordial leads. It may indicate problems with the right side of the heart, but a right bundle branch block type pattern with a normal axis and QRS duration is not uncommon in normal individuals.

Left bundle branch block

Septal depolarization is reversed so there is a change in the initial direction of the QRS complex in every lead. The complexes are widened and in V1 there is no initial positive wave, but a deep negative wave in which there may be a small upward inflection. In V6 there is a no initial negative wave and the complex has a characteristic 'M' shape. This often indicates heart disease and makes further interpretation of the ECG other than rate and rhythm impossible.

Bifascicular block

Is the combination of right bundle branch block and block of the left anterior or left posterior fascicle. Right bundle branch block with left anterior hemiblock is the commoner of the two and appears as an 'RSR' in V1 together with left-axis deviation. In the context of an acute myocardial infarction this may progress to complete heart block in some patients but generally does not require preoperative pacing. Right bundle branch block with left posterior hemiblock is much less common and appears as right bundle branch block with an abnormal degree of right-axis deviation; however, other causes for the right-axis deviation should be considered and it is a non-specific sign.

Trifascicular block

This is the term sometimes used to indicate the presence of a prolonged PR interval together with a bifascicular block.

Preoperative management

• First-degree heart block in the absence of symptoms is common. It needs no specific investigation or treatment.

• Second- or third-degree heart block may need pacemaker insertion. If surgery is urgent this may be achieved quickly by inserting a temporary transvenous wire prior to definitive insertion.

• Bundle branch, bifasicular, or trifasicular block (bifasicular with first-degree block) will rarely progress to complete heart block during anaesthesia and so it is not normal practice to insert a pacing wire unless there have been episodes of syncope.

Intraoperative heart block

• Atropine is rarely effective.

• If hypotension is profound then an isoprenaline infusion can be used to temporize: 1–10 μg/min (dilute 0.2 mg in 500 ml of 5% glucose or dextrose-saline and titrate to effect (2–20 ml/min), or 1 mg in 50 ml 5% glucose/ dextrose-saline at 1.5–30 ml/h).

- Transcutaneous pacing is rarely practical in theatre because of difficulty in siting the posterior pad. Oesophageal pacing is effective—the electrode is passed into the oesophagus like a nasogastric tube and connected to the pulse generator. The position can be adjusted until there is ventricular capture.

- Transvenous pacing is both more reliable and effective and relatively easy. A Swan–Ganz sheath of adequate size to pass the wire is inserted into the internal jugular or subclavian vein (this can be done while other equipment is being collected). A balloon-tipped pacing wire is then inserted to the 20 cm mark. The balloon is inflated and a pulse generator connected at 5 V. It can then be advanced—atrial capture is often seen followed by ventricular capture. When this happens the balloon is deflated and a further 5 cm of catheter inserted. If the 50 cm mark is reached the catheter is coiling up or not entering the heart. Deflate the balloon, withdraw to the 20 cm mark and try again.

Cardiac pacemakers

Pacemakers are frequently used for a variety of brady- and tachyarrythmias. The North American Society of Pacing and Electrophysiology and the British Pacing and Electrophysiology Group initiated a generic code for describing pacemaker function. The code consists of five letters or positions. The first three describe antibradycardia functions and are always stated. The fourth and fifth positions relate to additional functions and are often omitted if not present (e.g. VDD or 000MS).

- Position 1 refers to the chamber paced (V/A/D for ventricle, atrium or dual).
- Position 2 refers to the chamber sensed (V/A/D).
- Position 3 refers to response to sensing (T/I/D for triggered, inhibited or dual).
- Position 4 refers to programmability or rate modulation (P simple programmable, M multiprogrammable, R rate modulation).
- Position 5 antitachycardia functions (P pacing, S shock, D dual).

Examples

- VVI: ventricular demand pacing. The ventricle is sensed and paced if there is no spontaneous rhythm. AV synchrony is lost but the risk of pacemaker induced ventricular tachycardia is low.
- DDD: pacing and sensing in both chambers. An atrial impulse inhibits atrial output and anticipates a ventricle impulse. If this occurs it inhibits the ventricular output but if there is no AV conduction then it paces the ventricle.
- 000MS: is an implantable defibrillator.

Implications

- Patients with pacemakers should attend follow-up clinics. The most recent pacemaker check should confirm good function. A preoperative ECG will detect some problems but by no means all. Absence of all pacing spikes may represent appropriate sensing or total failure.
- Bipolar diathermy is safe with pacemakers. If conventional diathermy is necessary then the plate should be positioned so that most of the current passes away from the pacemaker and it should be used in short bursts. The pacing wires may act as aerials and cause heating where the wire contacts the endocardium. The pacemaker may detect the diathermy as ventricular activity and inhibit its output, but only for the duration of diathermy use. In an emergency a pacemaker can be changed to V00 (asynchronous - ventricular pacing) by placing a magnet over the box. However, this should only be done as a last resort as there is a risk of inducing ventricular fibrillation.
- Any pacemaker that has the facility to cardiovert or overpace should have this facility turned off for theatre to avoid erroneous discharge if diathermy noise is interpreted as a tachyarrhythmia. It is important that it is turned back on before the patient leaves the theatre area.

Valvular heart disease (see also p. 347–54)

Preoperative assessment may be the first time a significant valve lesion is diagnosed or a patient may already be under regular cardiological review pending possible cardiac surgery. In both cases the anaesthetist will need to assess the significance of the lesion and tailor the anaesthetic appropriately. Antibiotic prophylaxis will need to be considered (see p. 896).

Aortic stenosis

- Aortic stenosis greatly increases the risks of surgery. The decrease in systemic vascular resistance caused by most anaesthetic drugs results in a marked fall in BP because cardiac output is relatively fixed. This fall in BP reduces coronary perfusion of a left ventricle that is hypertrophied and may result in ischaemia, reduced contractility, and a vicious spiral of a further falling BP.

- The severity is best assessed by measuring the valve gradient by echocardiography or cardiac catheterization, but poor exercise tolerance and especially syncope suggest severe stenosis. The onset of left ventricular failure has a poor prognosis. The valve gradient should be interpreted with a measure of left ventricular function because with time the left ventricle will fail and the measured gradient will then start to fall. Less than 40 mmHg is mild, 40–80 mmHg is moderate, and > 80 mmHg is severe (untreated severe symptomatic stenosis has a 50% 1–year survival).

- Anaesthesia should be avoided if at all possible with severe stenosis. In other cases spinal anaesthesia should be avoided; epidural and general anaesthetic techniques can be used but it is most important to give drugs slowly with invasive BP measurement so that falls in systemic vascular resistance can be rapidly treated. Hypotension should be treated by an alpha agonist such as metaraminol to minimize the risk of ischaemia that can be induced by a tachycardia. A CVP line or other measure of left ventricular filling is also helpful to diagnose and appropriately treat hypotension.

Aortic regurgitation

- The anaesthesia-induced fall in systemic vascular resistance is better tolerated than with aortic stenosis. A fall in systemic vascular resistance decreases the regurgitant flow; conversely an increase in systemic vascular resistance (caused by pain or drugs, e.g. ketamine) may increase regurgitant flow and precipitate heart failure. A degree of tachycardia shortens diastole and therefore reduces regurgitation. As the ventricle is less hypertrophied it is less at risk from tachycardia-induced ischaemia. A heart rate of 90 beats/min may be optimal.

- The severity is best assessed by echocardiography or cardiac catheterization. This will also assess left ventricular function. Clinically, dyspnoea and pulmonary oedema suggest advanced disease and the diastolic BP falls in proportion to the severity of the valve lesion.

- Although vasodilation is well tolerated, an epidural may be safer than spinal as it can be slowly increased allowing appropriate measures if the BP falls. Vasopressors should be used carefully to avoid excessive increases in systemic vascular resistance. Invasive monitoring is desirable in advanced disease.

Mixed aortic valve disease

This may be very taxing for an anaesthetist because of the conflicting requirements of each aspect of the valve lesion. The predominant lesion should be determined by echocardiography or cardiac catheterization and the patient managed in the same way as if this was the only lesion.

Mitral stenosis

+ The majority are secondary to rheumatic fever. The greatest risk is developing pulmonary oedema which may be precipitated by tachycardia especially atrial fibrillation. The reduction in diastole and loss of the atrial kick greatly impairs left ventricular filling through the stenotic valve. Typically exercise tolerance falls over many years (although this may not be apparent in patients with arthritis awaiting orthopaedic surgery). There may also be acute crises due to intermittent atrial fibrillation or thromboembolism.

+ Severity is best assessed by echocardiography (valve orifice > 2 cm^2 is mild, 1–2 cm^2 is moderate and < 1 cm^2 is severe).

+ No anaesthetic technique has been shown to be safer. However, general anaesthesia often produces the most stable cardiovascular conditions. Central neuraxial blocks associated with marked falls in systemic vascular resistance are inappropriate in patients with relatively fixed cardiac outputs.

+ Invasive monitoring is desirable especially to guide fluid balance, but CVP poorly reflects left ventricular filling. Intra-operative tachycardia should be treated rapidly. Esmolol is rapidly effective and titratable. Any negative inotropic effects are easily outweighed by the benefits of controlling the rate. If the tachycardia is due to new atrial fibrillation then d.c. cardioversion should be considered.

+ Anticoagulation should be resumed as soon as possible after the operation as these patients are at risk of thromboembolism and this risk is higher postoperatively.

Mitral regurgitation

+ This may be due to a valve lesion, a dilated heart, or papillary muscle dysfunction. The haemodynamic considerations are the same but the aetiology (e.g. IHD) may have additional considerations. Mitral valve prolapse with regurgitation, inducible regurgitation (by squatting or squatting to standing), or valve thickening on echo should be treated as mitral regurgitation. Anaesthesia and alterations in systemic vascular resistance are well tolerated unless the regurgitation is very severe.

+ Severity is best assessed by echocardiography, but it should be realized that the left ventricular ejection fraction will be overestimated in the presence of mitral regurgitation.

+ Most anaesthetic approaches are well tolerated. Fluid overload is a major risk but less than with mitral stenosis. Monitoring and approach are largely dictated by the underlying aetiology.

Prosthetic valves

- A full cardiovascular assessment including an ECG, chest radiograph, and echo within the last 12 months are needed to assess the function of the valve.
- Antibiotic prophylaxis is needed for most surgery (see p. 896).
- Tissue valves do not require anticoagulation. If a patient is taking anticoagulants another explanation should be sought and managed appropriately.
- The risk of thromboembolism if anticoagulation is stopped with a mechanical heart valve is small (8/100 patient years). Therefore if reversal of all anticoagulation is vital (e.g. neurosurgery) this can be done for up to 7 days with only a small risk. For most surgery the consequences of increased bleeding are less severe. In these cases warfarin should be stopped 4 days before planned surgery. When the INR falls below 2.0, heparin should be started (either sodium heparin to keep APTR 2.5 or weight-adjusted LMWH). This can be stopped 3 h prior to surgery and resumed as soon after surgery as is safe but certainly within 7 days.

Endocarditis prophylaxis

See p. 896.

The patient with an undiagnosed murmur

If a patient presents for surgery and a previously undiagnosed murmur is noticed then this should be fully investigated and diagnosed before surgery takes place. This should include history, examination, ECG, chest radiograph, and echocardiography. Absence of a diastolic murmur or cardiac symptoms should not be assumed to infer that the valve lesion is minor.

If the patient has a truly life-threatening emergency that precludes full investigation then a clinical assessment of the valve lesion may be the only way to plan perioperative management.

Post cardiac transplant

The number of patients who receive heart or heart–lung transplants is increasing and their improved survival makes it increasingly likely that they present for non-cardiac surgery outside a specialist centre. Liaison with the transplant centre is often helpful especially for the results of the most recent investigations. The most important considerations relate to ongoing immunosuppression, altered cardiac (and pulmonary) physiology, and the direct effects of previous surgery.

Immunosuppression

- Immunosuppression predisposes to infection. Thus strict asepsis is required if invasive procedures such as CVP line insertion cannot be avoided. Any suggestion of pulmonary infection should be verified and aggressively treated before surgery.
- Anaemia and thrombocytopenia as well as leukopenia may be produced requiring treatment before surgery.
- Cyclosporin is associated with renal dysfunction and is the most likely cause of hypertension that affects 40% of heart–lung transplant recipients. It may also prolong the action of non-depolarizing muscle relaxants.
- Corticosteroid use may necessitate additional doses perioperatively (p. 98).

Pathophysiology of the heart transplant recipient

- The resting heart rate is increased (100–110 beats/min) in the absence of vagal tone on the donor heart sinoatrial node. Diastolic dysfunction is common early after transplant but also if rejection is developing. Coronary blood flow is increased due to a denervation although endothelial function (and therefore nitric oxide responsiveness) is normal. Cardiac output will eventually increase in response to increased metabolic demand but the response is slow. There is some evidence of sympathetic reinnervation after several years, which may increase the rapidity of this response. The Frank–Starling mechanism is normal. The high resting heart rate and slow response to sympathetic stimulation result in poor tolerance of sudden hypovolaemia.
- Disrupted pulmonary lymphatics makes these patients very susceptible to pulmonary oedema. Strict attention to maintaining euvolaemia is therefore vital.
- If pharmacological manipulation is required then direct-acting agents should be used: atropine has no effect on the denervated heart, the effect of ephedrine is reduced and unpredictable, and hydralazine and phenyl-ephrine produce no reflex tachy- or bradycardia in response to their primary action. Adrenaline, noradrenaline, isoprenaline, and beta-blockers act as expected.
- Sinus bradycardia and AV block are early signs of rejection, although rejection may be associated with any arrhythmia (heart–lung recipients usually present with pulmonary rather than cardiac rejection). Comparisons with previous ECGs is therefore important.

Direct effects of previous surgery

- Previous and often repeated use of central and peripheral vessels can make intravenous and arterial access difficult.
- Cough may be impaired due to a combination of phrenic and recurrent laryngeal nerve palsies. This increases the risks of sputum retention and postoperative chest infection.
- Heart–lung recipients will have a tracheal anastomosis. It is desirable to avoid unnecessary intubation but if it is necessary use a short tube and minimize tracheal cuff pressure. (NB: this may increase during prolonged nitrous oxide anaesthesia.)

Choice of technique

There is no evidence to support one technique above any other. Peripheral surgery under regional block is likely to be well tolerated. However, subarachnoid block may result in rapid vasodilation which is highly undesirable. If regional anaesthesia is not possible or desirable then either general or epidural anaesthesia are acceptable if administered with care and understanding.

Pericardial disease

Acute pericarditis

- This is usually a viral condition that presents with chest pain. The diagnosis is supported by widespread ST elevation on an ECG.
- It frequently occurs with a myocarditis which may increase the likelihood of arrhythmia and sudden death.
- Elective surgery should be postponed for at least 6 weeks.

Constrictive pericarditis

- This may be postinfective or secondary to an autoimmune disease such as systemic lupus erythematosus. The only effective treatment is pericardectomy which may be dramatically effective.
- Systolic function of the myocardium is well maintained but diastolic function is severely impaired. When exercise tolerance is impaired general anaesthesia has a significant risk.
- Tachycardia and reduced cardiac filling are poorly tolerated.
- Elevations in intrathoracic pressure, as occur during IPPV can result in profound hypotension.
- If anaesthesia is unavoidable and regional block is not possible then a spontaneously breathing technique is preferable to IPPV. Preload should be maintained and tachycardia avoided.

Congenital heart disease and non-cardiac surgery

Congenital heart disease (CHD) is common, 8 per 1000 births, with about 85% of these children reaching adult life. New surgical techniques, better intra-operative myocardial protection and advances in paediatric cardiac anaesthesia have led to marked improvements in survival rates for many forms of CHD.

Although many of these children and adults will have undergone corrective surgery, many will still have residual problems. A study in 1992 reported a 47% incidence of adverse perioperative events in CHD patients undergoing non-cardiac surgical procedures.

General considerations

When faced with a patient with CHD the anaesthetist must understand the physiological implications of the underlying cardiac defect. Operative procedures for CHD aim to improve the patient's haemodynamic status although complete cure is not always achieved. Paediatric cardiac surgical procedures can be divided into the following groups:

- Curative procedures: the patient is completely cured and has a normal life expectancy (e.g. persistent ductus arteriosus and atrial septal defect closure).
- Corrective procedures: the patient's haemodynamic status is markedly improved but their life expectancy may not have returned to normal (e.g. tetralogy of Fallot repair).
- Palliative procedures: these patients may have distinctly abnormal circulations and physiology but avoid the consequences of untreated CHD. Their life expectancy is not normal but many are expected to reach mid adulthood (e.g. Fontan procedures).

Preoperative assessment

Aim to gain a clear understanding of the anatomy and pathophysiology of the patient's cardiac defect.

- History: define the nature and severity of the cardiac lesion. Ask about symptoms of congestive cardiac failure (especially regarding limitation of daily activities). Consider the presence of abnormalities and syndromes associated with CHD and current medication.
- Examination: check for cyanosis, peripheral oedema, and hepato splenomegaly. Assess peripheral pulses and the heart and lungs for murmurs and signs of infection and failure. Cyanosed patients should have a brief neurological examination.
- Investigations: a recent chest radiograph and ECG. Record baseline SpO_2 on air. Laboratory tests obviously depend on the type of surgery proposed but most will require FBC, clotting screen, LFTs, and electrolytes. Some patients will need pulmonary function tests.
- Consult with the patient's cardiologist—information regarding recent echocardiography and catheter data should be available. Potential risk factors in the patient can be discussed along with potential treatment regimes, e.g. inotropes or vasodilators.

Factors indicative of high risk

- Recent worsening of cardiac failure or symptoms of myocardial ischaemia.
- Severe hypoxaemia with $SpO_2 < 75\%$ on air.
- Polycythaemia (haematocrit > 60%)
- Unexplained dizziness/syncope/fever or recent CVA.
- Severe aortic/pulmonary valve stenosis.
- Uncorrected tetralogy of Fallot or Eisenmenger's syndrome.
- The recent onset of arrhythmias.

In all patients with CHD consider whether the proposed surgery is necessary with regard to the potential risks; whether admission to ICU/HDU will be required, and whether the patient can or should be moved to a cardiac centre. High risk factors will affect these decisions.

Specific problems found in patients with CHD

- Myocardial dysfunction—some degree of ventricular dysfunction is common. This may be due to the underlying disease (e.g. hypoplastic left ventricle), or may be secondary (e.g. following poor intra-operative myocardial protection).
- Arrhythmias may be related to the original disease or be iatrogenic (surgery or medication). Some CHD patients develop heart block following cardiac surgery and have pacemakers *in situ*.
- Air emboli—all CHD patients should be considered at risk from air embolism. All intravascular lines should be free of air.
- Cyanosis can occur due to many causes, e.g. shunting of blood from the right side of the heart to the left (e.g. tetralogy of Fallot, Eisenmenger's syndrome) or due to general intracardiac mixing (e.g. complete atrioventricular septal defect). Cyanosis results in polycythaemia and an increased blood volume. Blood viscosity is increased with impaired tissue perfusion. There is often thrombocytopenia and a deficiency in fibrinogen leading to a bleeding tendency. These changes are coupled with an increase in tissue vascularity which worsens bleeding problems. Cyanosis can also lead to renal and cerebral thrombosis and renal tubular atrophy.
- Anticoagulants are taken by many CHD patients, most commonly daily aspirin or warfarin. Management of anticoagulation in the perioperative period can be difficult. Seek advice from the patient's cardiologist and a haematologist.
- Antibiotic prophylaxis—most CHD patients are at risk from endocarditis (see p. 896).
- Myocardial ischaemia developing in a patient with CHD is significant and should be investigated.

Specific CHD lesions

There are over 100 forms of CHD, but eight lesions account for 83% of all cardiac defects. These are ventricular septal defect (VSD), atrial septal defect (ASD), persistent ductus arteriosus (PDA), pulmonary stenosis (PS), tetralogy of Fallot (TOF), aortic stenosis (AS), coarctation of the aorta, and transposition of the great vessels (TOGV). In addition, many of the other lesions are managed palliatively by producing a Fontan circulation.

ASD (secundum type)

Patients are often asymptomatic. The ASD usually results in a left to right shunt and can be closed surgically or by the transcatheter route. In patients in whom the defect has not been closed one must be careful of paradoxical emboli.

ASD (primum type)

This is an endocardial cushion defect and the lesion may involve the atrioventricular valves. The more severe form, atrioventricular septal defect (AVSD), is associated with Down's syndrome and results in severe pulmonary hypertension if not treated in infancy. Surgical repair of these lesions occasionally results in complete heart block.

VSD

This represents the commonest form of CHD. Clinical effects depend on how many are present and their size. A small, single VSD may be asymptomatic with a small left to right shunt (pulmonary:systemic flow ratio < 1.5:1). In patients who have not had corrective surgery prevent air emboli and fluid overload and remember antibiotic prophylaxis.

Patients with a moderate sized, single VSD often present with mild CCF. They have markedly increased pulmonary blood flow (pulmonary:systemic flow ratio 3:1). If the lesion is not recognized these patients are at risk of pulmonary hypertension and shunt reversal.

Patients with a large VSD have equal pressures in their right and left ventricles and often present around 2 months of age with severe CCF. These patients require early operations. However, if they require anaesthesia for another procedure prior to their definitive cardiac operation they may present severe problems. They should be intubated for all but the most minor procedures, and one should try to avoid increasing the left to right shunt (e.g. avoid hyperventilation and unnecessarily high inspired oxygen levels). Care should be taken with fluid administration, and inotropic support is often required.

Patients with multiple VSDs often require pulmonary artery banding to protect their pulmonary circulation. This band will tighten as the child grows, resulting in cyanosis. The VSDs often close spontaneously and then the band may then be removed.

PDA

Patients with PDA may have a moderate left to right shunt and this can result in an elevated pulmonary vascular resistance rather like a moderately sized VSD. PDAs can be closed surgically or transcatheter.

Tetralogy of Fallot

These patients have pulmonary stenosis, a VSD, an overriding aorta and right ventricular hypertrophy. Total repair of TOF is now undertaken at around 3 to 8 months of age. Prior to complete repair, these patients may be treated medically with beta-blockade or surgically via a Blalock–Taussig (BT) shunt from a subclavian artery (usually the right) to the pulmonary artery. In patients without a BT shunt and prior to definitive surgery, the ratio of systemic vascular resistance (SVR) to pulmonary vascular resistance (PVR) determines both the systemic blood flow and blood oxygen saturation. If these patients require surgery prior to their repair they should be intubated and ventilated in order to maintain a low PVR. Cyanosis should be treated with hyperventilation, intravenous fluid, and systemic vasopressors such as phenylephrine.

Eisenmenger's syndrome

Patients with this syndrome have a markedly increased morbidity and mortality. They have an abnormal and irreversible elevation in PVR resulting in cyanosis and right to left shunting. The degree of shunting depends on the PVR:SVR ratio. Increasing the SVR or decreasing the PVR leads to better blood oxygen saturation rather like in patients with TOF. Desaturation episodes can be treated as for TOF above. Inotropic support may be required even for the shortest of procedures and an intensive care bed should be available. Avoid reductions in SVR (epidural/spinal anaesthesia) and rises in PVR (hypoxia/hypercarbia/acidosis/cold). Eisenmenger's patients should be managed in a specialist centre whenever possible.

Fontan repair

This is a palliative procedure, classically for patients with tricuspid atresia, but it may be performed for a number of different cardiac lesions including hypoplastic left heart syndrome. The Fontan procedure is not a specific operation but a class of operations that separate the pulmonary and systemic circulations in patients with an anatomical or physiological single ventricle. This separation is accomplished by ensuring that all superior and inferior vena caval blood flows directly into the pulmonary artery, bypassing the right ventricle and, usually, the right atrium. Thus, pulmonary blood flow is dependent solely on systemic venous pressure. S_pO_2 should be normal.

The Fontan circuit invariably leads to elevated systemic venous pressures which in time leads to liver congestion, protein-losing enteropathy, and a tendency for fluid overload with ascites and pleural and pericardial effusions. Hypovolaemia can rapidly lead to hypoxia and cardiovascular collapse. Patients require anticoagulation with warfarin.

Great care should be observed when anaesthetizing these patients. Intermittent positive pressure ventilation results in a significant fall in cardiac output and high ventilatory pressures may result in poor pulmonary perfusion. Fluid overload is poorly tolerated, as is hypovolaemia. Central venous pressure monitoring is helpful but is probably best instituted via the femoral venous route.

Adults with congenital heart disease

Anything but the most straightforward or emergency situation should be discussed and often referred to an appropriate cardiac centre. Lesions may have been left uncorrected, palliated, or had full anatomical correction.

Uncorrected disease

* A lesion with a large left to right shunt will cause progressive pulmonary hypertension leading to eventual shunt reversal (Eisenmenger's syndrome). Once irreversible pulmonary hypertension has developed surgical correction is not possible. These patients have high mortality for any surgery, even minor procedures. If surgery is absolutely necessary it should be performed in a specialist centre.
* Ventricular or atrial septal defects may be small and have no symptoms and little haemodynamic effect. With the exception of endocarditis prophylaxis a small ventricular or atrial septal defect presents no anaesthetic problems.

Palliated disease

- These patients have had operations that improve functional capacity and life expectancy but do not restore normal anatomy. Operations include Senning and Mustard for transposition of the great vessels (neonatal switch is now preferred) and Fontan for single ventricle syndromes (e.g. hypoplastic left heart and pulmonary atresia).
- A precise understanding of the underlying physiology is required to avoid disaster when anaesthetizing these patients. At present this is best provided in specialist cardiac centres or at least after seeking their advice.
- Patients with a Fontan circulation are surviving well into adulthood and consequently their numbers will increase in the practice of non-cardiac anaesthetists. Blood leaves a single ventricle, passes through systemic capillaries and then through pulmonary capillaries before returning to the heart. The consequences of this are that the measured CVP is, and needs to be, high to provide a pressure gradient across the pulmonary circulation. Any pulmonary hypertension is tolerated very badly because ventricular filling is reduced. The high venous pressure can result in life-threatening haemorrhage from mucosal procedures like adenoidectomy (or nasal intubation!).

Corrected disease

These patients have either had spontaneous resolution or complete surgical correction. Providing they have normal functional capacity they can be treated normally. Check for any associated congenital abnormalities.

Endocarditis prophylaxis

This is required for all patients with congenital cardiac disease except: isolated secundum atrial septal defect repaired without a patch more than 6 months ago or persistent ductus arteriosus ligated more than 6 months ago.

Chapter 3
Respiratory disease

Bruce McCormick and Iain Wilson

Effects of surgery and anaesthesia on respiratory function

Surgery

Respiratory complications after surgery are largely related to two factors:

- Site of surgical incision. Upper abdominal operations are associated with pulmonary complications in 20–40% of the general surgical population. The incidence with lower abdominal surgery is 2–5%. Following upper abdominal or thoracic surgery, there is a reduction in lung volume, shallow respiration, and a reluctance or inability to cough effectively. These changes often result in poor basal air entry and sputum retention, which may develop into atelectasis and/or infection. Effective postoperative analgesia, early mobilization, and physiotherapy may reduce their incidence and severity.

- Pre-existing respiratory dysfunction. Patients with underlying respiratory disease are at increased risk of developing problems during and after surgery. Complications are minimized if the underlying condition is identified and optimally controlled preoperatively. All patients benefit from a review of their medical therapy, early mobilization, and pre- and postoperative chest physiotherapy. Advice from a respiratory physician may be helpful to ensure optimal preoperative condition.

Anaesthesia

- FRC decreases by 15–20% (about 450 ml): loss of muscle tone on induction of anaesthesia causes the diaphragm to move cranially (loss of end-expiratory tone) and the rib-cage to move inward. The FRC may be reduced to 50% of the awake, supine value in the morbidly obese. Ketamine does not reduce muscle tone and consequently FRC is maintained during anaesthesia with this agent.

- Closing capacity is the lung volume at which airway closure begins. Under anaesthesia closing capacity is greater than FRC and airway closure occurs. This occurs more readily in smokers, the elderly and those with underlying lung disease.

- Immediately after induction chest CT shows atelectasis in the dependent zones of the lungs in over 80% of subjects. As a result, at least 10% of pulmonary blood flow is shunted or goes to areas of low V/Q ratio.

- Tidal volume and lung compliance decrease (moves down compliance curve) and airway resistance increases slightly.

- Intubation halves dead space by circumventing the upper airway. Alveolar dead space rises from 0 to about 70 ml.

- The response to hypercapnoea is blunted and the acute responses to hypoxia and acidaemia almost abolished by anaesthetic vapours at concentrations as low as 0.1 MAC.

- The diaphragm moves less after abdominal surgery (vital capacity falls by 50% after cholecystectomy, even in healthy patients).

- Most of these adverse changes are more marked in patients with lung disease, but usually improve within a few hours postoperatively. After major surgery they may last several days.

Further reading

Hall JC, Tarala RA, Tapper J, Hall J (1996). Prevention of respiratory complications after abdominal surgery: a randomised control trial. *British Medical Journal*, **312**, 148–52.

Hedenstierna G, Rothen HU (1996). Pulmonary gas exchange, effects of anaesthesia and of artificial ventilation. In *International practice of anaesthesia* (eds Prys-Roberts and Brown), Butterworth-Heinemann, Oxford.

Respiratory tract infections and elective surgery

- Patients who have respiratory tract infections producing fever and cough with or without chest signs on auscultation should not undergo elective surgery under general anaesthesia due to the increased risk of pulmonary complications postoperatively.

- Adult patients with simple coryza are not at significantly increased risk of developing postoperative pulmonary problems unless they have pre-existing respiratory disease or are having major abdominal or thoracic surgery. There is some evidence that the incidence of laryngospasm is increased in patients with a recent history of upper respiratory tract symptoms who are asymptomatic at the time of surgery.

- Compared with asymptomatic children, children with symptoms of acute or recent upper respiratory tract infection are more likely to suffer transient postoperative hypoxaemia ($S_aO_2 < 93\%$). This is most marked when intubation is necessary. See p. 812.

Further reading

Fennelly ME, Hall GM (1990). Anaesthesia and upper airway respiratory tract infections—a non-existent hazard? *British Journal of Anaesthesia*, **64**, 535–6.

Levy L, Pandit UA, Randel GI, Lewis IH, Tait AR (1992). Upper respiratory tract infections and general anaesthesia in children. *Anaesthesia*, **47**, 678–82.

Smoking

Smokers, both active and passive, have a six-fold increased risk of developing perioperative respiratory problems.

Implications of smoking for anaesthesia

- Cigarette smoke contains nicotine, a highly addictive substance, and at least 4700 other chemical compounds of which 43 are known to be carcinogenic. Long-term smoking is associated with serious underlying problems such as COPD, lung neoplasm, ischaemic heart disease, and vascular disorders.

- In the respiratory tract, mucus is produced in greater quantities yet cleared less efficiently due to impaired mucociliary clearance. The airways are hyper-reactive and there is impairment of both cell-mediated and humoral immunity. These changes make smokers more susceptible to respiratory events during anaesthesia and also to postoperative atelectasis or pneumonia, particularly after abdominal or thoracic surgery. Coexisting obesity increases these risks.

- Increased airway irritability increases events such as coughing, laryngospasm, and desaturation during induction with volatile anaesthetic agents (particularly isoflurane). Avoid by using a less irritant volatile (e.g. sevoflurane) and deepening anaesthesia slowly, or treat with an intravenous agent such as propofol.

- Maintaining spontaneous breathing via an ETT or LMA may be awkward due to airway irritation—try local anaesthesia to the vocal cords, opioids, relaxants, and IPPV.

Risk reduction

- At least 8 weeks' abstinence from smoking is required to decrease morbidity from respiratory complications to a rate similar to that of non-smokers.

- Smokers unwilling to stop preoperatively will still benefit by refraining from smoking for 12 h before surgery. During this time the effects of nicotine (activation of the sympathoadrenergic system with raised coronary vascular resistance) will wear off. The level of carboxyhaemoglobin (COHb), which may reach 5–15% in heavy smokers, will also fall.

- Raised COHb levels cause a left-shift of the oxygenation curve and therefore reduced oxygen carriage by the blood. COHb has a similar absorption spectrum to oxyhaemoglobin and causes pulse oximeters to give a falsely high oxygen saturation reading.

Further reading

Nel MR, Morgan M (1996). Smoking and anaesthesia revisited (editorial). *Anaesthesia*, **51**, 309–11.

Schwilk B, Bothner U, Schraag S, Georgieff M (1997). Perioperative respiratory events in smokers and non-smokers undergoing general anaesthesia. *Acta Anaesthesiologica Scandinavica*, **41**, 348–55.

Predicting postoperative pulmonary complications before surgery

The incidence of postoperative complications in surgical patients with pre-existing respiratory dysfunction can be reduced if these patients are identified preoperatively. Large and rigorous studies to identify risk factors for pulmonary complications are relatively lacking (in comparison to the large prospective studies of cardiac risk performed since the 1970s). Comparisons between studies are difficult: definitions of complications, patient groups, and surgical interventions differ greatly.

Spirometry was formerly considered highly important in the assessment of surgical patients and included in widely adopted guidelines. Recent evidence suggests that preoperative spirometry does not predict individual risk of pulmonary complications and should not be used alone to determine operability for non-thoracic surgery. Scoring systems which assess overall co-morbidity (ASA physical status grade, Goldman cardiac risk index, and Charlson co-morbidity index) are the best predictors of complications. Abnormal findings on examination or an abnormal chest radiograph reflect significant lung disease and are independent predictors of pulmonary complications.

Even in patients with severe pulmonary disease, surgery which does not involve the abdominal or chest cavities is inherently of very low risk for serious perioperative pulmonary complications.

Factors shown to predict perioperative pulmonary complications

Scoring systems which assess overall co-morbidity (ASA physical status grade, Goldman cardiac risk index, and Charlson co-morbidity index)

Increasing age (>60 years)

Smoking within 8 weeks

History of malignancy

Symptoms of chronic bronchitis

Body mass index >27

Upper abdominal and thoracic surgery

Abnormal clinical signs in chest

Abnormality on chest radiograph

$PaCO_2$ >6 kPa

Impaired cognitive function

Postoperative nasogastric intubation

Further reading

Lawrence VA, Dhanda R, Hilsenbeck SG, Page CP (1996). Risk of pulmonary complications following abdominal surgery. *Chest*, **110**, 744–50.

Zollinger A and Pasch T (1998). The pulmonary risk patient. *Bailliere's Clinical Anaesthesia*, **5**, 391–400.

Preoperative assessment of respiratory function

History

* Ask about hospital admissions with respiratory disease—particularly visits to intensive care.
* Determine patient's assessment of lung function and their compliance with treatments. Respiratory disease tends to fluctuate in severity and patients are usually best at determining their current state. Ideally, surgery is performed when the patient is optimally controlled.
* Note cough and sputum production (character and quantity)—with major surgery send a current sputum sample for C&S preoperatively.
* Note past and present cigarette consumption.
* Assess current treatment, reversibility of symptoms with bronchodilators, and steroid intake.
* Note any respiratory symptoms suggestive of cardiac disease (orthopnoea, PND).
* Dyspnoea can be described using Roizen's classification. Undiagnosed dyspnoea of grade II or worse may require further investigation (see below).

Roizen's classification of dyspnoea

Grade 0:	No dyspnoea while walking on the level at normal pace
Grade I:	'I am able to walk as far as I like provided I take my time'
Grade II:	Specific street block limitation—'I have to stop for a while after one or two blocks'
Grade III:	Dyspnoea on mild exertion—'I have to stop and rest going from the kitchen to the bathroom'
Grade IV:	Dyspnoea at rest

Examination

Abnormal findings on clinical examination of the respiratory system are predictive of pulmonary complications after abdominal surgery. Complications of respiratory disease (right heart failure) and its treatment (steroid effects) should be sought. Try to establish any contribution of cardiac disease to respiratory symptoms.

A formal assessment of exercise tolerance such as stair climbing correlates well with pulmonary function tests and provides a reliable test of pulmonary function. However, it also reflects cardiovascular status, cooperation, and determination and is an impractical assessment for those with limited mobility. A few patients present for surgery whilst receiving CPAP for sleep apnoea syndrome or BIPAP for chronic respiratory failure. Continue these perioperatively and decide the best place for the patients to be looked after.

Respiratory investigations

Peak flow

A useful test for COPD or asthma. When the patient maintains a daily record it will indicate current fitness. Normal values are shown on p. 1104. With peak flows of less than 200 litres/min effective coughing is difficult. Measured on ward using a peak flow meter (best of three attempts); technique is important.

Spirometry

Measured in the respiratory function laboratory or at the bedside using a bellows device. It has been widely used to assess risk in patients with significant respiratory disease scheduled for major surgery. However, recent evidence suggests that spirometry does not predict pulmonary complications, even in patients with severe COPD. Specific subgroups of patients may benefit from spirometry:

- those with equivocal clinical and radiological findings, or unclear diagnosis.
- patients in whom functional ability cannot be assessed because of lower extremity disability.

Spirometry also forms part of the assessment of patients for lung parenchymal resection (see p. 366).

In those with obstructive symptoms the reversibility with salbutamol should be tested. If time permits, and the patient has undertreated obstructive disease, a course of steroids (prednisolone 20–40 mg daily for 7 days) should be assessed for effectiveness.

Normally the forced vital capacity (FVC) is reported along with forced expiration in 1 s (FEV1), plus the ratio FEV1/FVC (as a percentage). The results of these tests are given with normal values calculated for that individual. A normal FEV1/FVC ratio is > 70% (see p. 1104).

There are no spirometric values which should be viewed as prohibitive for surgery. Despite poor preoperative spirometry, many series of patients undergoing thoracic and major non-thoracic surgery are being increasingly reported. A FEV1 less than 1000 ml indicates that postoperative coughing and secretion clearance will be poor and increases the likelihood of a period of respiratory support following major surgery.

Flow volume loops

These are measured in the respiratory function department. Peak flows at different lung volumes are recorded, and although more complex to interpret, loops are capable of providing more accurate information regarding ventilatory function. They can assess airway obstruction from both extrinsic (e.g. thyroid) and intrinsic (e.g. bronchospasm) causes. In addition they provide useful data about the severity of obstructive and restrictive respiratory disease.

Transfer factor

This measures the diffusion capability of carbon monoxide into the lung. It is reduced in lung fibrosis and other interstitial disease processes.

Blood gases

A baseline set of gases provides a guide to the patient's normal respiratory function and should be measured in anyone breathless on minimal exertion. Carbon dioxide retention will be detected and the efficiency of oxygenation assessed. Record the FiO_2 when gases are taken. Check for previous results in patients who have been hospitalized before. A resting $PaCO_2$ > 6.0 kPa is predictive of pulmonary complications and suggests ventilatory failure.

Chest radiograph

An abnormality predicts risk of pulmonary complication. Essential in any patients with significant chest disease or signs on examination scheduled for major surgery. Reveals lung pathology, cardiac size and outline, and provides a baseline should postoperative problems develop. Always try to obtain an erect PA film in the X-ray department.

Chest CT

Chest CT is required in a few patients with lung cysts/bullae to assess the size and extent of their disease more accurately than can be assessed on a normal chest radiograph. Anterior or posterior pneumothorax and interstitial disease such as lung fibrosis may be detected. Spiral CT chest investigations can detect pulmonary embolus and dissecting aortic lesions.

V/Q scan

A V/Q scan reports the likelihood of pulmonary embolus. In patients with abnormal chest radiographs this test is often difficult to interpret. Also useful in further assessment of patients for lung parenchymal resection to predict the effect of resection on overall pulmonary performance (resecting a non-ventilated/perfused lung will reduce shunt and should improve oxygenation).

Further reading

Lawrence VA, Dhanda R, Hilsenbeck SG, Page CP (1996). Risk of pulmony complications after elective abdominal surgery. *Chest*, **110**, 744–50.

Smetana GW (1999). Preoperative pulmonary evaluation. *New England Journal of Medicine*, **340**, 937–44.

Zollinger A, Pasch T (1998). The pulmonary risk patient. *Bailliere's Clinical Anaesthesia*, **5**, 391–400.

Postoperative care in respiratory disease

Important features of particular disease processes are outlined in the sections below; however, the postoperative care of all patients with respiratory disease is guided by the following principles:

Early mobilization and posture

+ Respiratory performance, functional residual capacity, and clearance of secretions are improved when sitting or standing compared with the supine position.
+ Early mobilization reduces the incidence of thromboembolic disease.

Regular clinical review

Regular review allows urgent investigation and aggressive therapy. Early detection of respiratory deterioration which may present in a non-specific way (confusion, tachycardia, fever, unwell) are of the utmost importance for rapid detection and resolution of problems. Seek the assessment and advice of the intensive care team early if the patient does not respond to treatment.

Physiotherapy

Incentive spirometry and breathing exercises aid clearance of secretions and reduce atelectasis.

Oxygen

+ Anaesthetic agents exert a dose-dependent depression on the sensitivity of central chemoreceptors, reducing the stimulatory effect of CO_2 on ventilation.
+ In patients with lung disease, depression of respiratory function can occur for up to 72 h postoperatively and is most common at night. Supplemental oxygen should be delivered for at least this period of time.
+ Patients who chronically retain carbon dioxide (advanced COPD) may be dependent on hypoxaemia for their main ventilatory drive due to down-regulation of central chemoreceptors. To prevent hypoventilation oxygen therapy should be controlled and delivered where adequate monitoring is available (ideally with serial arterial blood gas measurement). A preoperative measurement of PaO_2/SaO_2 and $PaCO_2$ is essential to establish a realistic target for each patient. Pulse oximetry cannot provide information about $PaCO_2$.
+ Humidified oxygen should be used and aids physiotherapy and sputum clearance.

Fluid balance

+ Accurate management and documentation of fluid balance is important. Adequate intravascular filling is essential to the maintenance of adequate perfusion of organs such as the kidneys and alimentary system.
+ Patients with lung disease are at increased risk of pulmonary oedema (a dilated right ventricle may mechanically compromise the function of the left ventricle). Fluid overload resulting in pulmonary oedema is poorly tolerated in these patients and a high index of suspicion should be maintained clinically.

- Readings from central venous catheters may be misleading in the presence of pulmonary hypertension or right ventricular failure (cor pulmonale).

Pain management

- Good analgesia is essential for the maintenance of respiratory function, compliance with physiotherapy, early mobilization, and minimizing the cardiac stress to patients with ischaemic heart disease.
- Regular paracetamol and, where not contraindicated, NSAIDs should be prescribed. NSAIDs should be used with caution in the elderly as renal function may be compromised.
- Patients with lung dysfunction may benefit from local or regional anaesthesia, thereby avoiding the sedating effects of opioid analgesics. Communication with the surgeon may allow surgical placement of catheters for regional anaesthesia (e.g. a paravertebral catheter for thoracotomy).
- The benefits of opioid-based analgesia (patient control, mobility, and avoidance of catheterization) should be weighed against the benefits of regional analgesia (avoidance of high-dose systemic opioids, preservation of respiratory function) and discussed with the patient preoperatively.
- Following major surgery, involve the pain management team early in the postoperative period. Patients should be seen at least daily by a member of the team.

Indications for postoperative admission to HDU/ICU

- Ideally admission to ICU or HDU should be planned preoperatively and discussed with the patient and consultant supervising the unit. Patients may require admission for ventilatory support (CPAP, BIPAP, invasive ventilation) or increased levels of monitoring and nursing care that are not available on the surgical ward.
- The precipitating reasons for admission to ICU or HDU may be predictable or unpredictable:

Predictable

- borderline or established failure of gas exchange preoperatively
- intercurrent respiratory infection (with urgent surgery)
- chest disease productive of large amounts of secretions (e.g. bronchiectasis)
- major abdominal or thoracic surgery
- major surgery not amenable to regional analgesia and necessitating systemic opioids
- long duration of surgery.

Unpredictable

- unexpected perioperative complications (e.g. fluid overload, haemorrhage, etc.)
- inadequate or ineffective regional analgesia with deterioration in respiratory function
- unexpectedly prolonged procedure
- acidosis

- hypothermia
- depressed conscious level/ slow recovery from anaesthetic/ poor cough.

Indications for minitracheostomy

- 'Minitracheostomy' describes devices available for cricothyroidotomy and insertion of a tube (typically 4 mm internal diameter) to facilitate tracheal suction via fine-bore catheters. It is useful in patients with a poor cough or excessive secretions and enables more effective physiotherapy. It is relatively ineffective at removing more tenacious secretions and may partially occlude the airway.
- Insertion carries the risks of haemorrhage and surgical emphysema. Use of minitracheostomy is declining.

Asthma

Asthma implies reversible airflow obstruction due to constriction of smooth muscle in the airways. Bronchial wall inflammation is a fundamental component and results in mucus hypersecretion and epithelial damage as well as an increased tendency for airways to constrict. Bronchoconstriction may be triggered by a number of different mechanisms.

Symptoms of asthma are most frequently a combination of shortness of breath, wheeze, cough, and sputum production. The presence of childhood symptoms, cough which wakes the patient at night, diurnal variation, specific trigger factors (especially allergic), absence of smoking history, and response to previous treatment may all be helpful in differentiating asthma from COPD.

Assessment

Patients and doctors frequently underestimate the severity of asthma, especially if it is longstanding.

* Assess exercise tolerance (e.g. breathless when climbing stairs, walking on flat, or when undressing) and general activity levels.
* Examination is often unremarkable but patients may have a hyperinflated chest, a prolonged expiratory phase and wheeze: there is little correlation between the presence or absence of wheeze heard with a stethoscope and the severity of underlying asthma.
* A single peak flow reading can be helpful but serial measurements are more informative. The response to bronchodilators should be measured.
* Spirometry will give a more accurate assessment and is easy to perform. Results of peak flow and spirometry are compared with predicted values based on age, sex, and height (see p. 1104).
* Blood gases are usually only necessary in assessing severe cases, particularly with impending major surgery.
* Patients with severe asthma (poorly controlled, frequent hospital admissions, previous ICU admission) should be considered for options such as additional medication or steroid cover. In general, patients with mild asthma (peak flow > 80% predicted and minimal symptoms) require little extra treatment prior to surgery.
* If seen before admission for surgery emphasize the need for good compliance with treatment prior to surgery. Consider doubling dose of inhaled steroids 1 week prior to surgery if there is evidence of poor control (> 20% variability in PEFR). If control is very poor, consider review by a chest physician and possibly a short (1 week) course of oral prednisolone (20–40 mg daily).
* Do not anaesthetize patients for elective surgery when the patient's asthma is less than optimally controlled. Viral infections are potent triggers of asthma so consider postponing elective surgery with a symptomatic upper respiratory tract infection.

Preoperatively

* Change inhaled bronchodilators to nebulized bronchodilators on admission.
* Add nebulized salbutamol 2.5 mg to premedication.

Medications used to treat asthma

Class of drug	Examples	Perioperative recommendation	Notes
Beta 2 agonists	Salbutamol, terbutaline, salmeterol	Convert to nebulized preparation	High doses may lower K^+
Vagolytic drug	Ipratropium	Convert to nebulized form	
Inhaled steroids	Beclomethasone, budesonide, flixotide	Continue with inhaled format	If patient on >1500 µg/day of beclomethasone, adrenal suppression may be present
Oral steroids	Prednisolone	Continue as IV hydrocortisone until taking orally	If >10 mg/day, adrenal suppression likely (p. 98)
Leukotriene inhibitor (anti-inflammatory effect)	Montelukast, zafirlukast	Restart when taking oral medications	
Mast cell stabilizer	Disodium cromoglycate	Continue by inhaler	
Phosphodiesterase inhibitor	Aminophylline	Continue where possible	Effectiveness in asthma debated. In severe asthma consider converting to an infusion perioperatively

- Clearly document any allergies or drug sensitivities, especially the effect of aspirin/NSAIDs on asthma.
- Ensure patients are prescribed prn nebulized bronchodilators after surgery.
- With major abdominal or thoracic surgery start chest physiotherapy pre-operatively.
- Treat anxiety with appropriate premedication.
- The incidence of perioperative bronchospasm and laryngospasm in asthmatic patients undergoing routine surgery is less than 2%, especially if they continue their routine medication. The frequency of complications is increased in patients over 50 years and in those with active disease (recent asthmatic symptoms or treatment for asthma).

Asthma drugs in the perioperative period

In patients with significant asthma undergoing major surgery:

- change salbutamol and ipratropium to nebulized form
- consider steroid supplementation if taking > 10 mg of prednisolone/ day or inhaled beclomethasone > 1.5 mg/day (p. 98)
- convert prednisolone to IV hydrocortisone (1 mg prednisolone equivalent to 5 mg hydrocortisone)
- aminophylline may be continued intravenously by infusion in critical patients (check levels 12-hourly), or given by suppository. It can also often be stopped!

Anaesthesia

- Most well-controlled asthmatics tolerate anaesthesia and surgery well, requiring minimal changes to anaesthetic technique.
- Poorly controlled asthmatics are at risk of perioperative respiratory problems (bronchospasm, sputum retention, atelectasis, infection, respiratory failure).
- Avoid histamine-releasing drugs (morphine, d-tubocurarine, atracurium, mivacurium).
- Intubation may provoke bronchospasm and should be carried out under adequate anaesthesia or opioid cover. Local anaesthetic to the cords may help.
- When asthma is poorly controlled, regional techniques are ideal for peripheral surgery. Spinal anaesthesia or plexus/nerve blocks are generally safe, provided the patient is able to lie flat comfortably.
- Patients with severe asthma (previous ICU admissions, brittle disease) undergoing major abdominal or thoracic surgery should be admitted to HDU/ICU for postoperative observation.

Severe bronchospasm during anaesthesia

See p. 848.

Postoperatively

- Following major abdominal or thoracic surgery good pain control is important and epidural analgesia is frequently the best choice, provided widespread intercostal blockade is avoided. When PCA is used pethidine is a better choice than morphine in symptomatic asthmatics. Oxygen should

Drugs considered safe for asthmatics

Induction	Propofol, etomidate, ketamine, midazolam
Opioids	Pethidine, fentanyl, alfentanyl
Muscle relaxants	Vecuronium, suxamethonium, rocuronium, pancuronium
Volatile agents	Halothane, isoflurane, enflurane, sevoflurane

be prescribed along with regular nebulizer therapy. Convert regular steroids to intravenous preparations. NSAIDs should be avoided in general (up to 10% of asthmatics may develop bronchospasm), but use them if they have been tolerated in the past.

• If there is increasing dyspnoea and wheeze following surgery consider which other conditions can result in wheeze. Left ventricular failure and pulmonary emboli are both potent triggers of bronchospasm. Also consider fluid overload and pneumothorax (recent central line?).

Further reading

Guidelines on the management of asthma (1993). *Thorax*, **48** (Supplement), S1–S24.
Hirshman CA (1991). Perioperative management of the asthmatic patient. *Canadian Journal of Anaesthesia*, **38**, R26–R32.
Warner DO et al. (1996). Perioperative respiratory complications in patients with asthma. *Anaesthesiology*, **85**, 460–7.

Chronic obstructive pulmonary disease (COPD)

COPD encompasses chronic bronchitis and emphysema. Chronic bronchitis is diagnosed on a history of a productive cough on most winter days of three consecutive years. Emphysema is a histological diagnosis of dilatation and destruction of the airways distal to the terminal bronchioles.

The majority of patients with COPD have been tobacco smokers for a significant period of their lives. Other factors associated with COPD include occupational exposure to dusts and atmospheric pollution, poor socio-economic status, repeated viral infections, α1-antitrypsin deficiency, and regional variation within the United Kingdom.

Symptoms of COPD usually start after the age of about 55 years. The most common symptom is shortness of breath but there is often a combination of shortness of breath, cough, wheeze, and sputum production. Symptoms are frequently severe by the time any medical help is sought. Patients frequently give a history of repeated exacerbations of respiratory symptoms during the winter months. The morning is usually the worst time for patients with both asthma and COPD.

An increasingly popular treatment of acute severe exacerbations of COPD is non-invasive ventilation via a full face or nasal mask. On occasions this technique may be used to assist severely affected patients through the postoperative phase of major surgery. Preoperative training is essential in conjunction with a respiratory unit.

Pathophysiology

The principal problems in COPD are the development of airflow obstruction and mucus hypersecretion, exacerbated by repeated viral and bacterial infections. Many patients have an element of reversible airflow obstruction. If this can be demonstrated it is managed as asthma. Progressive airflow obstruction may lead to respiratory failure.

Patients with predominant emphysema may be thin, tachypnoeic, breathless at rest, and, although hypoxic, develop CO_2 retention only as a late or terminal event. Patients with predominant chronic bronchitis are frequently overweight with marked peripheral oedema, poor respiratory effort, and CO_2 retention. These classical stereotyped pictures of 'pink puffer' or 'blue bloater' are relatively infrequently seen compared with the majority of patients who have a combination of features.

Assessment

- Establish exercise tolerance—ask specifically about hills and stairs. A formal assessment of exercise tolerance such as stair climbing correlates well with pulmonary function tests.
- Ensure any element of reversible airflow obstruction (asthma) is optimally treated. A trial of oral prednisolone may be worth considering, combined with a medical review.
- Pulmonary hypertension and right ventricular failure may follow severe or chronic pulmonary disease—optimize treatment of heart failure if present.
- Check spirometry to clarify diagnosis and assess severity (this is much more informative than peak flow in COPD).

- Check arterial blood gases if the patient has difficulty climbing one flight of stairs, is cyanosed, has an oxygen saturation of < 95% on air, or has any peripheral oedema.
- If the patient has a very poor exercise tolerance (less than one flight of stairs) and is undergoing a procedure that will make breathing painful or difficult postoperatively, consider whether ICU or HDU care would be appropriate postoperatively.
- Change to nebulized bronchodilators prior to surgery and continue for 24–48 h afterwards.

Anaesthesia

- See guidelines under asthma (see p. 59).
- Patients with severe COPD (particularly CO_2 retainers) are at a high risk of respiratory failure developing in the postoperative period following abdominal or thoracic surgery and may be sensitive to any respiratory depressant. Consider HDU/ICU for any on this group postoperatively.
- Some patients (particularly those who are obese, breathless, and require long operations) are unsuitable for a spontaneously breathing anaesthetic.

Postoperatively

- Mobilize as early as possible.
- Give regular physiotherapy to prevent atelectasis and encourage sputum clearance.
- Give oxygen as appropriate (see p. 54).
- If the patient becomes pyrexial with more copious or purulent sputum send a sample for culture and start an antibiotic. Oral amoxicillin, trimethoprim, or clarithromycin are usually sufficient to treat for mild exacerbations of COPD. If the patient is seriously unwell treat as postoperative pneumonia.
- Continue with nebulized salbutamol (2.5 mg four times a day) and ipratropium (500 μg four times a day) until fully mobile and change back to inhalers 24 h before discharge. Salbutamol may be given more frequently but there is no benefit from higher doses of ipratropium.
- If the patient is very slow to mobilize consider referral to a pulmonary rehabilitation programme if available.

Lung volume reduction surgery for COPD

This procedure has increased over the last few years. Lung volume reduction surgery is performed through a sternotomy and involves excision of 20 to 30% of each lung, aiming to improve respiratory mechanics in severe COPD. Improvements in FEV1 (forced expiration in 1 s) of 80%, reduction in total lung capacity and residual volume, marked relief of dyspnoea, and improved exercise tolerance and quality of life are described. Twenty per cent of patients exhibit no functional improvement.

Further reading

Cooper JD, Trulock EP, Triantafillou AN (1995). Bilateral pneumectomy (volume reduction) for chronic obstructive pulmonary disease. *Journal of Thoracic and Cardiovascular Surgery*, **109**, 106–19.

Wong DH, Weber EC, Schell MJ, Wong AB, Anderson CT, Barker SJ (1995). Factors associated with postoperative pulmonary complications in patients with severe chronic obstructive pulmonary disease. *Anesthesia and Analgesia*, **80**, 276–84.

Bronchiectasis

Bronchiectasis may be caused by genetic factors, e.g. cystic fibrosis, or acquired following damage to the lower respiratory tract, especially in severe early childhood infections. Most patients have a chronic productive cough, which may be present throughout the year. There is frequently a component of asthma associated with chronic inflammatory changes in the airways. Once established, bacterial infections can be difficult or impossible to eradicate. *Pseudomonas aeruginosa* is a common pathogen that may be present for many years and be associated with intermittent exacerbations of respiratory symptoms.

The mainstay of treatment for bronchiectasis is regular physiotherapy, frequent courses of appropriate antibiotics, and treatment of any asthmatic symptoms. In cystic fibrosis there is also malabsorption due to pancreatic insufficiency, so appropriate dietary advice and pancreatic supplements are essential.

Patients with bronchiectasis need to be as fit as possible before undergoing any major surgery which will inhibit their coughing and respiratory function. For elective surgery this may mean a planned admission for intravenous antibiotics and physiotherapy prior to surgery.

Preoperatively

- Before elective surgery the patient should be as fit as possible. Consultation with their chest physician may be helpful. A course of IV antibiotics and physiotherapy for 3–10 days immediately prior to surgery may be necessary.
- Ensure that the patient will receive physiotherapy immediately postoperatively if they have severe bronchiectasis. Contact on-call physiotherapist if necessary.
- Maximize bronchodilation: convert to nebulized bronchodilators.
- Increase dose of prednisolone by 5–10 mg/day if on long-term oral steroids.
- Send sputum sample for C&S before surgery. If antibiotics are needed postoperatively the most appropriate one may then be started.
- Prior to major surgery, consider starting IV antibiotics on admission. Use current or most recent sputum culture to guide appropriate prescribing. If in doubt assume that the patient has *Pseudomonas aeruginosa* in their sputum and use a combination such as ceftazidime and gentamicin, or imipenem and gentamicin.
- In patients with severe disease check spirometry and blood gases.
- Postpone elective surgery if the patient has more respiratory symptoms than usual.

Postoperatively

- Ensure that regular physiotherapy is available: three times daily and at night if severely affected.
- Adequate oxygenation, check SaO_2.
- Continue appropriate IV antibiotics for at least 3 days postoperatively or until discharged.
- Maintain adequate nutrition, especially if there is any malabsorption.
- Refer to chest physicians early if there is any deterioration in respiratory symptoms.

Cystic fibrosis

Pathophysiology

The basic defect is an abnormal epithelial chloride and sodium transport system encoded by a gene on chromosome 7. Patients experience chronic sinusitis, nasal polyps in 50% (polypectomy is a leading reason for anaesthesia in this group), and respiratory, cardiovascular, and gastrointestinal disease. Neonates may present for surgical treatment of meconium ileus. In the lung, viscid mucus causes plugging, atelectasis, and frequent chest infection (particularly *Pseudomonas*). Treatment is primarily clearance of secretions by postural drainage and antibiotic treatment of infections. Heart–lung transplant was first performed in 1985 and early series show a 78% 1-year survival. The perioperative complication rate in cystic fibrosis is about 10% (mostly pulmonary).

Perioperative management

- Exclude or treat active chest infection.
- Clinical signs can be misleading. Perform a chest radiograph. Look for bullae and pneumothorax.
- Spirometry: FEV1 may be prognostic.
- Almost all patients with cystic fibrosis have symptoms from their bronchiectasis and will require treatment as outlined above. Always inform the patient's cystic fibrosis physician of an admission to a surgical ward.
- Intubation allows bronchial toilet. Monitor for pneumothorax.
- Eighty per cent of cystic fibrosis patients have pancreatic malabsorption. Maintaining adequate nutrition after surgery is essential and the advice of an experienced cystic fibrosis dietician is essential.

Further reading

Walsh TS, Young CH (1995). Anaesthesia and cystic fibrosis. *Anaesthesia*, **50**, 614–22.

Restrictive pulmonary disease

Restrictive pulmonary disease may be caused by intrinsic lung disease (such as pulmonary fibrosis) or by extrinsic conditions in which the lung parenchyma is normal but there is a failure of the respiratory mechanism to provide an adequate air supply to the lung. Extrinsic conditions include disease of the chest wall (kyphoscoliosis, severe obesity) or other abdominal problems producing significant splinting of the diaphragm. Changes on the chest radiograph will be according to the underlying condition.

Pulmonary fibrosis

Pulmonary fibrosis makes patients breathless because they have lungs that are hard to inflate and have impaired ability to take up oxygen. Initially there is an inflammatory reaction centred on the alveoli, impairing gas exchange. Over a period of time, which can vary from days to years, collagen is formed in and around the alveoli causing more marked impairment of gas exchange and smaller, stiffer lungs.

Pulmonary fibrosis is the final response of the lung to a number of different stimuli. Causes include those associated with autoimmune disorders (e.g. rheumatoid arthritis, scleroderma), inhaled dusts (e.g. asbestos) or ingested substances, especially drugs (e.g. amiodarone, chemotherapy agents, paraquat poisoning). Allergic response to inhaled substances can cause fibrosis if exposure is prolonged, e.g. bird fancier's and farmer's lung. Pulmonary infections rarely trigger a fibrotic response. Treatment is usually with oral steroids but other immunosuppressive therapy may be used and young patients may be considered for lung transplantation if severely affected.

Preoperatively

Many patients are stable and only slowly deteriorate over some years. These patients may tolerate surgery relatively well.

- Check preoperative blood gases. A reduced PaO_2 reflects significant disease.
- Obtain lung function tests including spirometry, lung volumes, and gas transfer if these have not been done within previous 6–8 weeks.
- For those on steroids, increase dose starting with premedication and continuing an extra 5–10 mg of prednisolone per day until the patient goes home.
- Discuss seriously affected patients with a chest physician.

Postoperatively

- Ensure adequate additional oxygen, maintain $SaO_2 > 92\%$.
- Mobilize early.
- Treat any respiratory infection vigorously.
- Ensure patient is continuing to receive steroids in appropriate form.

Restrictive pulmonary disease due to chest wall conditions

Chest wall or thoracic spinal deformities result in inefficient respiration and a reduction of all lung volumes. Respiration is characterized by rapid shallow breaths and is easier in the sitting position. Blood gases often remain normal until late. CO_2 retention is a late sign and implies severe disease and incipient ventilatory failure. The significance of the condition may be assessed using spirometry.

Postoperatively sputum retention may be a major problem and good physiotherapy and analgesia are vital. Spinal disease will preclude certain regional anaesthetic techniques, such as epidural analgesia. Patients may develop respiratory failure with relatively minor postoperative problems and must be assessed regularly. A laparotomy in a patient who depends on their diaphragm for adequate ventilation because of underlying chest wall disease may cause respiratory failure to develop in the early postoperative period.

Perioperative plan

- Follow the principles described under pulmonary fibrosis.
- Consider ICU/HDU following major surgery.
- Vigorous physiotherapy pre- and postoperatively.
- Early involvement of the ICU team and respiratory physicians if deterioration occurs.
- May be suitable for elective training in CPAP/NIPPV techniques pre-operatively.

Sleep apnoea syndrome (see also page 511)

Sleep apnoea is defined as cessation of airflow at the mouth and nose for at least 10 s. Sufferers develop recurrent apnoea and hypoxaemia during sleep. Many are overweight, middle-aged men, who present with complaints of snoring with periods of apnoea, disturbed sleep, excessive daytime drowsiness, and headaches. The patient may develop systemic and pulmonary hypertension, congestive cardiac failure, and respiratory failure with CO_2 retention. Two types of sleep apnoea are recognized: obstructive sleep apnoea from obstruction of the upper airway, which affects 85% of sufferers, and central apnoea (due to intermittent loss of respiratory drive), which affects 10% of sufferers; 5% of patients have both types. Both conditions result in intermittent respiratory arrest during rapid eye movement (REM) sleep, which resolves when the patient responds to the hypoxia that develops. Patients frequently have marked daytime hypersomnolence because of repeated nocturnal arousal from hypoxia. The condition is diagnosed in a sleep laboratory by monitoring oxygen saturation and nasal airflow; additional tests including measurement of respiratory and abdominal muscle activity, EEG, and EMG activity (polysomnography) may be required in some patients.

In children obstructive sleep apnoea is most commonly associated with adenotonsillar hypertrophy, but the severity of obstructive sleep apnoea is not always proportional to the size of the tonsils and adenoids. Obstructive sleep apnoea should be considered in all children presenting for adenotonsillectomy and, if suspected, a full blood count (to detect polycythaemia), pulse oximetry, and ECG (looking for signs of cor pulmonale) should be performed. Three per cent of children presenting for adenotonsillectomy have features of right ventricular strain on their ECG and echocardiography is indicated in these patients to exclude right ventricular hypertrophy.

Treatment

- Weight reduction and management of associated conditions such as obstructive airway disease, hypertension, and cardiac failure may be successful.
- CPAP applied overnight by a nasal mask is often effective.
- A few patients require surgery to the upper airway. In children adenotonsillectomy may be indicated.

Operative risks

Patients with sleep apnoea syndrome are at risk of respiratory failure perioperatively as they are extremely sensitive to all sedative drugs, especially opioid analgesics. The risk of developing respiratory complications after major abdominal or thoracic surgery is high.

Preoperative care

In cases of suspected sleep apnoea:

- Take a history from the patient and, if possible, their sleeping partner. Ask the patient about daytime hypersomnolence and how easily they would fall asleep during common tasks such as reading, talking to someone, or driving.
- Ask the partner about snoring and whether any apnoeic spells have been noted at night; the patient is usually unaware of these but spouses may be very worried.

- Obesity and a collar size of more than 17 inches are risk factors for obstructive sleep apnoea.
- Consider a respiratory opinion in patients with peripheral oedema and oxygen saturation < 92%.

Previously diagnosed sleep apnoea

- Ensure that the patient is optimally treated for any associated medical conditions.
- If the patient is on inhalers, change to nebulized bronchodilators.
- Ensure that the patient will be able to continue taking their usual medication by an appropriate route postoperatively.
- If the patient is receiving CPAP at night, ensure that ward staff are familiar with setting it up.
- Examine the patient: heart failure and peripheral oedema suggest severe obstructive sleep apnoea.
- Measure blood gases and pulse oximetry to determine the normal PaO_2 and whether the patient retains CO_2.
- Contact the chest physiotherapist.
- Do not write up night sedation or sedative premedication.

Anaesthesia

- Airway maintenance, mask ventilation, and intubation may be difficult.
- Regional anaesthesia is often preferred to minimize the use of sedative agents.
- Regional techniques may also provide effective postoperative analgesia, avoiding the requirement for opioids.
- Consider the use of NSAIDs.

Postoperative care

- Patients are best managed in a high-dependency setting or even ICU.
- After major surgery some patients may need to be ventilated for a few hours until they are stable enough to wean from the ventilator.
- Continuous pulse oximetry should be used on the ward.
- The patient should be nursed sitting up whenever possible.
- There is debate about the optimum method of oxygen supplementation. Aim to maintain the oxygen saturation that the patient maintained preoperatively, titrating the oxygen to the minimum required. A few patients may develop CO_2 retention with oxygen therapy. This is best detected by blood gas analysis in those patients at risk who become difficult to wake or who develop signs of CO_2 retention.

Further reading

Boushra NN (1996). Anaesthetic management of patients with sleep apnoea syndrome. *Canadian Journal of Anaesthesia*, **43**, 599–616.

Warwick JP, Mason DG (1998). Obstructive sleep apnoea syndrome in children. *Anaesthesia*, **53**, 571–9.

Anaesthesia for patients after lung transplantation

Lung transplantation was first performed in 1963; outcomes have improved since the introduction of ciclosporin A in 1981.

Surgery may be indicated for complications related to transplant, complications of immunosuppressive treatment, the underlying condition (emphysema, α1-antitrypsin deficiency, pulmonary fibrosis, primary pulmonary hypertension, cystic fibrosis), or unrelated reasons.

Pathophysiology of the transplanted lung

- The transplanted lung is denervated—mucosal sensitivity and the cough reflex are suppressed below the anastomosis, and sputum clearance is impaired postoperatively.
- Hypoxic vasoconstriction is unimpaired.
- Lymphatic drainage is severed but then re-established 2–4 weeks post-transplantation. Transplanted lungs are at particular risk of pulmonary oedema, especially in the early postoperative period.
- In double lung transplant the heart may be denervated and has a higher resting heart rate (90–100 beats/min) and may be more susceptible to arrhythmias.

Anaesthetic management

- The interaction of immunosuppressive drugs (ciclosporin A, steroids, azathioprine) with anaesthetic drugs is more theoretical than clinical.
- Underlying disease may have effects on pulmonary function. There may be residual systemic disease.
- Monitor neuromuscular function and avoid high doses of opioid in order to achieve early extubation.
- Intubation should be performed to leave the tube just through the cords and the cuff carefully inflated and checked intra-operatively to minimize the risk of damage to the tracheal or bronchial anastomosis. If a double lumen tube is required it should be placed under direct vision using a fibrescope.
- Strict attention to fluid balance is required.
- Aim for early return of pulmonary function and extubation.
- Postoperative admission to intensive care is only indicated when anaesthesia is complicated by inadequate recovery of respiratory function, the surgical condition, or the presence of rejection or infection.

Chapter 4
Endocrine and metabolic disease
Gordon French, James Low, and
Jennifer Thompson

Diabetes mellitus[1]

Diabetes mellitus is present in 5% of the population, 80% of whom have non-insulin-dependent diabetes (NIDDM) and 20% have insulin-dependent diabetes (IDDM). Complications resulting from microangiopathy and neuropathy have important implications for anaesthesia. The severity and incidence of these may be related to the duration and control of the disease.

Insulin is necessary even when fasting to maintain glucose homeostasis and balance stress hormones (e.g. adrenaline). It promotes anabolism, wound healing, and polymorph phagocytic function, and prevents ketogenesis. Lack of insulin is associated with hyperglycaemia, osmotic diuresis, dehydration, hyperosmolarity, hyperviscosity, a predisposition to thrombosis, cerebral oedema, and increased rates of wound infection. Sustained hyperglycaemia is associated with an increased hospital stay and complication rates.

Diabetes is 'starvation in the midst of plenty'—a high blood glucose is combined with intracellular glucose depletion, which in turn results in ketosis. Perioperatively insulin is needed for transport of glucose into cells and to counter the catabolic effects of increased levels of stress hormone.

Preoperative assessment

- Cardiovascular: the diabetic is prone to hypertension, ischaemic heart disease, cerebrovascular disease, myocardial infarction and cardiomyopathy. Autonomic neuropathy can lead to tachy- or bradycardia and postural hypotension. Diabetics (especially IDDM) have three times the incidence of ischaemic heart disease, and this may be 'silent'. Perioperative mortality and morbidity is increased with underlying renal damage (microalbuminuria).
- Autonomic neuropathy (present in 50% of diabetics) increases the risk of unstable BP, myocardial ischaemia, arrhythmias, gastric reflux, and hypothermia during surgery.
- Renal: 40% of diabetics develop microalbuminuria, which is associated with hypertension, ischaemic heart disease, and retinopathy. This may be reduced by treatment with ACE inhibitors.
- Respiratory: diabetics are prone to perioperative chest infections, especially if they are obese and smokers.
- Airway: thickening of soft tissues (glycosylation) occurs, especially in ligaments around joints—the 'limited joint mobility syndrome'. If the neck is affected there may be difficulty achieving the 'sniffing the morning air' position or sufficient mouth opening for intubation.
- Gastrointestinal: 50% have delayed gastric emptying and are prone to reflux.
- Eyes: cataracts are common, especially in the elderly diabetic.
- Diabetics are prone to infections.
- Miscellaneous: diabetes may be caused or worsened by treatment with corticosteroids, thiazide diuretics, and the contraceptive pill. Thyroid disease, obesity, pregnancy, and stress can also affect diabetic control.

1   McAnulty GR, Robertshaw HJ, Hall GM. (2000). Anaesthetic management of patients with diabetes mellitus. *British Journal of Anaesthesia*, **85(1)**, 80–90.

• The diabetic patient is often the best judge of their insulin regime. High blood glucose levels are frequently found on admission to hospital, presumably stress related, and may settle spontaneously. The 'diabetic team' may have nurse specialists as well as medical staff who will advise on glucose control. Many patients are also familiar with sliding scale insulin regimes from previous hospital admissions.

General principles

The overall aims of perioperative diabetic management are:

• avoid hypoglycaemia which can cause irreversible cerebral damage
• avoid severe hyperglycaemia resulting in osmotic diuresis and severe dehydration (>14 mmol/litre)
• avoid large swings in glucose, i.e. maintain blood glucose in the range 6–10 mmol/litre
• supply cells with insulin so that intracellular glucose starvation does not occur, preventing ketoacidosis
• prevent hypokalaemia, hypomagnesaemia, and hypophosphataemia.

It is not necessary to admit diabetics 2 days before surgery, unless there are major problems with diabetic control. A glycosylated haemoglobin (HbsAc) >9% (normal 3.8–6.4%), suggests inadequate control of the blood glucose.

All general medications should be continued until and including the morning of surgery. For diabetic medications:

• Metformin should be stopped 2 days before major surgery as it can precipitate lactic acidosis.
• Chlorpropamide should ideally be stopped 3 days before surgery because of its long action. This is often not possible and should not pose a major problem if frequent blood glucose monitoring is undertaken.

In both these cases, a shorter acting drug such as glibenclamide should be substituted.

• An occasional patient may still be taking a long-acting insulin, e.g crystalline insulin zinc suspension. If possible, this should also be stopped several days before surgery and substituted with an intermediate- or short-acting insulin.
• Intermediate- and short-acting insulins and other oral hypoglycaemics can be continued up until the day of surgery, and then follow the regimes below.

The stress response of surgery will alter the patient's insulin requirements. Treatment will need to be adjusted according to:

• the nature of the surgery—the extent, length, and period until eating and drinking again
• whether the patient is IDDM or NIDDM
• the quality of their blood sugar control—should be 6–10 mmol/litre
• Insulin requirements usually reduce once the patient begins to recover from surgery.

Preoperative management

• Measure blood sugar preoperatively—4-hourly for IDDM and 8-hourly for NIDDM.

- Test urine for ketones and sugar.
- Place first on operating list.
- If diabetes is very poorly controlled but ketones are not present, start a sliding-scale insulin regime. If ketones are present, consider delaying non-urgent surgery and involving the diabetic team. If urgent surgery required use the 'Major surgery regime'.

Perioperative management

- In general, if the patient can be expected to eat and drink within 4 h of surgery, then it is classified as minor. All surgery other than minor is classified as major. The tables below give various regimes for both types of surgery.
- Patients with diet-controlled diabetes mellitus rarely need more than routine monitoring of their blood glucose levels (4-hourly). Consider an insulin infusion if the blood glucose is >17 mmol/litre or urinary ketones are present.
- Avoid prescribing Hartmann's solution to diabetics as the lactate may raise the blood sugar level.

Glucose and insulin infusions should be administered through the same cannula to prevent accidental administration of insulin without glucose. Both infusions should be regulated by volumetric pumps and a one-way valve included in the glucose line to prevent retrograde flow of insulin should the cannula become blocked (on unblocking a large amount of insulin could then be accidentally discharged into the patient).

Minor surgery. For patients whose random sugar is <10 mmol/litre on admission, will only miss one meal and are first on the list for minor surgery. (If blood sugar >10 mmol/litre follow as for major surgery).

Non-insulin-dependent diabetics	Omit oral hypoglycaemic
	Blood glucose measurement:
	1 h preop.
	at least once during operation
	postop. 2-hourly until eating
	then 8-hourly
	Restart oral hypoglycaemics with first meal
Insulin-dependent diabetics	Omit normal SC insulin if glucose <7 mmol/litre
	Give half normal insulin if glucose >7 mmol/litre
	Blood glucose measurement:
	1 h preop.
	at least once during operation
	postop. 2-hourly until eating
	then 4-hourly
	Restart normal SC insulin regime with first meal

Major surgery

Non-insulin-dependent and insulin-dependent diabetics	Check blood sugar and potassium preoperatively
	Omit oral hypoglycaemics or normal subcutaneous insulin
	Start intravenous infusion of 5% glucose (500 ml/4 h) or 10% glucose (500 ml/8 h) depending on fluid requirements. Dextrose 4%/saline 0.18% may also be used: If K+ <4.5 mmol/litre add 20 mmol of KCl to each litre
	Start a variable-rate insulin infusion (50 ml of 0.9% saline containing 50 units of soluble insulin—1 unit per ml) at 0800h on the day of surgery
	Blood glucose measurement: 2-hourly from start of infusion at least once during operation (hourly if op. >1 h) hourly postoperatively for 4 h then 2-hourly.
	If infusion not maintaining blood sugar within normal limits then the rates should be increased. Similarly patients on very high doses of insulin normally should be started on a higher rate
Postoperative	NIDDM—stop infusion and restart oral hypoglycaemics when eating and drinking IDDM—stop infusion when eating and drinking. Calculate the total daily dose (units) of insulin the patient was taking preoperatively and administer this as SC soluble insulin (Actrapid) divided into 3–4 daily doses. Adjust doses until blood sugar levels stable. Once stable restart normal regime

Intravenous insulin sliding scale

Blood glucose (mmol/litre)	Insulin infusion rate (unit/h)	Insulin infusion rate if blood glucose not maintained <10 mmol/litre (unit/h)
<4	0	0
4.1–9	1	2
9.1–13	2	3
13.1–17	3	4
17.1–28	4	6
>28	6 (check infusion running and call doctor)	8 (check infusion running and call doctor)

Anaesthetic technique

Standard intra-operative monitoring should be used. Check the blood glucose hourly. There are no particular contraindications to standard general anaesthetic techniques:

- Consider a rapid sequence induction if gastric stasis is suspected.
- If there is autonomic involvement administer all drugs slowly.
- Regional techniques may be particularly useful for extremity surgery and reduce the risk of undetected hypoglycaemia.
- Chart any pre-existing nerve damage before performing blocks.
- Autonomic dysfunction may exacerbate the hypotensive effect of spinals and epidurals.

Hypoglycaemia

Hypoglycaemia (blood glucose <4 mmol/litre) is the main danger to diabetics perioperatively. Fasting, recent alcohol consumption, liver failure, and septicaemia commonly exacerbate this. Characteristic signs are:

- Tachycardia, light-headedness, sweating, and pallor. This may progress to cause confusion, restlessness, incomprehensible speech, double vision, convulsions, and coma. If untreated, permanent brain damage will occur, made worse by hypotension or hypoxia.
- Anaesthetized patients may not show any of these signs. Monitor blood sugar regularly and suspect hypoglycaemia with unexplained changes in the patient's condition.
- Give 50 ml of 50% glucose (or any glucose solution available) intravenously and repeat blood sugar measurement. Alternatively give 1 mg of glucagon (IM or IV).
- 10–20 g (2–4 teaspoons) of sugar, by mouth or nasogastric tube, is an alternative.

Glucose insulin potassium regime ('GKI' or 'Alberti')[2]

This is an alternative simpler regime for major surgery, which does not require infusion pumps, but may provide less accurate control of blood sugar. The original regime as described by Alberti consists of:

- 500 ml of dextrose 10%
- add 10–15 units actrapid, plus 10 mmol potassium chloride per 500 ml bag
- infuse at 100 ml/h
- provides insulin 2–3 units/h, potassium 2 mmol/h, and glucose 10 g/h.

Dextrose 10% is not always available, so the following regime with 5% dextrose can be used:

- infusion of 5% glucose (500 ml bags) at the calculated rate for the patient's fluid maintenance requirements
- insulin and potassium should be added to each bag as per the table below
- the bag may be changed according to 2-hourly blood glucose measurements.

Blood glucose (mmol/litre)	Soluble insulin (units) to be added to each 500 ml bag	Blood potassium (mmol/litre)	KCl (mmol) to be added to each 500 ml bag
<4	5	<3	20
4–6	10	3–5	10
6.1–10	15	>5	None
10.1–20	20		
>20	Review	If potassium level not available, add 10 mmol KCl to each bag	

2 Alberti KGMM (1991). Diabetes and surgery. *Anesthesiology*, **74**, 209–11.

Acromegaly

This syndrome is caused by an excess of growth hormone, produced by a tumour of the anterior pituitary. These patients present several specific anaesthetic challenges.

Cardiovascular

Hypertension, ischaemic heart disease, arrhythmias, cardiac enlargement, and cardiomyopathy are often present. An ECG and careful clinical examination for signs of failure and valvular disease are essential. Echocardiography is valuable for those who are symptomatic or who have murmurs.

Airway

The patient may have a very large jaw, head, tongue, lips, and general hypertrophy of the mucosa of the larynx, trachea, and airway structures making intubation potentially difficult. Vocal cord thickening or strictures, glottic and subglottic stenosis, and chondrocalcinosis of the larynx may also complicate intubation. Sleep apnoea can occur as a result of these changes. Kyphosis makes positioning difficult and compromises respiratory function. Enlargement of the thyroid is also common.

- Snoring and daytime somnolence may indicate sleep apnoea.
- Careful airway assessment should be performed and consider direct/ indirect laryngoscopy preoperatively if vocal cord or laryngeal pathology is suspected.
- Awake fibreoptic intubation is the technique of choice for patients with anticipated difficult intubation but in reality is seldom required.
- Elective tracheostomy should be considered in those with severe respiratory obstruction.
- Consider ICU or HDU postoperatively, especially if the patient has a history of sleep apnoea or severe cardiovascular disease. Acromegalics may have a decreased central respiratory drive and opioid analgesia/ hypnotic sedatives should be used with caution, preferably in an HDU or ICU.

Endocrine

- Diabetes is common, caused by the excess growth hormone. Perform a preoperative blood sugar measurement and consider starting a sliding scale insulin regime.
- Hypothyroidism and hypoadrenalism may occur either posthyphophysectomy, or secondary to the expanding tumour, decreasing production of thyroid-stimulating hormone and ACTH.

Raised intracranial pressure

This may also be present.

Drugs

- Patients may be on somatostatin analogues (octreotide, lanreotide). These may cause gastrointestinal side-effects including vomiting and diarrhoea.
- Bromocriptine, a long-acting dopamine agonist, is often used to lower growth hormone levels. It can cause severe postural hypotension.

Miscellaneous

- Large hands and feet may present a problem in placing SpO_2 probes.
- Nerve compression syndromes are common so take care to protect vulnerable areas (the ulnar nerve at the elbow, the median nerve at the wrist, and the common peroneal nerve below the knee).
- Myopathy (especially proximal myopathy) may occur. Severe cases may have respiratory muscle involvement. Postoperative mobilization may be problematical.
- The patient's size makes positioning difficult, and long tables and beds may be needed.
- Large ETTs should be available (10 mm), but are not usually required
- Use extra padding to protect pressure areas.

Further reading

Hakala P, Randell T, Valli H (1998). Laryngoscopy and fibreoptic intubation in acromegalic patients. *British Journal of Anaesthesia*, **80**, 345–7.

Smith M, Hirsch NP (2000). Pituitary disease and anaesthesia. *British Journal of Anaesthesia*, **85**, 3–14.

Thyroid disease

Patients with thyroid disease may present for removal of an enlarged thyroid gland (goitre) or for non-thyroid related surgery.

Preoperative assessment

- Thyroid function: check that the patient is euthyroid. Surgery should be delayed if possible until this is achieved. Clinically a heart rate of less than 80 beats/min and no hand tremor are useful confirmatory signs.
- Respiratory obstruction can occur due to the anatomical position of the gland. Pay particular attention to the airway, noting any tracheal deviation. This is a particular problem when the gland extends retrosternally or is very large. Infiltrating carcinomas may make any neck movement difficult. A chest radiograph and thoracic inlet views are essential. If there is shortness of breath, dysphagia, or stridor (occurs with >50% compression), a CT or MRI scan will reveal the extent of the tracheal compression. An awake fibre-optic intubation or gas induction will probably be the safest course of action in this situation (see pp. 300, 870, 509). Explain the procedure but avoid atropine premedication if the patient is hyperthyroid or in atrial fibrillation.
- Refer patient to an ENT surgeon for indirect laryngoscopy. Pre-existing vocal cord palsy should be recorded.
- Superior vena caval obstruction can occur (distended neck veins that do not change with respiration).
- Look for other autoimmune disorders.

Pharmacology

- Carbimazole inhibits iodination of tyrosyl residues in thyroglobulin. Its main side-effect is granulocytopenia (0.1–1.2%).
- Propylthiouracil as above, plus reduces de-iodination of T4 to T3 in peripheral tissue.
- Lugol's iodine (iodine solution in potassium iodide): this decreases the secretion of thyroid hormone from the gland and decreases vascularity.
- Propranolol, a non-selective beta-blocker, decreases the peripheral conversion of T4 to T3. This action is not present in more cardioselective beta-blockers.

Thyrotoxicosis

- This typically presents with weight loss, hypertension, sweating, and cardiac arrhythmias (especially atrial fibrillation).
- Treatment is with carbimazole (30–45 mg orally daily for 6–8 weeks). Occasionally in severe cases with a large goitre, Lugol's iodine is substituted 10 days preoperatively to reduce gland vascularity.
- Beta-blockade (propranolol 30–60 mg 8-hourly) is also started if there are signs of tremor or palpitations. The adequacy of blockade can be determined by assessing the sleeping heart rate. Maintain beta-blockers perioperatively to reduce the possibility of thyroid storm (see below).

Thyroid crisis ('storm')

This is due to uncontrolled release of thyroid hormones in a thyrotoxic patient, especially if not well controlled with carbimazole. Acute illness, surgery, and trauma are potent triggers. Patients may present perioperatively with hyperpyrexia, tachycardia, or SVT (mimicking malignant hyperpyrexia), agitation, nausea and vomiting, diarrhoea, jaundice, or sudden mania. The condition can be fatal and needs urgent treatment.

- Identify the cause and treat on HDU/ICU.
- Give emergency drugs as follows:
  - Carbimazole 60–120 mg or propylthiouracil 600–1200 mg orally or down a nasogastric tube. Wait for 1 h for this to start working then give:
    - Lugol's solution (aqueous oral iodine solution) 0.3 ml 8-hourly, orally. If this is given before the carbimazole has time to work, it may cause further release of hormone!
    - Propanolol, up to 10 mg IV bolus and 20–80 mg 8-hourly orally or 1–5 mg 6-hourly IV. Esmolol may also be used acutely as a bolus of 0.5–1.0 mg/kg over 30 s, followed by an infusion of 50–300 µg/kg/min.
    - Hydrocortisone 100 mg 6-hourly IV.
    - Cooled intravenous fluids. Heart failure may be precipitated in the elderly. Consider CVP or a pulmonary artery flotation catheter.
    - Active cooling.
    - Plasma exchange or charcoal perfusion.
- It may be necessary to use IPPV to optimize oxygenation.
- Dantrolene has been used with success in doses of 1–10 mg/kg IV
- Some authorities suggest broad spectrum antibiotics

Hypothyroidism

- This is commonly due to autoimmune thyroid destruction, but may be secondary to pituitary or hypothalamic disease, previous thyroid surgery, or treatment with radioactive iodine.
- Cardiovascular complications include decreased blood volume, cardiac output, and heart rate with a predisposition to hypertension and ischaemic heart disease. Pericardial effusions also occur. Patients are thus susceptible to profound hypotension on induction of anaesthesia, which may be relatively resistant to the effects of catecholamine therapy.
- The low metabolic rate predisposes to hypothermia, and drug metabolism can be slow. Careful monitoring of the twitch response and reduced dosage of relaxants and opioids is advised.
- Delay surgery if possible to attain a euthyroid state. Joint management with an endocrinologist is suggested. The elderly are susceptible to heart failure with increasing cardiac work caused by thyroxine therapy. A suggested regime is:
  - l-thyroxine 100–200 µg daily, orally. Start with 25 µg in the elderly or patients with heart disease and increase at 3–4-weekly intervals. Suitable for elective surgery that can be delayed.
  - If surgery is urgent then liothyronine (T3), 50–100 µg IV slowly under ECG control, followed by 25 µg 8-hourly can be used. Its effects develop after a few hours and disappear 24–48 h after discontinuing therapy.

Hypothyroid coma

This can present following surgery, anaesthesia, or secondary to infection or trauma. It is characterized by mental deterioration, impaired thermoregulation, and may be fatal if not treated promptly. Treatment consists of:

• intravenous liothyronine (as above)
• hydrocortisone 100 mg 6-hourly
• IV fluids and antibiotics
• IPPV and active warming.

Hypoparathyroidism

If the parathyroids are also removed this can cause hypocalcaemia postoperatively. This can present with cramps, tetany, stridor, paraesthesia, mental confusion, or convulsions. Trousseau's and Chvostek's signs may be elicited. A prolonged QT interval (>0.44 s) may lead to arrhythmias, especially Torsades de pointes. Treat with calcium gluconate (10%) 10–20 ml IV, slowly with continual ECG monitoring (see parathyroid disease pp. 83–84).

Further reading

Farling PA (2000). Thyroid disease. *British Journal of Anaesthesia*, **85**, 15–28.
Ober KP (1995). Endocrine emergencies. *Medical Clinics of North America*, **79**, no.1.

Parathyroid disorders

The parathyroid glands are responsible for maintaining calcium homeostasis via the secretion of parathyroid hormone. Parathyroid hormone acts on the bones and kidneys to increase serum calcium and decrease serum phosphate. It stimulates osteoclasts directly, causing the release of calcium and phosphate into the extracellular fluid and simultaneously increasing phosphate excretion and calcium reabsorption in the kidney. Over- or undersecretion of parathyroid hormone therefore mainly affects these electrolytes.

Hyperparathyroidism

- Primary—usually an adenoma causing a high calcium level and low phosphate level.
- Secondary—complicates chronic renal failure. Parathyroid hyperplasia causes a normal or low calcium level and a high phosphate level.
- Tertiary—when parathyroid hyperplasia progresses to autonomous secretion, behaving like an adenoma. Excessive secretion of parathyroid hormone continues when the renal failure is corrected.

Diagnosis

- Primary hyperparathyroidism is diagnosed on the basis of a raised level of parathyroid hormone with high calcium. Tumours are very rarely palpable and are localized at surgery. No other investigations are required. Methylene blue (up to 1 mg/kg) is sometimes given immediately preoperatively to help localize the parathyroid gland.
- If hypercalcaemia recurs postoperatively, then formal sampling of venous drainage from the thymus and areas of the mediastinum is performed under radiological control. Exploration for recurrent disease may involve sternotomy or extensive neck dissection.
- Secondary hyperparathyroidism usually presents as excessive bone resorption (seen earliest in the radial aspect of the middle phalanx of the second digit) or soft tissue calcification of the vascular and soft tissues including kidneys, heart, lungs, and skin. Parathyroid hormone and serum phosphate are raised.

Clinical presentation

- Often very subtle, with 50% of cases being asymptomatic.
- Anorexia, nausea, vomiting, constipation, and weight loss.
- Polyuria, polydipsia, and renal calculi.
- Depression, poor memory, drowsiness.
- A shortened Q-T interval on the ECG.

Hypercalcaemic crisis

This is increasingly common amongst the elderly with undiagnosed hyperparathyroidism and in patients with malignant disease. Treatment includes:

- Rehydration, with 4–6 litres of fluid often required.
- Forced saline diuresis using saline and furosemide (frusemide) (40 mg, 4-hourly).

- If serum calcium is over 4.5 mmol/litre, this is life-threatening and can be rapidly but transiently lowered by 500 ml of 0.1 M neutral phosphate given over 6–8 h.
- Pamidronate 60 mg in 500 ml saline over 4 hours.
- Calcitonin, 3–4 units/kg IV followed by 4 units/kg SC 12-hourly.
- Dialysis is reserved for patients in renal failure.
- Invasive vascular monitoring should be considered as these patients are often elderly and LVF can occur.
- Steroids are useful in patients with malignancy: hydrocortisone 200–400 mg IV daily (can take several days to work).

Perioperative plan

- Patients are commonly hypovolaemic, therefore restore normal intra-vascular volume using 0.9% saline.
- If the patient has normal cardiovascular and renal systems, a normal ECG and a total serum calcium <3 mmol/litre, proceed with the operation.
- If the serum calcium is >3 mmol/litre or the ECG is abnormal or the patient has cardiovascular or renal impairment, then they should be delayed and treated.
- Careful monitoring of neuromuscular blockade should be undertaken if non-depolarizing muscle relaxants are used.

Hypoparathyroidism

- Parathyroidectomy is the commonest cause of hypoparathyroidism, but postradiotherapy and idiopathic cases also occur. Patients with a history of extensive neck surgery in the past should have serum calcium measured before proceeding with further surgery.
- Only ionized serum calcium is physiologically active. Measurement of ionized calcium is not affected by albumen level. However, about half the total calcium is bound to albumin and is inactive. A low serum albumin will therefore alter the total calcium measured. A state of dynamic equilibrium between the bound and unbound calcium serves to maintain a very stable concentration of ionized calcium.
- Ionized calcium should be corrected prior to elective surgery. Calcium gluconate 10% = 1 g (2.2 mmol) in 10 ml. Give 10 ml slowly and follow with 40 ml in 1 litre of normal saline over 8 h.
- Low serum magnesium is also common and can be treated with 1–5 mmol magnesium sulphate IV slowly.

To find the corrected total serum calcium (in mmol/litre) add 0.02 mmol for every 1 g albumin below 40 g.

In other words:

(40 – measured albumin) × 0.02 + measured serum calcium.

Normal total calcium = 2.2–2.5 mmol/litre.

Normal ionized calcium = 0.9–1.1 mmol/litre.

• Acute hypocalcaemia causing tetany can be treated with 10% calcium gluconate (10–20 ml) IV.

Further reading

Edwards R (1997). Thyroid and parathyroid disease. *International Anaesthesiology Clinics*, **35**, 63–83.
Mihai R, Farndon JR (2000). Parathyroid disease and calcium metabolism. *British Journal of Anaesthesia*, **85**, 29–43.

Addison's disease

Addison's disease is characterized by decreased or absent glucocorticoid secretion, usually combined with mineralocorticoid insufficiency. It can be primary or secondary and may present as an acute, chronic, or acute-on-chronic illness. The most common cause is autoimmune.

Clinical features
- Postural hypotension.
- Hypoglycaemia.
- Nausea, vomiting, diarrhoea, and weight loss.
- Decreased body hair.
- Pigmentation especially in areas exposed to the sun.
- Can be associated with pernicious anaemia, myasthenia gravis, and vitiligo
- May not be clinically obvious until a significant stress occurs, e.g. acute abdomen.

Investigations
- Low serum glucose.
- Low Na^+, raised K^+ and urea (it is difficult to diagnose Addison's disease with a normal plasma urea).
- Plasma ACTH—measure simultaneously with plasma cortisol at 08:00h. Even if cortisol is normal the ACTH will be elevated.
- Short Synacthen stimulation test—250 μg of Synacthen dissolved in 1 ml of sterile water is given intravenously. Serum cortisol is measured 30 min later. A serum cortisol >580 nmol/litre excludes the diagnosis.
- Plasma renin activity and aldosterone—plasma renin activity is usually high with a low aldosterone.

Treatment
- Hydrocortisone orally: 20 mg in the morning and 10 mg at night.
- Fludrocortisone to replace aldosterone: 0.1 mg PO daily.

Adrenal crisis
Adrenal crisis can be precipitated by any stress response where the adrenal glands are unable to increase glucocorticoid production to meet demand:
- Classically presents as hypotension, hyponatraemia, hyperkalaemia, and hypoglycaemia.
- Characteristically resembles hypovolaemic shock, but can also mimic septic shock with fever, peripheral vasodilatation, and a high cardiac output.
- Patients with primary adrenal insufficiency usually have a hypovolaemic picture (due to mineralocorticoid deficiency).

Management
- Admit to ICU/HDU.
- Hydrocortisone 200 mg IV should be given immediately, then 100 mg 6-hourly IM or 200 mg/24 h IV, until oral replacement is possible.

- Fluid resuscitation with CVP guidance. 0.9% saline is an appropriate fluid with 50% dextrose infused if hypoglycaemia occurs.

- Inotropes if hypotension persists. The choice of inotrope will depend on the clinical picture, i.e. noradrenaline if the patient has severe vaso-dilatation.

- Dexamethasone, 4 mg IV, can also be used if the diagnosis has not been confirmed. Hydrocortisone interferes with the cortisol assay but dexamethasone does not.

Perioperative management of patients with long-standing Addison's disease

- Give all medication up to the morning of surgery.

- 25 mg IV hydrocortisone should be given at induction.

- Small or intermediate cases should be managed as per perioperative steroids (p. 99).

- In major cases, hydrocortisone 200 mg/24 h should be used until the patient can be weaned back onto maintenance therapy.

- 4-hourly blood glucose and daily electrolytes.

- Joint care with an endocrinologist is advisable.

Relative adrenal insufficiency in the critically ill

- Relative hypoadrenalism in ITU patients is well described.

- Occurs in about 3–52% of septic patients.

- An abnormal response to a short Synacthen test is a poor prognostic indicator.

Further reading

Mackenzie JS, Burrows L, Burchard KW (1998). Transient hypoadrenalism during surgical critical illness. *Archives of Surgery*, **133**, 199–204.

Oelkers W (1996). Adrenal insufficiency. *New England Journal of Medicine*, **335**, 1206–11.

Weatherill D, Spence AA (1984). Anaesthesia and disorders of the adrenal cortex. *British Journal of Anaesthesia*, **56**, 741–9.

Conn's syndrome[3]

A syndrome associated with hypersecretion of aldosterone. This can arise from either a benign adenoma of the adrenal cortex (75%) or from bilateral adrenal hyperplasia (25%).

Clinical features

- Hypertension—usually mild.
- Hypokalaemia—often severe and aggravated by patients having been placed on thiazide diuretics to treat hypertension.
- Muscle weakness or paralysis especially in ethnic Chinese (secondary to hypokalaemia).
- Nephrogenic diabetes insipidus secondary to renal tubular damage.
- Hypovolaemia.
- Metabolic alkalosis.
- Impaired glucose tolerance in about 50% of patients.

Diagnosis

- The aldosterone (pg/ml):renin (ng/ml/h) ratio. This helps to overcome the confounding problems of posture, sodium intake and drugs. If the ratio is >400 then diagnose an aldosterone-secreting tumour. Secondary hyperaldosteronism has a raised serum aldosterone with a normal ratio.
- Important to distinguish between adenoma and hyperplasia as adenoma is usually treated surgically and hyperplasia medically.
- Arteriography, venous sampling, and MRI are all used

Preoperative assessment

- Spironalactone is usually given to reverse the metabolic and electrolyte effects. It also allows the patient to restore normovolaemia. Doses of up to 400 mg/day may be required.
- The patient should have normal serum potassium and bicarbonate.
- Hypertension is usually mild and well controlled on spironolactone, but features of end organ damage, e.g. LVH, should be excluded.
- Unilateral adrenalectomy can be done laparoscopically or via laparotomy and an appropriate method of analgesia should be discussed.
- Handling of the adrenal gland during surgery can cause cardiovascular instability but is not as severe as with a phaeochromocytoma.
- A short-acting alpha-blocker should be available (phentolamine 1 mg boluses IV).

Management of patients with Conn's syndrome for non adrenal surgery

- Such patients usually have bilateral glomerulosa hyperplasia.
- Hypertension is usually more severe and may require additional therapy (ACE inhibitors are useful).
- Ensure a normal serum potassium preoperatively.
- Perform cardiovascular assessment as for any hypertensive patient.

3 Winship SM, Winstanley JH, Hunter JM (1999). Anaesthesia for Conn's syndrome. *Anaesthesia*, **54**, 564–74.

Cushing's syndrome

Cushing's disease results from excess ACTH production by a pituitary adenoma and is more correctly called pituitary-dependent Cushing's syndrome. Cushing's syndrome is a collection of signs and symptoms due to an excessively high plasma cortisol. The most common cause of Cushing's syndrome is treatment with glucocorticoid drugs. Anaesthetists will see this syndrome in:

- Patients having pituitary or adrenal surgery to resect tumours causing a raised cortisol.
- Patients with malignant tumours. These occasionally secrete an ACTH-like hormone that causes profound Cushinoid features. Oat cell carcinoma of the lung is a common cause.
- Patients on high-dose steroid therapy .

Clinical features

- Moon face and truncal obesity.
- Proximal myopathy and osteoporosis.
- Easy bruising and fragile skin.
- Impaired glucose tolerance, diabetes.
- Hypertension and left ventricular hypertrophy.
- Hypernatraemia and hypokalaemia.
- Gastrointestinal reflux.
- Sleep apnoea.

Diagnosis

- Classical clinical features are often seen but will not differentiate the various causes of a raised cortisol level. Urinary free cortisol or lack of diurnal variation will confirm a pathological cause but will not define the aetiology.
- The 'short dexamethasone suppression test' (1 mg of dexamethasone is given at night and a cortisol sample taken in the morning) is a sensitive test to confirm abnormally raised serum cortisol. Serum cortisol will be suppressed in the morning if the HPA axis is working normally.
- Serum ACTH levels will help determine if adrenal or pituitary pathology is the cause.
- Very high ACTH levels suggest ectopic production, e.g. carcinoma of the lung, and very low levels suggest adrenal hypersecretion.
- The 'high dose dexamethasone suppression test' (2 mg is given 6-hourly for 48 h and serum cortisol measured) will cause a fall in early morning and urinary free cortisol on the second day in pituitary-dependent Cushing's syndrome, but not in ectopic or adrenal causes.
- Inferior petrosal venous sinus sampling following CRH stimulation is the final confirmatory test for pituitary Cushing's syndrome.
- MRI scan of the pituitary fossa.

Preoperative assessment

- 85% of patients are hypertensive and are often poorly controlled.

- ECG abnormalities (high-voltage QRS and inverted T waves) can make IHD difficult to exclude but will revert to normal after curative surgery. These ECG changes seem to be related to the Cushing's disease itself.
- Sleep apnoea is common and patients should be asked about daytime somnolence and snoring.
- 60% of patients have diabetes or impaired glucose tolerance and a sliding scale should be started before major surgery if glucose is >10 mmol.
- Gastro-oesophageal reflux is common and preoperative acid suppression therapy and rapid sequence induction should be considered.
- Venous access can be very difficult.
- Patients can be obese and appropriately sized blood pressure cuffs, operating tables, and supports should be ordered.

Further reading

Sheeran P, O'Leary E (1997). Adrenocortical disorders. *International Anesthesiology Clinics*, **35**, 85–98.

Smith M, Hirsch NP (2000). Pituitary disease and anaesthesia. *British Journal of Anaesthesia*, **85**, 3–14.

Phaeochromocytoma

This is a rare tumour arising from the chromaffin cells in the adrenal medulla or occasionally from other ganglia of the sympathetic nervous system. Tumours can secrete noradrenaline, adrenaline, or dopamine and the symptomatology of the patient will depend on which is the dominant catecholamine. Noradrenaline-secreting tumours usually present with refractory hypertension, whilst adrenaline- or dopamine-secreting tumours present with a variety of episodic signs and symptoms, ranging from tachycardia to panic attacks. 90% occur sporadically but 10% are part of a familial syndrome, e.g. multiple endocrine neoplasia (MEN) syndrome.

Clinical presentation

- Sustained hypertension is the most common presenting feature (85% of cases).
- Nausea, vomiting, headaches, trembling, and sweating can all occur.
- The overall picture depends on the type and proportion of catecholamines that are secreted.
- Dilated cardiomyopathy with LVF due to prolonged exposure to catecholamines is well recognized.
- Acute pulmonary oedema can occur at any time, especially if patients are incorrectly treated with beta-blockers.
- Raised serum glucose due to increased glycogenolysis and impaired insulin secretion should be excluded.

Diagnosis

- Measurement of free catecholamines in a 24-h urine collection to confirm the diagnosis.
- MRI scan to localize the tumour.
- Selective venous sampling.
- Recurrent tumours, metastasis, and tumours in abnormal sites can be identified with meta-iodobenzyl guanidine (MIBG). The tumour takes up this amine precursor. It is poor for localizing intra-adrenal tumours.

Perioperative management

This is discussed on p. 306.

Further reading

Prys-Roberts C (2000). Phaeochromocytoma—recent progress in its management. *British Journal of Anaesthesia*, **85**, 44–57.

Apudomas

These are tumours of amine precursor uptake and decarboxylation (APUD) cells. The cells synthesize and secrete polypeptides and amines which may cause systemic disturbance of, for example, insulin, glucagon, catecholamines, 5-HT, somatostatin, gastrin, and vasoactive peptide. APUD cells are present in the anterior pituitary gland, thyroid, adrenal medulla, gastrointestinal tract, pancreatic islet, carotid bodies, and lungs. Tumours of APUD cells include phaeochromocytoma, insulinoma, gastrinoma, carcinoid tumour, and VIPomas and may occur as part of the multiple endocrine neoplasia (MEN) syndrome.

Gastrinoma

- Excess production of gastrin by benign adenoma, malignancy, or hyperplasia of the D cells of the pancreatic islets. Leads to Zollinger–Ellison syndrome, severe peptic ulceration, and diarrhoea. May also have GI bleeds, perforation, electrolyte disturbance, and volume depletion.
- Treatment includes proton pump inhibitors, e.g. omeprazole, H_2 receptor antagonists, and octreotide.
- May present for surgery related to gastrinoma, e.g. perforation, or totally unrelated pathology.
- Antacid prophylaxis preoperatively and rapid sequence induction.
- Invasive pressure monitoring for major surgery.

VIPoma

- Very rare tumour, often small cell bronchogenic carcinoma. Secretion of vasoactive intestinal peptide (VIP) leads to Verner– Morrison syndrome characterized by watery diarrhoea, hypokalaemia, achlorhydria, and hypovolaemia.
- May present for tumour resection, or more often for unrelated pathology.
- Treat hypovolaemia, metabolic acidosis, and electrolyte imbalance with octreotide and glucocorticoids.
- Invasive pressure monitoring for major surgery.
- Frequent measurement of arterial blood gases to check acid base status and electrolytes.

Insulinoma

- Very rare pancreatic islet cell tumour, which secretes insulin leading to fasting hypoglycaemia.
- Patients often present for surgical excision of non-malignant tumours.
- Diazoxide, chlorothiazide, and octreotide may be used to inhibit insulin secretion.
- Prevent intra-operative hypoglycaemia.

Further reading

Owen R (1993). Anaesthetic considerations in endocrine surgery. In *Surgical endocrinology* (eds. J Lynn, SR Bloon), pp. 71–84. Butterworth-Heinemann, Oxford.

Carcinoid tumours

Carcinoid tumours are derived from argentaffin cells and produce peptides and amines. Most occur in the GI tract (75%), bronchus, pancreas, and gonads. Tumours are mainly benign, and of those that are malignant only about a quarter release vasoactive substances into the systemic circulation, leading to the carcinoid syndrome. Mediators are metabolized in the liver, therefore only tumours with hepatic metastases or a primary tumour with non-portal venous drainage lead to the carcinoid syndrome. To date about 20 different vasoactive substances have been identified including serotonin, bradykinin, histamine, substance P, prostaglandins, and vasoactive intestinal hormone.

Patients with an asymptomatic carcinoid tumour have simple carcinoid disease and do not present particular anaesthetic difficulties; however, patients with carcinoid syndrome can be extremely difficult to manage perioperatively.

Carcinoid syndrome

Patients may have symptoms related to:

- The primary tumour causing intestinal obstruction, pulmonary symptoms, e.g. haemoptysis, respiratory compromise, etc.
- Vasoactive peptides resulting in flushing (90%,) especially of the head, neck, and torso. Diarrhoea (78%) may lead to dehydration and electrolyte disturbances. Other symptoms include bronchospasm (20%), hypotension, hypertension, tachycardia, hyperglycaemia, and right heart failure (mediators metabolized in the lungs before reaching the left side) secondary to endocardial fibrosis affecting the pulmonary and tricuspid valves.

Patient preparation

- Treat symptomatically—antidiarrhoeals, bronchodilators, correction of dehydration and electrolyte imbalance, and treatment for heart failure if required.
- Prevent the release of mediators—octreotide 100 µg SC tds for 2 weeks prior to surgery and octreotide 100 µg IV slowly (diluted to 10 µg/ml) at induction.
- Avoid factors which may trigger carcinoid crises—catecholamines, anxiety, and drugs which release histamine, e.g. morphine.
- Perform echocardiography if cardiac involvement is suspected.

Anaesthetic management

- Best managed by teams/centres familiar with the difficulties.
- Major complications anticipated in the perioperative period include severe hypotension, severe hypertension, fluid and electrolyte shift and imbalance, and bronchospasm.
- Premedication—anxiolytic (benzodiazepine) and octreotide 100 µg (50–500 µg) SC 1 h preoperatively if not already treated , otherwise continue with preoperative regime.
- Monitoring—in addition to ECG and pulse oximetry, invasive blood pressure monitoring (preinduction as both induction and surgical manipulation of the tumour can cause large swings), central venous pressure monitoring, regular blood sugars, blood gases.

- Use a pulmonary artery flotation catheter if indicated due to cardiac complications.
- Induction—prevent pressor response to intubation (etomidate/ propofol and fentanyl). Suxamethonium is relatively contraindicated, as it may increase mediator release with fasciculations.
- Maintenance—inhalational with isoflurane, vecuronium or pancuronium, fentanyl, or low-dose epidural (avoiding hypotension as this may elicit bradykinergic crisis) for analgesia.
- Octreotide IV boluses 10–20 μg to treat severe hypotension.
- Avoid all histamine-releasing drugs and catecholamines.
- Labetalol, esmolol, or ketanserin can be used if required for hypertension.
- Postoperatively, ICU or HDU is required, patients may awaken very slowly (thought to be due to serotonin). Hypotensive episodes may occur, requiring further IV boluses of octreotide (10–20 μg). Wean octreotide over 7–10 days following tumour resection.

Further reading

Veall GRQ, Peacock JE, Bax NDS, Reilly CS (1994). Review of the anaesthetic management of 21 patients undergoing laparotomy for carcinoid syndrome. *British Journal of Anaesthesia*, 72, 335–41.

Porphyria

The porphyrias are a group of diseases in which there is an enzyme defect in the synthesis of the haem moiety leading to an accumulation of precursors that are oxidized into porphyrins. There are hepatic and erythropoietic varieties, but only three hepatic forms, inherited in an autosomal dominant manner (although with variable expression), affect the administration of anaesthesia:

- Acute intermittent porphyria (AIP). Common in Sweden—increased urinary porphobilinogen and d-aminolaevulinic acid.
- Variegate porphyria (VP). Common in Afrikaners—increased copro- and protoporphyrin in the stool. Dermal photosensitivity.
- Hereditary coproporphyria (HCP). Very rare, increased urinary porphyrins. Dermal photosensitivity.

Porphyric crises

- Acute porphyric crises may be precipitated by drugs, stress, infection, alcohol, menstruation, pregnancy, starvation, or dehydration.
- Symptoms include acute abdominal pain, vomiting, motor and sensory peripheral neuropathy, autonomic dysfunction, cranial nerve palsies, mental disturbances, coma, convulsions, pyrexia.

General principles

- Patients may never have had an attack, therefore a positive family history must be taken seriously.
- Patients may present with unrelated pathology, e.g. appendicitis.
- Symptoms may mimic surgical pathologies, e.g. acute abdominal pain, acute neurology.
- Any patient giving a strong family history of porphyria must be treated as potentially at risk. Latent carriers may exhibit no signs, be potentially negative to biochemical screening, but still be at risk from acute attacks.

Anaesthetic management

Many commonly used drugs are thought to have the potential to trigger porphyric crises. However, it is difficult to be definitive, as crises can also be triggered by infection or stress, which often occur simultaneously. Drugs which are considered to be definitely unsafe to use, probably safe, and controversial are documented in the table below. Up-to-date information is available in the British National Formulary, the Committee on the Review of Porphyrinogenicity (CORP)[4] or via the internet: www.leeds.ac.uk/ifcc/SD/porph/

Suggested anaesthetic techniques

- Premedication—important to minimize stress: use temazepam, droperidol, chloral hydrate.

4   CORP Secretariat, Lennox Eales Porphyria Laboratories, MRC/UCT Liver Research Centre, University of Cape Town Medical School, Observatory 7925, South Africa. Fax: 010–27–21–448–6815.

	Definitely unsafe	Probably safe	Controversial
Induction agents	Barbiturates, etomidate	Propofol	Ketamine
Inhalational agents	Enflurane	Nitrous oxide, ether, cyclopropane	Halothane, isoflurane, sevoflurane, desflurane
Neuromuscular blocking agents	Alcuronium	Suxamethonium, tubocurarine, gallamine, vecuronium	Pancuronium, atracurium, rocuronium, mivacurium
Neuromuscular reversal agents		Atropine, glycopyrrolate, neostigmine	
Analgesics	Pentazocine	Alfentanil, aspirin, buprenorphine, codeine, fentanyl, paracetamol, pethidine, morphine, naloxone	Diclofenac, ketorolac, sufentanil
Local anaesthetics	Mepivicaine, ropivacaine	Bupivacaine, prilocaine, procainamide, procaine	Cocaine, lidocaine (lignocaine)
Sedatives	Chlordiazepoxide, nitrazepam	Lorazepam, midazolam, temazepam, chlorpromazine, chloral hydrate	Diazepam
Antiemetics and H_2 antagonists	Cimetidine, metoclopramide	Droperidol, phenothiazines	Ondansetron, ranitidine
CVS drugs	Hydralazine, nifedipine, phenoxybenzamine	Adrenaline, α-agonists, β-agonists, β-blockers, magnesium, phentolamine, procainamide	Diltiazem, dizopyramide, sodium nitroprusside, verapamil
Others	Aminophylline, oral contraceptive pill, phenytoin, sulphonamides		Steroids

- Regional anaesthesia—bupivacaine is considered safe for epidural anaesthesia but in the context of any peripheral neuropathy, detailed preoperative examination and documentation is essential. In acute porphyric crises, regional anaesthesia should be avoided, as neuropathy may be rapid in onset and progressive.
- General anaesthesia—propofol is the induction agent of choice. Maintenance with nitrous oxide and/or propofol infusion. There are few data for isoflurane. Neuromuscular blockade—suxamethonium and vecuronium are considered safe (atracurium controversial). Fentanyl, morphine, and pethidine all considered safe.
- Monitoring—invasive blood pressure during acute crisis as hypovolaemia is common and autonomic neuropathy may cause labile blood pressure. Perform central venous pressure monitoring if clinically indicated.

Problems during anaesthesia

- Hypertension and tachycardia—treat with beta-blockers such as atenolol.
- Convulsions—treat with diazepam, propofol, or magnesium sulphate (avoid barbiturates and phenytoin).

Postoperative management

- ICU/HDU if a crisis is suspected.
- Remember that the onset of a porphyric crisis may be delayed for up to 5 days.

Treatment of acute porphyric crises

- Reverse factors which increase ALA synthetase. Give haem arginate 3 mg/kg IV once daily for 4 days (leads to negative feedback to ALA synthetase). Treat infection, dehydration, electrolyte imbalance, give glucose (20 g/h).
- Withdraw drugs which may have precipitated the crisis.
- Treat symptoms with 'safe' drugs.
- Monitor the patient appropriately.

Further reading

James MFM, Hift RJ (2000). Porphyrias. *British Journal of Anaesthesia*, **85**, 143–53.
Jensen NF, Fiddler DS, StriepeV (1995). Anaesthetic considerations in porphyrias. *Anaesthesia and Analgesia*, **80**, 591–9.

The patient on steroids

Steroids are used as replacement therapy in adrenocortical insufficiency or to suppress inflammatory and immunological responses. Patients on steroids requiring surgery may develop complications from their underlying disease, or from a potentially impaired stress response due to hypothalamic–pituitary–adrenal (HPA) suppression. Classically these patients were given additional large doses of steroids perioperatively; however, recent research suggests that much more modest physiological replacement doses are more than adequate in the majority of cases.

Hypothalamic–pituitary–adrenal suppression

- Endogenous cortisol production is of the order of 25–30 mg/24 h (following a circadian pattern). During stress induced by major surgery, it is in the range 75–100 mg/day. The increase is rapid and levels remain elevated for a variable period of time (up to 72 h following cardiac surgery).
- Low-dose steroid treatment <10 mg prednisolone per day usually carries little danger of HPA suppression.
- Treatment with >10 mg prednisolone (or equivalent) risks HPA suppression. This may occur after treatment via the oral, topical, parenteral, nebulized, or inhaled routes. These patients must be assumed to be suffering from an inability to mount a normal endogenous steroid response to stress and be supplemented accordingly.
- HPA suppression can be measured using various methods. In practice the short synacthen test is reliable, cheap, and safe. Patents are given 250 μg synacthen (synthetic corticotrophin) IV and serum cortisol is measured at 0, 30, and 60 min. Normal peak cortisol levels range from 420–700 nmol/litre and indicate the ability of the patient to mount a stress response. In patients where the result is equivocal, an insulin tolerance test can be performed under the advice and supervision of an endocrinologist.

Perioperative steroid replacement therapy

- Normal dose steroid <10 mg prednisolone/24 h: assume normal HPA therefore no extra supplementation required.
- Steroids stopped within last 3 months: assume still on previous dose and treat accordingly.
- Consider whether the surgery is minor, intermediate, or major and supplement accordingly.
- High-dose immunosuppression: it is imperative that these patients continue their usual dose of steroids, given IV if required, otherwise organ failure can ensue.
- Prednisolone 5 mg is equivalent to:
  - hydrocortisone 20 mg
  - methylprednisolone 4 mg
  - betamethasone 750 μg
  - dexamethasone 750 μg
  - cortisone acetate 25 mg
  - prednisone 5 mg
  - triamcinolone 4 mg.

Patient currently taking regular steroids		
<10 mg prednisolone/day	Assume normal hypothalamic–pituitary axis	No additional steroid cover required
>10 mg prednisolone/day	Minor surgery, e.g. hernia	Routine preoperative steroid or hydrocortisone 25 mg IV at induction
	Intermediate surgery, e.g. hysterectomy	Routine preoperative steroid plus hydrocortisone 25 mg IV at induction. Postoperative hydrocortisone 25 mg 6-hourly for 24 h
	Major surgery, e.g. cardiac	Routine preoperative steroid plus hydrocortisone 25 mg IV at induction. Postoperative hydrocortisone 25 mg 6-hourly for 48–72 h
High-dose immunosuppression	Should continue usual immunosuppressive dose until able to revert to normal oral intake, e.g. 60 mg prednisolone/24 h = 240 mg hydrocortisone/24 h	
Patient formerly taking regular steroids		
<3 months since stopped steroids	Treat as if on steroids	
>3 months since stopped steroids	No perioperative steroids necessary	

Complications of steroid therapy

Steroids have multisystemic adverse effects: diabetes, obesity, hypertension, and skin manifestations are particularly important. Also:

- CVS—hypertension
- renal—polyuria, nocturia
- CNS—depression, euphoria, psychosis, insomnia
- GI—peptic ulceration, pancreatitis
- ophthalmic—cataracts
- immune—increased susceptibility to infection
- skin—thin, easily bruised, poor healing
- endocrine—weight gain, diabetes, adrenal suppression, hypokalaemia
- musculoskeletal—osteoporosis, proximal myopathy, wasting.

Further reading

British National Formulary 39, March 2000.
Nicholson G, Burrin JM, Hall GM (1998). Perioperative steroid replacement. *Anaesthesia*, 53, 1091–104.

Potassium and anaesthesia

Potassium (K^+) is the major intracellular cation in the human body and plays a crucial role in the electrophysiology of cell membranes. Imbalances in potassium homeostasis can be of critical importance to the anaesthetist. Measurements of plasma potassium can be sent to the laboratory (note that a falsely elevated potassium will be seen with a haemolysed sample) or obtained more rapidly via a blood gas analyser.

Hypokalaemia

Plasma potassium less than 3.5 mmol/litre. This may reflect a total K^+ deficit of up to 500 mmol (i.e. 15–20% of total body K^+). An approximation of the deficit can be calculated by assuming that a decrease in the serum of 0.27 mmol/litre is equivalent to a total deficit of 100 mmol of potassium. Hypokalaemia can be caused by:

- Intercompartmental shift of potassium—alkalosis (0.1 increase in pH decreases K^+ by 0.6 mmol/litre), insulin administration, β_2 agonists, hypothermia.
- Increased potassium loss—diuretics, mineralocorticoid activity, renal tubular acidosis, ketoacidosis, ileal conduit, diarrhoea/vomiting, excess sweating, dialysis.
- Decreased potassium intake.

Clinical manifestations

- ECG changes—T wave flattening and inversion, prominent U wave, ST segment depression, prolonged PR interval
- dysrhythmias, decreased cardiac contractility
- skeletal muscle weakness, tetany
- ileus, polyuria, impaired renal concentrating ability
- decreased insulin secretion, growth hormone secretion, and aldosterone secretion
- negative nitrogen balance
- encephalopathy in patients with liver disease.

Treatment

The risks of replacement are not trivial, especially via the intravenous route. Some estimate of total deficit should be attempted.

- Oral replacement is safest, up to 200 mmol per day, e.g. potassium chloride (Sando-K) two tablets four times a day = 96 mmol K^+.
- IV replacement:
  - Essential for patients with cardiac manifestations or skeletal muscle weakness from hypokalaemia or where oral replacement is not appropriate.
  - Aim to increase K^+ to 4.0 mmol/litre if treating cardiac manifestations.
  - Maximum concentration for peripheral administration = 40 mmol/litre (greater concentrations than this can lead to venous necrosis).
  - 40 mmol KCl can be given in 100 ml normal saline over 1 h but only via an infusion device, with ECG monitoring, in HDU/ ICU/theatre environment and via a central vein.
  - Plasma K^+ should be measured at least hourly during rapid replacement.

Anaesthetic considerations

• The principal anaesthetic problem is the risk of arrhythmia.

• The rate of onset is important, chronic mild hypokalaemia is less significant than that of rapid onset.

• Ratio of intracellular to extracellular K^+ is of more importance than isolated plasma levels.

• Classically a K^+ under 3.0 mmol has led to postponement of elective procedures (some controversy exists about this in the fit, non-digitalized patient who may well tolerate chronically lower K^+ levels down to 2.5 mmol/litre without adverse events).

• Patients must be viewed individually and the decision to proceed should be based on the chronicity and level of hypokalaemia, the type of surgery, and any other associated pathologies.

• For emergency surgery, if possible replace K^+ in the 24 h prior to surgery. Aim for levels of 3.5–4.0 mmol/litre. If this is not possible use an IV replacement regime as documented above intra/perioperatively.

• May increase sensitivity to neuromuscular blockade, therefore need to monitor block.

• Increased risk of digoxin toxicity at low K^+ levels. Aim for K^+ of 4.0 mmol in a digitalized patient.

Hyperkalaemia

Plasma potassium greater than 5.0 mmol/litre (some laboratories suggest >5.5 mmol/litre). Hyperkalaemia can be caused by:

• Intercompartmental shift of potassium—acidosis, rhabdomyolysis, trauma, malignant hyperpryrexia, suxamethonium (especially with burns and denervation injuries), familial periodic paralysis.

• Decreased urinary excretion—renal failure acute or chronic, adrenocortical insufficiency or drugs (K^+ sparing diuretics, ACE inhibitors, ciclosporin etc.).

• Increased intake—IV administration, rapid blood transfusion.

Clinical manifestations

• The most important effects are on skeletal and cardiac muscle.

• ECG changes progressing through peaked T waves, widened QRS, prolonged PR interval, loss of P wave, loss of R wave amplitude, ST depression, ventricular fibrillation, asystole.

• ECG changes potentiated by low calcium, low sodium, and by acidosis.

• Muscle weakness at K^+ >8.0 mmol/litre.

• Nausea, vomiting, diarrhoea.

Treatment

Treatment should be initiated if K^+ >6.5 mmol/litre or ECG changes present. Unlike hypokalaemia, the incidence of serious cardiac compromise is high and therefore intervention is important. Treat the cause if possible.

• Insulin 15 units in 100 ml 20% dextrose IV over 30–60 min.

• Calcium 5–10 ml 10% calcium gluconate or 3–5 ml 10% calcium chloride (rapid onset, short lived).

• Bicarbonate 50 mmol IV (especially with acidosis).

- Ion Exchange Resin – calcium resonium 15 g PO / 30 g PR 8 hourly.
- Beta-agonists, consider salbutamol 5 mg nebulized.
- Dialysis or haemofiltration.

Anaesthetic considerations

Do not consider elective surgery. If surgery is essential:

- treat hyperkalaemia as above
- ECG monitoring
- avoid: suxamethonium, Hartmann's solution, acidosis, hypothermia
- control ventilation—mild hyperventilation may be beneficial
- monitor neuromuscular blockade, effects accentuated
- monitor K^+ regularly.

Further reading

Gennari FJ (1998). Hypokalaemia review article. *New England Journal of Medicine*, **339**, 451–8.

Tetzlaff JE, O'Hara JF Jr, Walsh MT (1993). Potassium and anaesthesia. *Canadian Journal of Anaesthesia*, **40**, 227–46.

Wong KC, Schafer PG, Schultz JR (1993). Hypokalaemia and anaesthetic implications. *Anaesthesia and Analgesia*, **77**, 1238–60.

Sodium and anaesthesia

Extracellular fluid volume is directly proportional to total body sodium (Na^+) content. Renal sodium excretion ultimately controls the extracellular fluid volume and total body sodium content. Imbalances in sodium homeostasis are common, and although the underlying mechanisms are poorly understood, the clinical manifestations can have significant implications for the anaesthetist.

The plasma sodium level is important, but it is equally important to evaluate the patient's state of hydration as sodium derangement can lead to hypo-/eu-/hypervolaemic states. Therefore, patients should be assessed clinically in conjunction with their plasma and urinary sodium levels.

Hyponatraemia

Plasma sodium less than 135 mmol/litre. This usually leads to a hypo-osmolar plasma. Hyponatraemia can be caused by:

- Water excess (hypervolaemic):
  - Intake greater than required (urinary Na^+ <10 mmol/litre), e.g. TURP syndrome, IV fluids, drinking to excess.
  - Reduced excretion (urinary Na^+ >20 mmol/litre), e.g. syndrome of inappropriate antidiuretic hormone (SIADH), tumours, CNS disorders such as head injury or CVA, IPPV, pneumonia, post-surgery.
  - Drugs, e.g. oxytocin.
- Water excess with sodium excess of a lesser magnitude (hypervolaemic):
  - Cardiac and hepatic failure (urinary Na^+ <10 mmol/litre).
  - Nephrotic syndrome.
- Water deficiency with sodium deficiency of a greater magnitude (hypovolaemic):
  - Renal loss (urinary Na^+ >20 mmol/litre), e.g. diuretics, post relief of urinary obstruction, hypoadrenalism, renal tubular acidosis, salt-losing nephropathy.
  - Other loss (urinary Na^+ <20 mmol/litre), e.g. diarrhoea and vomiting, pancreatitis.
- Redistribution of sodium and water (euvolaemic):
  - Sick cell syndrome—seen in the terminally ill, Na^+ redistributed to the intracellular compartment, possibly secondary to impaired Na^+/K^+ cell membrane transport.
  - Hyperglycaemia—leading to intra- to extracellular water movement.

Clinical manifestations

The general signs are those of dehydration and hypovolaemia in sodium deficiency. Specific symptoms include:

- The speed of onset of hyponatraemia is much more important in the manifestation of symptoms than the absolute Na^+ value.
- Rare if Na^+ >125 mmol/litre.
- Na^+ 125–130 mmol/litre mostly gastrointestinal symptoms.
- Na^+ <125 mmol/litre—neuropsychiatric symptoms, mortality high if untreated. Signs include nausea and vomiting, muscular weakness,

headache, lethargy, psychosis, raised intracranial pressure, seizures, coma, respiratory depression.

Treatment

Treatment depends on the clinical manifestations and speed of onset:

- Asymptomatic with long-standing hyponatraemia. Simple fluid restriction and reversal of precipitating factors.
- Asymptomatic with acute onset hyponatraemia—treat as above.
- Symptomatic (usually associated with rapid onset hyponatraemia):
  - Treatment required urgently in consultation with an endocrinologist.
  - Intravenous saline 0.9%, rate of correction controversial, but rapid correction can lead to central pontine myelinolysis, subdural haemorrhage, and cardiac failure. Therefore, aim for 5–10 mmol/litre/day. Aim to attain Na^+ no greater than 130 mmol/litre initially.
  - Diuretics may also be required, especially if seizures and/or cerebral oedema are present or if administration of saline does not bring about a spontaneous diuresis. Use mannitol 20% 500 ml or furosemide (frusemide) 20 mg IV.
  - SIADH—fluid restriction and demeclocyclidine 300–900 mg daily.
- Treat any underlying pathology concomitantly.

Anaesthetic implications

- No elective surgery if Na^+ <120 mmol/litre or if the patient shows signs of fluid balance disturbance, decreased levels of consciousness, seizures, or focal nervous system deficit.
- May need to deal with problem acutely intra-operatively, e.g. TURP syndrome (p. 628).

Hypernatraemia

Plasma sodium greater than 145 mmol/litre. Always reflects a hyperosmolar state. Hypernatraemia can be caused by:

- Sodium excess (hypervolaemic, urinary Na^+ >20mmol/litre)—hyperaldosteronism, Cushing's syndrome, iatrogenic, e.g. secondary to hypertonic saline, drugs such as sodium bicarbonate, TPN.
- Water depletion (euvolaemic urinary Na^+ variable)—renal, e.g. diabetes insipidus or other insensible loss, inadequate water intake, burns.
- Sodium deficiency with an even greater water deficiency (hypovolaemic, urinary Na^+ >20 mmol/litre):
  - renal loss, e.g. osmotic diuresis secondary to mannitol, glucose, urea
  - other (urinary Na^+ <10 mmol/litre), e.g. vomiting, diarrhoea, sweating, wound exudates, adrenocortical insufficiency.

Clinical manifestations

- May have features of dehydration.
- The rate of onset is important, slow onset is much better tolerated
- CNS symptoms are prominent because of the hyperosmolar state (cellular dehydration).
- Altered mental status, lethargy, irritability, restlessness.
- Seizures, muscle twitching, spasticity, hyperreflexia.

- Fever, nausea, vomiting, intense thirst.
- Intracranial haemorrhage as a result of cerebral dehydration.
- Prerenal failure secondary to decreased cardiac output.

Treatment

Correction should be achieved slowly over at least 48 h, as rapid correction may lead to cerebral oedema and convulsions.

- Treat the underlying cause if possible.
- Treat with oral fluids (water) if possible.
- Sodium excess (hypervolaemic): diuretics, e.g. furosemide (frusemide) 20 mg IV and 5% dextrose, dialysis if required.
- Water depletion (euvolaemia): estimate the total body water deficit, treat with 5% dextrose.
- Sodium deficiency (hypovolaemic): 0.9% saline until hypovolaemia corrected, then consider 0.45% saline.
- Diabetes insipidus—keep up with urinary fluid losses and give desmopresssin 1–4 μg daily (SC/IM/IV).

Anaesthetic implications

- No elective surgery if Na^+ >155 mmol/litre or hypovolaemic.
- Urgent surgery—use invasive central venous pressure monitoring if volume status is uncertain or may change rapidly intra-operatively, and be aware of dangers of rapid normalization of electrolytes.

Further reading

Kumar S, Berl T (1998). Sodium. *The Lancet*, **352**, 220–8.
Worthley LIG (1997). Fluid and electrolyte therapy. In *Intensive care manual* (ed. TE Oh), Butterworth-Heinemann, Oxford.

Obesity

- Body mass index (BMI) = mass (kg)/[height (m)]^2.
- Obesity is defined by a BMI >28 kg/m^2 and morbid obesity by BMI >35 kg/m^2.
- 17% of the UK population are obese and approximately 1% morbidly obese.
- Obesity is associated with hypertension, ischaemic heart disease, non-insulin-dependent diabetes mellitus, peripheral vascular disease, gallstones, and osteoarthritis.

Pathophysiology

- Obesity is associated with in increase in absolute blood volume, although this is low relative to body mass (occasionally only 45 ml/kg).
- Oxygen consumption is increased by metabolically active adipose tissue and the workload of supporting muscles.
- FRC is reduced in the awake obese patient and decreases significantly following induction, which may encroach upon the closing capacity.
- Oxygen desaturation occurs rapidly in the obese apnoeic patient.
- Pulmonary compliance is decreased by up to 35% (due to heavy chest wall and splinted diaphragm).
- Obesity hypoventilation syndrome (OHS) occurs with progressive obesity causing respiratory impairment. Carbon dioxide respiratory drive is lost and hypoxaemia, pulmonary hypertension, and polycythaemia can develop.
- Obstructive sleep apnoea (OSA) is also more common in the obese.
- Increased gastric volumes, raised intra-abdominal pressure, and a higher incidence of hiatus hernia pose a significant risk of aspiration.
- Insulin resistance may cause perioperative diabetes.
- Volume of distribution for drugs is altered due to a smaller proportion of total body water, greater proportion of adipose tissue, increased lean body mass, and increased blood volume and cardiac output.

Conduct of anaesthesia

- Calculate the BMI and assess venous access, risk of aspiration, and possibility of a difficult intubation/difficulty with mask ventilation. A BMI of 46 is associated with a 13% risk of difficult intubation. It is useful to assess the airway in both the erect and supine positions.
- Consider asking for assistance.
- A typical operating table will support 150 kg, but the tilting/tipping may not function.
- Thromboembolic events are twice as common and so thromboprophylaxis is important.
- Premedication with respiratory depressants should be used with caution. An H$_2$ blocker or proton pump inhibitor plus metoclopramide should be administered on the ward (± 30 ml sodium citrate 0.3 M in the anaesthetic room).

- The sphygmomanometer cuff width should be 20% greater than the diameter of the arm. Invasive blood pressure monitoring may be required.
- Fluid balance may be difficult to assess clinically and increased blood loss is common due to difficult surgical conditions.
- Full preoxygenation is essential.
- Intubation may be warranted for all but the briefest of procedures due to the risk of aspiration, and IPPV is often necessary because of the increased work of breathing and tendency to hypoventilation.
- Awake fibreoptic intubation may be indicated, although some use topical anesthesia and direct laryngoscopy. Traction on the breasts by an assistant or use of a polio blade may help.
- Reduced FRC can be increased by administering PEEP or large sustained manual inflations. Increasing the I:E ratio may reduce airway pressures.
- Aortocaval compression may occur in the supine position and table tilt may help. Avoid head-down positioning especially in spontaneous ventilation.
- Local anaesthetic doses for spinals and epidurals should be 75–80% of normal because engorged extradural veins and fat constrict these spaces.

Postoperative

- Postoperative mortality is twice that of the non-obese.
- Mobilize as soon as practical—ensure enough staff are available.
- Pulmonary atelectasis is common and lung capacities remain decreased for at least 5 days post abdominal surgery. To optimize the FRC/closing capacity ratio the obese patient should be nursed at 30–45 degrees head-up tilt for this period.
- Humidified oxygen and early, regular physiotherapy should be administered.
- Nocturnal nasal CPAP and continual pulse oximetry may be considered in OSA.
- PCA is more predictable than IM opioids because injections are frequently into subcutaneous fat.
- HDU care should be available for higher-risk patients with pre-existing respiratory disease especially those undergoing thoracic or abdominal surgery.

Further reading

Dominguez-Cherit G, Gonzalez R, Borunda D, *et al.* (1998). Anesthesia for morbidly obese patients. *World Journal of Surgery*, **22**, 969–73.

Shenkman Z, Shir Y, Brodsky J (1993). Perioperative management of the obese patient. *British Journal of Anaesthesia*, **70**, 349–59.

Chapter 5
Renal disease

Jonathan Purday

Chronic renal failure

Patients with chronic renal failure (CRF) usually have complex medical histories, take a multitude of drugs, and often have severe systemic complications which increase the risk of anaesthesia and surgery. The main causes of CRF include glomerulonephritis, diabetes mellitus, hypertension, cystic disease, and pyelonephritis/interstitial nephritis.

Preoperative

- Check for hypertension, diabetes mellitus, and ischaemic heart disease.
- The cause of CRF may have anaesthetic considerations.
- Check for symptoms and signs of fluid overload (dependent oedema, basal crepitations) or hypovolaemia (sitting and standing BP, JVP, thirst, skin turgor).

Investigations

- FBC: usually normochromic, normocytic anaemia due to uraemia affecting erythropoesis, decreased red cell survival, and increased bleeding tendency. Many patients maintain a haemoglobin of 8 g/dl. These patients should not be transfused and if symptomatic can be commenced on erythropoetin therapy. In the past blood transfusion has been shown to increase the survival of renal transplants. Recent surveys, which show a general increase in graft survival, have demonstrated far less effect, and therefore a policy of deliberate transfusion is now rarely used.
- Electrolytes: a recent serum K^+ is essential. If K^+ >6.0 mmol/litre dialysis will usually be required prior to surgery. Na^+ is often decreased due to increased water retention. Calcium is often decreased due to inadequate vitamin D.
- Coagulation: uraemia affects platelet function and leads to a prolonged bleeding time. INR and APTT are usually normal (DDAVP 0.3 µg/kg in 50 ml saline over 30 min may improve platelet function if necessary, in uncontrolled bleeding).
- ECG: may show ischaemic heart disease. Rarely signs of hyperkalaemia K^+ >6.5 mmol/litre (arrhythmias, widened QRS, peaked T waves) or hypokalaemia K^+ <3.0 mmol/litre (arrhythmias, U waves, flattened T waves and A/V block) may be seen. These are metabolic emergencies and need urgent treatment.

Perioperative care

- Many patients with CRF have an upper limb arteriovenous shunt for haemodialysis. Venous/arterial cannulation and non-invasive BP readings should be avoided in this arm for fear of damaging the shunt. Wrap the arm in cotton-wool as a reminder and for protection. When no other veins are available, short-term emergency cannulation of the fistula arm is acceptable (avoiding the fistula).
- Patients with or without a shunt may need further access in the future, at which time their survival may depend upon good vascular access. Avoid cannulation of the forearm and antecubital veins. Use veins in the back of the hand or ulna aspect of forearm as these are rarely used for fistulae.

Arterial lines should only be used when essential and the radial artery is preferred.

- Fluid and electrolyte balance must be carefully managed. CRF patients are very susceptible to further renal damage with dehydration. Find out their normal daily fluid allowance and plan accordingly.
- Many patients with some renal function benefit from a preoperative IV saline 0.9% infusion to maintain renal blood flow.
- All fluids containing K^+ should be avoided—generally use saline.
- For patients with K^+ >5.5 mmol/litre, suxamethonium and factors that cause acidosis (hypoventilation and respiratory obstruction) should be avoided due to the risks of increasing potassium further.
- If large fluid shifts are likely, CVP monitoring should be performed.
- Delayed gastric emptying and increased gastric acidity make gastric reflux and aspiration more likely. Give H_2 antagonists/proton pump inhibitors (cimetidine may cause confusion and should be avoided) and consider rapid sequence induction.
- Immunity is suppressed by uraemia and this is often exaggerated by immunosuppressants, therefore use strict asepsis for any invasive procedures.
- Universal precautions are particularly important as hepatitis B and C are common.

Postoperative

Ensure careful fluid balance, and avoid nephrotoxic drugs and accumulation of analgesics.

Drugs and renal disease

Most drugs are excreted by the kidneys. Therefore most drugs or their metabolites have the potential to accumulate in renal failure. Loading doses of drugs are unchanged but maintenance doses of drugs are usually reduced. If in doubt refer to the BNF.

Some drugs are directly nephrotoxic and can lead to a decrease in renal function. Many anaesthetic drugs and techniques can decrease renal blood flow, glomerular filtration rate, and urine output.

	Drugs safe in CRF	Drugs contraindicated in CRF
Premed	Lormetazepam, temezepam, midazolam	
Induction	Propofol, thiopental, etomidate	
Maintenance	Isoflurane, desflurane, halothane, propofol	Enflurane
Muscle relaxant	Atracurium, cisatracurium,	Pancuronium
Opioids	Alfentanil, remifentanil	Pethidine
Local anaesthetics	Bupivacaine, lidocaine (lignocaine)	
Analgesics	Paracetamol, codeine	NSAIDS

Special considerations

- Opioids: all have prolonged action in renal failure. Morphine and pethidine are both metabolized to active metabolites (morphine 6-glucuronide and norpethidine) by the liver. Norpethidine can cause convulsions. Fentanyl builds up in peripheral tissues rarely leading to delayed respiratory depression. Morphine and fentanyl can be used with care. Respiratory rate and pulse oximetry should be measured postoperatively and continuous oxygen prescribed. Build-up of metabolites can best be avoided by using a PCA system for administration, or use of regional block techniques. Drugs vary as to how well they are removed from the blood with dialysis and morphine may take some time to be removed.

- Sevoflurane: can be used for induction, but has been shown to produce inorganic fluoride with prolonged exposure. No evidence of nephrotoxicity has been found, but isoflurane is a safe alternative.

- Suxamethonium: will increase serum K^+ by 0.5 mmol/litre and is therefore contraindicated in hyperkalaemic patients but otherwise can be used.

- Vecuronium and rocuronium: can be used with extreme care in renal failure, but atracurium (or cisatracurium) is a better alternative due to Hofmann elimination.

- Local anaesthetic drugs have a shorter duration of action, particularly for infiltration, in the acidic tissues of renal failure. Therefore bupivacaine may have advantages over lidocaine (lignocaine). The increased risk of haemorrhage and haematoma formation must be considered before using spinal and epidural techniques.

- Reversal of neuromuscular blockade. The use of a nerve stimulator is recommended. Neostigmine, glycopyrrolate, and atropine can all be used but half-lives are likely to be doubled.

- Antibiotics are usually excreted by the kidney. The usual advice is a normal loading dose with a decreased maintenance but always check with the BNF. Aminoglycosides and vancomycin are nephrotoxic (particularly in combination with other risk factors, e.g. diuretics, dehydration, jaundice, etc.). It is best to avoid these antibiotics, if possible, but in severe infection, blood levels should be closely monitored.

Patients on haemodialysis

- Haemodialysis patients undergo dialysis for several hours, three or four times a week.
- These patients usually have an intravenous access catheter (short term) or an arteriovenous shunt. These shunts are extremely important and are at risk from accidental damage or clotting (see above).
- Haemodialysis patients should be dialysed a few hours before surgery to control potassium levels. Following dialysis, patients will be relatively hypovolaemic and may have residual anticoagulation effects (heparin used during dialysis).
- Expect a degree of vascular instability on induction. Intra-operatively use 0.9% saline to achieve normovolaemia as this can be removed by dialysis at a later date. Give IV fluids to replace losses, but do not use excessive fluid. Colloids such as modified gelatins can be used as normal.
- Delay haemodialysis for 1–2 days postoperatively if possible, to avoid heparin-induced bleeding.
- Remember suxamethonium may increase K^+ by 0.5–1 mmol/litre.

Patients on peritoneal dialysis

- In peritoneal dialysis a temporary (hard) or permanent (soft or 'Tenchkoff') catheter is inserted into the peritoneal cavity. Dialysis is carried out by the exchange of fluid across the peritoneal membrane. As dialysis is continuous these patients often have a more relaxed fluid restriction than haemodialysis patients.

- Peritoneal dialysis patients should have their dialysate drained prior to surgery for optimal respiratory function. They can often omit 24–48 h of dialysis but if they have bowel surgery they will need a short period of haemodialysis. It is often kinder to the patient to insert a venous dialysis catheter under general anaesthesia.

- Take care with the choice of cannulation sites (see above).

Transplanted patients

- These patients may still have a degree of CRF and a functioning fistula, but if the transplanted kidney is working well fluid balance is not normally a problem.

- Patients are at particular risk of infection as they are immunosuppressed and therefore strict asepsis must be applied.

- The transplant is at risk if immunosuppresion is withdrawn, therefore care must be taken during perioperative fasting.

- Long-term steroid treatment may lead to adrenal suppression, osteoporosis, and increased risk of GI bleeding. Steroid cover may be required (p. 98).

- Avoid haemodynamic compromise of the transplanted organ and any potentially nephrotoxic drugs. Remember that even if serum creatinine is normal, creatinine clearance and renal function may be compromised and therefore NSAIDs are best avoided.

- Beware prone positioning when the transplanted kidney can be damaged by supports.

Patients with raised creatinine

Creatinine is a breakdown product of skeletal muscle metabolism. Under normal circumstances it undergoes minimal tubular secretion and its clearance accurately reflects the glomerular filtration rate (GFR). However, tubular secretion occurs with increasing serum creatinine leading to an overestimate of GFR. The plasma creatinine shows a rectangular hyperbolic relationship with creatinine clearance (see diagram). This has several important ramifications:

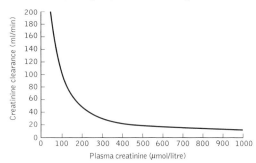

* GFR must be reduced by up to 50% before serum creatinine rises above normal levels.
* Small changes in serum creatinine in the low (normal) range imply a large change in GFR, making the test very sensitive.
* Individuals with different muscle mass will have very different curves and therefore each result must be determined in relation to this, and trends are most useful.
* The GFR does not always reflect overall renal function if an acute illness has caused a recent depression in GFR.
  Consider whether the raised creatinine represents acute renal impairment (possibly reversible), or CRF. If an acute onset is suspected:
* Optimize the preoperative metabolic state and consider IV saline the night before theatre to avoid dehydration.
* Insert a urinary catheter and monitor urine output hourly peri- and postoperatively (maintain >1 ml/kg/h).
* Have a low threshold for CVP insertion to monitor fluid balance.
* Take scrupulous care with fluid balance and blood pressure (avoid hypotension relative to the patient's normal value).
* Occasionally inotropes may be required to achieve an adequate BP.
* If urine output falls despite fluid loading (CVP 10–15 cmH$_2$O), try mannitol (0.5 g/kg) or furosemide (frusemide) (20–40 mg).
* Avoid NSAIDs and any potentially nephrotoxic drugs.
* Take care of arm vessels in case of future fistula.
* Contact the ICU or a renal physician to ascertain likely long-term plans for renal management—will dialysis be needed immediately postoperatively? If so a venous dialysis catheter can be inserted at the time of the anaesthetic.

Acute renal failure

Acute renal failure (ARF) commonly develops in the perioperative period and is associated with a high mortality (oliguric 50–80%, non-oliguric 10–40%). It is easily diagnosed in those with a rising creatinine, or oliguria. Occasionally, however, ARF may occur with relatively normal volumes of urine.

Risk factors for developing perioperative acute renal failure include:

- sepsis (especially abdominal)
- prolonged hypotension/hypovolaemia
- prolonged preoperative dehydration (orthopaedic/surgical patients)
- advanced age
- nephrotoxins—drugs, myoglobin
- diabetes mellitus
- renovascular surgery
- known chronic renal failure with raised serum creatinine (acute on chronic)
- a history of cardiac failure, hypertension, diabetes mellitus, rhabdomyolysis (crush syndrome), aortic surgery, pregnancy-induced hypertension
- urinary obstruction
- hepatorenal syndrome (see p. 132).

Nephrotoxic drugs	
Analgesics	Aspirin, NSAIDs
Antibiotics	Aminoglycosides, amphotericin B, vancomycin
ACE inhibitors	
Anti-neoplastic	Cisplatinum, methotrexate
Immunosuppressants	Ciclosporin
Psychiatric	Lithium
Radiocontrast agents	

Assessment of renal function

- Assess volume of urine being produced hourly (remember catheters can become blocked). Urinary electrolytes can help differentiate hypoperfusion (Na^+ <20 mmol/litre, urine osmolality >500 mosmol/kg) from acute tubular necrosis (ATN) (Na^+ >20 mmol/litre, urine osmolality <500 mosmol/kg). Remember that these results are meaningless if diuretics have been given.
- Serum creatinine is the main initial measurement of renal function (remember it is affected by body mass—see earlier) and increasing levels indicate worsening renal function. Serum urea is much less helpful as it also increases in dehydration, GI bleeding, sepsis, and diuretic administration, even with normal renal function.
- Electrolyte levels should be checked prior to surgery (exclude high serum K^+).

- Creatinine clearance is a useful marker of renal function. However, it needs a 24-h urine collection, and is rarely performed in the perioperative period.
- Abdominal ultrasound can be easily performed and will help differentiate chronic causes (two small kidneys) and obstructive causes. It can also estimate renal perfusion.
- If further assessment of renal function is required, dynamic renal scans examine perfusion and excretion from the kidney, but guidance should be sought from a nephrologist.

Perioperative considerations

- The main priority is the prevention/further deterioration of acute renal failure, plus maintenance of an adequate urine output (1–2 ml/kg/h)— 'non-oliguric renal failure'. Urinary catheterization should be considered early (i.e. presurgery).
- Preoperative rehydration is important in preventing ARF. Patients who are significantly dehydrated (e.g. bowel obstruction) need fluid deficit corrected prior to surgery, and this is often best judged by CVP monitoring (maintain CVP at 10–15 cmH$_2$O).
- The response to a fluid bolus (250–500 ml) over 10–15 min may help differentiate between hypovolaemia and acute tubular necrosis while more invasive monitoring is prepared.
- An adequate BP is important for renal perfusion. A mean arterial pressure of >70 mmHg (85 mmHg in hypertensive patients) should be maintained (use inotropes if necessary).
- The outcome from polyuric ARF is better than oliguric ARF, but no patient should be given furosemide (frusemide) until they have an adequate filling pressure and systemic arterial pressure.
- Furosemide (frusemide) is given initially as an IV bolus of 20–40 mg. In patients with established renal insufficiency (i.e. raised serum creatinine) give 250 mg over 1 h as an infusion.
- Consider mannitol (0.5–1 g/kg IV).
- Monitor serum K$^+$ 1–2-hourly if raised (most blood gas analysers give accurate levels).

Guidelines for renal replacement therapy

	Haemofiltration	Haemodialysis	Peritoneal dialysis
Time period	Continuous	Intermittent	Continuous
CVS stability	Stable	Unstable	Stable
Fluid removal	Good	Good	Poor
Urea removal	Reasonable	Good	Poor
Abdominal surgery	Indicated	Indicated	Contraindicated
Infection	Moderate risk	Moderate risk	High risk
Bleeding complications	Moderate	Moderate	Low

- In patients with established ARF, further acid–base deterioration should be avoided. Plan for perioperative renal replacement therapy (see Table).
- Any abdominal surgery or infection contraindicates peritoneal dialysis and a dialysis catheter should be inserted whilst the patient is still anaesthetized.

Postoperative care

- Avoid NSAIDs in all patients at risk of renal failure.
- Give appropriate IV fluids and avoid dehydration (consider CVP monitoring if not instituted).
- Closely monitor urine output.
- If oliguria occurs (<0.5 ml/kg/h) try a fluid challenge of 250– 500 ml 0.9% saline/gelofusine, or mannitol (0.5–1 g/kg IV). Consider CVP and adequate arterial pressure as previously.
- Intra-abdominal pressure if raised to more than 20 mmHg can lead to anuria by direct compression on the renal pelvises. Raised intra-abdominal pressure is found in up to 30% of emergency surgery cases and is especially common after massive intra-abdominal bleeding such as a leaking abdominal aneurysm repair.
- Intra-abdominal pressure can be measured via the bladder. Instil 50 ml saline into the bladder via a standard foley catheter, clamp off the drainage port, and measure pressure via a manometer line connected to a needle inserted into the catheter lumen. Remember that raised intra-abdominal pressure will also tend to cause falsely high reading of CVP pressures (hence the patient may be underfilled despite apparently adequate CVP).
- Bleeding may be a particular problem due to poor platelet function. Reverse any residual heparin (protamine 1 mg/100 units heparin slow IV) and consider cryoprecipitate and DDAVP (0.3 mg/kg IV over 30 min in 50 ml 0.9% saline). Conjugated oestrogen (0.6 mg/kg/day for 5 days) may also help.

Emergency management of raised serum potassium

Treatment

Treatment should be initiated if K^+ >6.5 mmol/litre or ECG are changes present. Unlike hypokalaemia, the incidence of serious cardiac compromise is high and therefore intervention is important. Treat the cause if possible.

- Insulin 15 units in 100 ml 20% dextrose IV over 30–60 min.
- Calcium 5–10 ml 10% calcium gluconate or 3–5 ml 10% calcium chloride (rapid onset, short lived).
- Bicarbonate 50 mmol IV (especially with acidosis).
- Ion exchange resin—calcium resonium 15 g PO/30 g PR 8-hourly.
- Beta-agonists, consider salbutamol 5 mg nebulized.
- Dialysis or haemofiltration.

Further reading

Bannister KM, Field MF (1996). Clinical physiology of the kidney: tests of renal function and structure. In *Oxford textbook of medicine (3rd edn)*, (eds. Weatherall, Ledingham, Warrell) pp. 3101–15. Oxford University Press, Oxford.

Bolsin SN (1996). Anaesthesia for patients with renal disease. In *International practice of anaesthesia* (eds. C Prys-Roberts, DR Brown), pp. 1781–6. Butterworth-Heinemann, Oxford.

El Nahas AM, Winearls CG (1996). Chronic renal failure. In *Oxford textbook of medicine (3rd edn)* (eds. Weatherall, Ledingham, Warrell), pp. 3294–306. Oxford University Press, Oxford.

Malbrain MLNG (1999). Abdominal pressure in the critically ill: measurement and clinical relevance. *Intensive Care Medicine*, 25, 1453–8.

Thadhani R, Pascuel M, Bonventre JV (1996). Acute renal failure. *New England Journal of Medicine*, 334, 1448–60.

Chapter 6
Hepatic disease

Jonathan Purday

Complications of liver disease

There are numerous causes of hepatic disease. The most common in the Western world is cirrhosis secondary to viral hepatitis or alcoholism. Patients with underlying hepatic disease often present to the anaesthetist and surgeon. Problems include:

- Bleeding. The liver is responsible for the production of clotting factors (all except factor VIII) and the prothrombin time is usually prolonged. This can be improved by daily vitamin K injections (10 mg IV slowly). Thrombocytopenia is common, as is defective platelet function. Bleeding is more likely to be secondary to thrombocytopenia than due to clotting factor deficiency. Both duodenal ulceration and oesophageal and gastric varices are common in patients with liver failure and bleeding can be torrential. Clotting studies and FBC must be carefully checked perioperatively and adequate provision must be made for the cross-match of blood, fresh frozen plasma, and platelets.

- Encephalopathy. In severe liver failure toxic products build up (particularly ammonia, due to deranged amino acid metabolism) leading to a progressive encephalopathy. This occurs in hyperacute hepatic failure (within 7 days), acute (7–28 days), and subacute (28 days to 6 months). This classification replaces fulminant hepatic failure where encephalopathy developed within 8 weeks of the precipitating illness. In cirrhosis this may be precipitated by sedatives, a high-protein diet (including GI bleed), infection, surgical operations, trauma, hypokalaemia, or constipation. The decreased level of consciousness may compromise the airway and intubation may be required if cerebral oedema develops.

Grades of hepatic encephalopathy

Grade 0	Alert and orientated
Grade I	Drowsy and orientated
Grade II	Drowsy and disorientated
Grade III	Rousable stupor, restlessness
Grade IV	Coma—unresponsive to deep pain

- Hypoglycaemia. The liver contains major stores of glycogen, a glucose precursor. Check blood glucose levels regularly. Give 10% dextrose infusions if <2mmol/litre. Monitor plasma K^+.

- Ascites. Fibrotic changes in the liver lead to portal hypertension, and in combination with salt and water retention and a low serum albumin, fluid accumulates in the peritoneal cavity. This can lead to respiratory failure, due to pressure on the diaphragm, and the ascites may need to be drained.

- Infection. Immune function is depressed and infections of the respiratory and urinary tract are common.

- Renal failure. This is often multifactorial. Combined liver and renal failure may result from:
  - a common pathomechanism (sepsis, toxic, immune, and genetic).
  - secondary due to decreased circulating blood volume or increased reno-

vascular resistance (prerenal), impaired renal tubular function, or hepatorenal failure. Hepatorenal failure is due to intrarenal arterial and arteriolar vasoconstiction and can only be diagnosed after exclusion of shock, sepsis, and nephrotoxic drugs.

Acute hepatic disease

Previously well patients with acute liver failure rarely present for anaesthesia and surgery (mortality rates of 10 and 100% have been described). More commonly, acute failure is due to decompensation of chronic liver disease. Hyperacute hepatic failure (encephalopathy within 7 days) paradoxically has the best prognosis.

Causes of acute liver failure

- Viral hepatitis: types A to G, cytomegalovirus, herpes simplex virus, and Epstein–Barr virus.
- Drugs: paracetamol excess, idiosyncratic reactions, halothane.
- Toxins: carbon tetrachloride, Amanita phalloides mushrooms.
- Others: acute fatty infiltration of pregnancy, HELLP syndrome, Wilson's disease, Reye's syndrome.

Patients with acute liver disease and encephalopathy have severe coagulopathy and active fibrinolysis, high cardiac output and reduced systemic vascular resistance, hypoglycaemia/hypokalaemia, and metabolic acidosis. They are also at risk of raised intracranial pressure. Due to the high perioperative mortality, patients should have all anaesthetics postponed (unless true emergency) until at least 30 days after liver function tests have returned to normal. Hepatitis B and C are highly contagious via parenteral inoculation to theatre personnel and universal precautions must be strictly adhered to.

Chronic hepatic disease

The commonest cause of chronic liver disease is cirrhosis, but chronic hepatitis is also widespread. Chronic hepatitis is any hepatitis lasting longer than 6 months and cirrhosis is hepatic fibrosis with regeneration nodules.

- Cirrhosis can be acquired (alcohol, viral hepatitis, drugs, secondary biliary, or veno-occlusive disease) or inherited (primary biliary, haemachromatosis, Wilson's, galactosaemia, sickle cell disease).

- Chronic hepatitis B develops in 3% of those infected. It is widespread in the Far East and Africa and infects 300 million people worldwide. Other high-risk groups include homosexuals, IV drug abusers, haemophiliacs, haemodialysis patients, and those in institutional care. It may progress to cirrhosis or hepatocellular carcinoma.

- Chronic hepatitis C develops in 75% of those infected. Risk groups are similar to hepatitis B and cirrhosis and hepatocellular carcinoma can develop. Blood products were previously responsible for many cases of hepatitis C but now all donors are screened.

- Other causes of chronic hepatitis include alcohol, autoimmune, metabolic, and drugs (isoniazid, methyldopa).

- Assessment of risk factors for surgery and anaesthesia is described by Child's classification. Common causes of mortality in the perioperative period include sepsis, renal failure, bleeding, and worsening liver failure with encephalopathy.

Surgical risk assessment: Child's classification as modified by Pugh

	Mortality		
	Minimal (<5%)	Modest (5–50%)	Marked (>50%)
Bilirubin (μmol/litre)	<25	25–40	>40
Albumin (g/litre)	>35	30–35	<30
PT (seconds prolonged)	1–4	4–6	>6
Ascites	None	Moderate	Marked
Encephalopathy (p. 122)	None	Grades 1 and 2	Grades 3 and 4
Nutrition	Excellent	Good	Poor

PT = prothrombin time.

Drug metabolism and liver disease

- The vast majority of drugs, including anaesthetic drugs, are metabolized by the liver.

- Most drugs are initially metabolized by the cytochrome P450 system. In Phase I they are either oxidized or reduced and in Phase II they are conjugated with a glucuronide, glycine, or sulphate to enhance water solubility and excretion in bile or urine.

- In early alcoholic liver disease the cytochrome P450 system is often induced, leading to rapid metabolism of drugs, whereas this is reversed in end stage disease.

- The liver has a large functional reserve and so these functions are usually preserved until end-stage disease.
- Pharmacodynamics and the sensitivity of target organs for sedatives and anaesthetics may be altered with coma easily induced in end-stage liver disease.

Causes of altered drug pharmacokinetics in liver failure

Liver problem	Pharmacological effect
Decreased portal blood flow in hepatic fibrosis	Decreased GI drug clearance
Hypoalbuminaemia	Increased free drug in plasma
Ascites and sodium and water retention	Increased volume of distribution
Biotransformation enzymes	Activity may increase or decrease
Reduced liver cell mass	Reduced activity
Obstructive jaundice	Decreased biliary excretion of drugs

Anaesthetic management of the patient with liver failure

Preoperative laboratory investigations

- Full blood count and clotting studies. The prothrombin time is a good marker of liver function.
- Electrolytes and creatinine. The urea is often falsely low due to decreased hepatic production.
- Glucose—hepatic stores of glycogen and glucose utilization are often affected.
- Liver function tests (see below).
- Arterial blood gases.
- Urinalysis.
- Hepatitis screening (although universal precautions should always be observed).

Assessment of liver function

- Serum liver function tests are rarely specific but prothrombin time (PT), albumin, and bilirubin are sensitive markers of overall liver function. Serial measurements are useful and indicate trends. It is important to avoid giving FFP, unless treating active bleeding, to avoid altering the PT time, which is an excellent guide to overall liver function.
- Liver transaminases (aspartate 'AST', alanine 'ALT') are sensitive to even mild liver damage and have no role in mortality prediction. Levels may decrease in severe disease.
- Alkaline phosphatase is raised with biliary obstruction.
- Immunological tests: antinuclear antibody is present in 75% of patients with chronic active hepatitis and smooth muscle antibody in nearly all cases of primary biliary cirrhosis. α-fetoprotein is a marker of hepatoma.
- Imaging techniques: ultrasound is the main initial investigation of obstructive jaundice. Other useful investigations include ERCP, CT, and MRI cholangiograms.
- Liver function tests (LFTs) must always be interpreted in consideration with a careful history and examination. The liver has a large reserve function and can often withstand considerable damage before LFTs become deranged.

Perioperative considerations

- Proton pump inhibitors or H2 antagonists should be used preoperatively. Rapid sequence induction will reduce the risks of gastric aspiration.
- Even in severe liver disease the problem is usually one of exaggerated effects of drugs on the CNS, rather than poor liver metabolism per se.
- Hepatic blood flow is often altered during anaesthesia and surgery by anaesthetic drugs (including α and β agonists/antagonists), positive pressure ventilation, PEEP, and surgical technique.
- In most cases anaesthesia reduces liver blood flow, particularly if halothane is used. However, isoflurane actually seems to improve hepatic blood flow.

Anaesthetic drugs in liver failure

	Drugs safe in liver failure	Drugs to be used with caution (may need reduced dosage)	Drugs contraindicated in liver failure
Premedication	Lorazepam	Midazolam, diazepam	
Induction	Propofol, thiopental, etomidate		
Maintenance	Desflurane, sevoflurane, isoflurane	Enflurane	Halothane (probably)
Muscle relaxants	Atracurium, cisatracurium	Pancuronium, vecuronium, suxamethonium	
Opioids	Remifentanil	Fentanyl, alfentanil, morphine, pethidine	
Analgesics	Paracetamol	NSAIDS, lidocaine (lignocaine), bupivacaine	

- Regional techniques can be used as long as coagulation is not too deranged, and it should be remembered that all local anaesthetics are metabolized by the liver.
- Isoflurane is the preferred volatile agents as enflurane, and particularly halothane, have marked effects in decreasing hepatic blood flow and inhibiting drug metabolism.

Physiological considerations

- Cardiovascular: liver disease causes various types of shunt, from cutaneous spider angioma to portapulmonary A/V shunts. These shunts lead to an increase in cardiac output, often by 50%. This is combined with a reduction in systemic vascular resistance and an increase in extracellular fluid due to an activated renin–angiotensin system. In contrast, some alcoholics may have a decreased cardiac output secondary to cardiomyopathy.
- Ascites: a common manifestation of liver disease. Water and sodium retention may be treated with potassium-sparing diuretics, e.g. spironolactone. A careful check of electrolytes is essential. Removal of ascites at operation will be followed by postoperative re-forming. This should be taken into account in fluid balance.
- Pulmonary: up to 50% of patients may have intrapulmonary shunting and V/Q mismatch, pleural effusions, and respiratory splinting of the diaphragm by ascites causing a decrease in PaO_2 not improved by increasing the FiO_2. Diuretics or paracentesis may improve ascites.
- Bleeding and clotting problems: both clotting factors and platelets are affected quantitatively and qualitatively. Coagulation should be carefully assessed preoperatively and adequate provision made for intra-operative blood products.

Postoperative liver dysfunction

Although postoperative jaundice is relatively common, significant liver dysfunction is relatively rare. Dysfunction has varied aetiology and often resolves without treatment. It should be remembered that hepatitis due to volatile agents is extremely rare and is largely a diagnosis of exclusion.

Causes of postoperative liver dysfunction or jaundice

Bilirubin overload (haemolysis)	Blood transfusion
	Haematoma resorption
	Haemolytic anaemia (sickle cell, prosthetic heart valve, glucose-6-phosphatase deficiency)
Hepatocellular injury	Exacerbation of pre-existing liver disease
	Hepatic ischaemia: hypovolaemia, hypotension, cardiac failure
	Septicaemia
	Drug-induced (antibiotics, halothane)
	Hypoxia
	Viral hepatitis
Cholestasis	Intrahepatic (benign, infection, drug-induced, e.g. cephalosporins, carbamazepine, erythromycin)
	Extrahepatic (pancreatitis, gallstones, bile duct injury)
Congenital	Gilbert's syndrome

- Common causes include hepatic oxygen deprivation from intra- and postoperative hypoxia and hypotension.
- Benign postoperative intrahepatic cholestasis mimics biliary obstruction and usually occurs after major surgery associated with hypotension, hypoxaemia, or multiple transfusions.
- The surgical procedure should also be considered, and significant haematoma resolution is a common cause.

Halothane hepatitis

- Halothane has been linked to postoperative liver dysfunction.
- Two syndromes are recognized:
  - The first is associated with a transient rise in liver function tests and low morbidity, often after initial exposure.
  - The second is thought to occur after repeated exposure and has an 'immune' mechanism with the development of fulminant hepatic failure (FHF) and high mortality. It is rare, with an incidence of 1 in 35 000 anaesthetics.
- Antibodies specific to FHF patients exposed to halothane are found in 70% of such patients. It is postulated that a halothane oxidative metabolite binds to liver cytochromes to form a hapten and induce a hypersensitivity reac-

tion. All patients exposed to halothane have altered liver proteins but it is unknown why only a few develop liver failure.

* There does appear to be a genetic susceptibility as shown by in vitro testing.
* Halothane has also been shown in several animal studies to significantly decrease liver blood flow, particularly during hypoxia.

Other inhalational anaesthetic agents

* The chance of an 'immune' reaction occurring to a volatile agent is thought to relate to the amount it is metabolized. Halothane is 20% metabolized.
* Enflurane is 2% metabolized and should therefore cause 10 times fewer reactions. Products of enflurane metabolism have been shown to alter liver proteins and there have been rare case reports linking enflurane with liver damage. There is a theoretical basis for cross-reactivity with previous halothane exposure.
* Isoflurane is 0.2% metabolized. There is, therefore, a theoretical risk of reaction and indeed there have been a few case reports. These, however, have been contested and isoflurane is considered safe for use in patients at risk of hepatic failure.
* Sevoflurane and desflurane also appear to be safe in liver failure.

Renal failure and the hepatorenal syndrome

Hepatorenal syndrome and acute tubular necrosis are common in patients with liver disease. Maintenance of an adequate urinary output with fluids is the mainstay of prevention. Once renal failure occurs, due to any cause, with a high creatinine level in the presence of cirrhosis, mortality is usually 100%.

- The hepatorenal syndrome is a functional renal failure which occurs spontaneously or more commonly due to fluid shifts particularly in patients with obstructive jaundice.
- The kidney is normal histologically and functions normally following a liver transplant or if transplanted into a recipient.
- All pathophysiological changes seen in ascites (renal sodium and water retention and plasma expansion) are present to an extreme form in the hepatorenal patient.
- Diagnostic criteria are:
    - urinary sodium <10 mmol/litre
    - urine:plasma osmolarity and creatinine ratios >1
    - normal CVP with no diuresis on central volume expansion
    - a patient with chronic liver disease and ascites.
- Worsening hepatorenal failure results in death, despite haemofiltration or dialysis, and can only be corrected by liver transplantation.

Prevention

- Preoperatively an IV infusion of 0.9% saline should be commenced to avoid hypovolaemia.
- Renal blood flow must be optimized by monitoring CVP and correcting any hypovolaemia.
- Remember that tense ascites may cause compression of the right atrium and falsely high CVP measurements.
- Mannitol is often used prophylactically to maintain urine output (0.5 g/kg over 30 min).
- Hypotension should be avoided intra-operatively and mean BP should be maintained within 10–20% of preoperative levels—particularly in the hypertensive patient.
- An adequate urine output of at least 1 ml/kg/h must be achieved.
- Avoid the use of any nephrotoxic drugs such as NSAIDs, and gentamicin in repeated doses.

Portal hypertension and oesophageal varices

- Portal hypertension commonly occurs with cirrhosis but can arise in any condition where there is disruption of pre-, intra-, or posthepatic blood flow.
- Portal hypertension causes enlargement of the anastomoses between the portal and systemic circulation leading to varices at the gastro-oesophageal junction, haemorrhoids, and dilated abdominal wall veins ('caput medusa').
- 30% of varices bleed and present as haematemesis or malaena.
- Mortality is up to 50% for the acute bleed, particularly in patients with advanced cirrhosis.

Treatment

- Initial management is to correct hypovolaemia, stop the bleeding, and try to avoid complications such as fluid and electrolyte imbalance, encephalopathy, and aspiration pneumonia.
- Two large-bore IVs and a CVP line should be inserted.
- Drugs that may cause or exacerbate the bleeding, e.g. aspirin, should be stopped.
- Early endoscopy is warranted to confirm the diagnosis (remember peptic ulceration and oesophageal and gastric erosions in up to 30% of cases) and control bleeding (band ligation appears more effective than sclerosant injection). However, 70% of patients will rebleed, most within 6 weeks.
- Vasoactive drugs (terlipressin 2 mg 6-hourly, vasopressin 0.2–0.4 units/min for 24–48 h) constrict vessels in the mesenteric beds but may cause coronary constriction and angina. GTN patches or infusion may help. Terlipressin causes less angina than vasopressin.
- Somatostatin (a hypothalamic hormone) 250 μg/h and octreotide (an analogue) 50 μg/h for 2 to 5 days (as well as terlipressin/vasopressin) in combination with endoscopic therapy may be more effective than either alone and should be started whilst waiting for an experienced endoscopist.
- Balloon tamponade with an oesophageal and gastric balloon can provide temporary haemostasis but should only be used where endoscopic and drug treatments have failed. There is a high risk of fatal complications (aspiration, oesophageal tear/rupture, and airway obstruction) and therefore this should only be used in HDU/ICU.
- 70% of cirrhotic patients who survive their first variceal bleed will rebleed, most within 6 weeks.
- Beta-blockade (propranolol 40–160 mg twice daily) can decrease portal pressure in the chronic situation and may decrease the rebleed rate from 70 to 50%, but may mask the early signs of hypovolaemia and exacerbate the hypotension during rebleeding.
- Portal-systemic shunting is now rarely performed as an emergency due to its high mortality. It can occasionally be performed after the first bleed, to lower portal pressure, but is contraindicated if there is any clinical or EEG evidence of encephalopathy.

- A transjugular intrahepatic portosystemic stent shunt (TIPSS) achieves shunting without the need for surgery but has a high thrombosis rate.
- Oesophageal staple transection can be used if endoscopic therapy fails or is unavailable. The effectiveness and mortality are similar to sclerotherapy. These patients are at increased anaesthetic risk from hypovolaemia, a full stomach, and liver impairment.

Further reading

Brown BR Jr. (1996). Risk assessment for anaesthesia in patients with liver disease. In *International practice of anaesthesia* (eds, C Prys-Roberts, DR Brown), pp. 1731–9. Butterworth-Heinemann, Oxford.

Clarke P, Bellamy MC (1999). Anaesthesia for patients with liver disease *The Royal College of Anaesthetists Bulletin*, **4**, 158–61.

Early management of bleeding oesophageal varices (2000). D*rug and Therapeutics Bulletin*, **38**, 37–40.

Strunin L (1996). Effects of anaesthetics and drugs on liver function. In *International practice of anaesthesia* (eds, C Prys-Roberts, DR Brown), pp. 1171–15. Butterworth-Heinemann, Oxford.

Chapter 7
Haematological disorders
Jonathan Purday

Anaemia

Anaemia, defined as a haemoglobin concentration below the normal for the age and sex, is common in patients undergoing surgery: usually due to blood loss (acute or chronic) but also from failure of production or haemolysis. Conventionally diagnosed when the haemoglobin (Hb) concentration is <13 g/dl in an adult male and <12 g/dl in an adult female.

Common causes of anaemia in the surgical patient are:

- Blood loss either acute or chronic.
- Bone marrow failure due to infiltration by tumour or suppression by drugs.
- Megaloblastic anaemias due to either folate or vitamin B_{12} deficiency.
- Complex anaemias with effects on production and breakdown, e.g. renal failure, rheumatoid arthritis, and hypothyroidism.
- Haemolytic anaemias are either inherited, e.g. the thalassaemias, sickle cell disease, and spherocytosis (see references), acquired, e.g. autoimmune (often drugs or infections), or physical (mechanical heart valves, DIC, and jogging).

Clinical

- Associated with fatigue, dyspnoea, palpitations, headaches, and angina. The severity often reflects the speed of onset more than the degree of anaemia because there is less time for adaptation.
- Symptoms of the commonest causes should be elicited, including relevant family history; always enquire about aspirin, NSAIDs, and alcohol.
- Respiratory and cardiovascular history may be worsened by the anaemia or make its impact greater.

Investigations

Measure Hb prior to surgery in appropriate patients (p. 7) including all those at risk of anaemia undergoing major surgery and anyone with other significant medical problems, especially heart or lung disease. Much can be deduced from the Hb and mean corpuscular volume (MCV) alone but in many instances a blood film gives additional useful information. Confirmatory tests such as ferritin, B_{12}, and folate levels, reticulocyte count, direct Coombs test, erythrocyte sedimentation rate, liver and renal function, and bone marrow should be requested as appropriate.

Preoperative preparation

Ideally, patients scheduled for elective surgery should have their FBC checked in the weeks approaching the operation so that abnormalities such as anaemia can then be investigated and corrected in time. When delay to surgery is possible it is more appropriate and far safer to treat the underlying cause and to raise the Hb slowly with simple, effective measures, e.g. oral iron, B_{12} injections. Transfusing a patient with pernicious anaemia may precipitate heart failure.

Perioperative blood transfusion (see also p. 911)

A better appreciation of the potential risks of allogeneic blood has led to a more conservative approach to transfusion support. Unfortunately, there are no evidence-based guidelines that set clear target levels for transfusion. In addition as Hb decreases cardiac output increases (decrease in blood viscosity) and oxygen delivery may be maintained.

- Although unsupported by clinical evidence, an Hb of 10 g/dl (haematocrit of 30%) is often quoted as the lowest acceptable level. This level has been criticized in recent years and there is increasing evidence that in fit patients lowering the transfusion trigger to 8 g/dl is not associated with increased morbidity but may actually improve it!
- Red cell transfusion is indicated if the haemoglobin level is <7 g/dl.
- Checking a HemoCue® reading gives comparable results to a Coulter® counter and can help to avoid a transfusion if above 8 g/dl.
- Each case must be assessed with a view to coexistent disease, expected intra-operative blood loss, and whether acute or chronic.
- For patients who may tolerate anaemia poorly, e.g. patients over the age of 65 or those with significant ischaemic heart or respiratory disease, consider raising the transfusion threshold to 9–10 g/dl.

Complications of blood transfusion

- Mismatch: most commonly due to giving the wrong blood to the wrong patient. The transfusion must be immediately stopped, the unit returned to transfusion and full blood, clotting and serum samples sent. Signs and symptoms of a transfusion reaction should be sought and a haematologist contacted.
- Transfusion reactions: acute allergic reactions with fever, sweating, tachy-cardia, and urticaria are not uncommon (2%). Provided there are no signs of a haemolytic reaction give antipyretics and antihistamines (paracetamol 1 g PO and chlorpheniramine 10 mg IV) and continue the transfusion. Haemolytic reactions are suggested by hypotension, back and chest pains, oliguria, and haemoglobinuria and should be treated as a mismatched transfusion. Anaphylactic shock may develop with hypotension, broncho-spasm, and urticaria and should be treated with urgent intravenous adrenaline boluses titrated to effect (see p. 857).
- Metabolic: acidosis, hyperkalaemia, and hypocalcaemia (from the citrate anticoagulant).
- Hypothermia: particularly in a large-volume transfusion unless the blood is adequately warmed (this can lead to poor platelet function and can exacerbate bleeding).
- Circulatory overload: particularly in patients with cardiac failure.
- Dilutional coagulopathy: clotting factors and platelets only survive a few days in stored blood.
- Cross-infection: the blood-borne viruses, e.g. HIV, hepatitis B and C (although screened, donors may donate prior to seroconversion), but also bacteria and malaria.
- Massive transfusion exacerbates all these problems but can also lead to acute lung injury after several days.

Group and save or cross-match?

- Once grouped and saved, blood can usually be cross-matched within half an hour.
- Patients who should be cross-matched include those patients who have a decreased preoperative Hb and those operations with a high chance of intra-operative blood loss.

Coagulation disorders

Abnormalities of coagulation are common in patients presenting for anaesthesia.

- Congenital disorders may not present until challenged by trauma or surgery in adult life.
- Acquired disorders are due to lack of synthesis of coagulation factors, increased loss due to consumption (such as disseminated intravascular coagulation) or massive blood loss, or the production of substances that interfere with their function.
- A family history may be elicited (haemophilia A and B—sex linked recessives; von Willebrand's disease—autosomal dominant with variable penetrance) but cannot be relied upon (absent in 30% of haemophiliacs).
- Response to previous haemostatic challenges (tonsillectomy, dental extractions) may indicate the severity of the coagulopathy, e.g. in severe haemophilia A (factor VIII <2%) bleeding occurs spontaneously; in mild haemophilia (factor VIII 5–30%) bleeding occurs only after trauma.
- Concurrent and past medical problems such as liver disease, malabsorption (vitamin K deficiency), infection, malignancy (DIC), autoimmune disease (systemic lupus erythematosus, rheumatoid arthritis) as well as medications (anticoagulants, aspirin, and NSAIDs) may be relevant.

Laboratory investigations

The usual screening tests of bleeding include a platelet count, prothrombin time/international normalized ratio (PT/INR), activated partial thromboplastin time (APTT), thrombin time (TT) and fibrinogen. Specific factor assays are dictated by the pattern of abnormalities in the initial screen and usually follow discussion with a haematologist. Circulating anticoagulants, e.g. antibodies to factor VIII or von Willebrand's factor, are often secondary to systemic lupus erythematosus, rheumatoid arthritis or malignancy. Management is difficult and surgery should be avoided if at all possible. Lupus anticoagulants are not uncommon, are often not associated with systemic lupus erythematosus, and may be of no clinical significance if transient, e.g. following viral infections.

Preoperative preparation

- An unexpected abnormality in the coagulation screen should be investigated before surgery by seeking advice from a haematologist.
- Anticoagulation guidelines—see p. 142.
- Previously untreated mild haemophilia requires strenuous efforts at avoiding blood products (use DDAVP or tranexamic acid instead, if appropriate), but if factor concentrates are necessary the treatment of choice is now recombinant material in accordance with established guidelines. Always involve a haemophilia specialist.
- Abnormalities due to liver disease or vitamin K deficiency—give daily vitamin K (phytomenadione) 10 mg slowly IV. FFP (15 ml/kg) may be needed in addition if the presenting symptom is bleeding.

Disorder	Platelet count	INR	APTT	TT	Fibrinogen	Other
Haemophilia A	Normal	Normal	↑	Normal	Normal	↓ VIII
Haemophilia B	Normal	Normal	↑	Normal	Normal	↓ IX
von Willebrand's disease	Normal (usually)	Normal	↑	Normal	Normal	↓ VIII, vWF, ↑ bleeding time
Liver disease	Normal or ↓	↑	↑	Normal	Normal or ↓	↓ V
Vitamin K deficiency	Normal	↑	↑	Normal	Normal	↓ II, VII, IX, X
DIC	Normal or ↓	↑	↑	Normal or ↑	Normal or ↓	↑ FDPs, d-dimers, ↓ II, V, VIII
Massive transfusion	↓	↑	↑	Normal or ↑	Normal or ↓	Normal FDPs
Heparin (unfractionated)	Normal (rarely ↓)	Normal or ↑	↑↑	↑	Normal	↑ anti-Xa
Heparin (LMWH)	Normal (rarely ↓)	Normal	Normal	Normal	Normal	↑ anti-Xa
Warfarin	Normal	↑↑	↑	Normal	Normal	↓ II, VII, IX, X
Lupus anticoagulant	Normal	Normal or ↑	↑↑	Normal	Normal	DRVVT +ve, cardiolipin antibody

Abbreviations: INR = international normalized ratio. APTT = activated partial thromboplastin time. TT = thrombin time. vWF = von Willebrand's factor. DIC = disseminated intravascular coagulation. LMWH = low-molecular-weight heparin. FDPs = fibrin degradation products. DRVVT = dilute Russell's viper venom time.

Perioperative management of coagulation failure

Acute DIC is probably the commonest cause of a significant coagulation abnormality in the surgical setting especially in the peri- and postoperative phase. It is associated with infections (especially Gram-negative bacteraemia), placental abruption, amniotic fluid embolism, major trauma, burns, hypoxia, hypovolaemia, and severe liver disease. Haemorrhage, thrombosis, or both may occur. Chronic DIC is associated with aneurysms, haemangiomas, and carcinomatosis. The laboratory abnormalities are variable, depending on the severity of the DIC, and reflect both consumption of platelets and coagulation factors as well as hyperplasminaemia and fibrinolysis.

- Treatment should be aimed primarily at removal or control of the underlying cause whilst support is given to maintain tissue perfusion and oxygenation.

- Abnormal coagulation parameters in the presence of bleeding or the need for an invasive procedure are indications for haemostatic support. Transfusion of platelets (for advice see under thrombocytopenia, p. 145) and FFP (15 ml/kg initially or 4 units in an average adult) should help restore platelets, coagulation factors, and the natural anticoagulants, antithrombin-III and protein C. Cryoprecipitate (10 units initially) may also be necessary if the fibrinogen level cannot be raised above 1 g/litre by FFP alone.

- The indications for heparin and concentrates of antithrombin and protein C are not established. Antifibrinolytics such as tranexamic acid are generally contraindicated in DIC. Intramuscular injections, aspirin, and NSAIDs should be avoided in any patient at risk of bleeding; the intravenous and subcutaneous routes are acceptable.

- Massive transfusion of stored blood perioperatively may cause significant coagulation disorders due to the lack of factors V, VIII, and XI. DIC, which can be precipitated by shock, is often also present. In addition thrombocytopenia is a frequent occurrence. Therapy consists of replacement FFP and platelets as guided by coagulation tests.

Guidelines for fresh frozen plasma administration (see p. 920)

- The usual dose is 12–15 ml/kg which raises the coagulation levels by 12–15%.

- FFP takes 20 min to thaw. The infusion should be commenced within 2 h of thawing and be complete within 4 h of thawing.

- Definite indications for use are life-threatening haemorrhage with overdose of coumarin anticoagulants or vitamin K deficiency and acute DIC.

- Conditional indications include massive blood transfusion (bleeding is usually secondary to thrombocytopenia) and liver disease.

Anticoagulants

The main indications for anticoagulation are:
- To prevent stroke in atrial fibrillation.
- To prevent stroke with mechanical heart valves.
- For the treatment and prevention of venous thrombosis and pulmonary emboli.

Warfarin
- An oral anticoagulant that results in the liver synthesizing non-functional coagulation factors II, VII, IX, and X as well as proteins C and S, by interfering with vitamin K metabolism. Prolongs the prothrombin time and monitoring is achieved by comparing this with a control—as the international normalized ratio (INR).
- It is recommended that the INR be between 2 and 3 for most indications. However, in mechanical heart valves, or for the recurrence of thrombosis or pulmonary emboli, an INR of 2.5–3.5 is required (see also p. 1088).
- Reversal of a high INR can be achieved in several ways depending on the circumstances. In the absence of bleeding, omitting a dose is usually sufficient. If there is minor bleeding or a grossly raised INR give a small intravenous dose of vitamin K (2–5 mg). Life-threatening bleeding requires slow intravenous vitamin K (10 mg) and either coagulation factor concentrate or FFP. The last two cases must be discussed with a haematologist.
- It should be remembered that warfarin pharmacokinetics and dynamics can be affected by a multitude of other drugs and the reader is referred to the references and the BNF for a fuller discussion. The important anaesthetic interactions include:
  - Potentiation (by inhibition of metabolism): Alcohol, amiodarone, cimetidine, ciprofloxacillin, cotrimoxazole, erythromycin, indometacin, metronidazole, omeprazole, paracetamol.
  - Inhibition (by induction of metabolism): barbiturates, carbamazepine.
  - In addition drugs that affect platelet function can increase the risk of warfarin-associated bleeding, e.g. aspirin and NSAIDs.

Heparin
- A parenterally active anticoagulant that acts by potentiating antithrombin; can be used for both prophylaxis and treatment of thromboembolism.
- Unfractionated heparin is given by IV bolus or infusion, and SC for prophylaxis. It is monitored by the prolongation of the APTT.
- It has a narrow therapeutic window with complex pharmacokinetics and great interpatient variation in dose requirements.
- Protamine sulphate can counteract heparin (1 mg IV neutralizes 100 units of heparin). It should be given slowly to avoid hypotension to a maximum of 50 mg—a higher dose is itself anticoagulant.
- LMWH has recently been introduced. It is replacing unfractionated heparin for both prophylaxis and treatment of thromboembolism. Administered once daily by subcutaneous injection it needs no monitoring.

Anticoagulation in the perioperative period

Patients on warfarin are at increased risk of perioperative thromboembolism if the drug is stopped and are at increased risk of bleeding if the drug is continued. Therefore a balance must be achieved between these two conflicting approaches. The risks of each will vary depending on the underlying reason for anticoagulation, the risks of bleeding postoperatively, the period of immobility, and the use of other prophylaxis such as compression stockings and foot pumps. There are no randomized controlled trials to compare different regimes so the following is a suggested regime based on current evidence.

The following points should be considered:

- Some minor surgery including skin, dental, and ocular surgery can be performed without stopping warfarin.
- It takes 4 days from stopping warfarin for the INR to reduce below 1.5 (the level thought to be safe for surgery).
- After warfarin therapy is restarted it takes about 3 days for the INR to reach 2.0.
- Although there is good evidence that surgery increases the risk of venous thromboembolism there is no evidence for increased risk of arterial embolism with atrial fibrillation or mechanical heart valves.
- Additional methods of prevention of venous thromboembolism include graduated compression stockings and intermittent pneumatic compression devices.
- For recommendations for regional anaesthesia (spinal and epidural anaesthesia) during anticoagulation see p. 998.

Recommendations for preoperative and postoperative anticoagulation after stopping warfarin

- Warfarin should be stopped 4 days prior to surgery to allow the INR to decrease below 1.5. This is if the INR is normally between 2 and 3. It may take longer if the INR is higher.
- The INR should be checked the day prior to surgery and once the INR is <2 alternative pre- and postoperative prophylaxis should be considered, and continued postoperatively until the INR is >2, according to the following table:

Indication	Preoperative	Postoperative
Acute venous thromboembolism		
Month 1	IV heparin	IV heparin
Months 2 and 3	Nothing extra	IV heparin
>Month 3	Nothing extra	SC heparin
Recurrent venous thromboembolism	Nothing extra	Nothing extra
Acute arterial thromboembolism		
Month 1	IV heparin	IV heparin*
Mechanical heart valves	Nothing extra	SC heparin
Non-valvular atrial fibrillation	Nothing extra	SC heparin

*Only if the risks of bleeding are low.

- In patients at high risk for thromboembolism a continuous IV infusion of unfractionated heparin should be started at 1000 units/h and adjusted to keep the APTT between 1.5 and 2.5. This should be stopped 6 h prior to surgery and restarted 12 h afterwards. This should be continued until warfarin therapy is restarted and the INR >2.0.
- For many patients in whom the risk of postoperative thromboembolism is not high enough to warrant IV heparin (and its increased risk of bleeding) the use of SC LMWH is recommended. Again this should be continued until warfarin is restarted and the INR >2.0.
- In emergency surgery there is too little time to withdraw warfarin and specialist haematological advice should be sought. Fresh frozen plasma (10–15 ml/kg) and vitamin K 1–2 mg IV slowly can be given, but this may lead to difficulty in regaining anticoagulant control postoperatively.

Aspirin

- Long-term, low-dose aspirin is a mainstay of secondary prevention in patients with thromboembolic disease.
- If aspirin is to be stopped it takes 7–9 days for platelet function to return to normal.
- There are few published trials looking at perioperative bleeding.
- In coronary artery bypass grafting aspirin increases perioperative bleeding but increases graft patency.
- In transurethral prostatectomy aspirin considerably increases perioperative bleeding.
- Minor surgery to skin or cataract surgery does not require aspirin to be stopped.

In conclusion, aspirin should be stopped for at least 7 days prior to surgery, when the risks of perioperative bleeding are high (major surgery) or where the risks of even minor bleeding are significant (retinal and intracranial surgery). This risk of bleeding again must be balanced against the possibility of precipitating a thromboembolic event, particularly in patients with unstable angina.

Thrombocytopenia

Thrombocytopenia may be due to:

- Failure of platelet production, either selectively (hereditary, drugs, alcohol, viral infection) or as part of general marrow failure (aplasia, cytotoxics, radiotherapy, infiltration, fibrosis, myelodysplasia, megaloblastic anaemia).
- Increased platelet consumption, with an immune basis (ITP, drugs, viral infections, systemic lupus erythematosus, lymphoproliferative disorders) or without an immune basis (DIC, TTP, cardiopulmonary bypass).
- Dilution, following massive transfusion of stored blood to bleeding patients.
- Splenic pooling (hypersplenism).

Note that platelet function can be impaired by renal failure and aspirin.

Laboratory features

Unexpected thrombocytopenia should always be confirmed with another sample and a blood film.

- The blood film will exclude pseudothrombocytopenia due to platelet clumping (caused by EDTA anticoagulant with a prevalence of 0.1%) and may provide diagnostic clues such as leukaemic cells, leucoerythroblastic picture, giant platelets (e.g. May–Hegglin anomaly), large platelets (e.g. ITP), small platelets (e.g. Wiskott–Aldrich syndrome), red cell fragmentation (DIC, TTP).
- Abnormal coagulation associated with thrombocytopenia suggests the possibility of DIC or liver disease or rarely von Willebrand's disease type IIB.
- The bone marrow will distinguish marrow failure from other causes of thrombocytopenia.
- Platelet antibody tests have not been shown to be important for routine diagnosis and management, but may be useful in special circumstances, e.g. anti-HPA-1A in neonatal alloimmune thrombocytopenia.

Clinical features

Spontaneous bleeding is rare above a platelet count of 50×10^9/litre. Minor bleeding (purpura, epistaxis) may occur below this level. Serious spontaneous haemorrhage (GI bleeding, haematuria, cerebral haemorrhage) is unlikely above a count of 10×10^9/litre unless there is concurrent coagulopathy or infection. For a given degree of thrombocytopenia the risk of bleeding is lower in ITP than in marrow failure, probably because young platelets in ITP are larger.

Preoperative preparation

- Unexplained thrombocytopenia should be investigated before elective surgery, as the appropriate precautions will be determined by the underlying cause.
- Minor procedures such as bone marrow biopsy may be performed without platelet support provided adequate pressure is applied to the wound.
- For procedures such as insertion of central lines, transbronchial biopsy, liver biopsy or laparotomy, the platelet count should be raised to at least 50×10^9/litre.

- For lumbar puncture, epidural anaesthesia, and operations in critical sites such as the brain or eyes, the platelet count should be raised to 100×10^9/litre.
- In ITP, platelet transfusions should be reserved for major haemorrhage. Preparation for surgery entails the use of steroids or high-dose immunoglobulins initially.

Platelet transfusions

A standard adult therapeutic dose of 6 units contains $>240 \times 10^9$/litre of platelets and will on average raise the platelet count by $(20–40) \times 10^9$/litre in an adult, providing there are no complicating risk factors such as sepsis or splenomegaly.

Platelets must be given either through a fresh blood-giving set or through a special platelet-giving set (usually sent with them).

Perioperative and postoperative management

- Efforts directed at minimizing trauma and achieving surgical haemostasis pay dividends.
- Monitor platelet count and give platelets as necessary to maintain a safe level until wound healing is well advanced.
- If microvascular bleeding continues despite a platelet count of $>50 \times 10^9$/litre suspect DIC. If confirmed by coagulation tests give FFP and cryoprecipitate as appropriate.
- Intramuscular injections and analgesics containing aspirin or NSAIDs should be avoided.
- Remember that with renal failure and aspirin abnormal platelet function may cause bleeding with normal platelet counts. DDAVP 40 μg in 50 ml 0.9% saline over 30 min may improve platelet function in renal failure.

Sickle cell disease

The term sickle cell disease (SCD) refers to the group of clinically significant haemoglobinopathies which have in common the inheritance of sickle haemoglobin, either in the homozygous state (HbSS, sickle cell anaemia) or in combination with another haemoglobin β chain abnormality such as haemoglobin C (HbSC disease), haemoglobin D (HbSD disease) or β-thalassaemia (HbS/β-thal). It is estimated that there are now over 10 000 patients with SCD in Britain. SCD is endemic in parts of Africa, the Mediterranean, the Middle East, and India. The highest incidence is from equatorial Africa, therefore all black patients should have a sickle test preoperatively.

Susceptibility to sickling is proportional to the concentration of HbS. In the heterozygous state (sickle cell trait) sickling is uncommon as the HbS concentration is <50%. HbC and HbD in association with HbS enhance the sickling process while HbF impedes it. Hypoxia, hypothermia, pyrexia, acidosis, and dehydration (often associated with infection) are known to precipitate sickle crises. The pathology of SCD is primarily a result of vaso-occlusion by sickled red cells leading to haemolysis and tissue infarction.

Clinical features

- The manifestations of SCD do not become apparent before 3–4 months of age when the main switch from foetal to adult haemoglobin occurs.

- There is great variability, not only between patients, but also within individual patients at different periods of life. Many remain well most of the time.

- Vaso-occlusive crises are the most common cause of morbidity and mortality. The presentation may be dramatic with acute abdomen, 'acute chest syndrome', stroke, priapism, and painful dactylitis. By the time patients reach adulthood most will have small, fibrotic spleens. A less acute complication is proliferative retinopathy due to retinal vessel occlusion and neovascularization (more common in HbSC disease).

- Aplastic crises are characterized by temporary shutdown of the marrow manifested by a precipitous fall in the Hb and an absence of reticulocytes. Infection with parvovirus B19 and/or folate deficiency are often responsible.

- Sequestration crises occur mainly in children. Sudden massive pooling of red cells in the spleen can cause hypotension and severe exacerbation of anaemia with fatal consequences unless transfusion is given in time.

- Haemolytic crises, manifest by a fall in Hb and rise in reticulocytes and bilirubin, usually accompany vaso-occlusive crises. Chronic haemolysis leads to gallstones in virtually all patients with SCD though many remain asymptomatic.

Laboratory features

- The Hb is usually 6–9 g/dl, much lower than symptoms suggest. Reticulocytes are almost always increased and the film shows sickled cells and target cells. Howell–Jolly bodies are present if the spleen is atrophic. Leucocytosis and thrombocytosis are common reactive features. In sickle cell trait the Hb and film are normal.

- Screening tests for sickling which rely on deoxygenation of HbS are positive in both HbSS and HbAS.
- Hb electrophoresis distinguishes SS, AS, and other haemoglobinopathies. Quantitation of the HbS level is important in certain clinical situations (e.g. crises) where a level of <30% is aimed for. It is not necessary to wait for the results of electrophoresis before embarking on emergency surgery; a positive sickle test and the blood picture usually allow distinction between SCD and sickle cell trait. A mixed race patient always has sickle cell trait.

Management

- As no effective routine treatment exists for SCD, care is directed toward prophylaxis, support, and treatment of complications. Folic acid supplements, pneumococcal/HIB vaccinations and penicillin prophylaxis are recommended from an early age, preferably within a comprehensive care programme.
- For crises—rest, rehydration with oral/IV fluids, antibiotics if infection is suspected, maintain PaO_2, keep warm, prompt and effective analgesia.
- Blood transfusions may be life saving, but the indications are limited. Exchange transfusions have a limited role in some vaso-occlusive crises (acute chest syndrome, stroke). Always discuss with a haematologist. Recent studies comparing preoperative exchange transfusions to achieve an HbS level of <30% with a conservative regime of a preoperative Hb between 9 and 11 g/dl have found no increase in complications.

Preoperative preparation

Always seek expert advice from a haematologist well before surgery. A sample for group and antibody screening should be sent well in advance as previously transfused sickle cell patients often have red cell antibodies.

Perioperative and postoperative care

Special attention must be given to the potential problems of hypoxia; dehydration, infection, acidosis, hypothermia, and pain associated with anaesthesia and surgery in both SCD and sickle cell trait patients. These considerations must be continued well into the postoperative period.

- Dehydration must be avoided by allowing oral fluids as late as possible and giving pre- and postoperative IV fluids.
- Hypoxia can be avoided by measuring pulse oximetry and giving prophylactic oxygen.
- Prophylactic antibiotic cover should be considered.
- Positive pressure ventilation may be required to achieve normocarbia and avoid acidosis.
- Hypothermia should be avoided by warming the operating room, using a fluid warmer, and the use of a Bair Hugger®. Core temperature should be monitored.
- Regional anaesthesia is not contraindicated and tourniquets can be used if limbs are meticulously exsanguinated prior to inflation.

Haemoglobin SC disease

- Results from double heterozygosity for HbS and HbC.
- Affects 0.1% of American blacks.
- Intermediate in severity between sickle cell disease and trait.
- Patients develop anaemia, splenomegaly, jaundice, aseptic necrosis of the femoral head, hepatic disease, retinal disease, and bone marrow and splenic infarcts.
- Myocardial necrosis has been described after general anaesthesia.
- Management principles are as for sickle cell disease.

Rare blood disorders

Hereditary spherocytosis

- An autosomal dominant condition in which erythrocytes have a smaller surface to volume ratio and are abnormally permeable to sodium.
- The inflexible red cells are phagocytized in the spleen resulting in a microspherocytic anaemia with marked reticulocytosis. The cells' increased osmotic fragility is diagnostic.
- Splenomegaly is common. Splenectomy leads to a 50–70% increase in red cell survival.
- Splenectomy should not be performed in children under 10 years of age, and should be followed by pneumococcal, meningococcal, and HIB vaccine and lifelong oral penicillin, to help avoid infection.
- There are no particular anaesthetic considerations.

Glucose-6-phosphate dehydrogenase (G6PD) deficiency

- X-linked trait with variable penetrance in American blacks and people from the Mediterranean.
- The disease may afford some protection against malaria and is prevalent in endemic areas.
- The G6PD enzyme is responsible for the production of NADPH, which is involved in the cell's defence against oxidative stresses such as infections (usually viral, but also septicaemia, malaria, and pneumonia) or oxidative drugs (aspirin, quinolones, chloramphenicol, isoniazid, probenacid, primaquine, quinine, sulphonamides, naphthalene, and vitamin K).
- Additionally, drugs producing methaemoglobinaemia, such as nitroprusside and prilocaine, are contraindicated, as patients are unable to reduce methaemoglobin, thereby diminishing oxygen-carrying capacity.
- Classically, ingestion of broad (fava) beans results in haemolysis (favism).
- Usually the haemolysis of red cells occurs 2 to 5 days after exposure, causing anaemia, haemoglobinaemia, abdominal pain, haemoglobinuria, and jaundice.
- Diagnosis is made by demonstration of Heinz bodies and red cell G6PD assay.
- Treatment includes discontinuation of the offending agent and transfusion may be required.

Thalassaemias

Thalassaemias are due to absent or deficient synthesis of α- or β-globin chains of haemoglobin. The severity of these disorders is related to the degree of impaired globin synthesis.

- The hallmark of the disease is anaemia of variable degree.
- Diagnosis is confirmed by haemoglobin electrophoresis and/or globin chain analysis.
- The disease is prevalent in peoples of Mediterranean (mainly β), African (α and β) and Asian (mainly α) extraction.
- Patients with α-thalassaemia have mild or moderate anaemia.

- Those with severe β-thalassaemia, also called thalassaemia major, are transfusion dependent.
- Since there is no iron excreting mechanism, iron from transfused blood builds up in the reticuloendothelial system, until it is saturated, when iron is deposited in parenchymal tissues, principally the liver, pancreas, and heart.
- Preoperative preparation should include assessment of the degree of major organ impairment (heart, liver, pancreas) secondary to iron overload.
- High-output congestive cardiac failure with intravascular volume overload is common in severe anaemia and should be treated preoperatively by transfusion.
- Previous transfusion exposure may cause antibody production and therefore cross-matching may be prolonged.
- The exceedingly hyperplastic bone marrow of the major thalassaemias may cause overgrowth and deformity of the facial bones leading to airway problems and making intubation difficult.

Hypercoagulability syndromes

Polycythaemia

Refers to a pattern of red blood cell changes that usually results in a haemoglobin >17.5 g/dl in males and >15.5 g/dl in females (this is accompanied by a corresponding increase in the red cell count 6.0 and 5.5×10^{12}/litre and a haematocrit of 55% and 47% respectively).

Causes of polycythaemia	
Primary	Polycythaemia vera
Secondary	Due to compensatory erythropoietin increase: high altitude, cardiovascular diseases, especially congenital cyanotic respiratory disease and alveolar hypoventilation, heavy smoking, methaemoglobinaemia
	Due to inappropriate erythropoietin increase: renal diseases (hydronephrosis, cysts, carcinoma), massive uterine fibromyomata, hepatocellular carcinoma, cerebellar haemangioblastoma
Relative	'Stress' or 'spurious' polycythaemia. Dehydration or vomiting. Plasma loss: burns, enteropathy

Polycythaemia vera

- Presenting features include headaches, dyspnoea, chest pain, vertigo, pruritis, epigastric pain, hypertension, gout, and thrombotic episodes (particularly retinal).
- The spleen is often enlarged.
- The platelet count is raised in 50% of cases.
- Differential diagnosis is with other causes of polycythaemia. These can be excluded by history, examination and blood tests including bone marrow aspiration, arterial blood gases, and erythropoietin levels.
- Therapy is aimed at maintaining a normal blood count by venesection and myelosuppression with drugs.
- Thrombosis and haemorrhage are a frequent cause of death and 30% develop myelofibrosis and 15% acute leukaemia.

Essential thrombocythaemia

- Megakaryocyte proliferation and overproduction of platelets are the dominant features with a sustained platelet count above 1000×10^9/litre.
- Closely related to polycythaemia vera with recurrent haemorrhage and thrombosis.
- Recurrent haemorrhage and thrombosis are the principal clinical features.
- Abnormal large platelets or megakaryocyte fragments may be seen on a blood film.
- Differential diagnosis is from other causes of a raised platelet count.
- Platelet function tests are consistently abnormal.
- Radioactive phosphate or alkylating agents are used to keep platelet counts down.

Causes of a raised platelet count	
Reactive	Haemorrhage, trauma, postoperative
	Chronic infection
	Malignancy
	Chronic iron deficiency
	Connective tissue diseases, e.g. rheumatoid arthritis
	Postsplenectomy with continuing haemolytic anaemia
Endogenous	Essential thrombocythaemia
	Polycythaemia vera, myelosclerosis, or chronic granulocytic leukaemia

Antiphospholipid syndrome

This is a rare, but increasingly recognized syndrome, when arterial or venous thrombosis or recurrent miscarriage occurs with positive laboratory tests for antiphospholipid antibody and/or lupus anticoagulant (LA). This syndrome may present with another autoimmune disease such as systemic lupus erythematosus (secondary) or as a primary disease. The main feature of the disease is thrombosis, with a spectrum from subacute migraine and visual disturbances to accelerated cardiac failure and major stroke. Arterial thrombosis helps distinguish this from other hypercoagulable states.

Diagnosis

Paradoxically the LA leads to a prolongation of coagulation tests such as the APTT but detailed testing is needed before the diagnosis can be confirmed.

Perioperative considerations

Patients may present for surgery because of their complications (miscarriage, thrombosis) or for incidental procedures. Initially patients are started on aspirin but after a confirmed episode of thrombosis, they usually remain on lifelong warfarin. The high risk of thrombosis in these patients means that if warfarin needs to be stopped for surgery, intravenous heparin should be commenced both pre- and postoperatively.

Anaesthesia and surgery in the hypercoagulable patient

- There are no published guidelines, but it seems prudent that elective patients who are polycythaemic should be venesected to a normal blood count to decrease the risk of perioperative thrombosis.
- Antithrombotic stockings and intermittent compression devices should be used with SC heparin.
- Haematological advice may be required.

Porphyria

See p. 95.

Further reading

Davies SC, Roberts-Harewood M (1997). Blood transfusion in sickle cell disease. *Blood Review*, **11**, 57–71.

Guidelines for the clinical use of red cell transfusions (2001). *British Journal of Haematology*, **113**, 24–31.

Guidelines on oral anticoagulation: third edition. (1998). *British Journal of Haematology*, **101**, 374–87.

Guidelines on therapeutic products to treat haemophilia and other hereditary coagulation disorders. (1997). *Haemophilia*, **3**, 63–77.

Kearon C, Hirsch J (1997). Management of anticoagulation before and after elective surgery. *New England Journal of Medicine*, **336**, 1506–11.

Mallett SV et al. (2000). Reducing red blood cell transfusion in elective surgical patients: the role of audit and practice guidelines. *Anaesthesia*, **55**, 1012–24.

McClelland DBL (ed.) (1996). *Handbook of transfusion medicine, 2nd edn.* HMSO Publications, London.

Spahn DR, Cassutt M (2000). Eliminating blood transfusions. *Anesthesiology*, **93**. 242–55.

Vichinsky EP et al. (1995). A comparison of conservative and aggressive transfusion regimens in the perioperative management of sickle cell disease. *New England Journal of Medicine*, **333**, 206–13.

White RH, McKittrick T, Hutchinson R, Twitchell J (1995). Temporary discontinuation of warfarin therapy: changes in the international normalized ratio. *Annals of Internal Medicine*, **122**, 40–2.

Jehovah's Witnesses

The Jehovah's Witness religious movement is 120 years old. There are an estimated 6 million Jehovah's Witnesses worldwide.

Most Jehovah's Witnesses will not accept a transfusion of blood nor its derivatives. This includes fresh frozen plasma (FFP), packed cells, white blood cells, and platelets. This policy was introduced in 1945, and since 1961 members who accept prohibited blood components have been expelled. However, in June 2000 a directive was issued stating that the organization would no longer expel individuals who did not comply with the policy of refusal of blood.

Absolute rules regarding specific blood products do not exist. Individual Witnesses may accept the use of certain blood components (e.g. albumin, immunoglobulins, haemophiliac preparations) on a personal basis.

Cardiac bypass may be accepted provided that the extracorporeal circuit is primed with crystalloid and the patient's blood is not stored as a part of the procedure. Perioperative cell salvage is acceptable to many Jehovah's Witnesses provided the equipment is arranged in a closed circuit that is constantly linked to the circulation and there is no storage of the patient's blood. Some Jehovah's Witnesses permit removal of blood in the anaesthetic room with reinfusion when surgical blood loss has ended (acute normovolaemic haemodilution), provided the blood remains in contact with the patient's circulation.

Administration of blood or blood products to a competent patient who has refused blood transfusion against their wishes is unlawful and may lead to criminal and/or civil proceedings for assault against the doctor.

In emergency situations when the doctor has not been able to ascertain the status of the patient with regard to blood transfusion the doctor has an obligation to act in the best interests of the patient. This may include the administration of blood or blood products. The doctor must make a detailed entry in the case notes as to what has been said and get the next-of-kin to countersign the entry. It is preferable that the consultant makes these decisions. If time permits, opinions of relatives or associates that the patient would not accept a blood transfusion must be verified if possible. Evidence of an advance directive should be sought. Contact with the patient's GP may be worthwhile as some Witnesses may leave a copy of their advance directive with him or her.

The care of children of Jehovah's Witnesses (aged less than 16 years) may present particular difficulty. If the parents refuse permission for blood transfusion it may be necessary to apply for a legal 'Specific Issue Order' via the High Court (in Scotland the Sheriff's Court) in order to administer a blood transfusion without parental consent. In England and Wales there is a judge who is always on call in London. The Senior Manager on call for the hospital should know how to contact him. A statement will be prepared for the judge and faxed to the court. It needs to be proven that the child's need for treatment is so overwhelming for his/her welfare that the parents' wishes must be overridden.

In an emergency situation, when there is not time to proceed via the court, blood should be transfused. Courts are likely to uphold this medical decision.

Anaesthetists have the right to refuse to anaesthetize Jehovah's Witnesses for elective surgery. However, the anaesthetist is obliged to provide care in emergency cases, and must respect the patient's wishes.

Clinical management

- Early communication with the anaesthetic department is essential. Apart from minor surgery a consultant anaesthetist should be available who is prepared to manage the patient.
- Meet the patient as early as possible preoperatively with the results of relevant investigations to ascertain the degree of limitation of normal routine management.
- There is a specific consent form that Jehovah's Witnesses must sign.
- At the preoperative visit establish which treatments are acceptable. Many Jehovah's Witnesses have signed an 'advance directive' which stipulates which treatments they will accept. Make the patient aware of the risks of non-acceptance of blood and blood products.
- Specifically discuss and document:
  - whether acute normovolaemic haemodilution is acceptable
  - if perioperative cell salvage may be used.
- Involve the local Hospital Liaison Committee in the discussions. Representatives can help avoid confrontation and assist the understanding of both parties. The address of the local committee may be obtained by contacting Hospital Information Services (Britain): Tel.: 0208 906 2211; Fax: 0208 343 0201; E mail: his@wbts.org.uk
- Preoperative anaemia should be investigated and treated. Oral iron supplements can be used to improve iron stores (ferrous sulphate 200 mg twice daily). The use of recombinant erythropoietin β has been described (initial dose 20 units/kg SC three times per week). Remember that the clinical response takes up to a month. Discussion of an individual case with a haematologist may be useful.
- Major operations can sometimes be staged to limit acute blood loss.
- Choice of anaesthetic and operative technique should be chosen to minimize blood loss (e.g. regional anaesthesia and the use of tourniquets).

Intra-operative management

- Minimize bleeding by careful patient positioning to avoid venous congestion, tourniquets where appropriate, meticulous haemostasis, and the use of controlled hypotensive anaesthesia where appropriate.
- Consider the use of invasive monitoring, even when the medical condition of the patient or the nature of the operation would not usually warrant it— in patients who are very anaemic it is very important to maintain cardiac output to maximize oxygen delivery.
- Consider the use of systems for intra-operative cell salvage if the operative field is not contaminated by bacteria or malignant cells. Use of cell salvage in life-threatening obstetric haemorrhage is controversial because of the concern of precipitating disseminated intravascular coagulation. Its use has been advocated in life-threatening obstetric haemorrhage in Jehovah's Witnesses.
- Drugs such as tranexamic acid (1 g three or four times a day) and aprotinin have been used to reduce fibrinolysis and increase coagulability. Desmopressin (0.3–0.4 μg/kg) has been recommended to boost factor VIII levels.

Postoperative care

* Have a low threshold for admission to HDU/ICU.

* Treat postoperative oozing aggressively. Remember simple measures such as direct compression. Early re-exploration is mandatory.

* Following massive blood loss patients should be electively ventilated to reduce oxygen demand. Augment oxygen delivery with inotropes if indicated. Consider intravenous iron sucrose (Venofer® 100–200 mg IV) three times per week, folinic acid (15 mg/day), recombinant erythropoetin β (20 units/kg SC three times per week) and parenteral nutrition.

* Surface cooling has been advocated to reduce oxygen consumption and increase oxygen delivery as the amount of dissolved oxygen in the plasma increases with decreasing temperature. However, hypothermia impairs haemostasis, which may be disadvantageous.

* Hyperbaric oxygen therapy has been described. Referral may be considered if an appropriate facility is available. However, few hyperbaric chambers can take a ventilated intensive care patient.

Further reading

Baker CE, Kelly GD, Perkins GD (1998). Perioperative care of a Jehovah's Witness with a leaking abdominal aortic aneurysm. *British Journal of Anaesthesia*, **81**, 256–9.

Catling SJ, Williams A, Fielding AM (1999). Cell salvage in obstetrics: an evaluation of the ability of cell salvage combined with in line leucocyte depletion to remove amniotic fluid from operative blood loss at caesarian section. *International Journal of Obstetric Anaesthesia*, **8**, 79–84.

Muramoto O (2001). Bioethical aspects of the recent changes in the policy of refusal of blood by Jehovah's Witnesses. *British Medical Journal*, **322**, 37–9.

The Association of Anaesthetists of Great Britain and Ireland (1999). *Management of anaesthesia for Jehovah's Witnesses.*

Chapter 8
Bone, joint, and connective tissue disorders

Paul Marshall

Rheumatoid arthritis

Rheumatoid arthritis (RA) is a multisystem disorder mainly involving joints. It affects up to 3% of females and 1% of males. Patients are frequently frail, in chronic pain, and taking medication with adverse effects. Disease-modifying antirheumatic drugs may have immunosuppressant effects. Airway problems are common.

Preoperative assessment

Articular

- Temperomandibular. Assess mouth opening as it may be limited.
- Cricoarytenoid. Fixation of the cricoarytenoid joints may lead to voice changes, hoarseness, or even rarely to stridor from glottic stenosis. Minimal oedema may lead to airway obstruction postoperatively.
- Atlantoaxial subluxation (AAS) occurs in approximately 25% of severe rheumatoids, but of these only a quarter will have neurological signs or symptoms. Enquire about tingling hands or feet, neck pain, and assess the range of neck movement. Excessive movement during anaesthesia can lead to cervical cord compression.
  - Anterior AAS. Comprises 80% of all AAS. C1 forward on C2 from destruction of transverse ligament. Significant if there is a gap of >3 mm between the odontoid and the arch of the atlas in lateral flexion radiographs. Atlantoaxial flexion is potentially hazardous.
  - Posterior AAS. This is rare. C1 backward on C2 resulting from destruction of the odontoid peg. Can be seen on lateral extension radiographs. Atlantoaxial extension (e.g. from direct laryngoscopy) is potentially hazardous.
  - Vertical AAS. Arises from destruction of lateral masses of C1. The odontoid moves upwards through foramen magnum to compress cervicomedullary junction.
  - Lateral AAS. Uncommon. Arises from involvement of the C1/C2 facet joints. More than 2 mm difference in lateral alignment is significant. Requires a frontal open mouth odontoid view to assess.
- Subaxial subluxation:
  - More than 2 mm loss of alignment is significant.
  - Look for this particularly if patient has undergone previous fusion at a higher level.
- Other joints. Assess joint deformities with a view to positioning and possible anaesthetic technique (if planning an axillary block can the patient abduct their arm?). Manual dexterity may be important if planning to use standard PCA apparatus after surgery. Special adaptations are available, e.g. trigger by blowing.

Non-articular

- Cardiovascular. Asymptomatic pericardial effusion is relatively common. Myocardial and valvular involvement are rare.
- Respiratory. Pulmonary fibrosis (methotrexate may contribute). Pleural involvement is usually asymptomatic. Pulmonary nodules can occur.

* Anaemia—usually normochromic anaemia of chronic disease, drug-associated bone marrow depression, and NSAID-associated blood loss.
* Renal. Amyloid or interstitial nephritis may occur. Asymptomatic renal impairment is common. Drug effects may contribute.
* Nervous system. Peripheral neuropathy. This may be aggravated by pressure effects when positioned on the operating table. Neurological symptoms and signs may arise from cord or root compression in the neck.
* The skin and veins are fragile.

Investigations

* All patients should have FBC, creatinine and electrolytes, ECG, and chest radiograph.
* Cervical spine radiographs. The role of preoperative cervical spine flexion/extension views is controversial and interpretation is difficult. The automatic reordering of radiographs in all patients seems unnecessary, particularly if it will not alter management. Flexion/extension views are mandatory in all patients with neurological symptoms or signs, and in those with persistent neck pain. Stabilization surgery may be necessary before other elective surgery is undertaken. Preoperative cervical spine radiographs may help determine management in some patients with severe disease requiring intubation but only after review of previous radiographs, case notes, and anaesthetic charts. Specialist radiological advice may be required. Unless it is certain that the cervical spine is stable, therefore, all rheumatoid patients should be treated as if they might have an unstable spine. This may involve awake fibreoptic intubation or manual in-line stabilization when undertaking direct laryngoscopy or LMA insertion.
* Pulmonary function tests should be carried out for patients with unexplained dyspnoea or radiological abnormalities.
* An ENT opinion should be sought and nasendoscopy performed if there is hoarseness or symptoms and signs of respiratory obstruction.
* Echocardiography is needed if there is valvular or pericardial involvement and in symptomatic cardiac disease.

Drugs in the perioperative period

* Consider steroid supplementation (p. 98).
* NSAIDs. Aspirin has irreversible effects on platelet function and should be stopped 10 days prior to surgery. Other NSAIDs should usually be continued to enable early mobilization, but should be stopped if there is excessive bleeding, shock, or deterioration in renal function.
* Disease-modifying antirheumatoid drugs (DMARDs). These drugs include gold, penicillamine, and immunusuppressant drugs such as methotrexate and azathioprine. Leflunomide is a recently introduced DMARD with an improved safety profile. The potential for these drugs to contribute to increased infection and reduction in wound healing has to be balanced against the likelihood of flare-ups of the disease and delayed mobilization if the drugs are with-drawn before surgery. In practice these drugs are commonly only omitted for a day or two following surgery as there is little evidence that omitting them preoperatively reduces postoperative complications and in particular wound infections. However, if there is leucope-

nia (e.g. with azathioprine) withdrawal of the drugs for 2–3 weeks before surgery may be advisable (consult with rheumatologist).

• DVT prophylaxis (see p. 11). Early mobilization.

• Gastrointestinal agents. Patients on H_2 antagonists, e.g. ranitidine and prostaglandin analogues, should continue prior to and after surgery.

Anaesthesia

• Take care of the neck and maintain it in a neutral position at all times when the patient is anaesthetized, especially on transfer and turning. Use manual in-line stabilization during airway manipulation whilst the patient is unconscious (unless it is certain that the spine is stable). If intubation is necessary consider fibreoptic intubation (p. 882), particularly if there is posterior AAS (rare) and/or predicted difficulty (p. 866). If direct laryngoscopy is undertaken together with manual in-line stabilization use a gum elastic bougie initially. If this is difficult have a low threshold for converting to awake fibreoptic intubation early on.

• Ensure careful positioning and padding/protection of vulnerable areas on the operating table. Note the position before induction, then try to maintain this during surgery.

• Regional techniques may be difficult. Patient discomfort from prolonged immobilization may favour general anaesthesia perhaps in combination with regional catheter techniques.

• Normothermia is especially important, as hypothermia may increase the risk of wound infections.

Postoperative

• Adequate pain control allows early mobilization. PCA is often impractical due to impaired hand function.

• Continue NSAIDs unless contraindicated.

• Physiotherapy and mobilization are important.

• Continue DVT prophylaxis until the patient is fully mobile.

• Maintain fluid intake and monitor renal function.

• Restart DMARDs to avoid exacerbation of joint immobility.

Further reading

Campbell RSD, Wou P, Watt I (1995). A continuing role for pre-operative cervical spine radiography in rheumatoid arthritis? *Clinical Radiology*, **50**, 157–9.

Macarthur A, Kleiman S (1993). Rheumatoid cervical joint disease—a challenge to the anaesthetist. *Canadian Journal of Anaesthesia*, **40**, 154–9.

Matti MV, Sharrock NE (1998). Anesthesia in the rheumatoid patient. *Rheumatic Diseases Clinics of North America*, **24**, 19–34.

Ankylosing spondylitis

Inflammatory arthritis of the sacroiliac joints and spine, leading to ankylosis and 'bamboo spine'. It is associated with HLA B27 in more than 90% of cases. The male to female ratio is about 4:1. Important anaesthetic implications are both articular and non-articular.

Articular

- Progressive kyphosis and fixation of the spine may preclude an intubating position. Severe cases will be impossible to intubate using conventional means and tracheostomy may also be impossible. Atlantoaxial subluxation and myelopathy can occur rarely. There may be limited mouth opening from temperomandibular involvement. Consider awake fibreoptic intubation.

- Axial skeletal involvement may make centroneuraxis block difficult or impossible. Spinal anaesthesia using a paramedian approach appears to be the most practical technique for neuraxial block. There may be an increased risk of epidural haematoma in patients with ankylosing spondylitis possibly as a result of associated trauma in attempts to place a catheter.

- Limited chest expansion may lead to postoperative pulmonary complications. Effective external cardiac massage may be impossible.

- Deformity leads to difficulty with positioning, particularly if a prone position required.

Non-articular

- Fibrosing alveolitis may occur, exacerbating postoperative hypoxia.

- Aortic regurgitation is present in 4% of cases. Mitral valve involvement and conduction defects are rare.

- Amyloid may cause renal involvement.

Further reading

Schelew BL, Vaghadia H (1996). Ankylosing spondylitis and neuraxial anaesthesia—a 10 year review. *Canadian Journal of Anaesthesia*, **43**, 65–8.

Sinclair JR, Mason RA (1984). Ankylosing spondylitis. The case for awake intubation. *Anaesthesia*, **39**, 3–11.

Systemic lupus erythematosus

This is a chronic multisystem disease commonest in young females, especially in pregnancy. It is characterized by the presence of numerous antibodies including antinuclear antibody and immune mediated tissue damage. Although joints may be affected there is no deformity or bony erosion and no specific airway implications. The main anaesthetic implications are cardiovascular disease, renal disease, and coagulation status.

Preoperative assessment

- Skin and joint involvement are common.
- Cardiovascular problems are relatively common and include myocarditis (15%), pericarditis (60%), and non-bacterial endocarditis affecting the mitral and aortic valves.
- Raynaud's phenomenon is common.
- Respiratory system: patchy atelectasis, pleurisy, and fibrosing alveolitis may occur.
- Neurological: cranial and peripheral nerve lesions may occur, secondary to arteritis and ischaemia. Depression, psychosis, and fits.
- Renal involvement occurs in 60% of patients usually in the form of nephrotic syndrome. Progressive renal failure and hypertension may also occur.
- Haematological: clotting disorders or hypercoagulable states can occur. Patients with systemic lupus erythematosus should have both full blood count and clotting status checked. Immune thrombocytopenia or circulating anticoagulants (e.g. antibodies to factor VIII) may be present. Up to a third of patients with systemic lupus erythematosus may demonstrate features of antiphospholipid syndrome. This is a hypercoagulable state which paradoxically may be associated with the presence of lupus anticoagulant and a prolonged APTT. Since a prolonged APTT may indicate either a clotting disorder or a hypercoagulable state further haematological advice should be sought. The anaemia of chronic disease is common and may be aggravated by blood loss (see p. 152).
- Oral and pharyngeal ulceration are common.
- Drugs; steroids and other immunosuppressant drugs are used.

Anaesthesia

- There may be absolute or relative contraindications to neuraxial blocks in patients taking anticoagulants or in patients with coagulopathy associated with systemic lupus erythematosus. Cases should be considered individually. Contraindications include platelets <100 000 × 10⁹/litre or INR >1.5 (see p. 998). The presence of a peripheral nerve lesion may be a relative contraindication to neuraxial block.
- Maintenance of normothermia may reduce the risk of infection as well as lessening the impact of Raynaud's phenomenon if present.
- If there is cardiac or renal involvement consider hourly urine output and invasive monitoring.
- Steroid supplementation (p. 98).

Further reading

Davies SR (1991). Systemic lupus erythematosus and the obstetrical patient—implications for the anaesthetist. *Canadian Journal of Anaesthesia*, **38**, 790–5.

Madan R, Khoursheed M, Kukla R, al-Mazidi M, Behbehani A (1997). The anaesthetist and the antiphospholipid syndrome. *Anaesthesia*, **52**, 72–6.

Scoliosis

Progressive lateral curvature of the spine with added rotation. Scoliosis may be idiopathic (about 75%) or secondary to other conditions with anaesthetic implications, for example

- Muscular dystrophies
- Poliomyelitis
- Cerebral Palsy
- Friedrich's Ataxia

Preoperative Assessment

Scoliosis may be progressive and lead to an increasing restrictive ventilatory defect which in turn leads to hypoxia, hypercarbia and pulmonary hypertension. Corrective surgery may be carried out in the teens to arrest these changes, or the surgery may be non spinal.

- Formal respiratory function tests including vital capacity and oxygen saturation on air are mandatory in severe cases (>65 degree curvature).
- Look for evidence of pulmonary hypertension and right heart failure. Some muscular dystrophies may be associated with primary cardiac abnormalities. Consider echocardiography.
- Avoid sedative premedication in patients with poor respiratory reserve.
- Plan for high dependency or intensive care in complex cases.

Anaesthesia

- Regional catheter techniques where possible (usually in combination with general anaesthesia) may reduce postoperative opioid requirements.
- Monitor neuromuscular function.
- Patients with muscular dystrophies may be susceptible to MH (see p. 199). Avoid suxamethonium and known triggers.

Further reading

Gibbons PA, Lee IS (1985). Scoliosis and anesthesia. *International Anesthesiology Clinics*, 23, 149–61.

Achondroplasia

The commonest form of dwarfism is caused by premature ossification of bones combined with normal periosteal bone formation giving a characteristic appearance of short limbs and a relatively normal cranium. The following should be noted:

• The larynx may be small and intubation is occasionally difficult. Have a range of tube sizes and a difficult intubation trolley available.

• Foramen magnum stenosis is common. Avoid hyperextension during intubation.

• Central and peripheral venous access is often difficult. Consider femoral vein cannulation.

• Use an appropriately sized blood pressure cuff.

• Obstructive sleep apnoea is common.

• Restrictive ventilatory defects may occur and can lead to pulmonary hypertension.

• Regional techniques may be difficult.

• The back may be normal. The epidural space is often narrowed.

• The volume of local anaesthetic needed for an epidural is reduced. It is difficult to predict the volume needed for a one-shot spinal. Use an incremental spinal or epidural catheter technique.

• The patient is of normal intelligence. Take care to treat on age rather than size.

Further reading

Berkowitz ID, Raja SN, Bender KS, Kopits SE (1990). Dwarfs: pathophysiology and anesthetic implications. *Anesthesiology*, 73, 739–59.

Morrow MJ, Black IH (1998). Epidural anaesthesia for Caesarian section in an achondroplastic dwarf. *British Journal of Anaesthesia*, 81, 619–21.

Chapter 9
Neuromuscular disorders

Andrew Teasdale

Epilepsy

Surgery and anaesthesia in epilepsy

The aim is avoidance of perioperative seizure by avoiding interference with drug therapy (maintaining GI function) and avoiding metabolic disturbance (maintaining hydration, glucose, and electrolyte balance). Prolonged starvation should be avoided and the anaesthetic technique should seek to minimize surgical stress and gastrointestinal dysfunction.

Preoperative assessment

- The nature, timing, and frequency of any seizure should be recorded preoperatively. The effect of the condition on lifestyle and on ability to hold a driving licence should be recorded.
- A full drug history should be taken. The effect of dose timing and a missed dose should be recorded.
- If prolonged postoperative GI dysfunction is anticipated, formulate a plan for nasogastric or parenteral anticonvulsant therapy.
- A plan for postoperative analgesia should be formulated with the patient.

Conduct of anaesthesia

- Avoid prolonged preoperative starvation.
- Sedative premedication, if necessary, may be achieved with benzodiazepines. Long-acting drugs such as diazepam (10 mg PO) or lorazepam (2–4 mg PO) are useful.
- Maintain antiepileptic therapy up to the point of surgery.
- All commonly used anaesthetic agents are anticonvulsant in conventional dosage (see table)—whilst all have been used in epileptics without ill effect, it is prudent to use actively anticonvulsant drugs to avoid the adverse physiological and social consequences of a fit in a previously well controlled patient.
- Thiopental is powerfully anticonvulsant in the therapeutic range.
- Muscle relaxation is best achieved by drugs without a steroid nucleus (e.g. atracurium, cisatracurium) since enzyme induction by all commonly used antiepileptic agents (especially phenytoin, barbiturates, and carbamazepine) may lead to reduced activity and shorter action of agents such as pancuronium and vecuronium.
- Avoidance of hyperventilation (and consequent hypocarbia) is essential since hypocarbia reduces cerebral blood flow and worsens pre-existing abnormal EEG activity.
- Regional anaesthesia is useful since earlier return to oral intake is possible. Maximum local anaesthetic doses should be kept in mind.
- Antiemetic medication should be with agents unlikely to cause dystonia (e.g. domperidone 30–60 mg PR, cyclizine 50 mg IV/IM, ondansetron 4 mg IV).
- Any epileptiform activity in the recovery period should be described and recorded. The misdiagnosis of postoperative shivering or confusion as epilepsy may have profound implications for the patient since driving privileges may be withdrawn.

Drug issues

The following anaesthetic and allied drugs should be used with caution in epileptics:

Drug	Notes
Methohexitone	Reported to produce seizures in children. Increased EEG evidence of spike activity during administration. No longer marketed in the UK
Ketamine	Avoided because of cerebral excitatory effects although has been used without incident in many epileptics
Etomidate	Associated with a high incidence of myoclonus (not centrally mediated). May be confused with epileptic activity
Antiemetics: phenothiazines (e.g. prochlorperazine), central dopamine antagonists (e.g. metoclopramide), butyrophenones (e.g. droperidol)	High incidence of dystonic reactions may lead to confusion with epileptic activity
Inhalational agents: enflurane	Associated with abnormal EEG activity after administration—especially in presence of hyperventilation
Neuromuscular blockers: steroid based (e.g. vecuronium, pancuronium)	Pharmacodynamic resistance due to enzyme activation

Propofol

Propofol is reported to be associated with abnormal movements both during induction and emergence from anaesthesia. Although in most cases this is unlikely to represent true seizure activity (EEG studies fail to demonstrate epileptiform activity during these episodes), it is also likely that patients with controlled epilepsy or previously undetected seizure foci may be prone to seizure during the rapid emergence from propofol anaesthesia. Propofol is widely used for sedation during 'awake' craniotomy for epilepsy surgery. Profound suppression of abnormal EEG activity is usually noted during its infusion. It has also been reported to be useful in status epilepticus in ITU.

Caution is advised in the administration of propofol to epileptics (particularly those holding driving licences) unless there is overwhelming clinical need for its administration. Co-induction with benzodiazepine (e.g. midazolam 2 mg IV) may reduce its potential to produce abnormal movements and reduce the potential for postoperative seizure.

Day case anaesthesia

All epileptics should be warned of the possibility of perioperative convulsions no matter how minor the procedure to be undertaken. Local and regional techniques should be used where possible. In general, those with well-controlled epilepsy (seizure free for over 1 year or nocturnal fits only) can be considered for day case anaesthesia.

Driving and epilepsy

At present, United Kingdom law mandates the withdrawal of a driving licence from an epileptic until 12 months from the last seizure. The implications of a single fit in the postoperative period on a previously well-controlled epileptic cannot be overstated. Up-to-date advice on fitness to drive is available from the DVLA (Driver and Vehicle Licensing Agency: www.dvla.gov.uk).

What if oral or nasogastric therapy is not possible?

The following drugs are available in parenteral or rectal formulations. In general, intramuscular administration of antiepileptic medication should be avoided because of unpredictable absorption postoperatively and the irritant nature of the formulations.

Drug levels should be measured during parenteral therapy or after changing the route of administration.

Drug	Notes
Carbamazepine	125 mg rectal, equivalent to 100 mg oral. Maximum 1 g daily in four divided doses
Phenobarbital	200 mg IM repeated 6-hourly. Child 15 mg/kg. Intravenous administration associated with sedation. Slow infusion of dilute preparation recommended
Phenytoin	Loading dose 15 mg/kg IV at rate of no greater than 50 mg/min. Maintenance dose (same intravenous as oral) twice daily. Infusion usually under ECG and BP control
Sodium valproate	Intravenous dose same as oral dose, twice daily. Dose to be injected intravenously over 3–5 min
Fosphenytoin	A prodrug of phenytoin. Less irritation and cardiovascular instability on injection. Absorbed very slowly after IM injection although non-irritant. Dose—same dose and frequency as oral phenytoin
Clonazepam	Intravenous infusion in high-dependency area only— facilities for airway control available. Child (any age) 500 μg. Adult 1 mg

Cerebrovascular disease

Cerebrovascular disease is manifest by either global cerebral dysfunction (multi-infarct dementia) or focal ischaemic disorder ranging from transient ischaemic attack to major stroke. Stroke is the third leading cause of death in the industrialized world (after heart disease and cancer).

Cerebrovascular disease is associated with hypertension, diabetes, obesity, and smoking. The incidence rises with age. Medical treatment revolves around the treatment of the underlying disorder, cessation of smoking, and antiplatelet/anticoagulant therapy. The use of low-dose aspirin prophylaxis is gaining wide acceptance and popularity.

Assessment of the patient with cerebrovascular disease

* Measure blood pressure (both arms) and test blood glucose. The therapeutic aims are for normotension and normoglycemia.
* Take a full drug history.
* Antihypertensive drugs can as a rule continue to the time of operation.
* Warfarin should be discontinued and substituted with heparin if necessary.
* Aspirin is only discontinued if the consequences of haemorrhage are great (e.g. tonsillectomy, neurosurgery, etc.).
* Document the nature of any ischaemic events and any residual neurological deficit. These may range from transient blindness (amaurosis fugax) to dense hemiplegia. This will help in differentiating new lesions from pre-existing deficits that may require urgent therapy.
* Ask about precipitating events. Vertebrobasilar insufficiency is most likely to be precipitated by postural changes and neck positioning. Avoidance of precipitating neck positions is mandatory.

Transient ischaemic attacks (TIA)

* These are defined as focal neurological deficits that occur suddenly and last for several minutes to hours but never more than 24 h. Residual neurological deficit does not occur.
* They are thought to be related to embolism of platelet and fibrin aggregates released from areas of atherosclerotic plaque. The risk of stroke in untreated patients is said to be around 5% per annum with a mortality of around 30% per episode.
* Patients with a history of TIA should be investigated and assessed by a specialist vascular service if practical. Doppler flow studies, with or without angiography, are indicated in all cases.
* Delay of all but emergency surgery is warranted until Doppler studies are performed. If surgery has to be undertaken, the principles of anaesthesia should be followed as outlined below.

Who needs carotid endarterectomy?

* At present only those with history of TIA with good recovery and a surgically accessible lesion of either greater than 80% stenosis or 'ragged' plaque are routinely considered for surgery. Crescendo TIA is considered by some as an indication for urgent surgery.

- Consensus opinion at present is against surgery in those with asymptomatic carotid bruit.

Cerebrovascular event (CVE or stroke)

- This may be caused by:
  - cerebral thrombosis
  - cerebral embolism
  - intracranial haemorrhage.
- The underlying cause is usually related to cerebrovascular disease secondary to advanced age, smoking, diabetes, and hypertension.
- 10% of stroke in the industrialized world is due to intracranial haemorrhage.
- Haemorrhage may occur into a tumour or vascular malformation.
- Embolization may originate from the heart or extracranial vessels.
- All may lead to deficits ranging from minor limb weakness to complete hemiplegia and death.
- Therapeutic goals and anaesthetic management are shared with those of TIA.

When to operate

- Operation within 6 weeks of a cerebral event is associated with an up to 20-fold increase in risk of postoperative stroke.
- Hemiplegia of less than 6–9 months' duration is associated with exaggerated hyperkalaemic response to suxamethonium.
- It therefore seems prudent to delay all but life-saving surgery for at least 6 weeks following a cerebral event and preferably to wait at least 6 months before considering elective surgery.

Anaesthetic management of patients with cerebrovascular disease

- Ensure that antihypertensive medication (with the possible exception of ACE inhibitors) is continued to the time of operation.
- ACE inhibiters are associated with non-specific kininase inhibition and may predispose to profound, resistant hypotention under anaesthesia.
- Thromboprophylaxis is advisable unless contraindicated (e.g. low-dose unfractionated heparin).
- Ensure that pressor and depressor agents are available prior to induction to treat unwanted changes in blood pressure. Use agents with which you are familiar. Maintain blood pressure as close as practical to preoperative levels to maintain cerebral blood flow:
  - useful pressors are ephedrine/metaraminol
  - useful depressors are labetalol, esmolol, GTN.
- Blood pressure may 'swing' excessively during surgery. This is due to a relatively rigid vascular system and relative hypovolaemia due to antihypertensive therapy. Intravenous fluid replacement should be proactive rather than reactive, with large-bore IV access and invasive central pressure monitoring if large fluid shifts are expected.
- Ensure that neck positioning is neutral and avoids movements associated with syncope (gained from the history).

- Induction of anaesthesia may result in dangerous hypotension followed by extreme hypertension on intubation. Gentle intravenous induction is indicated. Cover for intubation may be provided by:
  - opioid (e.g. alfentanil 500–1000 μg IV)
  - beta-blocker (e.g. labetalol 50 mg slow IV)
  - lidocaine (lignocaine) 1–1.5 mg/kg IV.
- Avoid hyperventilation. Hypocapnia is associated with reduced cerebral blood flow and therefore cerebral ischaemia. Normocarbia should be the goal of intra-operative ventilation.
- Examine the patient early in the postoperative period to determine any change in neurological status. New neurological signs will require urgent referral to a neurologist/vascular surgeon and urgent treatment if possible.

Parkinson's disease

Parkinsonism is a syndrome characterized by: tremor, akinesia, rigidity, and postural instability. The aetiology of Parkinson's disease is unknown, but Parkinsonism may be precipitated by drugs (especially neuroleptic agents), or be post-traumatic/postencephalitic.

Pathophysiology

Parkinsonism is due to an imbalance of the mutually antagonistic dopaminergic and cholinergic systems of the basal ganglia. Pigmented cells in the substantia nigra are lost, leading to reduced dopaminergic activity. There is no reduction in cholinergic activity. Drug therapy of Parkinsonism is aimed at restoring this balance by either increasing dopamine or dopamine-like activity or reducing cholinergic activity within the brain.

Medical treatment

Drug therapy in Parkinsonism is limited by severe side-effects (nausea and confusion), especially in the elderly. Up to 20% of patients will remain unresponsive to drug therapy.

Dopaminergic drugs

- l-dopa is an inactive form of dopamine, which needs conversion by decarboxylases to dopamine within the brain to be effective. It is the therapy of first choice in idiopathic Parkinsonism. It is more useful in patients with bradykinesia and rigidity than tremor, and is usually administered with decarboxylase inhibitors (e.g. benserazide, carbidopa) that do not cross into the brain, reducing peripheral conversion of dopamine and thus reducing dose and side-effects.

- Monoamine oxidase B inhibitors (MAO-B inhibitors; e.g. selegiline) act by reducing central breakdown of dopamine. Selegiline has fewer drug interactions than the non-specific MAO inhibitors, but may cause a hypertensive response to pethidine and dangerous CNS excitability with SSRI and tricyclic antidepressants (see p. 207).

- Ergot derivatives such as bromocriptine, cabergoline, lisuride, and pergolide act by direct stimulation of dopamine receptors. They are usually reserved for adjuvant therapy in those already on l-dopa or those intolerant of the side-effects of l-dopa.

- Entacapone is an adjuvant agent capable of reducing the dose of l-dopa and increasing the duration of its effect. It is usually reserved for those experiencing 'end of dose' deterioration after long-term dopaminergic therapy.

- Other adjuvant dopaminergic agents are ropinirole, pramipexole, amantadine, apomorphine, and tolcapone.

- There are no parenteral dopaminergic agents currently available for use in Parkinsonism.

Anticholinergic (antimuscarinic) drugs

- The most commonly used agents in this group are benztropine, procyclidine, benzhexol, and orphenadrine. These agents are indicated as first-line therapy only when symptoms are mild and tremor predominates. Rigidity and sialorrhoea may be improved by these agents but bradykinesia will not be affected. This class of drugs is useful for drug-induced Parkinsonism but not in tardive dyskinesia.

- Parenteral formulations exist for procyclidine and benztropine, making these useful for acute drug induced dystonias.

Surgical therapy

Surgery for treatment of Parkinson's induced disability is increasing in popularity. It is normally performed in the awake patient using stereotactic guided probes:

- Thalamotomy is used in those with tremor as the predominant disability, especially if the tremor is unilateral. Anterior thalamotomy is sometimes used for rigidity.
- Pallidotomy is primarily for those with rigidity and bradykinesia, although the tremor (if present) may also be reduced.

Drug issues

Most patients with severe disease are on several maintenance drugs and drug interactions are a potential hazard (see p. 178).

Anaesthetic considerations

Ideally, patients with severe disease should be under the care of a physician with a special interest in Parkinson's disease and the perioperative care should involve them.

The following assessment is of particular interest:

- A history of dysphagia or excessive salivation (sialorrhoea) is evidence of increased risk of aspiration and possible failure to maintain an airway in the perioperative period. Gastro-oesophageal reflux is common in this group of patients.
- Postural hypotension may be evidence of both dysautonomia and drug-induced hypovolaemia and should warn of possible hypotension on induction of anaesthesia or position changes during surgery.
- Drug-induced arrhythmias, especially ventricular premature beats, are common although they are usually not clinically significant.
- Respiratory function may be compromised by bradykinesia and muscle rigidity as well as by sputum retention. Chest radiograph, lung function tests, and blood gases may be indicated.
- Difficulty in voiding may necessitate urinary catheterization. Postoperative urinary retention may be a potent cause of postoperative confusion.
- The severity of the underlying disease should be determined and other likely problems anticipated, e.g. akinesia, muscle rigidity, tremor, confusion, depression, hallucinations, and speech impairment.

Conduct of anaesthesia

- Treatment for Parkinsonism should be continued up to the start of anaesthesia. Distressing symptoms may develop as little as 3 h after a missed dose.
- Premedication is usually unnecessary unless distressing sialorrhoea is present. Antisialogogue treatments include atropine (10 μg/kg IM up to 1 mg) or glycopyrrolate (200–400 μg IM).

Drug interactions in Parkinsonism

Class of drug	Interaction	Notes
Analgesics:		
pethidine	Hypertension and muscle rigidity with selegiline	May resemble malignant hyperpyrexia
synthetic opiates, e.g. fentanyl, alfentanil	Muscle rigidity	More apparent in high doses
Inhalational agents	Potentiates l-dopa induced arrhythmias	Avoid use of halothane if ventricular arrhythmia present on preop. ECG
Antiemetics: e.g. metoclopramide, droperidol, prochlorperazine	May produce extrapyramidal side-effects or worsen Parkinson symptoms	For management of PONV see p. 179. Metoclopramide may increase plasma concentration of l-dopa
Antipsychotics: e.g. phenothiazines, butyrophenones, piperazine derivatives	May produce extrapyramidal side-effects or worsen Parkinson symptoms	Better to use 'atypical antipsychotics' such as sulpiride, clozapine, risperidone, etc.
Antidepressants: tricyclics (e.g. amitriptylene)	Potentiate l-dopa induced arrhythmias (tricyclics only)	
serotonin reuptake inhibitors (e.g. fluoxetine)	Hypertensive crises and cerebral excitation with selegiline (tricyclics and SSRIs)	
Antihypertensives (all classes)	Marked antihypertensive effect in treated and untreated Parkinsonism. Related to postural hypotension and relative hypovolaemia	Most marked with clonidine and reserpine

- The presence of preoperative sialorrhoea or dysphagia is a sign of gastrointestinal dysfunction. Airway control with intubation by rapid sequence induction may be indicated.
- Maintain normothermia to avoid shivering.
- There is no evidence that any anaesthetic technique is superior to any other.
- Analgesia: intravenous morphine is useful if regional or local analgesia is not possible (PCA may prove difficult for the patient). Oral analgesia may be difficult to administer with coexisting dysphagia (a nasogastric tube may be necessary).

Postoperative considerations

- In principle, the more disabled the patient preoperatively, the greater the need for postoperative high-dependency and respiratory care.
- Postoperative physiotherapy should be arranged if rigidity is disabling.
- Nasogastric tube insertion may be needed if GI dysfunction is present to allow early return of oral medication.
- Prolonged GI dysfunction postoperatively may lead to severe disability since no parenteral dopaminergic therapy is currently available.

Antiemetics

- Domperidone (10–20 mg 4–6-hourly PO or 30–60 mg 4–6-hourly PR). The drug of first choice for PONV in Parkinson patients. It does not cross the blood–brain barrier to a significant degree and is thus not associated with significant extrapyramidal effects.
- Serotonin antagonists ondansetron 4 mg IV or granisetron 1 mg IV slowly, may be useful rescue agents in PONV if domperidone alone is ineffective.
- Antihistamine derivatives (e.g. cyclizine 50 mg IV/IM).

Further reading

Anesthesia and Parkinson's disease (1996). *International Anesthesiology Clinics*, **34**, 133–50.

Severn AM, Parkinsonism and the anaesthetist (1988). *British Journal of Anaesthesia*, **61**, 761–70.

Anaesthesia in spinal cord lesions

There are approximately 40 000 patients in the United Kingdom with spinal cord injuries. Most are young adults who may present for a variety of surgical interventions. Fertility in affected females approaches that of the non-injured population and obstetric services are regularly required.

Pathophysiology of spinal cord injury

Spinal shock can be divided into three distinct phases:

* The initial phase: very short (minutes) period of intense neuronal discharge caused by direct cord stimulation. This leads to extreme hypertension and arrhythmias, with risk of left ventricular failure, myocardial infarction, and pulmonary oedema. Early treatment with steroids during this phase may improve neurological outcome (refer to section on trauma management).

* Spinal shock: follows rapidly from the initial phase and is characterized by hypotension and bradycardia due to loss of sympathetic tone as well as probable myocardial dysfunction. It is most common after high cord lesions (above T7). There is associated loss of muscle tone and reflexes below the level of the lesion. Vagal parasympathetic tone continues un-opposed, leading to a tendency to profound bradycardia and even asystole with tracheal suctioning or intubation. This phase may last from 3 days to 8 weeks. Paralytic ileus is common during this phase.

* Reflex phase: as neuronal 'rewiring' occurs distal to the cord lesion, efferent sympathetic discharge returns, along with muscle tone and reflexes.

Autonomic dysreflexia

This is characterized by a massive, disordered autonomic response to stimulation below the level of the cord lesion. It is rare in lesions lower than T7. The incidence increases with higher lesions and is most common in those with cervical lesions. It may occur within 3 weeks of the original injury but is unlikely to be a problem after 9 months. The dysreflexia and its effects are thought to arise because of a loss of descending inhibitory control on regenerating presynaptic fibres and interneurons, leading to chaotic reflex action and massive release of catecholamines, especially noradrenaline.

Hypertension is the most common feature of this reflex disorder but is by no means universal. Features include headache, flushing, pallor (may be manifest above the level of lesion), nausea, anxiety, hypertension, sweating, bradycardia, and penile erection. Less commonly pupillary changes or Horner's syndrome occur. Dysreflexia may be complicated by seizures, pulmonary oedema, coma, or death and should be treated as a medical emergency. The stimulus required to precipitate the condition varies but is most commonly:

* urological—bladder distension, urinary tract infection, catheter insertion, etc.
* obstetric—labour, cervical dilation, etc.
* bowel obstruction/faecal impaction
* acute abdomen
* fractures
* rarely minor trauma to skin, cutaneous infection (bedsores).

Management

- Discover the cause if possible and treat.
- If no apparent cause, examine carefully for unrevealed trauma or infection, catheterize and check for faecal impaction.

If simple measures fail to control hypertension then treatment options include:

- Nifedipine 10–20 mg SL
- Phentolamine 2–10 mg IV repeated if necessary
- Transdermal GTN
- Clonidine (150–300 μg by slow IV infusion) is useful if there is associated hypertension and spasticity.
- Beta-blockers are indicated only if there is associated tachycardia (bradycardia is more common—see above). A useful drug is esmolol (10 mg IV repeated until symptoms are controlled) but beware of reflex bradycardia.

Systemic complications of spinal cord lesions

- Reduced blood volume (up to 60 ml/kg, a reduction of approximately 20%).
- Abnormal response to the Valsalva manoeuvre with continued drop in blood pressure (no plateau) and no overshoot with release of pressure.
- Profound postural hypotension with gradual improvement after initial injury (never to normal). Changes in cerebral autoregulation reduce its effect on CBF and consciousness in the non-anaesthetized patient.
- Lesions above C3—apnoea.
- Lesions at C3/4/5—possible diaphragmatic sparing, some respiratory capacity. Initial lesions may progress in height with shock and oedema, with recovery as the oedema improves, leading to a marked improvement in respiratory capacity.
- Below C5—phrenic sparing, intercostal paralysis. Recruitment of accessory muscles is necessary to improve respiratory capacity (this may take up to 6 months).
- Paralysis of abdominal muscles severely affects the ability to force expiration, reducing the ability to cough.
- The FVC is better in the horizontal or slight head-down position due to increased diaphragmatic excursion. Abdominal contents push the diaphragm higher in this position leading to improved muscle contraction (Starling's law).
- Bronchial hypersecretion may occur immediately after high lesions with resolution after several weeks.
- Poor thermoregulation due to isolation of central regulatory centres from information pathways, inability to use muscle to generate heat and altered peripheral blood flow. This may lead most commonly to hypothermia but occasionally to hyperthermia in hot climatic conditions.
- Muscle spasms and spasticity occur due to intact reflexes below the level of the lesion. They are caused by even minor stimuli such as light touch. They may be violent enough to injure the patient and may be severe enough to interfere with surgery and physiotherapy. Baclofen and diazepam may be necessary, the former increasingly via epidural infusion.

- Reduced bone density leading to increased risk of fractures. There is heterotopic calcification around the joints in up to 20% of patients.
- Poor peripheral perfusion leading to pressure sores and difficult venous access.
- Anaemia, usually mild unless associated with chronic illness such as decubitus ulcers.
- There is a tendency to thrombosis and therefore pulmonary embolism. Some centres warfarinize tetraplegics 5 days after initial presentation.
- There is delayed gastric emptying in tetraplegics—up to five times longer.

Suxamethonium in chronic spinal cord lesions

- After upper motor neuron denervation, the motor endplate effectively extends to cover the entire muscle cell membrane. With administration of suxamethonium, depolarization occurs over this extended endplate, leading to massive potassium efflux and potential cardiac arrest.
- Recommendations vary as to the period of potential risk of this phenomenon. It would be prudent to avoid use of suxamethonium from 72 h following the initial injury. There are no reports of clinically significant hyperkalaemia with suxamethonium after 9 months.
- If rapid sequence induction with suxamethonium is considered essential during the high-risk phase then potassium flux may be reduced by precurarization (e.g. 5–10 mg atracurium) and methods of treating hyperkalaemia should be available (calcium, bicarbonate, insulin/dextrose).

Conduct of anaesthesia

Spinal shock phase

Surgery during this phase is usually confined to the management of life-threatening emergencies and coexisting injury. Anaesthesia should reflect this.

- Severe bradycardia or even asystole may complicate intubation. Atropine (300 μg IV) or glycopyrrolate (200 μg IV) prior to intubation should prevent this.
- Extreme care should be taken if cervical spine injury is suspected.
- Preloading with fluid (500–1000 ml crystalloid) will reduce hypotension on induction.
- Central line insertion may be necessary to manage fluid balance and guide appropriate inotrope therapy.

Reflex phase

Previous anaesthetic history is vital—many procedures in these patients are multiple and repeated. Pay close attention to the following:

- Is there a sensory level and is it complete? (Risk of autonomic dysreflexia)
- If complete, is the proposed surgery below the sensory level? (Is anaesthesia necessary?)
- Has there been spinal instrumentation? (Potential problems with spinal/epidural)
- Is the cervical spine stable/fused/instrumented? (Potential intubation difficulty)
- Is postural hypotension present? (Likely to be worsened by anaesthesia)

- Is there a history of autonomic dysreflexia (paroxysmal sweating and/or headache) and if so, what precipitated it?
- In cervical lesions, what degree of respiratory support is necessary?
- Are there contractures, pressure sores? (Care with positioning and pressure areas)

Investigations

- FBC—potential anaemia.
- Urea and electrolytes—potential renal impairment.
- Liver functions—possible impairment with chronic sepsis.
- Lung function tests (FVC)—mandatory with all cervical lesions due to potential respiratory failure.

Is anaesthesia necessary?

In principle, if the planned procedure would require anaesthesia in a normal patient, it will be required for a cord-injured patient.

- Minor peripheral surgery below a complete sensory level is likely to be safe without anaesthesia.
- Even with minor peripheral surgery, minimal stimulation may provoke muscular spasm that may require anaesthesia to resolve. Local anaesthetic infiltration may prevent its occurrence.
- Care should be taken in those with high lesions (T5 and above) undergoing urological procedures or with a history of autonomic dysreflexia.
- If the decision is made to proceed without anaesthesia, intravenous access is mandatory and ECG, NIBP, and pulse oximeter should be applied.
- An anaesthetist should be present on 'standby' for such procedures.

General anaesthesia

- Monitoring should be applied prior to induction and blood pressure measured before and after every position change. Invasive monitoring should be performed with the same considerations as for the non-cord injured patient.
- Despite theoretical risk of gastro-oesophageal reflux there appears to be no increased risk of aspiration. If intubation is necessary for the desired procedure, anticholinergic pretreatment is recommended.
- Those with cervical cord lesions are likely to require assistance with ventilation under general anaesthesia. If IPPV is performed in tetraplegics, blood pressure may drop precipitously. Fluid preloading and vasopressors (ephedrine) may be required.
- With the exception of paralysis to facilitate intubation, neuromuscular blockade is unlikely to be necessary if the surgery is below sensory level unless troublesome muscular spasm is present.
- Care should be taken to preserve body temperature (wrapping or forced air warming blankets). Position with respect to pressure areas.
- Fluid management may be difficult as blood volume is usually low, and with high cord lesions, reflex compensation for blood loss is absent. Fluid preloading coupled with aggressive replacement of blood losses with warmed fluid is recommended.

Regional anaesthesia

Advantages

- Prevents autonomic dysreflexia.
- Unlikely to cause cardiovascular instability since sympathetic tone is already low prior to blockade.
- No reported effect of spinal injection of local anaesthetics or opioids on neurological outcome.
- Avoids risks of general anaesthesia.
- In general, spinal anaesthesia is performed more commonly than epidural anaesthesia as it is technically easier and more reliable in prevention of autonomic dysreflexia. Use standard doses of local anaesthetic agents (bupivacaine 'heavy' or plain). Intrathecal opiates appear to confer no advantage.

Disadvantages

- May be technically difficult to perform. Spinal anaesthesia is usually possible but epidural techniques are likely to fail in the presence of spinal instrumentation or previous spinal surgery due to obliteration of the epidural space.
- There is difficulty in determining the success or level of blockade in complete lesions. Incomplete lesions are tested in the same way as for normal patients and it is theoretically possible to test the level by testing abolition of spasms provoked by ethyl chloride spray or by observation of relaxation of spasticity.

Postoperative care

- Tetraplegics are best nursed supine or only slightly head up due to improved ventilatory function in this position.
- Temperature should be closely monitored and hypothermia actively treated.
- Analgesia should be provided by conventional means according to the type and level of surgery.
- Dysreflexia may occur and require drug treatment after removal of precipitating causes (such as pain and urinary retention)—for treatment, refer to the section above.

Obstetric anaesthesia

Effect of pregnancy on spinal cord injury

- Exaggerated postural hypotension and worsened response to caval occlusion.
- Reduced respiratory reserve with increased risk of respiratory failure and pneumonia. Increased oxygen demand.
- Worsening of pre-existing anaemia due to haemodilution.
- Labour is a potent cause of autonomic dysreflexia in those with lesions above T5 (dysreflexia may be the first sign of labour in such patients).

Effect of spinal injury on pregnancy

- Increased risk of infection (urinary and pressure sores).
- Increased risk of premature labour (increasing risk with higher level injury).
- Increased risk of thromboembolic complications.
- Labour pains will not be felt in complete lesions above T5.
- Lesions between T5 and T10 will be aware of some contractions.

Management of labour

- All cord-injured patients should be reviewed early in pregnancy and a plan formulated for the likely need for analgesia. The relative risks and difficulties of epidural catheter insertion should be predicted and discussed with the patient. A plan for anaesthesia in the event of Caesarean section should also be formulated and recorded in the patient notes.
- Epidural analgesia is usually possible in those with high cord lesions without vertebral instrumentation at the level of catheter insertion.
- Spinal anaesthesia is usually possible for elective Caesarean section and may be achievable with both single-shot or microcatheter techniques, irrespective of the presence of spinal instrumentation.
- General anaesthesia may proceed with the precautions outlined above.

Epidural analgesia in labour

- The most effective preventive measure for autonomic dysreflexia is adequate epidural analgesia. Those with high lesions may have an epidural commenced prior to induction of labour.
- Hypotension is not usually a problem after adequate fluid preloading (at least a litre of crystalloid or colloid). However, hypotension from any cause should be treated aggressively in those with high lesions due to the lack of compensatory mechanisms and a tendency to progressive hypotension.
- Aortocaval compression should be avoided by careful positioning for the same reasons.
- Autonomic dysreflexia has been reported up to 48 h after delivery. If successful block is achieved it would appear prudent to leave the epidural in situ for this time to restart analgesia if required.
- Failure to establish adequate epidural blockade may necessitate drug treatment of autonomic dysreflexia (see above).

Further reading

Hambly PR, Martin B (1998). Anaesthesia for chronic spinal cord lesions *Anaesthesia*, **53**, 273–89.

Myasthenia gravis

Myasthenia gravis is caused by autoimmune disruption of postsynaptic acetylcholine receptors at the neuromuscular junction. In symptomatic patients up to 80% of functional receptors are lost, leading to weakness and marked fatigability. The disease may occur at any age but is most common in young adult women. It may be associated with thymus hyperplasia with approximately 15% of affected patients having thymomas.

Clinically important manifestations of the disease range from mild ptosis to bulbar palsy and respiratory insufficiency. Patients are usually maintained on anticholinesterase medication (pyridostigmine) and occasionally steroids. Other treatments include immunosuppressants, thymectomy, and plasmapheresis in patients with resistant or life-threatening weakness.

All patients with myasthenia are exquisitely sensitive to the effects of non-depolarizing neuromuscular blocking agents:

- Non-depolarizing drugs should be used sparingly. Monitor the response with a nerve stimulator. Initial doses of around 10–20% of the normal dose are usually adequate.

- Newer short- and intermediate-acting non-depolarizing drugs such as atracurium, mivacurium, or vecuronium are preferable to the longer-acting drugs.

- Plasmapheresis depletes plasma esterase levels, thus prolonging the effect of drugs eliminated by these enzyme systems (suxamethonium, mivacurium, ester-linked local anaesthetics).

- Suxamethonium may have an altered effect and patients may be resistant to depolarization due to reduced receptor activity, requiring increased dose. This, in conjunction with treatment-induced plasma esterase deficiency, leads to an increased risk of non-depolarizing (Phase II) block.

Preoperative assessment

- Assess the degree of weakness and the duration of symptoms. Those with isolated ocular symptoms of long standing are unlikely to have progressive disease. Those with poorly controlled symptoms should have their condition optimized unless this is precluded by surgical urgency.

- Any degree of bulbar palsy is predictive of the need for both intra- and postoperative airway protection.

- Perform lung function tests—FVC <50% predicted (or <2.9 litres) or those who have coexisting respiratory disease are more likely to require postoperative ventilation.

- Take a full drug history and determine the effect that a missed dose of anticholinesterase has on the patient. Those with severe disease may undergo rapid deterioration following a single missed dose.

- Maintain anticholinesterase therapy up to the time of induction. Although theoretical inhibition of neuromuscular blockade is possible, this has never been reported.

- Premedication should be minimal.

- Facilities for postoperative ventilation should be available.

Rapid sequence induction

- Suxamethonium may be used if indicated—doses of 1.5 mg/kg are usually effective.
- If doubt exists as to the difficulty of intubation, awake techniques may be useful.
- If suxamethonium is used, do not use any neuromuscular blockade drug until muscle activity has returned and no fade is present.

Perioperative considerations

- All but short, minimally invasive procedures will require ventilation as the respiratory depressant effects of all drugs may be accentuated.
- Avoid any neuromuscular blockade if possible. Intubation and ventilation may be performed using non-paralysing techniques.
- If muscle relaxants are necessary use reduced doses (10% normal) under nerve stimulator control (placed and tested before blockade). Careful titration of dose to effect is necessary.
- Reversal of neuromuscular blocking drugs should be achievable with standard doses of neostigmine if preoperative symptom control has been good (see below). Avoidance of reversal is preferred since further doses of anticholinesterase may introduce the risk of overdose (cholinergic crisis). Drugs with spontaneous reversal such as atracurium are optimal.
- Consider inserting a nasogastric tube for postoperative anticholinesterase therapy if early return to oral intake is not predicted.
- Extubation should only be performed when full return of muscular activity and consciousness allows. The best predictive test for safe extubation is a sustained head lift of >5 s. Those with bulbar palsy need special care and may require airway protection until the return of bulbar function.

Postoperative considerations

- Postoperative ventilation is likely to be required following major body cavity surgery.
- Analgesia may be provided by any appropriate means. Regional techniques are especially useful.
- Rapid return of therapy is mandatory—via nasogastric tube if necessary.
- In the event of gastrointestinal failure and inability to provide oral or nasogastric anticholinesterase therapy, parenteral therapy is indicated (see p. 188).

Preoperative predictors of postoperative need for ventilation

- Duration of disease of greater than 6 years.
- A history of coexisting chronic respiratory disease.
- Dose requirements of pyridostigmine >750 mg/day less than 48 h prior to surgery.
- A preoperative vital capacity of less than 2.9 litres.

Signs of impending respiratory failure
Stridor (may be due to vocal cord adductor weakness)
Inability to cough (vocal cord weakness and reduced vital capacity)
Generalized muscle weakness (inability to sustain hand grip or head lift)
The best monitors of postoperative respiratory capacity are: repeated peak flow measurement (cheap, easy, and reliable if used as trend) and vital capacity measurement (requires special equipment and training). These are best done regularly (hourly initially) and interpreted according to trend
Blood gases and peripheral saturation may remain normal up to the point of respiratory failure and are thus not reliable monitors of postoperative respiratory capacity

Anticholinesterase therapy

An easy conversion for oral pyridostigmine to parenteral (IV, IM, or SC) neostigmine is to equate every 30 mg of oral pyridostigmine to 1 mg of parenteral neostigmine. If oral therapy is contraindicated for a prolonged period, conversion to a subcutaneous or intramuscular neostigmine regime is indicated. For doses see below.

Principles of perioperative cholinesterase management

- Maintain oral cholinesterase therapy up to the point of surgery.
- Reversal of neuromuscular blockade is possible with neostigmine if indicated by nerve stimulator—in general, no twitches on train of four means no reversal possible.
- Dosage of neostigmine should be used under nerve stimulator control, starting with a 2.5–5 mg bolus and increasing if necessary with a 1 mg bolus every 2–3 min to a maximum equivalent dose to the oral pyridostigmine dose (1:30). For example, if the pyridostigmine dose is 120 mg 3–4-hourly, then the maximum neostigmine dose should be 4 mg (to be repeated after 2–4 h if necessary).
- Resume oral anticholinesterase therapy as soon as practical.
- If oral therapy is not possible, commence parenteral neostigmine in the doses outlined above.

Thymectomy

Consensus now favours thymectomy in all adults with generalized myasthenia gravis. Remission rates are high and improvement of symptoms is almost universally attainable (96% gain benefit regardless of preoperative characteristics). The best results are achieved in those with normal or hyperplastic thymus, although those with thymoma (benign or locally invasive) also derive major benefit

The approach most used is trans-sternal, allowing best access to perform the required anterior mediastinal exenteration. Transcervical approaches provide less satisfactory access for surgery. Thoracoscopic thymectomy is gaining acceptance, although its reputed benefit of reduced complications and need for postoperative ventilation is yet to be proven.

Anaesthetic management follows the same general principles outlined in this chapter, although all patients need postoperative care in HDU or require

Specific drugs of interest in myasthenia gravis

Drug	Interaction	Notes
Non-depolarizing neuromuscular blocking agents	Marked sensitivity	Avoid use if possible. Start with 10% normal dosage. Always monitor neuromuscular function. Use short- and intermediate-acting agents only
Suxamethonium	Resistance to depolarization and delayed onset of action	No reported clinical ill effects of using 1.5 mg/kg. Delayed recovery in patients with induced esterase deficiency (plasmapheresis, anticholinesterase treatment). Follow with non-depolarizing agents only when full recovery of neuromuscular function is noted
Inhalational anaesthetic agents	All inhalational agents reduce neuromuscular transmission by up to 50% in myasthenia	May be useful by avoiding neuromuscular blocking agents
Intravenous anaesthetic agents	No discernible clinical effect on neuromuscular transmission	Total intravenous anaesthesia with propofol may be useful if neuromuscular function is precarious prior to surgery
Local anaesthetic agents	Prolonged action and increased toxicity in ester-linked agents with anticholinesterase therapy and plasmapheresis. Exacerbation of myasthenia reported	Use minimum dosage required for adequate block. Monitor respiratory function as with general anaesthesia
Drugs dependent on esterases for elimination	Prolonged effect and increased toxicity if patient on plasmapheresis or (theoretically) anticholinesterase therapy	Suxamethonium, remifentanil, mivacurium, ester-linked local anaesthetics, esmolol etc.
Antibiotics	Neuromuscular blocking effects may become clinically important	Avoid use of aminoglycosides (e.g. gentamicin). Similar effects reported with erythromycin and ciprofloxacin
Miscellaneous	All the following agents have a reported effect on neuromuscular transmission: procainamide, beta-blockers —especially propranolol, phenytoin	

Specific drugs of interest in myasthenia gravis (*continued*)

Drug	Dosage	Notes
Pyridostigmine	Adult: 30–120 mg at suitable interval (usually 4–6-hourly). Do not exceed total daily dose of 720 mg Child: <6 years initial dose 30 mg; 6–12 years initial dose 60 mg. Total daily dose 30–360 mg Neonate: 5–10 mg every 4 h, 30–60 min before feeds	Useful duration of action. No parenteral preparation available. Less powerful and slower onset than neostigmine
Neostigmine (by mouth)	Adult: 15–30 mg PO at suitable intervals (up to 2-hourly). Total daily dose 75–300 mg Child: <6 years initial dose 7.5 mg PO; 6–12 years initial dose 15 mg PO. Total daily dose 15–90 mg Neonate: 1–5mg PO 4hrly, 30 minutes before feeds	More marked GI effects than pyridostigmine. Useful if parenteral therapy indicated but more likely to require antimuscarinic (atropine or glycopyrrolate) cover if used by this route
Neostigmine (by subcutaneous or intramuscular injection)	Adult: 1–2.5 mg at suitable interval (usually 2–4-hourly) Total daily dose 5–20 mg Child: 200–500 µg as required Neonate: 50–250 µg 4-hourly 30 min before feeds	
Edrophonium	Adult: 2 mg by intravenous injection followed after 30 s by 8 mg if no adverse reaction Child: 20 µg/kg IV followed by 80 µg/kg after 30 s if no adverse reaction	Usage limited by ultra short duration of action and cost to diagnosis of myasthenia and differentiation of myasthenic and cholinergic crises
Distigmine	Adult: 5 mg daily half an hour before breakfast. Maximum 20 mg daily	Very long acting with risk of cholinergic crisis due to dosage accumulation. Not recommended in small children or neonates

ventilation for a short period in the early postoperative period. Fewer than 8% of sternotomies for thymectomy require ventilation for more than 3 h postoperatively. Almost all patients will require a degree of muscle relaxation if preoperative preparation has been optimal and postoperative analgesia can be achieved satisfactorily with epidural or PCA.

Eaton–Lambert syndrome

Eaton–Lambert syndrome (myasthenic syndrome) is a proximal muscle weakness associated with cancer (most often small cell carcinoma of the lung).

- The condition is thought to be due to a reduction in the release of acetylcholine (prejunctional failure).
- It is not reversed by anticholinesterase therapy and muscle weakness is improved by exercise.
- Associated dysautonomia may be manifest as dry mouth, impaired accommodation, urinary hesitance, and constipation.

Anaesthetic implications

Unlike myasthenia gravis, patients with myasthenic syndrome are sensitive to both depolarizing and non-depolarizing neuromuscular agents. Reduced doses should be used if the disease is suspected. Maintain a high index of suspicion in those undergoing procedures related to diagnosis and management of carcinoma of the lung.

Further reading

Baraka A (1992). Anaesthesia and myasthenia gravis. *Canadian Journal of Anaesthesia*, **39**, 476–86.

Krucylak PE, Naunheim KS (1999). Preoperative preparation and anesthetic management of patients with myasthenia gravis. *Seminars in Thoracic and Cardiovascular Surgery*, **11**, 47–53.

Wainwright AP, Brodrick PM (1987). Suxamethonium in myasthenia gravis. *Anaesthesia*, **42**, 950–7.

Dystrophia myotonica[1]

Dystrophia myotonica (myotonic dystrophy, myotonia atrophica) is the most common of the dystonias (1 in 20 000), the others being myotonia congenita and paramyotonia. It is an autosomal dominant trait, presenting in the second or third decade of life.

The disease leads to a persistent contraction of skeletal muscle following stimulation and is characterized by prefrontal balding and cataracts. The main clinical features are related to muscular atrophy, especially of facial, sternomastoid, and peripheral muscles.

Clinical features

- Muscle contraction is not affected by neuromuscular blocking agents (with the exception of suxamethonium—see below) or regional anaesthesia.
- Progressive deterioration/atrophy of skeletal, cardiac, and smooth muscle over time leads to a deterioration in cardiorespiratory function and a possibly severe cardiomyopathy.
- Further respiratory deterioration occurs due to degeneration of the central nervous system, leading to central respiratory drive depression.
- Progressive bulbar palsy, leading to difficulty in swallowing/clearing secretions and a proneness to aspiration.
- Degeneration of the cardiac conduction system causes dysrhythmia and atrioventricular block.
- There is mitral valve prolapse in approximately 20% of patients.
- Mental deterioration after the second decade.
- Endocrine dysfunction leading to diabetes mellitus, hypothyroidism, adrenal insufficiency, and gonadal atrophy.
- Death usually occurs in the fifth or sixth decade.
- Pregnancy may aggravate the disease and Caesarean section is more common due to uterine muscle dysfunction.
- Therapy is supportive with the use of antimyotonic medications such as procainamide, phenytoin, quinine, and mexiletine.

Conduct of anaesthesia

Preoperative evaluation

- Respiratory: clinical examination supplemented by spirometry and blood gases if indicated.
- Cardiac: signs of heart failure and check ECG for conduction problems. Some patients may have a cardiomyopathy that improves with exercise.
- Presence of bulbar palsy indicated by difficulty in swallowing or clearing secretions.
- Inability to cough may necessitate postoperative ventilation or tracheostomy.
- Gastric emptying may be delayed—premedication with an antacid (ranitidine 150–300 mg PO) or a prokinetic (metoclopramide 10 mg PO) may be indicated.
- There is a weak association between myotonic dystrophy and malignant hyperpyrexia (see p. 199).

Perioperative

- Suxamethonium produces prolonged muscle contraction (and potassium release) and should be avoided. The contraction may make intubation, ventilation, and surgery difficult.
- Non-depolarizing drugs are safe to use, but do not always cause muscle relaxation. Use of a nerve stimulator may provoke muscle contraction, leading to misdiagnosis of tetany.
- Reversal with neostigmine may also provoke contraction. Non-depolarizing agents with short action and spontaneous reversal (atracurium, mivacurium) are preferred.
- Intubation and maintenance of anaesthesia can often be achieved without the use of any muscle relaxant.
- Invasive arterial monitoring is indicated for significant cardiovascular impairment.
- Even small doses of induction agents can produce profound cardiorespiratory depression.
- Bulbar palsy mandates intubation under general anaesthesia.
- Regional anaesthesia does not prevent muscle contraction. Troublesome spasm may be helped by infiltration of local anaesthetic directly into the affected muscle. Quinine (600 mg IV) or phenytoin (3–5 mg/kg IV slowly) have been effective in some cases.
- High concentrations of inhaled anaesthetics should be avoided because of their effect on myocardial contraction and conduction.
- Patient warmth must be maintained. Postoperative shivering may provoke myotonia.

Postoperative care

- High-dependency care is indicated after anything but minor peripheral surgery. Discharge to low-dependency areas should only be considered if the patient is able to cough adequately and maintain oxygenation on air or simple supplemental oxygen.
- Analgesia is best provided, if possible, by regional or local block to avoid the systemic depressant effects of opiates.

Myotonia congenita

This develops in infancy and early childhood and is characterized by pharyngeal muscle spasm leading to difficulty in swallowing. It improves with age and patients have a normal life expectancy.

Paramyotonia

This is extremely rare. It is characterized by cold-induced contraction, only relieved by warming the affected muscle. Anaesthetic management is the same as for myotonic dystrophy. Patient warmth is paramount.

Imison AR (2001) Anaesthesia and myotonia – an Australian experience. *Anaesthesia and Intensive Care* **29**, 34–7.

Multiple sclerosis

Multiple sclerosis is an acquired disease of the central nervous system characterized by demyelinated plaques within the brain and spinal cord. The onset of symptoms usually occurs in early adulthood with 20–30% following a benign course and 5% a rapid deterioration. It is most common in geographical clusters within Europe, North America, and New Zealand.

Symptoms range from isolated visual disturbance and nystagmus to limb weakness and paralysis. Respiratory failure due to both respiratory muscle failure and bulbar palsy may be a feature in end-stage disease. Symptoms are characterized by symptomatic episodes of variable severity with periods of remission for several years. Permanent weakness and symptoms develop in some patients, leading to increasingly severe disability.

The disease is incurable, but steroids and interferon have been associated with improved symptom-free intervals. Most patients suffer from associated depression. Baclofen and dantrolene are useful for painful muscle spasm.

Demyelinated nerve fibres are sensitive to heat. A temperature rise of 0.5 °C may cause a marked deterioration in symptoms.

Conduct of anaesthesia

* Preoperative evaluation must include a history of the type of symptoms suffered and a detailed neurological examination. This will allow comparison with postoperative state to elucidate any new lesions.

* Respiratory function may be compromised. Bulbar palsy will lead to increased risk of aspiration and reduced airway reflexes in the post-anaesthetic period.

* General anaesthesia does not affect the course of multiple sclerosis.

* Regional anaesthesia does not affect neurological symptoms, but it may be medicolegally prudent to avoid nerve blockade in a limb susceptible to symptoms.

* Central neuraxial blockade has been associated with recurrence of symptoms. However, this is reduced by use of minimal concentrations of local anaesthetic/opioid in combination. Epidural analgesia for labour is not contraindicated as long as local anaesthetic concentration is kept to a minimum.

* Suxamethonium is associated with a large efflux of potassium in debilitated patients and should be avoided.

* Response to non-depolarizing drugs is normal although caution and reduced dosages are indicated in those with severe disability.

* Careful cardiovascular monitoring is essential since autonomic instability leads to marked hypotensive responses to drugs and sensitivity to hypovolaemia under anaesthesia.

* Temperature homeostasis is important and should be monitored in all patients. Pyrexia must be avoided and should be treated aggressively with antipyretics (paracetamol 1g PR/PO), tepid sponging, and forced air blowers. Hypothermia may delay recovery from anaesthesia.

Muscular dystrophy

The muscular dystrophies comprise a range of congenital muscular disorders characterized by progressive weakness of affected muscle groups. They can be classified according to inheritance:

- X-linked:
  - Duchenne's
  - Becker's.
- Autosomal recessive:
  - limb-girdle
  - childhood
  - congenital.
- Autosomal dominant:
  - facioscapulohumeral
  - oculopharyngeal.

Duchenne's muscular dystrophy

This is the most common and the most severe form.

Clinical features

- Sex-linked recessive trait, clinically apparent in males.
- Onset of symptoms of muscle weakness at ages 2–5 years.
- The patient is usually confined to a wheelchair by 12 years.
- Death usually by 25 years due to progressive cardiac failure or pneumonia.
- Cardiac: myocardial degeneration leading to heart failure and possible mitral valve prolapse. Evidence of heart failure is often apparent by 6 years (reduced R wave amplitude and wall motion abnormalities). Isolated degeneration of the left ventricle may lead to right outflow obstruction and right heart failure.
- Respiratory: progressive respiratory muscle weakness, leading to a restrictive ventilation pattern, inadequate cough, and eventual respiratory infection and failure.
- Axial muscle weakness leads to severe kyphoscoliosis.
- Disease progression may be tracked by serum creatinine kinase levels. These are elevated early in the disease but reduce to below normal as muscles atrophy.

Other muscular dystrophies (Becker's, facioscapulohumeral, and limb girdle dystrophy) are less severe than Duchenne's dystrophy, with onset at a later age and slower progression of the disease. Isolated ocular dystrophy is associated with a normal lifespan.

Conduct of anaesthesia

- Evidence of cardiac and respiratory disease should be sought.
- Reduced gut muscle tone leads to delayed gastric emptying and increased risk of aspiration.

- Antacid premedication (H_2 receptor blocker or proton pump inhibitor) with a prokinetic such as metoclopramide may be useful to reduce risk of aspiration.
- An antisialogogue such as glycopyrrolate 4.5 μg/kg IV may be needed if secretions are a problem.
- Careful intravenous induction of anaesthesia with balanced opioid/ induction agent.
- Potent inhalational anaesthetics should be used cautiously in these patients because of the risk of myocardial depression.
- Suxamethonium should be avoided because of potassium efflux and potential cardiac arrest.
- Non-depolarizing neuromuscular blockers are safe although reduced doses are required. Nerve stimulator monitoring should be used.
- Malignant hyperpyrexia has been associated with muscular dystrophy. The association appears to be weak although a high index of suspicion should be maintained at all times.
- Respiratory depressant effects of all anaesthetic drugs are enhanced and postoperative respiratory function should be monitored carefully. Those with pre-existing sputum retention and inadequate cough are at high risk of postoperative respiratory failure and may need prolonged ventilatory support.
- Regional analgesia is useful to avoid opiate use and potential respiratory depression after painful surgery. Caudal epidural may be technically easier to perform than lumbar epidural in those with kyphoscoliosis.

Guillain Barré syndrome

Guillain Barre syndrome is an immune-mediated progressive demyelination disorder characterized by acute or subacute proximal skeletal muscle paralysis. The syndrome is often preceded by limb paraesthesia/back pain and in more than half of affected patients by a viral illness. No single viral agent has been implicated. One-third of patients will require ventilatory support. The more rapid the onset of symptoms, the more likely the progression to respiratory failure. Impending respiratory failure may be evidenced by difficulty in swallowing and phonation due to pharyngeal muscle weakness. Inability to cough is a terminal sign. Autonomic dysfunction is common.

More than 85% of patients achieve a full recovery, although this may take several months. The use of steroids in the management of this condition remains controversial.

Conduct of anaesthesia

* Respiratory support is likely to be necessary, both during surgery and in the postoperative period.
* Autonomic dysfunction leads to potential severe hypotension during induction of anaesthesia, initiation of positive pressure ventilation, and postural changes under anaesthesia or recovery. Hydration should be maintained with wide-bore intravenous access and pressor agents (ephedrine 3 mg bolus IV) prepared prior to induction. Tachycardia due to surgical stimulus may be extreme and atropine may elicit a paradoxical bradycardia.
* Suxamethonium should be avoided due to potential catastrophic potassium efflux. The risk of hyperkalaemia may persist for several months after clinical recovery.
* Non-depolarizing muscle relaxants may not be needed, and should be used cautiously.
* Epidural analgesia is useful and may avoid the need for systemic narcotic analgesia. Epidural opioids have been used to manage distressing paraesthesias in these patients.

Motor neurone disease (amyotrophic lateral sclerosis)

This is a degenerative disorder of upper and lower motor neurones in the spinal cord. It manifests initially with weakness, atrophy, and fasciculation of peripheral muscles (usually those of the hand) and progresses to axial and bulbar weakness. Progression is relentless, with death from respiratory failure usually occurring within 3 years of diagnosis.

Patients remain mentally competent up to the point of terminal respiratory failure, leading to ethical and moral difficulty in the provision of long-term ventilation.

Conduct of anaesthesia

- Bulbar palsy increases the risk of sputum retention and aspiration. Intubation may be necessary. Many patients with advanced disease will have a long-term tracheostomy for airway protection and episodes of mechanical ventilation.
- Respiratory support is likely to be necessary, both during surgery and in the postoperative period.
- Autonomic dysfunction leads to potentially severe hypotension during induction of anaesthesia, initiation of positive pressure ventilation, and postural changes under anaesthesia or recovery. Hydration should be maintained with wide-bore intravenous access if necessary and pressor agents (e.g. ephedrine 3 mg bolus IV) prepared prior to induction.
- Suxamethonium should be avoided due to potential catastrophic potassium efflux.
- Non-depolarizing agents should be used in reduced dosage if necessary and their action monitored with a nerve stimulator.

Malignant hyperthermia

Aetiology

Malignant hyperthermia (MH) is a disorder of skeletal muscle, inherited as an autosomal dominant condition. It is associated with loss of normal Ca^{2+} homeostasis at some point in the excitation–contraction coupling system. An abnormality anywhere along this complex process can cause the clinical features seen in MH. This explains why differing chemical agents trigger MH and also the heterogeneity seen in DNA studies.

Worldwide about 50% of MH families have been shown to be linked to the ryanodine receptor (RYR1) on chromosome 19q. This is a Ca^{2+} efflux channel on the sarcoplasmic reticulum. Fifteen causative RYR1 mutations have been found to date. Three other probable sites on chromosomes 1, 3, and 7 have also been linked to MH.

Epidemiology

- Incidence is about 1 in 10–15 000 of the general population, although it is difficult to estimate. All races are affected.

- Previously mortality figures were very high (70–80%). Now they are very low (2–3%) due to better monitoring and awareness of MH as well as the availability of dantrolene.

- New MH susceptible cases (probands) continue to occur, about 20 per year in the United Kingdom, although there is an increase in the number of negative probands due to the increased index of suspicion.

- More commonly seen in young adults, especially males (maybe lifestyle rather than true sex difference).

- Occurs more frequently in minor surgical procedures, e.g. dental/ENT, when suxamethonium and inhalational agents are regularly used.

- Previous uneventful anaesthesia does not preclude MH, even when triggering agents must have been used. 75% of MH probands have had previous anaesthesia prior to the MH crisis.

Clinical presentation

The presentation of MH varies considerably and no one sign is unique to MH. The clinical diagnosis is therefore often difficult. It can be a florid dramatic life-threatening event or have an insidious onset.

- The clinical signs fall into two groups:
  - muscle: including muscle rigidity, hyperkalaemia, high CK, myoglobinuria
  - increased metabolism: including tachycardia, increased CO_2 production, metabolic acidosis. Often described as a 'metabolic storm'.

- The two most important early signs are an unexplained increasing $ETCO_2$ and a concomitant tachycardia.

- It is important to exclude other more common causes, e.g. 'light anaesthesia', respiratory/ventilatory problems.

- If there is unexplained, unexpected increasing $ETCO_2$ together with a tachycardia then suspect MH and proceed to 'Treatment of a crisis'.

- Masseter muscle spasm (MMS) is also an early warning sign (see below).
- Increase in temperature is a late sign of MH.
- Rarely MH patients may present 2–3 days postoperatively with massive myoglobinuria leading to renal failure due to severe muscle damage.

Treatment of a crisis

See p. 855.

Masseter muscle spasm (MMS)

- MMS occurs during induction of anaesthesia after the administration of depolarizing muscle relaxants, e.g. suxamethonium. Inhalational agents are unlikely to cause MMS at induction but may produce MMS as part generalized muscle rigidity during the course of anaesthesia.
- MMS is a subjective sign, difficult to define, and often not fully investigated. MMS may be the only sign of MH even with continued exposure to inhalational agents.
- Suspect MMS if jaw stiffness occurs at a time when relaxation would have been expected to occur. Significant MMS will be severe enough to hinder intubation and persists for at least 2 min. Suxamethonium can produce short-lived MMS in normal patients.
- If significant MMS occurs treat as potentially MH.
- If possible abandon surgery, if not convert to 'MH safe' technique (volatile free), allow approximately 15 min to ensure that the patient is stabilized. Monitor $ETCO_2$, temperature, and consider an arterial line.
- Investigations that are particularly useful are the initial and 24-h creatine kinase (CK) and examination of the first voided specimen for myoglobinuria, indicating evidence of muscle damage.
- Prolonged severe muscle stiffness greatly in excess of the 'normal scoline pains' may occur.
- About 30% of patients who have MMS apparently as the sole sign are MH susceptible but other signs may have been present but not recorded (have usually been missed rather than absent).
- Additional MH signs increase the likelihood of MH significantly: 50–60% if metabolic signs present, 70–80% if muscle signs present.
- MMS maybe the first indication of a previously unsuspected muscle disease, particularly the myotonic conditions. Perform resting CK and EMG. Consider neurological opinion.

Diagnosis of MH susceptibility

- When the clinical diagnosis is suspected refer the patient to an MH unit with all the clinical details/anaesthetic chart/laboratory results. The timing of the various events is important.
- The patient and the family should be warned of the potential implications of MH in the meantime.
- Unless MH can be clearly excluded on clinical grounds the patient will be offered muscle biopsy (in vitro contracture testing) to confirm or refute the diagnosis.
- MH is not a diagnosis to be made without follow-up arrangements and explanations to the patient.

• Guidelines for diagnostic DNA testing for MH have been published. A new proband will be screened by muscle biopsy and DNA. If a causative mutation is found in the confirmed MH proband, the family may then be offered DNA screening, otherwise routine muscle biopsy will be offered. Family members not showing the causative mutation in the proband will still need a muscle biopsy. It is hoped that MH centres will manage this process, so that an up to date centralized register about the best way to screen each family can be maintained.

Diagnostic muscle biopsy

• In vitro contracture testing (IVCT) is the standard diagnostic screening test, using the European MH Group protocol. Living muscle samples are exposed to halothane and caffeine separately under preset conditions. This is an open invasive procedure usually performed under a 3 in 1 femoral nerve block or occasionally general anaesthesia (propofol/fentanyl/nitrous oxide/oxygen) in which eight muscle fibres about 3–4 cm long are removed from the vastus medialis. The patient needs to travel to the MH centre for this to be done.

• The diagnosis is considered positive if the muscle produces a contracture in response to halothane and/or caffeine.

• The most important diagnosis for the patient is the MH-negative one. It is accepted that in order to ensure the accuracy of the MH-negative diagnosis there is the potential for 'false positive' results. Combined results from European MH centres indicate the IVCT has a 99% sensitivity and 93.6% specificity.

• Once the clinical diagnosis has been confirmed in the proband the family is then offered screening. The purpose of family screening is to identify the small number of MH-susceptible patients in the family rather than label the whole family. Only a small proportion of the family will need to be screened.

• Family screening is organized on the basis of the autosomal dominant inheritance, so that relatives with a 50% chance, i.e. parents, children, and siblings, are offered screening in the first instance.

• Children are not screened until they are 10–12 years old.

• The MH centre can provide written information, warning cards, and discs for susceptible patients.

Anaesthesia for a known or suspected MH-susceptible patient

• MH patients can only be identified from their history. Preoperative questioning about their personal and family anaesthetic history is therefore essential.

• MH-susceptible patients should not be denied necessary surgery on the grounds of MH alone.

• The extra risk of avoiding suxamethonium and the anaesthetic vapours needs to be evaluated for each particular patient and circumstance. In most cases this would not pose any additional risk but will do so in patients with airway problems, e.g. rapid sequence induction, when inhalational induction would be the usual technique of choice, and the prevention of awareness.

- It is not absolutely essential to screen suspected patients beforehand, providing that proper individual assessment has been made of the risks involved, as family screening can take some considerable time to organize. For uncomplicated elective surgery, it is probably wise to screen the patient first, for their own long-term benefit and that of their descendants.
- General anaesthesia must be performed in a main hospital site not in the dental surgery or small outlying hospital.
- Local anaesthetics are safe for MH patients, so can be used in dental surgeries etc.
- Regional techniques are the method of choice if appropriate, with or without sedation (benzodiazepines, low-dose propofol).
- General anaesthesia can be undertaken using propofol infusion, opioids, or regional blockade, spontaneous ventilation or IPPV using non-depolarizing neuromuscular blocking agents.
- The MH centre can always be contacted for confirmation of history, biopsy results, advice etc.

MH 'triggering' agents

- Agents that are absolutely contraindicated are suxamethonium and all the anaesthetic vapours.
- Phenothiazines have been implicated in the past, as have drugs which increase catecholamine levels, e.g. antidepressants. No patient has ever been referred to the Leeds Unit because of an MH crisis in response to these agents. They can be used with caution.

Anaesthesia for the MH susceptible patient	
MH 'triggering' agents	Avoid suxamethonium and all the anaesthetic vapours
MH 'safe' agents	All induction agents including ketamine, all analgesics, all non-depolarizing agents, all local anaesthetics (preferably plain solutions). Atropine/gylcopyrrolate/neostigmine. Ephedrine and other vasopressors. Metoclopramide/droperidol. Nitrous oxide, benzodiazepines
Monitoring	ECG, NIBP, ETCO2, core temperature. Check temp 2 h preop. to establish the baseline and 4–6 h postop.
Anaesthetic equipment	If no vapour-free machine is available, remove the vaporizers and blow both the anaesthetic machine and the ventilator with oxygen for 20–30 min. Use fresh clean tubing/masks/ET tubes, etc. If possible select a ventilator with little inner tubing, e.g. Nuffield Penlon
Dantrolene	This is not required prophylactically, as no reaction should occur. It is unpleasant for the patient and markedly prolongs the action of non-depolarizing muscle relaxants. However, it should be readily available

Patient with a known family history of MH

- Establish family history and the relationship of your patient to the proband or other tested family members, together with their names.
- The MH centre will then be able to identify the correct family and advise on the individual's risk of MH, whether it is appropriate to be tested, etc. Depending on the family, it may not be appropriate to screen your patient first but rather a relation nearest to a known MH individual. This may exclude the risk of MH in your patient without further need of testing.
- If anaesthesia needs to be conducted urgently and the family information cannot be confirmed, treat as potentially MH susceptible.

Suspicious previous anaesthetic history

- Postoperative pyrexia. If the intra-operative and immediate recovery period were uneventful MH is not implicated. If the timing of pyrexia cannot be established, treat as potentially MH.
- Unexplained/unexpected cardiac arrest/death during anaesthesia has a 50% chance of being due to MH.
- Postoperative severe myoglobinuria (red/black urine), which may even present as renal failure in a fit healthy patient, could be due to MH or a muscle problem.
- Take a thorough history of the event, if possible obtain the records even if at another hospital. If surgery is urgent treat as MH susceptible and resolve the problem afterwards otherwise seek further advice from the MH centre.

Obstetric patients

Mother MH susceptible

Discuss options with the obstetric anaesthetist prior to the estimated date of delivery to formulate plans in case of emergency. Treat with MH safe agents. Regional techniques are preferable for both labour and instrumental deliveries. Ephedrine can be used to maintain blood pressure. Syntocinon and ergometrine can be used. Should general anaesthesia be essential a rapid-onset non-depolarizing muscle relaxant should be used (e.g. rocuronium) and general anaesthesia maintained with a propofol infusion. It is essential to anticipate airway problems and consider other options, e.g. awake intubation.

Father MH susceptible

The mother should not be given MH triggering agents which can cross the placenta. Avoid inhalational agents until after delivery of the baby. Suxamethonium can be used as it is highly charged and does not cross the placenta to any great extent.

The baby should be treated as potentially MH susceptible if it requires surgery as it has a 50% chance of being affected.

Associated conditions

- Central core disease (CCD) is a non-progressive inherited condition causing peripheral muscle weakness and occasionally musculoskeletal and cardiac problems. It is the only condition known to be associated with MH, but this is not invariable. CCD patients should be treated as potentially MH susceptible but offered screening because of the discordant association.

Other muscle diseases are not thought to be related to MH but clearly cause anaesthetic problems in their own right.

- Heat stroke and King–Denborough syndrome remain controversial.
- Neurolept malignant syndrome and sudden infant death syndrome are not associated with MH.

MH Centres and the British MH Association (BMHA)

- There is only one MH centre in the United Kingdom: Dr P. J. Halsall, MH Investigation Unit, Clinical Sciences Building, St James's University Hospital, Leeds LS9 7TF. Tel: 0113 2065274; Fax: 0113 2064140; Hotline: 07947 609601 (usually available for medical emergencies only).

- The British MH Association (BMHA) is a charitable patient support group which provides the 'hotline', warning cards/discs and translations for travel abroad, newsletters, as well as fundraising for research. Secretary Mrs A. Winks, 11 Gorse Close, Newthorpe, Nottingham NG16 2BZ. Tel: 01773 717901.

- There are 22 MH centres in Europe. Contact the European MH Group Secretary Dr P. J. Halsall (address above) for further details or the EMHG website: www.emhg.org.

- For USA and Canada contact MHAUS 39 East State St, PO Box 1069, Sherburne, NY 13460, USA. Tel: in North America, 1–800-MH-Hyper, outside North America, 1–315–464–7079; www.mhaus.org. Hotline: 1–800–98-MHAUS.

- For Australia contact Dr Neil Street, Anaesthetic Dept, The New Children's Hospital, Westmead, NSW, PO Box 3515 Parramatta 2124. Tel: (02)9845 0000; Fax: (02) 9845 3489.

- For New Zealand contact Dr Neil Pollock, Anaesthetic Dept, Palmerston North Hospital, Mid Central Health, Palmerston North, NZ. Tel: (06) 3569169; Fax: (06) 3508566.

Further reading

Ellis FR, Halsall PJ, Christian AS (1990). Clinical presentation of suspected malignant hyperthermia during anaesthesia in 402 probands. *Anaesthesia*, **45**, 838–41.

Guidelines for the treatment of an MH crisis. A poster published by the Association of Anaesthetists of Great Britain and Ireland. Bedford Square London.

Halsall PJ, Ellis FR (1996). Malignant hyperthermia. *Current Anaesthesia and Critical Care*, **7**, 158–66.

MacLennan DH, Phillips MS (1992). Malignant hyperthermia. *Science*, **256**, 789–94.

Urwyler A, Deufel T, McCarthy TV, West SP for the European MH Group (2001). Guidelines for the molecular genetic testing of susceptibility to malignant hyperthermia. *British Journal of Anaesthesia*, **86**, 283–7.

Chapter 10
Psychiatry

Suzie Tanser

General considerations

Approximately 20% of people in the United Kingdom suffer from psychiatric ill health and approximately 1% will have a major disorder. Many of these people may present for surgery, either for coexisting disease or as a result of deliberate self-harm. Psychiatric disorders often coexist with alcohol or drug abuse (see pp. 220, 222). History taking may be difficult and relatives or carers may need to be present for the preoperative assessment. Consent to surgery or anaesthesia can only be given by a competent adult (see p. 4). The majority of patients with psychiatric disorders can give consent normally.

Psychiatric patients are often surprisingly strong and if confused by unfamiliar faces or surroundings may become aggressive. Sedative premedication should be considered and adequate personnel should always be present for induction and emergence in patients at risk. Many patients will be on long-term medication and this should be continued throughout the perioperative period whenever possible. Many psychiatric drugs have the potential to interact with anaesthetic agents.

Schizophrenia

Prevalence 2–4 per 1000. The presence of any one of Schneider's 'first-rank symptoms' in the absence of physical disease. First-rank symptoms include auditory hallucinations, thought withdrawal, insertion or broadcasting, delusional perceptions, somatic passivity and feelings. Chronic schizophrenia is characterized by 'negative symptoms' such as withdrawal, catatonic disturbances, and lack of emotion. It commonly begins in late adolescence in either sex and any social group. In the acute phase patients may be highly delusional and/or aggressive and may not be able to give informed consent. Controlled schizophrenics may be completely lucid and rational but care must be taken to ensure that their medication is continued where possible. Some chronic schizophrenics have predominantly negative symptoms and may be withdrawn and difficult to communicate with.

Manic-depressive disorders

An abnormality of mood. Can be bipolar (mania and depression) or unipolar. In the depressive phase verbal memory may be impaired and communication difficult. When in the manic phase there may be disinhibition, flight of ideas, delusions of power, and memory distubances. There is a wide spectrum of disease ranging from severe depression through normal stable mood to severe mania.

Neuroses and personality disorders

These represent the largest proportion of psychiatric disorders attending psychiatric outpatients (75%). Includes anxiety, obsession, hysteria, and hypochondriacal neuroses. The anxiety or obsession can impede normal functioning and cause considerable distress. Catecholamine levels may be very high or the patient may suffer from hyperventilation. These patients require a great deal of reassurance and premedication is often required to smooth induction.

Tricyclic antidepressants

* Used for treating severe or endogenous depression. May also be used to treat panic disorders, neuralgia, and nocturnal enuresis in children.
* Properties include alpha 1 antagonist, anticholinergic, antidopaminergic, and antihistaminic effects.
* Side-effects include antimuscarinic (dry mouth, blurred vision, constipation, tachycardia), alpha 1 blockade (hypotension), plus other effects such as hyponatraemia (possibly due to secretion of antidiuretic hormone), ECG changes, arrhythmias, and blood dyscrasias. Characteristic ECG changes include increased P-R interval, wide QRS complexes, and decreased T wave amplitude.
* Interactions with anaesthetic drugs are common, but generally predictable. Increased catecholamine concentration at central sites may lead to increased anaesthetic requirements and exaggerated response to endogenous and exogenous catecholamines. The threshold for ventricular dysrhythmias may be lowered. Where possible, catecholamine administration and drugs causing catecholamine release (e.g. ephedrine) should be avoided. If augmentation of blood pressure is necessary, direct-acting agents such as methoxamine may be used with caution. If hypertensive episodes occur, alpha-blockers such as phentolamine may be used. Anticholinergic drugs that cross the blood–brain barrier such as atropine should be avoided as these may precipitate confusional states postoperatively.

Lithium

Lithium carbonate is used for the treatment of bipolar depression. It resembles sodium, will permeate voltage-sensitive ion channels, and may accumulate inside cells causing partial depolarization. It may interact with anaesthetic agents that have their effects on sodium channels. Where levels are above the therapeutic range there may be prolonged recovery from barbiturates and an increased duration of action of non-depolarizing muscle relaxants. Levels should be monitored and maintained between 0.4 and 1 mmol/litre. Toxicity is associated with tremor, convulsions, and renal impairment and made worse by sodium depletion and dehydration.

Selective serotonin reuptake inhibitors (SSRI)

* Introduced in 1987 these are now the most commonly prescribed antidepressant drugs.
* They are highly selective for inhibitors of serotonin reuptake and are considerably less toxic than tricyclics.
* Cardiovascular side-effects are rare. Bradycardias have occasionally been reported and, in patients with coronary artery disease, SSRIs may precipitate coronary artery vasoconstriction.
* Inappropriate ADH secretion has been reported in elderly patients and may present with severe hyponatraemia.
* Nausea, vomiting, and diarrhoea are common side-effects due to inhibition of serotonin in the GI tract.
* Platelet aggregation may occasionally be impaired.
* The 'serotonin syndrome' results from increased synaptic levels of serotonin in the brainstem and spinal cord. It presents as confusion, agitation,

coma, rigidity, myoclonus, autonomic instability, fevers, DIC, renal failure, and arrythmias. It may be precipitated by the addition of drugs such as monoamine oxidase inhibitors, tricyclic antidepressants, pethidine, or pentazocine. Avoidance of these drugs is recommended. Treatment is supportive. SSRIs are metabolized by the cytochrome P-450 system and so may interact with other drugs metabolized by the same system, e.g. warfarin (increased bleeding time). Interactions with the benzodiazepines (increased sedation) have also been reported.

- Acute withdrawal may precipitate a syndrome of anxiety, agitation, and increased sweating.

Monoamine oxidase inhibitors (MAOI)

- Used for refractory depression.
- These drugs inhibit the oxidative metabolism of catecholamines at central sites. Older MAOIs were non-selective (inhibiting both MAO-A and MAO-B oxidase enzymes) and irreversible. Newer types are selective for the MAO-A enzyme and cause reversible inhibition (reversible inhibitor of monoamine oxidase A or 'RIMA').

  - MAO-A preferentially deaminates serotonin, noradrenaline, and adrenaline.
  - MAO-B deaminates all non-polar aromatic amines such as phenylethylamine.
  - Tryamine and dopamine are metabolized by both forms of the enzyme.
  - Both enzymes are present in neural and non-neural tissue with a preponderance of type A in the brain and type B in the liver and lungs.

- Non-selective MAOIs have anticholinergic effects, may cause postural hypotension, and are associated with a number of serious side-effects:

  - Inhibition of non-neural MAO is responsible for the 'cheese' reaction—a hypertensive crisis induced by eating foods rich in tyramine. Indirectly acting sympathomimetics such as ephedrine and metaraminol can be

Drug interactions with MAOIs (current therapy or cessation within past 2 weeks)

Drugs to be avoided	Reason	Suitable alternative treatment
Pethidine	Hyperpyrexia, hypotension/ hypertension	Morphine, fentanyl
Ephedrine, metaraminol	Hypertension	Phenylephrine, noradrenaline
Pancuronium	Releases stored noradrenaline	Vecuronim, atracurium
Suxamethonium	Phenelzine only, due to decreased pseudocholinesterase activity	Mivacurium, rocuronium
Tricyclic antidepressants	Hypertensive episodes	Atypical antidepressants

Generic and proprietory names of common psychiatric drugs

Generic name	Proprietory name
Tricyclic antidepressants	
Amitriptyline	Lentizol, Tryptizol, Triptafen
Amoxapine	Asendis
Clomipramine	Anafranil
Dothiepin	Prothieden
Doxepin	Sinequan
Imipramine	Tofranil
Lofepramine	Gamanil
Nortriptyline	Allegron, Motipress, Motival
Protryptiline	Concordin
Trimipramine	Surmontil
SSRIs	
Fluoxitine	Prozac
Fluvoxamine	Faverin
Citalopran	Cipramil
Paroxetine	Seroxat
Sertraline	Lustral
MAOI non-selective	
Phenelzine	Nardil
Isocarboxazid	Isocarboxazid
Tranylcypromine	Parnate
MAOI-A (RIMA)	
Moclobemide	Manerix
MAOI-B	
Selegiline	Eldepryl, Zelapar

potentiated in the same way and should be avoided. Hypertensive crises can be treated with alpha-blocking agents (e.g. phentolamine) or directly acting vasodilators. Noradrenaline or methoxamine are the vasopressors of choice.

- An adverse interaction is also seen with pethidine, secondary to blockade of 5-HT uptake. This reaction is potentially fatal and manifests itself as agitation, hypertension, hyperthermia, convulsions, and coma. Other opiates have been safely used including morphine, fentanyl, alfentanil, and remifentanil.
- Pancuronium should be avoided as it releases stored adrenaline.
- Interactions persist for up to 2 weeks after cessation of therapy.
- Tranylcypromine is the most hazardous due to stimulant action.
- Phenelzine has been shown to decrease pseudocholinesterase concentration and there have been isolated reports of a prolonged action of suxamethonium. This appears to be unique to phenelzine.

- It is no longer recommended that these drugs be stopped preoperatively due to risks associated with recurrence of depression, but care should be taken to avoid interactions with the anaesthetic drugs listed above.

- The new generation of selective MAO-A inhibitors (reversible inhibition of monoamine oxidase type A, RIMAs) are being increasingly used. They have a short half-life, are well tolerated, have no anticholinergic effects, and do not cause postural hypotension. They have no central excitatory side-effects, no interactions with tricyclics, and a clinically insignificant response to ingested tyramine. They may still cause an excitatory response to pethidine so it should be avoided. Indirectly acting sympathomimetics (e.g. ephedrine, metaraminol) should also not be used.

- Selegiline is a selective MAO-B inhibitor used in the treatment of Parkinson's disease. Interactions are fewer than with the MAO-A inhibitors, but pethidine is best avoided and vasopressors used with care.

Further reading

Kam P, Chang G (1997). Selective serotonin reuptake inhibitors. Pharmacologiy and clinical implications in anaesthesia and critical care medicine. *Anaesthesia*, 52, 982–8.

Stack CG, Rogers P, Linter S (1988). Monoamine oxidase inhibitors and anaesthesia—a review. *British Journal of Anaesthesia*, **60**, 222–7.

Ure D, Gillies M, James K (2000). Safe use of remifentanil in a patient treated with the monoamine oxidase inhibitor phenelzine. *British Journal of Anaesthesia*, **84**, 414–16.

McFarlane HJ (1994). Anaesthesia and the new generation monoamine oxidase inhibitors. *Anaaesthesia*, **49**, 597–9.

Chapter 11
Miscellaneous problems

Down's syndrome

Down's syndrome (trisomy 21) is the commonest congenital abnormality, with an incidence of 1.6 per 1000 births. Anaesthesia and surgery carry a higher morbidity and mortality than in the general population.

General considerations

In addition to the characteristic dysmorphic features and impaired global development, Down's syndrome is associated with disorders of many organ systems:

+ Congenital cardiac defects (in up to 40%)—predominantly endocardial cushion defects and ventricular septal defects.
+ Eisenmenger's syndrome (pulmonary hypertension with right-to-left shunt) may complicate the perioperative management of the older child particularly if there is associated obstructive sleep apnoea.
+ Recurrent respiratory tract infection due to relative immune deficiency and a degree of upper airway obstruction (tonsillar/adenoidal hypertrophy).
+ Atlantoaxial instability (in up to 30% of individuals)—subluxation/dislocation tendency due to bony abnormality of the atlas and axis and laxity of the transverse atlantal ligament.
+ Epilepsy (in up to 10% of individuals).
+ Obesity and potentially difficult venous access.

Preoperative assessment

+ Careful airway assessment for potential difficult airway maintenance and intubation (relatively large tongue, crowding of midfacial structures, high arched narrow palate, micrognathia, short broad neck).
+ Cardiorespiratory assessment for signs and symptoms of congenital cardiac defects, pulmonary hypertension, and chest infections.
+ Symptoms of atlantoaxial instability (abnormal gait, clumsiness, hyper-reflexia, clonus, hemi/quadriparesis, extensor plantars, neurogenic bladder, ataxia, and sensory loss), although atlantoaxial instability is frequently asymptomatic.

Investigations

Patients have usually been fully investigated by the paediatric team:

+ Full blood count (incidence of polycythaemia and leukaemia is 20 times that seen in the general population). Urea and electrolytes and thyroid function tests (hypothyroidism in up to 40%).

Preoperative investigations as per clinical findings and surgical procedure planned:

+ ECG as routine.
+ Chest radiograph if there are cardiorespiratory problems.
+ Echocardiography if signs or symptoms are suspicious of a cardiac defect.
+ Lateral cervical spine radiographs are indicated only if there are neurological signs or symptoms, and current opinion would suggest that routine screening is inappropriate.

Preparation

* Optimize cardiac and respiratory function.
* Reduced threshold for arranging HDU/ICU for postoperative care due to the high incidence of perioperative complications.
* Patients are often uncooperative and a sedative premedication to prevent struggling during induction is often helpful, e.g. oral midazolam (0.5 mg/kg) or temazepam (0.5 mg/kg) in the older age group. Exercise caution if problems with airway obstruction exist.
* Establish rapport with parents and carers.
* EMLA/Ametop cream should be applied if intravenous induction is planned.
* Inhalational induction with sevoflurane/halothane is useful, especially in uncooperative patients with difficult intravenous access. IM ketamine (5–10 mg/kg) is also an option.
* Drying agents may be useful if hypersalivation is problematic. Caution should be exercised when giving atropine as exaggerated sensitivity to both mydriatic and cardiac effects have been reported. Consider a reduced dosage or using an alternative agents, e.g. glycopyrrolate.
* There is a high incidence of gastro-oesophageal reflux. Give reflux prophylaxis (ranitidine) if symptomatic.

Perioperative considerations

* Potential difficult airway maintenance and intubation.
* Take care to avoid excessive movements of the neck, especially during laryngoscopy and positioning for surgery.
* There is increased incidence of subglottic stenosis in children with Down's syndrome—a smaller tracheal tube than would have been predicted by age is frequently required.
* No abnormal responses to anesthetic drugs have been substantiated.
* Prone to hypoventilation—IPPV often preferable to spontaneous ventilation.
* Prophylactic antibiotics for cardiac defects should be given prior to predictable bacteraemic events.
* Strict asepsis—relative immune deficiency and increased susceptibility to infections.
* Universal precautions—increased incidence of hepatitis B and C.
* Postoperative pain management may be problematic. Consider regional blocks wherever possible. PCA can be used successfully in appropriate patients.

Postoperative considerations

* Patients who are compromised and those undergoing major surgery should be managed on HDU/ICU postoperatively.
* Parents/carers are indispensable in the recovery period as Down's syndrome patients are often agitated postoperatively and may be very difficult to manage.

- Associated hypotonia (up to 75%) may affect the ability to maintain an adequate airway following anaesthesia and patients should be carefully observed.
- Patients are prone to atelectasis and respiratory tract infections especially following abdominal and thoracic surgery—humidified oxygen, regular physiotherapy, adequate analgesia, and close monitoring are required.
- The duration of postoperative ventilation, intensive care, and hospital stay all tend to be longer than the general population.

Further reading

Mitchell V, Howard R, Facer E (1995). Clinical review: Down's syndrome and anaesthesia. *Paediatric Anaesthesia*, 5, 379–84.

Anaesthesia for the elderly

Anaesthesia and surgery in the elderly population are associated with increased morbidity and mortality. Specific factors to consider include:

- Degenerative disease of all types is commoner in geriatric patients. History may be unreliable and hospital notes occasionally formidable.
- Cardiovascular: ischaemic heart disease is common, with reduced ventricular compliance, contractility, and reduced cardiac output. Blood flow to the kidneys and brain may be reduced, with impaired autoregulation. Atherosclerosis may be widespread, resulting in a less compliant arterial tree and systemic hypertension. The physiological response to cardiovascular disturbance may be blunted, due to reduced baroreceptor sensitivity and impaired autonomic function. Atrial fibrillation is common.
- Respiratory: pulmonary elasticity, lung and chest wall compliance, TLC, FVC, FEV_1, VC, and inspiratory reserve are all reduced, with an increase in residual volume. Although FRC is unchanged, closing capacity falls progressively with age, leading to airway collapse, VQ mismatch, and hypoxaemia. Atelectasis, pulmonary embolism, and chest infection are all more common in elderly patients, the latter in part due to ineffective mucociliary activity. PAO_2 and PaO_2 decrease with age (PAO_2 =13.3 – age/30 kPa, or PAO_2 = 100 – age/ 4 mmHg).
- Renal system: glomerular filtration is reduced. Muscle bulk decreases with age resulting in reduced creatinine production, hence even a modest rise in serum creatinine may represent significant renal impairment. Tubular function is also impaired, with reduced renal concentrating ability and reduced free water clearance. Fluid balance is more critical, as responses to both fluid loading and dehydration are impaired.
- Pharmacology: pharmacokinetics are altered, with reduced hepatic and renal blood flow and a reduction in total body water. Pharmacodynamics may also be altered, with increased sensitivity to many agents, especially CNS depressants. MAC decreases steadily with age (4–5% per decade after 40 years—for example, the MAC of isoflurane is approximately 0.92 at 80 years of age). Plasma proteins are often reduced, resulting in reduced protein binding of drugs and metabolites, thereby increasing free drug levels and possible toxic effects.
- Nervous system: in addition to autonomic dysfunction, cerebrovascular disease is common, and hearing, vision, and memory may be impaired. Confusion is more likely, both pre- and postoperatively.
- Nutrition: malnutrition is common in the elderly, and is associated with increased morbidity and mortality. Trials of nutritional supplementation show reduced length of hospital stay and reduced minor postoperative complications, but without a decrease in mortality. Consider oral protein supplementation, nocturnal nasogastric feeding, or even TPN in those with significant malnutrition.

Preoperative considerations

- Full and thorough assessment—significant cardiac, respiratory, and renal disease may have been previously undetected. An ECG is required for all patients. Note cognitive function and the level of social support.

- In patients who have sustained a fracture, actively seek an underlying medical cause for a fall, e.g. arrhythmias, myocardial infarction, transient ischaemic attack, CVE, pulmonary embolus, GI bleed.
- Assessment of exercise tolerance and functional ability is important. This may be misleading, however, as patients tend to live within their functional reserve.
- Dehydration is common. Many patients do not drink adequately when confined to bed. Consider prescribing preoperative IV fluids.

Perioperative considerations

- Arm–brain circulation time is increased, and dose requirements for induction agents are drastically reduced. Titrate drugs slowly against effect, and inject into a running IV infusion.
- Use fluid warmers/body warming devices whenever possible. Elderly patients have a reduced basal metabolic rate and are susceptible to heat loss as a result of impaired thermoregulation.
- Regional anaesthesia may have some advantages over general anaesthesia, including fewer thromboembolic complications, confusion, and respiratory upset postoperatively. However, hypotension is more commonly seen in elderly patients undergoing spinal/epidural anaesthesia due to impaired autonomic function and reduced compliance of the arterial tree. General anaesthesia may be best for those who require precise control of their blood pressure. Regional anaesthesia for hip fractures may reduce mortality at 1 month, but regional and general anaesthesia appear to produce comparable results for longer-term mortality.
- Careful perioperative fluid balance. Consider measuring the CVP when large fluid shifts are expected. Patients are more often 'underfilled' than 'overloaded'. Regular review is essential following major surgery.

Postoperative considerations

- Prescribe postoperative oxygen therapy following abdominal or thoracic surgery, in the presence of cardiovascular or respiratory disease, in situations when there has been significant blood loss, and when opioid analgesia has been prescribed. Nasal cannulae are often better tolerated.
- Postoperative analgesia: consider prescribing a regular simple analgesic such as paracetamol, and use NSAIDs with caution (the complications of NSAID use are more prevalent in the elderly). Intramuscular and subcutaneous opioids may be unreliably absorbed due to variable tissue perfusion, and an elderly confused patient may have difficulty using a PCA. Regional techniques or an IV opioid infusion (with appropriate supervision) may be the most appropriate method of pain relief.
- Early and frequent physiotherapy and mobilization are extremely important.

Further reading

Dickson RE, Patey RE (1999). Perioperative management of the elderly trauma patient. *Hospital Medicine*, **60**, 425–9.

Parker MJ, Urwin SC, Handoll HHG, Griffiths R (2000). General versus spinal/epidural anaesthesia for surgery for hip fractures in adults (Cochrane Review). *The Cochrane Library*, **issue** 3.

Latex allergy

Background

Latex is the sap of Hevea brasiliensis (the rubber tree). It is a complex mixture of polyisoprene particles in a phospholipoprotein envelope and a serum containing sugars, lipids, nucleic acids, minerals, and proteins. Latex is made heat stable and elastic by vulcanization (heating in the presence of sulphur). Chemicals such as accelerators and antioxidants are also added to enhance strength, stretch, and durability.

Latex is found in many of the products used in the operating environment, including gloves, urinary catheters, syringes, drug vial stoppers, intravenous giving sets, intravenous cannulas, injection ports, masks, airways, endotracheal tubes, rebreathing bags, bellows, and circuits. Many pieces of surgical equipment also contain latex, including drains, bulb irrigation syringes, vascular tags, and rubber shod clamps.

Epidemiology

Development of latex sensitivity is dependent on previous exposure. There are certain groups at particular risk of developing latex sensitivity:

- Health care workers: estimates have put the risk of developing latex sensitivity at between 5 and 17%, depending on the degree and nature of exposure; the actual figure may well prove to be much higher (up to 50%).
- Rubber industry workers: there is an increased incidence of positive skinprick tests to latex, and chronic respiratory symptoms associated with eosinophilia in this population.
- Neural tube defects (including spina bifida): the reported incidence of latex sensitivity due to recurrent bladder catheterizations is estimated at between 20 and 65%.
- Fruit allergy: an association between latex and fruit allergy has been described, and cross-reactivity demonstrated with certain fruit allergens (banana, avocado, passion fruit, tomato, grape, celery, kiwi fruit, chestnut).

Spectrum

- Irritant contact dermatitis: non-allergic irritant contact dermatitis occurs due to damage of the skin from irritation of an exogenous substance.
- Contact dermatitis: a type IV (delayed) hypersensitivity reaction based on allergic sensitization. Presents with an eczematous eruption, which can then progress to lichenificaton and scaling on chronic exposure. Mediated by T lymphocytes exposed to chemicals added in the vulcanizing process such as the accelerators (thiurams and thioureas) and antioxidants (benzothiazoles).
- Type I hypersensitivity: IgE-mediated type I hypersensitivity has been attributed to water-soluble proteins in latex and starch powder-bound proteins. Clinical manifestations may result from exposure to latex via a variety of routes including skin, mucous membranes, inhalation, and intravenous. The three main presentations are:
  - Contact urticaria: particularly in health care workers, typically 10–15 min following, and usually at the site of, exposure. This may be the initial step in the progression to more severe reactions.

• Asthma and rhinitis: characterized by bronchial obstruction and secretions. Starch powder used as a lubricant for gloves has been implicated here.

• Anaphylaxis, vascular collapse, and shock: this is most commonly encountered intra-operatively and although intravenous and mucus membrane inoculation are the most common triggers, anaphylaxis has been described with donning of gloves and indirect contact with individuals who use latex gloves.

Clinical features of latex anaphylaxis

A careful history with particular reference to risk factors is important pre-operatively to give an indication of potential problems.

Onset is normally delayed by 20–60 min following exposure to the antigen and progressively worsens over 5–10 min. The reaction presents with hypotension, rash, and bronchospasm (rash may be absent). It may be difficult to exclude anaphylaxis from anaesthetic drugs since this presents in a similar manner and is treated in the same way (see p. 857). Subsequent analysis of serum mast cell tryptase confirms anaphylaxis and skin-prick testing will determine the causative factor.

Management of elective surgery

• The prophylactic use of antihistamines and corticosteriods has not been established.

• The patient should be scheduled first on the operating list (latex can remain in the air).

• Items to be particularly careful of include BP cuff, gloves, urinary catheters, anaesthetic reservoir bag/face masks, syringes, elastic in disposable hats/TEDS/underpants, IV giving sets, drug vials with latex stoppers.

• Many companies are now moving towards latex-free equipment, but each theatre suite should have a list detailing which equipment is guaranteed latex free.

• The LMA (Intavent) is latex free.

• If uncertain about the BP cuff, wrap plastic sheeting around the arm prior to placement.

• Most ETTs and airways are latex free.

Every department should have a latex-free trolley containing the following:

• Non-latex gloves. Note that 'hypoallergenic' gloves are non-standardized and are often made from latex. Gloves used in patients allergic to latex should be made of synthetic rubber such as neoprene or polyvinyl chloride, e.g. 'Derma Prene' Ansell Medical or 'Neotech' Biogel.

• Latex-free equipment including masks and airways (plastic), endotracheal tubes (PVC), reservoir bags (neoprene), valves (silicon), IVI tubing, bellows, and circuits.

• Latex-free (or glass) syringes.

• Latex-free (or Teflon) intravenous cannulas.

• Barrier protection for placement between latex-containing items and the patient's skin (e.g. Webril).

• Drugs for treatment of anaphylaxis and latex-free resuscitation equipment.

Further reading

Kam PC, Lee MS (1997). Latex allergy: an emerging clinical and occupational health problem. *Anaesthesia*, **52**, 570–5.

Woods JA, Lambert S (1997). Natural rubber latex allergy: spectrum, diagnostic approach, and therapy. *Journal of Emergency Medicine*, **15**, 71–85.

Anaesthesia for drug misusing patients

General points

* In the United Kingdom around 1in 4 of the population aged over 16 has taken an illegal drug at some stage (10 million people).
* Misuse of street drugs is not isolated to inner cities and areas of social deprivation.
* Consider drug misuse in all patients requiring emergency surgery and anaesthesia. An accurate drug history is unlikely to be forthcoming.
* Drug misuse may contribute to a reduced conscious level even if other causes are present (especially trauma).
* Drug addicts are exposed to high risks of infective complications associated with intravenous drug abuse. HIV (6% in London) and viral hepatitis (up to 60%) are commonest. Bacterial endocarditis is rare but serious, and associated with pulmonary abscesses, embolic phenomena from vegetations, and vasculitis.
* Drugs in common use fall into four groups (see table). Combinations of drugs are common, often with alcohol.

Street drugs in common use

Drug	Clinical signs
Cannabis	Tachycardia, abnormal affect (e.g. euphoria, anxiety, panic or psychosis), poor memory and fatigue (chronic use)
Stimulants—cocaine, amphetamines, ecstasy	Tachycardia, labile blood pressure, excitement, delirium, hallucinations, hyperreflexia, tremors, convulsions, mydriasis, sweating, hyperpyrexia exhaustion, coma
Hallucinogens—LSD, phencyclidine, ketamine	Sympathomimetic, weakly analgesic, altered judgement and perceptions, toxic psychosis, dissociative anaesthesia
Opioids—morphine, heroin, opium	Euphoria, respiratory depression, hypotension, bradycardia constipation pinpoint pupils, coma

Anaesthesia

* High index of suspicion—especially in trauma.
* Difficult venous access—intravenous drug users may be able to direct you to a patent vein. May need central venous cannulation or cut-down for relatively minor procedures. Consider gas induction.
* Take full precautions against infection risk.
* Plan postoperative analgesia with patient preoperatively—see below.
* Resistance to opioids.

Opioid misusing patient

- Patients who are misusing opioids should expect the same quality of analgesia as other patients. Combinations of regional nerve blocks and NSAIDs may avoid the need for opioids.
- If opioids are the only method of providing analgesia they should be administered in the same way as for normal patients with doses titrated to effect (see p. 988 for a suitable dosing regime).
- A small group of 'ex-addicts' will have great fears about being prescribed opioids if they have been 'cured' of their addiction. This should not become an obstacle to treating postoperative pain, but opioids should clearly not be given without first obtaining consent.
- Do not attempt detoxification perioperatively! Opioid addicted surgical patients should be supported by specialist addiction services during the perioperative period (usually contactable via the local psychiatric services).

Cocaine and crack cocaine

- Cocaine toxicity is mediated by central and peripheral adrenergic stimulation. Presenting symptoms include tachycardia, hypertension, aortic dissection, arrhythmias, accelerated coronary artery disease, coronary spasm, infarction, and sudden death. Intracerebral vasospasm can lead to stroke, rigidity, hyperreflexia, and hyperthermia. Inhalation of cocaine can cause alveolar haemorrhage or pulmonary oedema.
- Psychiatric symptoms range from a feeling of elation and enhanced physical strength to full toxic paranoid psychosis.
- Patients needing surgery following ingestion of cocaine may need intensive care management whilst they are stabilized. Most of the life-threatening side-effects of cocaine are due to vasospasm and can be reversed using combinations of vasodilators, antiarrhythmic agents and alpha/beta-blockers titrated against effect using full invasive monitoring.
- Combination local anaesthetic/vasoconstrictors (or any vasopressor) should be avoided. Tachycardia or hypertensive crisis may result. If vasopressors are required in theatre use very small doses and titrate against response.
- Intra-arterial injections of cocaine have lead to critical limb and organ ischaemia. Successful treatment has included regional plexus blockade, intravenous heparin, stellate ganglion block, intra-arterial vasodilators or urokinase, and early fasciotomy.

Ecstasy (3,4, methylenedioxymethamphetamine (MDMA))

- Approximately 20 people die from taking ecstasy annually in the United Kingdom.
- Hyperthermia (>39 °C), disseminated intravascular coagulation, and dehydration are common features.
- Hyperthermia has been linked to a combination of dehydration and hyperactivity. Excessive ADH release may also cause hyponatraemia leading to coma. Treatment involves carefully monitored fluid and electrolyte replacement.

Further reading

Cheng DCH (1994). The perioperative care of cocaine abusing patients. *Canadian Journal of Anaesthesia*, **41**, 883–7.

Anaesthesia and chronic alcohol abuse

Anaesthetists may assist in the management of patients who have ingested alcohol acutely or chronically:

* trauma (vehicle related, violence, domestic accidents, child abuse)
* complications of drinking (coma, GI bleeding, portal hypertension, pancreatitis)
* unrelated surgical procedures in alcoholics.

Physical complications of alcohol abuse

* Acute intoxication and coma. Blood alcohol concentration >400 mg/ 100 ml risks respiratory arrest and carries a 5% mortality.
* Alcoholic liver disease. Earliest form is reversible fatty liver progressing to alcoholic hepatitis, characterized by abdominal pain, weight loss, jaundice, and fever. Histological changes can be reversed by abstinence. Alcoholic cirrhosis is characterized by jaundice, ascites, portal hypertension, and hepatic failure. Cirrhosis is irreversible but abstinence may result in stabilization and increased life expectancy.
* Pancreatitis.
* Upper gastrointestinal bleeding—gastritis, erosive gastric ulcers, and Mallory–Weiss oesophageal tears. Oesophageal varices in those with severe liver disease and portal hypertension.
* Cardiac arrhythmias including atrial fibrillation (may complicate binge drinking and chronic misuse). Ventricular arrhythmias.
* Ischaemic heart disease and hypertension. Modest alcohol intake may offer cardioprotection. Alcoholic cardiomyopathy is characterized by a dilated hypokinetic left ventricle with a decreased ejection fraction. Patients may present with congestive cardiac failure and oedema, exacerbated by low serum albumin. Cardiac failure is a feature of heavy alcohol ingestion.
* Hypoglycaemia may complicate acute alcohol intoxication, alcoholic liver disease, and pancreatic disease. More common in children and adolescents.
* Ketoacidosis may present after binge drinking in association with vomiting and fasting. Blood alcohol concentrations may not be elevated at the time.
* Convulsions are most commonly seen 7–48 h after cessation of drinking. Typically tonic–clonic with loss of consciousness. Several fits over a period of a few days are common. Normally self-limiting unless associated with trauma or sustained unconsciousness. Hypokalaemia and hypomagnesaemia predispose to convulsions. Exclude other causes such as intracranial bleeds, tumours, or abscesses.
* Anaemia (macrocytic—direct toxic alcohol effect; megaloblastic—folate deficiency; iron deficiency—poor diet, upper GI blood loss). Neutropenia (due to marrow toxicity or folate deficiency). Thrombocytopenia.
* Immunodeficiency with increased prevalence of respiratory infections (including TB).
* Skin diseases: psoriasis, eczema, rosacea, fungal infections, and acne are commoner in heavy drinkers.

Pharmacological considerations

Patients with acute alcohol ingestion are partially anaesthetized and reduced concentrations of volatile agents are required to produce anaesthesia (and respiratory and cardiac side-effects). Chronic exposure to alcohol induces tolerance to some anaesthetic agents. Serious liver pathology may result in depressed metabolism and drug clearance, which increases drug half-life (see liver failure p. 127).

Preoperative assessment

- Quantify excessive drinking and lifestyle. History of other drug misuse.
- Ask about weight loss and history of GI bleeding.
- Recurrent chest infections (smoking, repeated pulmonary aspiration, reduced ciliary activity).
- Examine for hypertension, cardiac failure, arrhythmias, fetor, spider naevi, ascites, jaundice, bruising, malnutrition, neglect, tremor, peripheral neuropathy, psychosis, encephalopathy, convulsions (withdrawal).

Investigations

- FBC (increased MCV, iron deficiency, bone marrow depression).
- Blood alcohol concentration.
- Glucose and electrolytes (hypokalaemia, hypernatraemia, and hypomagnesaemia).
- Liver enzymes: raised γ-glutamyl-transpeptidase and aminotransferases. Albumin is often reduced.
- Coagulation may be abnormal due to clotting factor deficiency (reduced synthesis of factors II, V, VII, X, and XIII).
- ECG: conduction defects, bifid T wave, ST changes (similar to digoxin changes), arrhythmias (commonly AF).
- Echocardiogram if suspicion of alcoholic cardiomyopathy: dilated LV, decreased ejection fraction, reduced LV function.
- Chest radiograph may show aspiration pneumonia, TB, or lung cancer.

Preoperative management

- Avoid non-emergency surgery in the presence of acute alcohol toxicity.
- If emergency surgical intervention is unavoidable, ensure adequate rehydration with careful attention to electrolyte and blood glucose disturbances. Give intravenous vitamins (e.g. Pabrinex slow IV twice daily for up to 7 days).
- Correct clotting abnormalities. Treat anaemia with appropriate transfusion.
- Patients with liver failure require intensive care if surgery is planned.

Anaesthetic management

- Patients with GI bleeding and cirrhosis are in danger of developing hepatic failure. Insert a gastric tube (with care in the presence of varices) to stop digestion of blood.
- Regional anaesthesia may avoid the need for large doses of sedative opioids (see below).

Postoperative management

- Anticipate alcohol withdrawal symptoms. Most patients can tolerate 24–48 h abstinence perioperatively. With major surgery it is often easiest not to complicate management by attempting alcohol withdrawal perioperatively.

- If problems occur, an infusion of ethanol 5% (add 50 g ethanol to 1 litre 0.9% saline or 5% dextrose) can be used to prevent alcohol withdrawal in the immediate perioperative period. Alternatively, oral or nasogastric administration of alcoholic drinks may be appropriate (within limits)!

- Alternatively treat with chlordiazepoxide (10–50 mg four times a day) if the patient can take oral medication or chlormethiazole if intravenous therapy is required. An infusion of chlormethiazole 0.8% (8 mg/ml) is initially given at 3–7.5 ml (24–60 mg)/min until the patient is lightly sleeping, and then reduced to 0.5–1 ml (4–8 mg)/min to maintain sedation. Overdosage with chlormethiazole can cause profound respiratory depression and should be used with great care if other sedatives/opioids are being used. Manage these patients in HDU. This should not be a reason to provide inadequate analgesia.

Further reading

Chick J (1993). Alcohol problems in the general hospital. *British Medical Bulletin*, **50**, 200–10.

Chapter 12
Rare syndromes

Graham Hocking

Aaskog–Scott syndrome

Characteristics: Cervical spine hypermobility/odontoid anomaly, mild/moderate short stature, cleft lip/palate, skin and skeletal anomalies/laxity, interstitial pulmonary disease.

Key points: Intubation may be difficult.

Reference: Teebi AS *et al.* (1993). Aarskog syndrome: report of a family with review and discussion of nosology. *American Joournal of Medical Genetics*, **46**, 501–9.

Achalasia of the cardia

Characteristics: Motor disorder of the distal two-thirds of the oesophagus, failure of relaxation, dysphagia and regurgitation, risk of malignant change.

Key points: Increased risk of gastric reflux.

Achondroplasia (see also p. 167)

Characteristics: Dwarfism, normal size trunk, short limbs, disproportionately large head, flat face, possible small larynx, bulging skull vault and kyphoscoliosis, spinal stenoses in the canal and foramen magnum can occur. See Dwarfism.

Key points: Possible difficult intubation, care on neck flexion (cord compression), central neural blocks may have unpredictable spread (use smaller amounts), increased risk of obstructive sleep apnoea.

References: Kalla GN et al. (1986). Anaesthetic management of achondroplasia. *British Journal of Anaesthesia*, 58, 117–19.

Wardall GJ, Frame WT (1990). Extradural anaesthesia for caesarian section in achondroplasia. *British Journal of Anaesthesia*, **64**, 367–70.

Acromegaly (see also p. 78)

Characteristics: Enlarged jaw/tongue/larynx, may have nerve entrapment syndromes, respiratory obstruction including sleep apnoea, diabetes mellitus, hypertension, cardiac failure, thyroid, and renal impairment.

Key points: Difficult intubation and maintenance of the airway, narrow cricoid ring may be present, associated organ dysfunction, perioperative glucose intolerance.

Reference: Seidman PA *et al.* (2000). Anaesthetic complications of acromegaly. *British Journal of Anaesthesia*, **84**, 179–82.

Albers–Schonberg disease (marble bones)

See Osteopetrosis.

Alagille's syndrome (syndromic bile duct paucity)

Characteristics: Paucity of interlobular bile ducts, chronic cholestasis, cardiac/musculoskeletal/ocular/facial abnormalities.

Key points: Coagulopathy, pathological fractures, retinopathy, neuropathies (vitamin deficiencies). Pretreat with vitamin K. Splenomegaly may cause thrombocytopenia. Full CVS assessment (stenosis/ hypoplasia common). Sagittal spinal cleft, cerebellar ataxia, document pre-existing peripheral neuropathy, gastric reflux risk (abdominal distension).

Reference: Choudhry DK *et al.* (1998). The Alagille's syndrome and its anaesthetic considerations. *Paediatric Anaesthesia*, **8**, 79–82.

Albright's osteodystrophy (pseudohypoparathyroidism)

Characteristics: Resistance of target tissues to parathyroid hormone. Short

stature, round face, short neck, diabetes mellitus, hypocalcaemia.
Key points: Neuromuscular irritability and convulsions can occur.

Albright's syndrome

Characteristics: Defective regulation of cAMP, multiple unilateral bone lesions, skin pigmentation, sexual precocity in females, bony deformity (including skull) and fractures, spinal cord compression. Acromegaly, thyrotoxicosis, Cushing's syndrome may coexist. See Acromegaly.
Key points: Identify endocrine abnormalities, may need larger than expected ETT. Cardiac arrhythmias may occur, bony deformity may complicate regional blocks.
Reference: Langer RA *et al.* (1995). Anesthetic considerations in McCune–Albright syndrome: case report with literature review. *Anesthesia and Analgesia*, **80**, 1236–9.

Alport syndrome

Characteristics: Hereditary nephropathy, predominantly affecting males, characterized by nephritis progressing to renal failure. Other features include sensorineural deafness, myopia, and thrombocytopenia with giant forms of platelets.
Key points: Check renal function and clotting, hypertension.
Reference: Kashtan CE *et al.* (1999). Alport syndrome: an inherited disorder of renal, ocular, and cochlear basement membranes. *Medicine*, **78**, 338–60.

Alstrom syndrome

Characteristics: Obesity from infancy, nystagmus, sensitivity to light, progressive visual impairment with blindness by age 7, sensorineural hearing loss, diabetes mellitus and renal failure in early adult life, cardiac disease.
Key points: Problems associated with obesity/organ dysfunction.
Reference: Russell-Eggitt LM *et al.* (1998). Alstrom syndrome: report of 22 cases and literature review. *Ophthalmology*, **105**, 1274–80.

Alveolar hypoventilation

Characteristics: Central hypoventilation due to midbrain lesion or severance of the spinal tracts from the midbrain (Ondine's curse). Periods of prolonged apnoea, hypoxia, hypercarbia (see p. 000 on sleep apnoea, etc.).
Key points: Abnormal respiratory drive, care with O_2 supplements if relying on hypoxic drive, re-establishing spontaneous ventilation may be difficult. Consider regional techniques, postoperative respiratory failure, cor pulmonale, polycythaemia, autonomic dysfunction.
References: Wiesel S, Fox GS (1990). Anaesthesia for the patient with central alveolar hypoventilation syndrome. *Canadian Journal of Anaesthesia*, **37**, 122–6.
Strauser LM *et al.* (1999). Anesthetic care for the child with congenital central alveolar hypoventilation syndrome (Ondine's curse). *Journal of Clinical Anesthesia*, **11**, 431–7.

Amyloidosis

Characteristics: Abnormal deposition of hyaline material in tissues. Macroglossia, unexpected cardiac or renal failure can occur, associated with other pathologies.
Key points: Assess to detect systems affected. Risk of postoperative organ failure.
Reference: Welch DB (1982). Anaesthesia and amyloidosis. *Anaesthesia*, **37**, 63–6.

Amyotonia congenita

See Spinal muscular atrophy.

Amyotrophic lateral sclerosis (see also p. 198)

Characteristics: Progressive degeneration of lower motor neurons, motor nuclei of the brainstem, descending pathway of the upper motor neurons. Atrophy and weakness involving most of the skeletal muscles including tongue, pharynx, larynx, and chest wall muscles. Fasciculation occurs. Sensation normal.

Key points: Impaired ventilation, altered response to muscle relaxants, aspiration risk (laryngeal incompetence), sensitive to respiratory depressants.

Reference: Rowland LP, Schneider NA (2001). Amyotrophic lateral sclerosis. *New England Journal of Medicine*, **344**, 1688–700.

Analbuminaemia

Characteristics: Deficiency of albumin.

Key points: Sensitivity to all protein-bound drugs. Titrate drugs carefully.

Reference: Dammacco F *et al.* (1980). Analbuminemia: report of a case and review of the literature. *Vox Sang*, **39**, 153–61.

Andersen's disease

See Glycogen storage disease IV.

Andersen's syndrome

Characteristics: Triad of potassium-sensitive periodic paralysis, ventricular arrhythmias, and dysmorphic features.

Key points: Long QT, spontaneous attacks of paralysis with acute changes in K^+, baseline level may be hypokalaemia/normokalaemia/ hyperkalaemia.

Reference: Sansone V *et al.* (1997). Andersen's syndrome: a distinct periodic paralysis. *Annals of Neurology*, **42**, 305–12.

Anhidrotic/hypohydrotic ectodermal dysplasia (Christ–Siemens–Touraine syndrome)

Characteristics: Characterized by hypodontia, hypotricosis, and hypohidrosis.

Key points: Difficult intubation, heat intolerance, recurrent cheat infections (poor mucus formation).

Reference: Sugi Y *et al.* (1999). Anesthetic management of a patient with hypohidrotic ectodermal dysplasia *Masui*, **48**, 888–90.

Ankylosing spondylitis (see also p. 163)

Characteristics: Asymmetric oligoarthropathy, total vertebral involvement, cardiomegaly, aortic regurgitation, cardiac conduction abnormalities, pulmonary fibrosis. Bamboo spine.

Key points: Difficult airway and central neural blockade.

References: Schelew BL, Vaghadia H (1996). Ankylosing spondylitis and neuraxial anaesthesia—a 10-year review. *Canadian Journal of Anaesthesia*, **43**, 65–8.

Wittmann FW, Ring PA (1986). Anaesthesia for hip replacement in ankylosing spondylitis. *Journal of the Royal Society of Medicine*, **79**, 457–9.

Antley–Bixler syndrome

Characteristics: Autosomal recessive disorder, multiple bone and cartilaginous abnormalities. Significant craniosynostosis, midface hypoplasia, choanal stenosis or atresia, femoral bowing, radiohumeral synostosis, multiple joint contractures. CVS, renal, and GI malformations have also been described.

Key points: Potential difficult airway, extremity deformities may complicate vascular access and positioning.

Reference: LeBard SE, Thiemann LJ (1998). Antley–Bixer syndrome: a case report and discussion. *Paediatric Anaesthesia*, **8**, 89–91.

Apert's syndrome

Characteristics: Craniosynostosis, high forehead, maxillary hypoplasia, relative mandibular prognathism, cervical synostosis, visceral malformations, congential heart anomalies.

Key points: Airway difficulties, assess for other organ involvement and raised ICP.

References: Ciceri G *et al.* (1997). Anesthesia in Apert syndrome. *Minerva Anestesiol.*, **63**, 167–9.

Nargozian C (1991). Apert syndrome. Anesthetic management. *Clinics in Plastic Surgery*, **18**, 227–30.

Arnold–Chiari malformation

Characteristics: Group of congenital hindbrain anomalies causing downward displacement of pons and medulla with variable neurological sequelae.

Key points: Preoperative assessment of CNS function and response to neck movement and ICP. Careful neuroanaesthetic (usual potential problems).

Reference: Semple DA, McClure JH (1996). Arnold–Chiari malformation in pregnancy. *Anaesthesia*, **51**, 580–2.

Arthrogryposis (congenital contractures)

Characteristics: Skin and subcutaneous tissue abnormalities, contracture deformities, micrognathia, cervical spine and jaw stiffness. 10% have associated congenital heart disease.

Key points: Difficult airway and venous access, sensitive to thiopental, hypermetabolic response is probably not MH.

References: Hopkins PM *et al.* (1991). Hypermetabolism in arthrogryposis multiplex congenita. *Anaesthesia*, **46**, 374–5.

Nguyen NH *et al.* (2000). Anaesthetic management for patients with arthrgryposis multiplex congenita and severe micrognathia. *Journal of Clinical Anesthesia*, **12**, 227–30.

Asplenia syndrome

Characteristics: Complex congenital heart defects, asplenia, and visceral anomalies.

Key points: Cardiac failure, frequently hiatus hernia and reflux, recurrent pneumonias.

Reference: Uchida K *et al.* (1992). Anesthetic management of an infant with a single ventricle (asplenia syndrome) for non-cardiac surgery. *Masui*, **41**, 1793–7.

Ataxia-telangiectasia

Characteristics: Progressive cerebellar ataxia, conjunctival telangiectases, progressive neurological degeneration. Recurrent chest and sinus infections, malignancies (leukaemias), sensitive to X-rays/radiotherapy (cellular damage), premature aging.

Key points: Recurrent chest infections, bronchiectasis.

Reference: Gatti RA *et al.* (1991). Ataxia-telangiectasia: an interdisciplinary approach to pathogenesis. *Medicine*, 70, 99–117.

Axenfeld–Reiger syndrome

Characteristics: Ocular and dental defects, maxillary hypoplasia, heart defects, short stature, mental deficiency

Key points: Potential airway problems.

Reference: Asai T *et al.* (1998). Difficult airway management in a baby with Axenfeld–Reiger syndrome [letter]. *Paediatric Anaesthesia*, 8, 444.

Bartter syndrome

Characteristics: Growth retardation, hypertrophy and hyperplasia of the juxtaglomerular apparatus, ADH antagonism by protaglandins, hyperaldosteronism, hypokalaemic alkalosis, normal BP, diminished response to vasopressors, platelet abnormalities.

Key points: Maintain CVS stability, control serum K^+, meticulous fluid balance, caution with renally excreted drugs. Central neural anaesthesia may be hazardous (stature, clotting, pressor response).

Reference: Abston PA, Priano LL (1981). Bartter's syndrome: anesthetic implications based on pathophysiology and treatment. *Anesthesia and Analgesia*, 60, 764–6.

Behçet's syndrome

Characteristics: Chronic multisystem vasculitis of unknown aetiology. Diagnosed by triad of recurring iritis, mouth ulceration, genital ulceration. Vasculitis may involve other organ systems.

Key points: Possible altered fibrinolysis, previous oral ulceration/ scarring may complicate airway management, full assessment of other organ function, minimize needle punctures (diffuse inflammatory skin reaction), autonomic hyper-reflexia may occur with spinal cord involvement.

References: Lee LA (2001). Behcet disease. *Seminars in Cutaneous Medicine and Surgery*, 20, 53–7.

Turner ME (1972). Anaesthetic difficulties associated with Bechet's syndrome. *British Journal of Anaesthesia*, 44, 100.

Beckwith–Wiedemann syndrome (infantile gigantism)

Characteristics: Macroglossia, microcephaly, omphalocele, perinatal/postnatal gigantism, neonatal hypoglycaemia (hyperinsulinism), possible congenital heart disease (ASD/VSD/PDA/ hypoplastic LV).

Key points: Abnormal airway anatomy, congenital heart disease, and severe hypoglycaemia. Extubate awake.

References: Suan C *et al.* (1996). Anaesthesia and the Beckwith– Wiedemann syndrome. *Paediatric Anaesthia*, 6, 231–3.

Gurkowski MA, Rasch DK (1989). Anesthetic considerations for Beckwith–Wiedemann syndrome. *Anesthesiology*, 70, 711–12.

Bernard–Soulier syndrome (giant platelet syndrome)

Characteristics: Congenital lack of membrane glycoprotein GP1b, reduced numbers of huge platelets, prolonged bleeding time.

Key points: Severe bleeding tendency, possibly improves with age, platelet infusions may be needed.

Blackfan–Diamond syndrome (congenital red-cell aplasia)

Characteristics: Congenital hypolastic anaemia, growth retardation, congestive cardiac failure.

Key points: Hepatosplenomegaly (may reduce FRC), hypersplenism, thrombocytopenia.

Reference: Willig TN *et al.* (2000). Diamond–Blackfan anemia. *Current Opinion in Haematology*, 7, 85–94.

Bland–White–Garland syndrome

Characteristics: Anomalous origin of left coronary artery from the pulmonary trunk, chronic myocardial ischaemia, subendocardial fibrosis, LV dilatation, valvular insufficiency (papillary muscle damage), congestive cardiac failure.

Key points: Perioperative myocardial failure, often difficult to wean from ventilation.

Reference: Kleinschmidt S *et al.* (1996). The Bland–White–Garland syndrome. Clinical picture and anaesthesiological management. *Paediatric Anaesthesia*, 6, 65–8.

Bloom's syndrome

Characteristics: Rare autosomal recessive disorder due to chromosome breakage and recombination, short stature, photosensitive, facial telangiectasic erythema, predisposition to malignant diseases.

Key points: Potential difficulties with mask fit and laryngoscopy, limit X-rays to minimum (may damage cells).

Reference: Aono J *et al.* (1992). Anesthesia for a patient with Bloom's syndrome. *Masui*, 41, 255–7.

Buerger's disease (thromboangiitis obliterans)

Characteristics: Peripheral vascular disease with ulceration, Raynaud's phenomenon, hyperhidrosis, bronchitis and emphysema.

Key points: Non-invasive BP may over-read.

Bullous cystic lung disease

Characteristics: Non-communicating lung cysts may be more compliant than normal lung.

Key points: Risk of rupture with IPPV causing pneumothorax. Avoid N2O. High-frequency jet ventilation has been used successfully.

Reference: Normandale JP, Feneck RO (1985). Bullous cystic lung disease. *Anaesthesia*, 40, 1182–5.

Burkitt's lymphoma

Characteristics: Undifferentiated lymphoblastic lymphoma most commonly affecting the jaw (also abdominal organs, breasts, testes).

Key points: May be difficult intubation.

Reference: Palmer CD *et al.* (1998). Anaesthetic management of a child with Burkitt's lymphoma of the larynx. *Paediatric Anaesthesia*, 8, 506–9.

Cantrell's pentalogy

Characteristics: Defect of the supraumbilical abdominal wall, agenesis of the lower part of the sternum and anterior portion of the diaphragm, absence of diaphragmatic part pericardium, cardiac malformation (VSD/ASD).

Key points: Check for right to left shunting, avoid pressure to lower thorax/abdomen, lungs may be hypoplastic.

Reference: Laloyaux P *et al.* (1998). Anaesthetic management of a prematurely born infant with Cantrell's pentalogy. *Paediatric Anaesthesia*, 8, 163–6.

Carpenter's syndrome

Characteristics: Cranial synostosis with small mandible, congenital heart disease (PDA/VSD), obesity, umbilical hernia and mental retardation, cerebrospinal malformations (narrowed foramen magnum, hypoplastic posterior fossa, kinked spinal cord).

Key points: Difficult intubation and system anomalies.

Reference: Islek I *et al.* (1998). Carpenter syndrome: report of two siblings. *Clinical Dysmorphology*, 7, 185–9.

Central core myopathy

See Congenital myopathy.

Cerebrocostomandibular syndrome

Characteristics: Micrognathia, cleft palate, rib defects/microthorax, mental deficiency, early death from respiratory complications.

Key points: Difficult intubation, tracheal anomalies.

Reference: Smith KG, Sekar KC (1985). Cerebrocostomandibular syndrome. Case report and literature review. *Clinical Pediatrics*, 24, 223–5.

Chagas' disease (American trypanosomiasis)

Characteristics: Many assymptomatic cases, malaise, anorexia, fever, unilateral oedema, hepatomegaly, cardiac failure, chronic myocarditis, megacolon/megaoesophagus.

Key points: Gastric reflux risk and associated organ dysfunction.

Reference: Saraiva RA *et al.* (1980). Cardiovascular response to anaesthesia in Chagas' disease. *Tropical Doctor*, 10, 62–5.

Charcot–Marie–Tooth disease (peroneal muscular atrophy)

Characteristics: Chronic peripheral neuromuscular denervation with subsequent atrophy, spinal and lower limb deformities, hyperkalaemia, may affect respiratory muscles (restrictive pattern).

Key points: Evidence suggests MH risk is low, suxamethonium should probably be avoided, pulmonary complications.

Reference: Antognini JF (1992). Anaesthesia for Charcot–Marie–Tooth disease: a review of 86 cases. *Canadian Journal of Anaesthesia*, 39, 398–400.

CHARGE association

Characteristics: Coloboma, Heart anomaly, choanal Atresia, Retardation, Genital, and Ear anomalies.

Key points: Difficult intubation (micrognathia), look for congenital heart anomaly.

Reference: Davenport SLH *et al.* (1986). The spectrum of clinical features in CHARGE syndrome. *Clinical Genetics*, 29, 298–310.

Chediak–Higashi syndrome (immunodeficiency, with some albinism)

Characteristics: Autosomal albinism, photophobia, nystagmus, weakness, tremor, thrombocytopenia.

Key points: Susceptible to infection, bleeding potential.

Reference: Ulsoy H *et al.* (1995). Anesthesia in Che'diak–Higashi syndrome—case report. *Middle East Journal of Anesthesiology*, **13**, 101–5.

Cherubism

Characteristics: Tumourous mandibular and maxillary lesions, intraoral masses.

Key points: Difficult intubation, profuse bleeding, can get acute respiratory distress, tracheostomy may be needed.

Reference: Maydew RP, Berry FA (1985). Cherubism with difficult laryngoscopy and tracheal intubation. *Anesthesiology*, **62**, 810–12.

Chronic granulomatous disease

Characteristics: Rare genetically transmitted disorder, recurrent life-threatening infections with catalase-positive micro-organisms, excessive inflammatory reactions lead to granuloma formation, multiple organ system involvement including pulmonary granulomata.

Key points: Regurgitation and aspiration risk (GI granulomata), long-term prophylactic antibiotics.

Reference: Wall RT *et al.* (1990). Anesthetic considerations in patients with chronic granulomatous disease. *Journal of Clinical Anesthesia*, **2**, 306–11.

Cockayne's syndrome

Characteristics: Rare autosomal recessive condition, failure of DNA repair, dysmorphic dwarf, mentally retarded infant/child. (See Dwarf.)

Key points: Problems with airway management, increased risk of gastric aspiration, hypertension, hepatic deficiencies, osteoporosis, deafness, blindness, and other effects of premature ageing (see Progeria) may be encountered.

References: Wooldridge WJ *et al.* (1996). Anaesthesia for Cockayne syndrome. Three case reports. *Anaesthesia*, **51**, 478–81.

Congenital adrenal hyperplasia (adrenogenital syndrome)

Characteristics: Congenital disorders leading to defects in cortisol biosynthesis, increased ACTH and disordered androgens, mineralocorticoids.

Key points: May mimic pyloric stenosis in neonate, electrolyte abnormalities, adequate perioperative fluid and steroid therapy.

Congenital analgesia

Characteristics: Rare hereditary disorder leading to self-mutilation, defective thermoregulation.

Key points: Careful positioning, vasomotor control and possible sensitivity to anaesthetic drugs.

Reference: Layman PR (1986). Anaesthesia for congenital analgesia. A case report. *Anaesthesia*, **41**, 395–7.

Congenital myopathy (central core disease) (see also p. 203)

Characteristics: Non-progressive extremity weakness (lower > upper), difficulty rising from sitting, increased lumbar lordosis, most test positive for MH in vitro, ptosis.

Key points: Avoid MH trigger factors. Ventilatory weakness, sensitive to muscle relaxants.

Reference: Shuaib A *et al.* (1987). Central core disease. *Medicine*, **66**, 389.

Conradi–Hunermann syndrome (chondrodysplasia punctata)

Characteristics: Epiphyseal calcifications, short stature, hypertelorism, saddle nose, short neck, tracheal stenosis and scoliosis, renal and congenital heart disease.

Key points: Ventilatory failure due to airway and thoracic deformities, renal impairment, skin protection (use patient's creams/ padding), attention to thermoregulation (lose heat quicker).

Reference: Yorozu T *et al.* (1989). Anaesthetic management of a patient with
    Conradi's syndrome (chondrodysplasia punctata). A case report. *Masui*, **38**, 1092–5.

Core syndrome

See Congenital myopathy.

Cornelia de Lange syndrome

Characteristics: Duplication/partial trisomy chromosome 3, psychomotor retardation, skeletal craniofacial deformities, VSD, GI anomalies.

Key points: Cardiorespiratory function, possible difficult airway, gastric reflux risk, susceptible to infections, possible increased MH risk.

Reference: Corsini LM *et al.* (1998). Anaesthetic implications of Cornelia de Lange
    syndrome. *Paediatric Anaesthesia*, **8**, 159–61.

Costello syndrome

Characteristics: Mental and growth retardation, cardiac arrhythmias, cardio-myopathy, talipes, scoliosis. (See Cutis laxa.)

Key points: Gastric reflux, arrhythmias.

Reference: Dearlove O, Harper N (1997). Costello syndrome [letter]. *Paediatric
    Anaesthesia*, **7**, 476–7.

CREST syndrome

Characteristics: Form of scleroderma, widespread necrotizing angiitis with granulomas, Calcinosis, Raynaud's phenomenon, oesophageal dysfunction, Sclerodactyly, Telangiectasis.

Key points: Multiple organ involvement, airway difficulties, gastric reflux risk, arrhythmias, nerve compression syndromes, contractures, pulmonary fibrosis.

Cretinism

Characteristics: Congenital hypothyroidism, neurological and intellectual damage, muscle weakness, cardiomyopathy.

Key points: Intubation problems (macroglossia), sensitive to anaesthetic drugs, respiratory complications, steroid cover, glucose and electrolyte abnormalities.

Creutzfeldt–Jacob disease (CJD) (see also p. 518)

Characteristics: Progressively fatal encephalopathy of infective origin, seizures, variable neurological signs, multiple brain cavities (status spongiosis). (See also New variant Creutzfeldt–Jacob disease.)

Key points: Muscular incoordination, malnutrition

Reference: MacMurdo SD *et al.* (1984). Precautions in the anesthetic management
    of a patient with Creutzfield–Jacob disease. *Anesthesiology*, **60**, 590–2.

Cri-du-chat syndrome

Characteristics: Inherited disease resulting in mental retardation, abnormal cry (due to abnormal larynx), laryngomalacia, microcephaly, micrognathia, macroglossia, spasticity, congenital heart disease (30%).

Key points: Potential airway problems, long curved epiglottis, narrow diamond shaped epiglottis, hypotonia (possible airway obstruction by soft tissues), temperature instability.

Reference: Brislin RP *et al.* (1995). Anaesthetic considerations for the patient with cri du chat syndrome. *Paediatric Anaesthesia*, 5, 139–41.

Crouzon's disease

Characteristics: Craniosynostosis, hydrocephalus, raised ICP, maxillary hypoplasia, mandibular prognathism, prominent nose, coarctation can occur.

Key points: Airway difficulties, postoperative respiratory obstruction. Assess for other organ involvement and ICP. Correction procedures can bleed profusely.

Reference: Payne JF, Cranston AJ (1995). Postoperative airway problems in a child with Crouzon's syndrome. *Paediatric Anaesthesia*, 5, 331–3.

Cutis laxa (elastic degeneration)

Characteristics: Defective elastin crosslinking probably related to copper deficiency, extreme laxity of facial and trunk skin, no retraction after stretching, fragile skin and blood vessels.

Key points: Pendulous pharyngeal/laryngeal mucosa may obstruct airway, respiratory infections and emphysema common, careful positioning.

Cystic hygroma

Characteristics: Benign multilocular lymphatic tumour of neck/oral cavity/tongue causing local pressure symptoms, including airway compromise.

Key points: Potential airway problems. Partially obstructed airway in awake patient may totally obstruct on induction, oral intubation often impossible (enlarged tongue), tracheostomy may be complicated with submandibular involvement.

Reference: Sharma S *et al.* (1994). Cystic hygroma: anaesthetic considerations and review. *Singapore Medical Journal*, 35, 529–31.

Dandy–Walker syndrome

Characteristics: Congenital obstruction to foraminae of Luschka/ Magendi. Progressive head enlargement, hydocephalus, craniofacial abnormalities, cardiac, renal, skeletal malformations, altered medullary respiratory control.

Key points: Usually require CSF shunt, control ICP, risk of respiratory failure, postoperatively consider ICU (recurrent apnoea).

Reference: Ewart MC, Oh TE (1990). The Dandy–Walker syndrome. Relevance to anaesthesia and intensive care. *Anaesthesia*, 45, 646–8.

Delleman syndrome (oculocerebrocutaneous syndrome)

Characteristics: Somatic mutation of autosomal dominant gene only compatible with life in mosaic form. Multiple brain, skin, eye, bony abnormalities.

Key points: Determine severity of abnormalities, seizures can occur under general anaesthetic (consider if there are unexplained autonomic changes), aspiration pneumonitis, hydrocephalus, vertebral anomalies, possible difficult intubation, postoperative apnoea monitoring.

Reference: Sadhasivam S, Subramaniam R (1998). Delleman syndrome: anesthetic implications. *Anesthesia and Analgesia*, 87, 553–5.

Dermatomyositis (polymyositis)

Characteristics: Inflammatory myopathy, skeletal muscle weakness may result in dysphagia/aspiration/recurrent pneumonia, myocarditis and occult cancer occur.

Key points: Restricted mouth opening, enhanced/delayed effect of muscle relaxant, pulmonary complications (aspiration pneumonia and lung fibrosis), cardiomyopathy (arrhythmias and cardiac failure), anaemia, steroid supplementation.

Reference: Ganta R *et al.* (1988). Anaesthesia and acute dermatomyositis/ polymyositis. *British Journal of Anaesthesia*, **60**, 854–8.

DiGeorge syndrome (velocardiofacial syndrome 'CATCH 22' syndrome)

Characteristics: Cardiac abnormalities, Abnormal facies, Thymic hypoplasia, Cleft palate, Hypocalcaemia , 22affected chromosome.

Key points: Immune deficiency, recurrent chest infections, upper airway problems/stridor, gastro-oesophageal reflux, hypo-tonia, obstructive apnoea, hyperventilation induced seizures (low calcium).

References: Flashburg MH et al. (1983). Anesthesia for surgery in an infant with DiGeorge syndrome. *Anesthesiology*, 58, 479–81.

Pike AC, Super M (1997). Velocardiofacial syndrome. *Postgraduate Medical Journal*, **73**, 771–5.

Dubowitz' syndrome

Characteristics: Retarded growth, microcephaly, craniofacial deformations and dysmorphia of the extremities. Psychomotor development varies between normal and retarded, thin hair, cryptorchism, hyperactivity.

Key points: Possible difficult intubation, thorough assessment since the condition may involve the cutaneous, ocular, dental, digestive, musculoskeletal, urogenital, cardiovascular, neurological, haematological, and immune systems.

References: Gomirato G (1992). Dubowitz' syndrome with special characteristics. *Panminerva Medica*, 34, 141–4.

Tsukahara M, Opitz JM (1996). Dubowitz syndrome: review of 141 cases including 36 previously unreported patients. *American Journal of Medical Genetics*, **63**, 277–89.

Dwarfism

Characteristics: Manifestation of over 55 syndromes. Disproportionate short stature (cf. 'midgets'—proportionate). Atlantoaxial instability, spinal stenosis and/or compression, difficult airway management, thoracic dystrophy (ventilatory problems and frequent pneumonias), scoliosis and kyphoscoliosis, congenital cardiac disease.

Key points: Evaluate and protect the cervical spine, document any pre-existing neurological deficit if central blockade considered, difficult airway, ventilatory difficulty and weaning.

Reference: Walts LF *et al.* (1975). Anaesthesia for dwarfs and other patients of pathological small stature. *Canadian Anaesthesia Society Journal*, 22, 703.

Dygue–Melchior–Clausen's syndrome

Characteristics: Autosomal recessive, mental retardation, small stature (short vertebral column) with thoracic kyphosis, protruding sternum, reduced articular mobility, microcephaly.

Key points: Difficult intubation.

Reference: Schlaepfer R (1981). Dyggve–Melchior–Clausen syndrome. *Case report and review of the literature Helvetica Paediatrica Acta*, **36**, 543–59.

Dysautonomia (Riley–Day syndrome)

Characteristics: Inherited disease, abnormally active parasympathetic nervous system with sporadic sympathetic storms, highly emotional, bouts of sweating, unexplained fluctuations in BP.

Key points: Autonomic instability, salivation, poor thermoregulation, regurgitation. Sensitivity to respiratory depressants with reduced hypercapnic drive (need IPPV). Reduced pain sensitivity. Volatile agents can cause hypotension and bradycardia.

References: Axelrod FB *et al.* (1988). Anesthesia in familial dysautonomia. *Anaesthesiology*, **68**, 631–5.

Challands JF, Facer EK (1998). Epidural anaesthesia and familial dysautonomia (the Riley–Day syndrome). Three case reports. *Paediatric Anaesthesia*, **8**, 83–8.

Eaton–Lambert syndrome

See Myasthenic syndrome.

Ebstein's abnormality (tricuspid valve disease)

Characteristics: Congenital heart defect, downward displacement of deformed tricuspid valve, atrialization of RV, may be no obvious clinical signs.

Key points: Risk of SVT during induction.

Reference: Takahashi K *et al.* (1992). Anesthesia for cesarean section in a patient with Ebstein's anomaly. *Masui*, **41**,1163–7.

Edward's syndrome (trisomy 18)

Characteristics: Craniofacial anomalies, congenital heart disease, mental/physical delays, only less severe cases survive.

References: Bailey C, Chung R (1992). Use of the laryngeal mask airway in a patient with Edward's syndrome [letter]. *Anaesthesia*, **47**, 713.

Miller C, Mayhew JF (1998). Edward's syndrome (trisomy 18) [letter]. *Paediatric Anaesthesia*, **8**, 441–2.

Ehlers–Danlos syndrome

Characteristics: Group of conditions arising from defective cross-linking of collagen. Variable features depending upon the tissue distribution of different collagens, extensible fragile skin, joint laxity and hypermobility, recurrent dislocations, prolonged or spontaneous bleeding, rupture of cerebral and other vessels, bowel perforation, ocular abnormalities, kyphoscoliosis, spontaneous pneumothorax.

Key points: Careful positioning and padding, beware of undiagnosed pneumothorax, intubation may cause severe tracheal bruising.

References: Dolan P *et al.* (1980). Anesthetic considerations for Ehlers–Danlos syndrome. *Anesthesiology*, **52**, 266–9.

Vicente Guillen R *et al.* (1986). Anesthesia in Ehlers–Danlos syndrome. *Rev. Esp. Anestesiol. Reanim.*, **33**, 446–7.

Eisenmenger's syndrome (pulmonary hypertension, VSD, right ventricular failure)

Characteristics: Cyanotic congenital heart disease, usually uncorrectable, pulmonary hypertension/VSD/RV failure, medical therapy may prolong life (thirties), high mortalilty in pregnant patients due to reductions in SVR and increased shunt (termination has been advocated).

Key points: Prevent increases in R to L shunt (caused by e.g. increased PVR/reduced SVR such as from volatiles, histamine release, etc.), avoid dehydration, consider pancuronium (sympathetic stimulation beneficial), air from infusions/syringes can cross VSD, risk of asystole under GA, slow equilibration of inhaled gases.

Reference: Foster JM, Jones RM (1984). The anaesthetic management of the Eisenmenger syndrome. *Annals of the Royal College of Surgeons of England*, **66**, 353–5.

Ellis–Van Creveld disease (chondroectodermal dysplasia)

Characteristics: Dwarfism, pulmonary/cardiac (ASD/VSD/single atrium) abnormalities, polydactyly. (See Dwarfism.)

Key points: Underlying anomalies, respiratory failure.

Reference: Wu CL, Litman RS (1994). Anaesthetic management for a child with the Ellis–van Creveld syndrome. A case report. *Paediatric Anaesthesia*, **4**, 335–7.

Epidermolysis bullosa

Characteristics: Rare autosomal recessive disease. Extreme bullae formation of skin and mucosa, typical dystrophic nails and flexion contractures of the joints lead to deformities. Carious teeth and small mouth caused by scarred contractures of the lips are characteristic.

Key points: Avoid trauma to skin and mucous membranes (e.g. care with positioning, electrodes, tape, padding below BP cuff, longest acceptable inflation interval), keep upper airway manipulations to a minimum, consider postoperative ICU.

References: Hagen R, Langenberg C (1988). Anaesthetic management in patients with epidermolysis bullosa dystrophica. *Anaesthesia*, **43**, 482–5.

Yasui Y et al. (1995). Anesthesia in a patient with epidermolysis bullosa. *Masui*, **44**, 260–2.

Erythema multiforme

Characteristics: Acute self-limiting condition of skin and mucous membranes, concentric rings of erythematous papules/bullae (epidermal necrosis); severe cases (Stevens–Johnson syndrome) can be fatal.

Key points: Beware postintubation laryngeal oedema, consider whether the cause is drug related.

Fabry's syndrome

Characteristics: Alpha-galactosidase deficiency leading to deposition of glycosphingolipid in many organs, ischaemic heart disease, neurological disorder, renal failure, hypohidrosis.

Key points: Assess CVS, CNS, and renal condition. Document existing neurological deficit prior to regional techniques. Monitor and control core temperature.

Reference: Watanabe H (1995). The anesthetic management of a patient with Fabry's disease. *Masui*, **44**, 1258–60.

Factor V Leiden mutation

Characteristics: Resistance to anticoagulant effect of protein C.

Key points: High risk of PE, careful control of anticoagulation.

Familial dysautonomia

See Dysautonomia.

Familial periodic paralysis

Characteristics: Muscular weakness related to K$^+$ changes (absolute K$^+$ value is not important).
Key points: See Hypokalaemic familial periodic paralysis.
Reference: Ahlawat SK, Sachdev A (1999). Hypokalaemic paralysis. *Postgraduate Medical Journal*, 75, 193–7.

Fanconi's anaemia

Characteristics: Congenital aplastic anaemia, defective DNA regeneration.
Key points: Sensitive to X-rays, limit exposure.

Fanconi syndrome (renal tubular acidosis)

Characteristics: Generalized defect in proximal tubular function resulting in phosphate wasting, glycosuria, aminoaciduria, bicarbonate wasting, excess potassium loss, polydipsia, polyuria, muscle weakness and acidosis, dwarfing, and osteomalacia. Usually secondary to other disease.
Key points: Correct and maintain careful fluid/electrolyte balance.
Reference: Joel M, Rosales JK (1981). Fanconi syndrome and anesthesia. *Anesthesiology*, 55, 455–6.

Farber's disease (lipogranulomatosis)

Characteristics: Ceramidase deficiency, hoarse cry, painful swollen joints, periarticular nodules, pulmonary infiltrates, mental handicap, thickened heart valves, cardiomyopathy, renal/hepatic failure, usually die by 2 years (airway problems).
Key points: Difficult intubation, laryngeal granulomata may complicate intubation, postextubation laryngeal oedema/bleeding, risk of postoperative renal/hepatic failure. Anatomical neck deformity may complicate urgent tracheostomy.
Reference: Asada A *et al.* (1994). The anesthetic implications of a patient with Farber's lipogranulomatosis. *Anesthesiology*, 80, 206–9.

Felty's syndrome

Characteristics: Hypersplenism in rheumatoid arthritis.
Key points: Pancytopenia, haemolysis due to red cell sequestration, increased plasma volume.

Fibrodysplasia ossificans (myositis ossificans)

Characteristics: Progressive bony infiltration of tendons/muscles/ fascia/ aponeuroses leading to joint ankylosis throughout the body. Permanent ankylosis of the jaw may be precipitated by minimal soft tissue trauma.
Key points: Difficulties with intubation, possibility of atlantoaxial subluxation, restrictive pulmonary disease, cardiac conduction abnormalities.
References: Newton MC et al. (1990). Fibrodysplasia ossificans progressiva.*British Journal of Anaesthesia*, 64, 246–50.
Nussbaum BL *et al.* (1996). Fibrodysplasia ossificans progressiva: report of a case with guidelines for pediatric dental and anesthetic management. *ASDC J. Dent. Child.*, 63, 448–50.

Fibromatosis (including juvenile and hyaline forms)

Characteristics: Large cutaneous nodules (especially head/neck/lips), joint contractures, gingival hypertrophy, osteolytic lesions.

Key points: Potential airway problems.

Reference: Norman B *et al.* (1996). Anaesthesia and juvenile hyaline fibromatosis. *British Journal of Anaesthesia*, **76**, 163–6.

Fraser syndrome (cryptophthalmos—'hidden eye')

Characteristics: Cryptophthalmos, laryngeal atresia/hypoplasia, fixed posterior arytenoids, genitourinary abnormalities, cleft lip and palate, possible association with congenital heart disease/neurological abnormalities.

Key points: Airway problems, underlying cardiac/renal disease.

Reference: Jagtap SR *et al.* (1995). Anaesthetic considerations in a patient with Fraser syndrome *Anaesthesia*, **50**, 39–41.

Freeman–Sheldon (craniocarpotaral dysplasia or 'whistling face') syndrome

Characteristics: Progressive congenital myopathy, multiple deformities of face, hands, and feet, microstomia with pursed lips.

Key points: Difficult intubation (micrognathia/neck rigidity/anterior larynx), postoperative respiratory complications, difficult venous access, possible MH risk.

References: Munro HM *et al.* (1997). Freeman–Sheldon (whistling face) syndrome. Anaesthetic and airway management. *Paediatric Anaesthesia*, **7**, 345–8.

Vas L, Naregal P (1998). Anaesthetic management of a patient with Freeman Sheldon syndrome. *Paediatric Anaesthesia*, **8**, 175–7.

Friedreich's ataxia

Characteristics: Autosomal recessive progressive ataxia with additional myopathy. Myocardial degeneration with failure and arrhythmias, respiratory failure, diabetes, peripheral neuropathy.

Key points: Previously quoted to be sensitive to suxamethonium although recent evidence does not support this.

Reference: Bell CF *et al.* (1986). Anaesthesia for Friedreich's ataxia. Case report and review of the literature. *Anaesthesia*, **41**, 296–301.

Gaisbock's syndrome

Characteristics: Relative polycythaemia due to decreased plasma volume, middle-aged obese smoking hypertensive men.

Key points: Risk of arterial thrombotic episodes, myocardial/cerebral ischaemia, consider venesection to normal haematocrit.

Gardner's sydrome (multiple polyposis)

Characteristics: Multiple colonic polyps (risk of malignant change), soft tissue tumours, osseous neoplasms.

Key points: Laryngeal polyps may be present.

Gaucher's disease

Characteristics: Autosomal recessive disorder of lipid catabolism, glycosphingolipids accumulate, leading to end-organ dysfunction, three variants differ in onset and CNS involvement.

Key points: CNS dysfunction, seizures, gastro-oesophageal reflux, chronic aspiration, possible upper airway obstruction (bulbar involvement/infiltration of the upper airway), hypersplenism, thrombocytopenia and anaemia.

References: Kita T et al. (1998). Anesthetic management involving difficult intubation in a child with Gaucher disease. Masui, 47, 69–73.

Tobias JD et al. (1993). Anesthetic considerations in the child with Gaucher disease. Journal of Clinical Anesthesia, 5, 150–3.

Gilbert's disease

Characteristics: Asymptomatic familial unconjugated non-haemolytic hyperbilirubinaemia.

Key points: Perioperative jaundice may be precipitated by stress/ surgery/ starvation.

Reference: Taylor S (1984). Gilbert's syndrome as a cause of postoperative jaundice. Anaesthesia, 39, 1222–4.

Glanzmann's disease (thrombasthenia)

Characteristics: Lack of membrane protein GPIIb and GPIIIa, normal number and sized platelets, defective aggregation, no clot retraction.

Key points: Moderately severe bleeding diathesis, platelet transfusions sometimes ineffective.

Glomus jugulare tumours

Characteristics: Highly vascular benign tumour of glomus body. Invades locally, may affect cranial nerves, causing progressive deafness and tinnitus.

Key points: Sudden severe haemorrhage during excision (?hypotensive technique), may need to sacrifice local structures (carotid etc.). Consider cerebral protection measures.

References: Braude BM et al. (1986). Management of a glomus jugulare tumour with internal carotid artery involvement Anaesthesia, 41, 861–5.

Mather SP, Webster NR (1986). Tumours of the glomus jugulare. Case report and anaesthetic management for the combined two-stage operation. Anaesthesia, 41, 856–60.

Glucagonoma

Characteristics: Rare tumour of alpha cells of pancreatic islets. Marked increases of blood glucagon and glucose levels, potential for significant metabolic and myocardial dysfunction.

Key points: Control of blood glucose—large amounts of glucagon can be released during tumour handling, careful evaluation of nutrition, fluid and electrolytes. Thromboembolic prophylaxis.

References: Nicoll JMV, Catling SJ (1985). Anaesthetic management of glucagonoma. Anaesthesia, 40, 152–7.

Sanders WC, Wolpert LA (1991). Anesthesia for glucagonoma resection. Journal of Clinical Anesthesia, 3, 48–52.

Glucose-6-phosphate-dehydrogenase deficiency (see also p. 50)

Characteristics: Predominantly males, attacks of haemolytic anaemia precipitated by infections and some drugs (including aspirin, vitamin K, chloramphenicol).

Key points: Chronic anaemia (increased 2,3-DPG) of 5–10 g/dl, may benefit from splenectomy.

Glycogenoses (glycogen storage diseases)

Type I (Von Gierke's disease)

Characteristics: Mental retardation, hepatosplenomegaly, renal enlargement, stomatitis, hypoglycaemic convulsions, bleeding diathesis, lactic acidosis and leucopenia.

Key points: Tendency to hypoglycaemia during fasting, cautious attention to the metabolic and homeostatic derangements, abdominal distension may affect ventilation.

Reference: Shenkman Z *et al.* (1996). Anaesthetic management of a patient with glycogen storage disease type 1b. *Canadian Journal of Anaesthesia*, **43**, 467–70.

Type II (Pompe's disease)

Characteristics: Wide spectrum of severity from neonatal acyanotic cardiac death to normal life expectancy. Features include cardiomegaly, progressive cardiac failure, outflow obstruction, generalized hypotonia, neurological deficits, macroglossia, normal glucose tolerance.

Key points: Macroglossia, cardiomyopathy, postoperative respiratory insufficiency, potential exaggerated hyperkalaemic response to suxamethonium.

Reference: McFarlane HJ, Soni N (1986). Pompe's disease and anaesthesia. *Anaesthesia*, **41**, 1219–24.

Type III (Forbes' disease)

Key points: Perioperative hypoglycaemia.

Type IV (Andersen's disease)

Characteristics: Hepatosplenomegaly, muscular hypotonia, severe growth retardation, cirrhosis and death before 3 years.

Key points: Hepatic dysfunction, muscle relaxants generally unnecessary, reduced doses of intravenous drugs, prone to heat loss and perioperative hypoglycaemia.

Type V (McArdle's disease)

Key points: Muscle weakness, cardiac failure.

Goldenhar syndrome (oculoauriculovertebral syndrome, hemifacial microsomia)

Characteristics: Eye and ear abnormalities, micrognathia, maxillary hypoplasia, cleft/high arched palate, cervical synostosis, congenital heart anomalies (Fallot/VSD).

Key points: Difficult intubation, cardiorespiratory and craniovertebral anomalies, atropine-resistant bradycardia.

Reference: Madan R *et al.* (1990). Goldenhar's syndrome: an analysis of anaesthetic management. A retrospective study of seventeen cases. *Anaesthesia*, **45**, 49–52.

Golz–Gorlin syndrome (focal dermal hypoplasia)

Characteristics: Dental/facial asymmetry, stiff neck, hypertension.

Key points: Difficult airway.

References: Ezri T *et al.* (1994). Anaesthesia for Golz–Gorlin syndrome [letter]. *Anaesthesia*, **49**, 833.

Holzman RS (1991). Airway involvement and anesthetic management in Goltz's syndrome. *Journal of Clinical Anesthesia*, **3**, 422–5, discussion 426.

Goodpasture's syndrome

Characteristics: Severe repeated intrapulmonary haemorrhages with fibrosis, hypertension, anaemia, renal failure.
Key points: Restrictive lung defect, renal failure.

Gorham syndrome ('disappearing bone disease')

Characteristics: Massive osteolysis—replacement of bone by fibrovascular tissue, pathological fractures, lymphangiomatosis, respiratory and neurological deficits, relapsing pleural effusions, chylothorax/pericardium. Poor prognosis. Most common in second/third decade but can occur at any age.
Key points: Respiratory function assessment, check cervical spine (often involved), avoid suxamethonium (may cause/worsen pathological fractures). Consider ICU respiratory support postoperatively.
Reference: Szabo C, Habre W (2000). Gorham syndrome: anaesthetic management. *Anaesthesia*, 55, 157–9.

Groenblad–Strandberg disease

See Pseudoxanthoma elasticum.

Haemochromatosis (bronze diabetes and haemosiderosis)

Characteristics: Iron deposits in liver, pancreas, joints, skin, and heart.
Key points: Cirrhosis, diabetes, arthritis, late cardiac failure, may be having weekly venesections.

Haemolytic uraemic syndrome

Characteristics: Typical triad of renal failure, haemolytic anaemia and thrombocytopenia. Multisystem disorder may also involve CVS, respiratory, CNS, and hepatic systems.
Reference: Johnson GD, Rosales JK (1987). The haemolytic uraemic syndrome and anaesthesia. *Canadian Journal of Anaesthesia*, 34, 196–9.

Haemorrhagic telangiectasia (Osler–Weber–Rendu syndrome)

Characteristics: Familial telangiectasia of mucous membranes (nose/oropharynx/viscera/skin), repeated haemorrhages, may have pulmonary AV fistulae, GI bleeding.
Key points: Avoid trauma to mucous membranes, bleeding difficult to control, IV access and line complicated (poor tissues).
Reference: Waring PH *et al.* (1990). Anesthetic management of a parturient with Osler–Weber–Rendu syndrome and rheumatic heart disease. *Anesthesia and Analgesia*, 71, 96–9.

Hallermann–Streiff syndrome

Characteristics: Oculomandibulodyscephaly and dwarfism. (See Dwarfism.)
Key points: Direct laryngoscopy may be difficult and hazardous (brittle teeth, temporomandibular joint dislocation).

Hallervorden–Spatz disease

Characteristics: Rare progressive disorder of basal ganglia, myotonia and dystonic posturing, scoliosis, dementia, trismus.
Key points: Difficult intubation, volatile agents relieve the posturing (returns after discontinuation).
References: Roy C *et al.* (1983). Anesthetic management of a patient with Hallervorden–Spatz disease. *Anesthesiology*, 58, 382–4.

Keegan MT *et al.* (2000). Anesthetic management for two-stage computer-assisted, stereotactic thalamotomy in a child with Hallervorden–Spatz disease. *Journal of Neurosurgical Anesthesiology*, **12**, 107–11.

Hand–Schuller–Christian disease (histiocytic granulomata)

Characteristics: Diabetes insipidus, hepatic failure, pancytopenia, respiratory failure.

Key points: Intubation difficulties, small larynx, electrolyte problems, may be on steroids.

Hartnup's disease

Characteristics: Defective tubular/jejunal reabsorption of most neutral amino acids leading to tryptophan malabsorption and nicotinamide deficiency, pellagra, psychiatric disorders.

Key points: Cerebellar ataxia

Hay–Wells syndrome

Characteristics: Maxillary hypoplasia.

Key points: Difficult intubation.

Hecht–Beals syndrome (trismus pseudocamptodactyly or Dutch–Kennedy syndrome)

Characteristics: Aracnodactyly, kyphoscoliosis, restricted mandible, multiple joint contractures, crumpled ears.

Key points: Airway difficulties (LMA beneficial), ventilatory defect, mitral valve prolapse, aortic root dilatation.

References: Nagata O *et al.* (1999). Anaesthetic management of two paediatric patients with Hecht–Beals syndrome. *Paediatric Anaesthesia*, **9**, 444–7.

Vaghadia H, Blackstocki D (1988). Anaesthetic implications in trismus psuedocamtodactyly (Dutch–Kennedy or Hecht–Beals) syndrome. *Canadian Journal of Anaesthesia*, **35**, 80–5.

Henoch–Schonlein purpura

Characteristics: Abnormal vascular reaction, normal platelets, nephritis (30%).

Key points: Haemorrhagic risk, renal failure.

Hepatolenticular degeneration (Kinnier–Wilson disease)

Characteristics: Defective copper metabolism, hepatic failure, epilepsy, trismus, weakness.

Key points: Sensitive to muscle relaxants.

Holt–Oram syndrome (hand–heart syndrome)

Characteristics: Rare disorder combining congenital anomalies of heart and upper limbs. Hypoplastic thumbs, hypoplastic clavicles, cardiac anomalies (ASD/VSD/occasionally others), hypoplastic vasculature, arrhythmias and sudden death.

Key points: Potentially difficult venous access (especially central), arrhythmias frequent even with normal anatomy, often previous cardiac surgery.

Reference: Shono S *et al.* (1998). Holt–Oram syndrome. *British Journal of Anaesthesia*, **80**, 856–7.

Homocystinuria

Characteristics: Homocystine excreted in urine, mental handicap, Marfan-like syndrome. (See Marfan's syndrome.)

Key points: Venous/arterial thrombotic episodes, pulmonary embolisms (requiring heparinisation), hypoglycaemia, renal failure.

Reference: van den Berg M, Boers GHJ (1996). Homocystinuria: what about mild hyperhomocystinaemia? *Postgraduate Medical Journal*, 72, 513–18.

Hunter syndrome (mucopolysaccharidosis II)

Characteristics: Widespread accumulation of mucopolysaccharides in tissues.

Key points: Airway problems, may need smaller ETT.

Reference: See Further reading.

Huntington's chorea/juvenile Huntington's disease

Characteristics: Similar conditions, progressive degenerative involuntary movement disorder, choreoathetoid movements, dysphagia, depression and apathy lead to cachexia.

Key points: Risk of regurgitation and pulmonary aspiration, possible associated autonomic neuropathy, poor respiratory function, avoidance of precipitating convulsions and clonic spasms, malnourishment, exaggerated response to thiopentone and suxamethonium.

References: Cangemi CF, Miller RJ (1998). Huntington's disease: review and anesthetic case management. *Anesthesia Progress*, 45, 150–3.

Gupta K, Leng CP (2000). Anaesthesia and juvenile Huntington's disease. *Paediatric Anaesthesia*, 10, 107–9.

Hurler syndrome (gargoylism, mucopolysaccharidosis I)

Characteristics: Most severe of the mucopolysaccaridoses, death at early age. All have similar appearance (gargoylism), short stature, typical facies, short neck, chest deformity and protruberant abdomen, increased muscle tone. Cardiac involvement (aortic and mitral incompetence).

Key points: Difficult intubation due to macroglossia and increased secretions. Prone to chest infections, generally die from pneumonia or cardiac complications.

Reference: See Further reading.

Hutchinson–Guilford syndrome (premature ageing syndrome)

See Progeria.

Hyperviscosity syndrome (Waldenstom's macroglobulinaemia, multiple myeloma)

Key points: Thrombotic risk, preop plasmapheresis may be needed.

Hypokalaemic familial periodic paralysis

Characteristics: Attacks of severe muscle weakness and flaccid muscle paralysis with low serum K^+.

Key points: Perioperative attack may compromise spontaneous ventilation, avoid drugs known to cause K^+ shifts (e.g. beta-agonists), risk of arrhythmias, sensitive to muscle relaxants.

References: Ahlawat SK, Sachdev A (1999). Hypokalaemic paralysis. *Postgraduate Medical Journal*, 75, 193–7.

Viscomi CM *et al.* (1999). Anesthetic management of familial hypokalemic periodic paralysis during parturition. *Anesthesia and Analgesia*, 88, 1081–2.

Hypoplastic left heart syndrome

Characteristics: LV hypoplasia, mitral valve hypoplasia, aortic valve atresia, hypoplasia of ascending aorta. Previously 100% mortality.

Key points: Survival depends upon PDA, balance of PVR and SVR (both circulations in parallel supplied by single ventricle), control of pulmonary blood flow, VF may occur with surgical manipulation.

Reference: Hansen DD, Hickey PR (1986). Anesthesia for hypoplastic left heart syndrome: use of high-dose fentanyl in 30 neonates. *Anesthesia and Analgesia*, **65**, 127–32.

Ichthyosis

Characteristics: Hyperkeratotic plates of flaky/fissured skin.

Key points: Difficulty placing and securing catheters/cannulas/ electrodes (consider bandaging).

Reference: Smart G, Bradshaw EG (1984). Extradural analgesia and ichthyosis. *Anaesthesia*, **39**, 161–2.

Idiopathic thrombocytopenic purpura

Characteristics: Thrombocytopenia <50 000 cells/mm3, petechiae.

Key points: Avoid heparin or aspirin. May be on steroids, consider platelet infusions, beware rebound thrombosis after splenectomy, minimize airway trauma, avoid regional blocks.

Isaacs' syndrome (continuous muscle fibre activity syndrome, neuromyotonia, quantal squander)

Characteristics: Autoimmune condition, continuous involuntary muscle fibre activity, delayed relaxation, fasciculation, ataxia, incoordination.

Key points: Anticonvulsants effective, regional blocks acceptable, probable exaggerated response to muscle relaxants.

Reference: Morgan PJ (1997). Peripartum management of a patient with Isaacs' syndrome. *Canadian Journal of Anaesthesia*, **44**, 1174–7.

Ivemark syndrome

Characteristics: Asplenia, complex cardiac pathology, abnormal abdominal viscera.

Key points: CVS assessment.

Jervell–Lange–Nielsen syndrome

Characteristics: Congenitally prolonged QT interval and enlarged T wave, deafness, prone to ventricular arrhythmias/cardiac arrest.

Key points: Select drugs and techniques known to minimize catecholamine levels, consider pacemaker insertion/beta-block (for CVS stability).

Reference: Ryan H (1988). Anaesthesia for caesarean section in a patient with Jervell–Lange–Nielsen syndrome. *Canadian Journal of Anaesthesia*, **35**, 422–4.

Jeune's syndrome (asphyxiating thoracic dystrophy)

Characteristics: Pulmonary hypoplasia, severe thoracic defect preventing normal intercostal function, renal dysfunction, myocardial dysfunction in older patients.

Key points: CVS, respiratory and renal dysfunction. Minimize ventilator pressures.

Reference: Borland LM (1987). Anesthesia for children with Jeune's syndrome (asphyxiating thoracic dystrophy). *Anesthesiology*, **66**, 86.

Joubert syndrome

Characteristics: Abnormality of respiratory control (brainstem/ cerebellar hypoplasia), hypotonia, ataxia, mental retardation.

Key points: Sensitive to respiratory depressant effects of anaesthetic agents (including. N_2O), spontaneously breathing general anaesthetic problematic, avoid opioids, close postoperative observation.

References: Habre W *et al.* (1997). Anaesthetic management of children with Joubert syndrome. *Paediatric Anaesthesia*, 7, 251–3.

Matthews NC (1989). Anaesthesia in an infant with Joubert's syndrome. *Anaesthesia*, 44, 920–1.

Kartagener's syndrome

Characteristics: Situs inversus, sinusitis, brochiectasis (defective cilia), immunoincompetence.

Key points: Dextrocardia (reverse ECG lead position/defibrillator paddles etc.). CVS and RS function. Preoperative physiotherapy, humidify gases, right lateral displacement (obstetrics).

Reference: Ho AM, Friedland MJ (1992). Kartagener's syndrome: anesthetic considerations. *Anesthesiology*, 77, 386–8.

Kawasaki disease (mucocutaneous lymph node syndrome)

Characteristics: Acute childhood (<5 years) febrile illness, coronary arteritis associated with aneurysms/thrombotic occlusions/IHD/ sudden death.

Key points: Depend upon stage of illness, degree of CVS dysfunction determines technique, invasive lines have a higher incidence of complications, accelerated atherosclerosis.

Reference: Waldron RJ *et al.* (1993). Kawasaki disease and anaesthesia. *Anaesthesia and Intensive Care*, 21, 213–17.

Kearns–Sayer syndrome

Characteristics: Extremely rare mitochondrial myopathy, ophthalmic complications, cardiac conduction abnormalities common (range from bundle branch block to third degree AV block), generalized CNS degeneration. (See Progressive external ophthalmoplegia.)

Key points: Sensitive to induction agents and muscle relaxants. Inhalation induction + deep intubation has been recommended. Risk of complete heart block. Depressed respiratory drive (care with opioids etc.).

Reference: Lauwers MH *et al.* (1994). Inhalation anaesthesia and the Kearns–Sayre syndrome. *Anaesthesia*, 49, 876–8.

Kelly–Paterson syndrome

See Plummer–Vinson syndrome.

Kenny–Caffey syndrome

Characteristics: Proportional dwarfism, macrocephaly, eye anomalies, dysmorphic facies, mandibular hypoplasia, episodic hypocalcaemic tetany, may be associated with Mournier–Kuhn syndrome.

Key points: Difficult airway (if mandibular hypoplasia), hypocalcaemia, anaemia, thoracic and skeletal abnormalities.

Reference: Janke EL *et al.* (1996). Anaesthetic management of the Kenny–Caffey syndrome using the laryngeal mask. *Paediatric Anaesthesia*, 6, 235–8.

King Denborough disease

Characteristics: Slowly progressive myopathy, short stature, kyphoscoliosis, pectus carinatum, cryptorchidism, characteristic facial appearance.

Key points: Malignant hyperpyrexia risk.

References: Watsubo T *et al.* (2001). Anesthetic management of the King-Denborough syndrome. *Masui*, **50**, 390–3.

Klinefelter syndrome

Characteristics: Chromosomal abnormality 47XXY. Poor sexual development, tall stature, reduced intelligence, vertebral collapse from osteoporosis.

Key points: May have reduced muscle bulk and power. Care during positioning.

Klippel–Feil syndrome

Characteristics: Three main types which differ in severity. Congenital fusion of cervical and/or thoracic vertebrae. Short neck, limited range of motion, possible cervical cord compression, syncope on sudden rotation of head, kyphoscoliosis, cardiac, respiratory, and genitourinary anomalies.

Key points: Skeletal/organ anomalies, difficult intubation, keep neck in neutral axis (basilar insufficiency).

Dresner MR, Maclean AR (1995). Anaesthesia for caesarean section in a patient with Klippel–Feil syndrome. The use of a microspinal catheter. *Anaesthesia*, **50**, 807–9.

Hunter J, Lee C (1995). Emergency anaesthesia in a patient with Klippel–Feil syndrome. *British Journal of Hospital Medicine*, **54**, 273–4.

Klippel–Trenaunay syndrome (angio-osteohypertrophy)

Characteristics: Generalized haemangiomas, soft tissue hypertrophy, bone overgrowth and/or arteriovenous malformations. (See Proteus syndrome.)

Key points: Possible airway/respiratory problems, high output cardiac failure, consumptive coagulopathy, pulse oximeter may under-read if placed on a limb with large A-V fistula (pulsatile venous flow).

References: Christie IW *et al.* (1998). Central regional anaesthesia in a patient with Klippel–Trenaunay syndrome. *Anaesthesia for Intensive Care*, **26**, 319–21.

Ezri T et al. (1996). Anaesthetic management for Klippel–Trenaunay–Weber syndrome. *Paediatric Anaesthesia*, **6**, 81.

Kneist's syndrome

Key points: Difficult intubation due to stiff neck.

Reference: Felius GM *et al.* (1985). Kniest syndrome and anesthesia. *Rev. Esp. Anestesiol. Reanim.*, **32**, 127–9.

Kugelberg Welander syndrome (spinal muscular atrophy type III)

See Spinal muscular atrophy.

Larsen's syndrome

Characteristics: Multiple congenital dislocations, flattened face, prominent forehead.

Key points: Subglottic stenosis, unstable cervical spine, difficult intubation, chronic respiratory disease from kypho-scoliosis.

Reference: Lauder GR, Sumner E (1995). Larsen's syndrome: anaesthetic implications. Six case reports. *Paediatric Anaesthesia*, **5**, 133–8.

Laurence–Moon–Biedl syndrome

Characteristics: Obesity, polydactyly, mental retardation, paraparesis, renal anomalies.

Key points: Renal failure, CVS assessment, diabetes insipidus.

Leber's disease

Key points: Idiopathic hypoventilation, sensitive to sedatives/analgesics. (See Alveolar hypoventilation.)

Reference: Hunter AR (1984). Idiopathic alveolar hypoventilation in Leber's disease. *Anaesthesia*, **39**, 781–3.

Leigh's syndrome

Characteristics: Necrotizing encephalomyelopathy in children.

Key points: Hypotonia, seizures, aspiration.

Reference: Ward DS (1981). Anesthesia for a child with Leigh's syndrome. *Anesthesiology*, **55**, 80–1.

Leopard syndrome

Characteristics: Rare inherited progressive disorder, similar to Noonan syndrome, Lentigines, ECG abnormalities, Ocular hypertelorism, obstructive cardiomyopathy, Pulmonary valve stenosis, Abnormal male genitalia, Retarded growth, Deafness.

Key points: CVS assessment will determine technique, cardiomyopathy may be occult.

Reference: Rodrigo MR *et al.* (1990). 'Leopard syndrome'. *Anaesthesia*, **45**, 30–3.

Leprechaunism

Characteristics: 'Gnome' facies, cutis laxa, adipose tissue atrophy, dwarfism, extreme wasting, dysphagia requiring parenteral feeding, abnormal endocrine state, mentally defective. (See Dwarfism and Cutis laxa.)

Key points: Maintain blood sugar during starvation (hyperinsulinism).

Reference: Cantani A (1987). A rare polydysmorphic syndrome: leprechaunism. Review of 49 cases reported in the literature. *Annals of Genetics*, **30**, 221–7.

Lesch–Nyhan syndrome (hyperuricaemia)

Characteristics: Disorder of purine metabolism, hyperuricemia, spasticity, choreoathetosis, dystonia, self-injurious behaviour, aggression, normal cognitive function, possible atlantoaxial instability.

Key points: Sudden unexplained death, seizures, abnormalities in respiration, apnoea, absent adrenergic pressor response—severe bradycardia, caution with exogenous catecholamines, increased incidence of vomiting/regurgitation, chronic pulmonary aspiration.

Reference: Larson LO, Wilkins RG (1985). Anesthesia and the Lesch–Nyhan syndrome. *Anesthesiology*, **63**, 197–9.

Letterer–Siwe disease (histiocytosis-X)

Characteristics: Histiocytic granulomata in viscera/bones, similar clinical course to acute leukaemia.

Key points: Pancytopenia, anaemia, purpura, haemorrhage, pulmonary infiltration, hepatic involvement, tooth loss.

Lipodystrophy (total lipoatrophy)

Characteristics: Generalized loss of body fat, fatty fibrotic liver, portal hypertension/splenomegaly, nephropathy, diabetes mellitus.
Key points: Hepatic failure, hypersplenism, anaemia, thrombocytopenia and possible renal failure.

Lowe syndrome (oculocerebrorenal syndrome)

Characteristics: Metabolic acidosis due to renal-tubular dysfunction, mental retardation, convulsions, glaucoma/cataracts, abnormal skull shape, bone fragility.
Key points: Renal failure, hypotonia, hypocalcaemia.
Reference: Watoh Y (1992). A series of anesthesia for a child with Lowe's syndrome. *Masui*, **41**, 1004–7.

Mafucci syndrome

Characteristics: Progressive condition, enchondromatosis and multiple soft tissue haemangiomata (including airway/cervical spine), increased risk of malignancy, intracranial lesions.
Key points: Anaemia, coagulopathy, increased risk of epidural haematoma (spinal lesions), assess for raised ICP, pathological fractures, GI bleeding. May be sensitive to vasodilating drugs.
Reference: Chan SK *et al.* (1998). Anaesthetic implications of Maffucci's syndrome. *Anaesthesia and Intensive Care*, **26**, 586–9.

Mandibulofacial dysostosis (Treacher–Collins syndrome)

Characteristics: Mandibulofacial dysostosis characterized by deafness, hypoplasia of facial bones (mandible, maxilla, and cheek bone), antimongoloid slant of palpebral fissures, coloboma of the lower lid and bilateral anomalies of auricle. May be associated with other cardiovascular malformations.
Key points: Potential difficult airway, postoperative pharyngeal/ laryngeal oedema may develop. Sleep apnoea, respiratory distress, and sudden death all reported.
Reference: Rasch DK *et al.* (1986). Anaesthesia for Treacher–Collins and Pierre–Robin syndromes: a report of three cases. *Canadian Anaesthesia Society Journal*, **33**, 364–70.

Maple syrup urine disease

Characteristics: Branched chain ketoacid decarboxylase deficiency, failure to thrive, fits, cerebral degeneration, neonatal acidosis.

Marchiafava–Michaeli syndrome

Key points: Autoimmune haemolytic anaemia, paroxysmal nocturnal dyspnoea, venous thromboembolism.

Marfan's syndrome

Characteristics: Inherited disorder of connective tissue metabolism. Tall with long/thin fingers, easy joint dislocation, high arched palate, emphysema, pectus excavatum, cataracts and retinal detachment, spontaneous pneumothorax, coronary thrombosis, dissecting aneurysms, aortic/mitral regurgitation, kyphoscoliosis.

Key points: Associated abnormalities, minimize laryngoscopic response, control BP, central blocks acceptable.

Reference: Gordon CF, Johnson MD (1993). Anesthetic management of the pregnant patient with Marfan syndrome. *Journal of Clinical Anesthesia*, 5, 248–51.

Maroteaux–Lamy syndrome (mucopolysaccharidosis IV)

Characteristics: Kyphoscoliosis, hepatosplenomegaly, recurrent chest infections, myocardial involvement.

Key points: Cardiac failure by 20 years, chronic respiratory infection, poor lung reserve, hypersplenism, anaemia, thrombocytopenia.

Reference: See Further reading.

Marshall–Smith syndrome

Characteristics: Accelerated bone maturation, dysmorphic facial features, airway abnormalities, death in early infancy from respiratory complications, generally die in infancy.

Key points: Airway difficulties including possible atlantoaxial instability/ laryngomalacia/tracheomalacia. Facemask ventilation may be impossible, maintain spontaneous breathing if possible, consider elective use of nasopharyngeal airway during induction/ emergence.

References: Antila H *et al.* (1998). Difficult airway in a patient with Marshall–Smith syndrome. *Paediatric Anaesthesia*, 8, 429–32.

Dernedde G (1998). Anaesthetic management of a child with Marshall–Smith syndrome. *Canadian Journal of Anaesthesia*, 45, 660–3.

Meckel's syndrome (Mekel–Gruber syndrome)

Characteristics: Microcephaly, micrognathia, congenital cardiac disease, polycystic kidneys.

Key points: Difficult intubation, may have cleft epiglottis, renal failure, encephalocele/cleft palate may be present.

Meig's syndrome

Characteristics: Large ovarian cyst in peritoneal space, respiratory distress, and poor nutrition.

Key points: Pleural effusion drainage, intravascular volume correction.

Reference: Hirota M *et al.* (1995). Perioperative management of patients with Meigs syndrome. *Masui*, 44, 874–9.

Menkes' disease

Characteristics: Suppression of copper-dependent enzymes resulting from copper deficiency, kinky hair, convulsions, mental retardation, bone and connective tissue lesions, and hypothermia.

Key points: Seizures, gastro-oesophageal reflux, airway complications (poor pharyngeal motor tone).

Reference: Tobias JD (1992).Anaesthetic considerations in the child with Menkes' syndrome. *Canadian Journal of Anaesthesia*, 39, 712–15.

Merrf syndrome

Characteristics: Mitochondrial encephalomyopathy, mixed seizures, myoclonus, progressive ataxia, spasticity, mild myopathy, growth retardation, deafness, dementia.

Mikulicz's syndrome

Characteristics: Salivary and lachrymal gland enlargement.
Key points: Glandular tissue may complicate airway management, anticholinergics probably best avoided.

Miller–Fisher syndrome

Characteristics: Variant of Guillain Barre syndrome (p. 197).

Millers syndrome

Characteristics: Rare congenital disorder with facial features similar to Treacher–Collins syndrome. Limb abnormalities, congenital heart disease (ASD/VSD/PDA).
Key points: As for Mandibulofacial dysostosis. Consider early tracheostomy for airway maintenance (especially if repeated procedures planned), difficult venous access, gastric reflux.
Reference: Stevenson GW (1991). Anaesthetic management of Miller's syndrome. *Canadian Journal of Anaesthesia*, **38**, 1046–9.

Moebius syndrome

Characteristics: Multiple cranial nerve palsies, orofacial malformations, limb anomalies, and a high incidence of other anomalies, including congenital cardiac disease, spinal anomalies, corneal abrasions, and peripheral neuropathies.
Key points: Difficult or failed intubation, potential for problems with aspiration of oral secretions due to salivary drooling (consider antisialogogue premedication).
Reference: Ferguson S (1996). Moebius syndrome: a review of the anaesthetic implications. *Paediatric Anaesthesia*, **6**, 51–6.

Morquio syndrome (mucopolysaccharidosis IV)

Characteristics: Short stature, short neck, hypoplastic odontoid leads to atlantoaxial instability (compression of long tracts and paraplegia can occur), prominent sternum, loss of muscle tone, hypermobility and loose skin, aortic incompetence.
Key points: Difficult airway due to short neck and instability, potential narrowed lumen (infiltration), respiratory and cardiac failure in early adult life, end organ dysfunction, sleep apnoea.
Reference: Tobias JD (1999). Anesthetic care for the child with Morquio syndrome: general versus regional anesthesia. *Journal of Clinical Anesthesia*, **11**, 242–6. (See Further reading.)

Moschkowitz disease (thrombotic thrombocytopenic purpura)

Characteristics: Haemolytic anaemia, thrombocytopenia, small vessel disease, neurological symptoms, renal disease.
Key points: Assess renal function, bleeding risk.

Mournier–Kuhn syndrome

Characteristics: Diffuse tracheobronchomegaly, communicating paratracheal cysts.
Key points: Intubate trachea and pack pharynx if mechanical ventilation needed.
Reference: Sane AC et al. (1992). Tracheobronchiomegaly. The Mournier–Kuhn syndrome in a patient with Kenny–Caffey syndrome. *Chest*, **102**, 618–19.

Moya–moya disease (in the German literature 'Nishimoto–Takeuchi–Kudo–Suzuki's disease')

Characteristics: Severe stenosis of internal carotid arteries, fine network of vessels around basal ganglia.

Key points: Neurological deterioration can follow general anaesthetic—optimize cerebral perfusion (control of BP, CO_2 etc.).

Reference: Bingham RM, Wilkinson DJ (1985). Anaesthetic management in Moya–moya disease. *Anaesthesia*, **40**, 1198–202.

Mucopolysaccharidoses

Characteristics: Metabolic disease characterized by abnormal accumulation and excretion of mucopolysaccharides, see individual syndromes (Hunter, Hurler, Morquio, Maroteaux–Lamy, and Scheie syndromes) for full details.

References: Moores C *et al.* (1996). Anaesthesia for children with mucopolysaccharidoses. *Anaesthesia and Intensive Care*, **24**, 459–63.

Multiple myelomatosis

Characteristics: Neoplastic proliferation of plasma cells characterized by immunoglobulin disorders.

Key points: Renal failure, haemorrhagic tendency, increased susceptibility to infections, pathological fractures (care positioning), hyperviscosity syndrome, anaemia, and hypercalcemia.

Reference: Wake M (1995). Anesthetic experiences in 3 patients with multiple myeloma. *Masui*, **44**, 1282–4.

Myasthenic syndrome (see also p. 191)

Characteristics: Paraneoplastic condition causing defective acetylcholine release at neuromuscular junctions, proximal muscle weakness in ocular and/or bulbar muscles, post tetanic facilitation.

Key points: Muscle weakness, sensitive to muscle relaxants, risk of respiratory complications, autonomic dysfunction, impaired oesophageal motility.

References: Seneviratne U, deSilva R (1999). Lambert–Eaton myasthenic syndrome. *Postgraduate Medical Journal*, **75**, 516–20.

Telford RJ, Holloway TE (1990). The myasthenic syndrome: anaesthesia in a patient treated with 3,4 diaminopyridine. *British Journal of Anaesthesia*, **64**, 363.

Myositis ossificans

Characteristics: Bony infiltration of tendons, facia, muscle, aponeuroses.

Key points: Airway problems if neck involved. Thoracic involvement reduces compliance, asphyxia and aspiration.

Myotonia congenita (Thomsen's disease) (see also p. 192)

Characteristics: Muscular disorder, widespread dystrophy and/or hypertrophy, more myotonia than other muscle diseases, palatopharyngeal dysfunction, cardiomyopathy.

Key points: Aspiration risk, strong association with MH, myotonia not responsive to muscle relaxants. Can be precipitated by cold, surgery, diathermy, anticholinesterases. Suxamethonium may cause myotonia with difficult intubation/ventilation.

Reference: See Further reading.

Nance Insley syndrome (otospondylomegaepiphyseal dysplasia 'OSMED')

Characteristics: Disrupted cartilaginous growth leading to midface hypoplasia, disproportionate short stature and short limbs. Progressive sensorineural deafness, cleft palate, micrognathia, joint contractures, vertebral abnormalities.

Key points: Possible difficult airway.

Reference: Denton R (1996). Anaesthetic problems in the Nance Insley syndrome. *Anaesthesia*, 51, 100–1.

Nemaline myopathy

Characteristics: Congenital myopathy, non-progressive hypotonia and symmetrical muscle weakness (including skeletal and diaphragm but sparing cardiac and smooth), skeletal deformities, facial dysmorphism.

Key points: Airway difficulties, poor respiratory function (restrictive), chronic aspiration, abnormal drug responses (including relaxants), rarely cardiomyopathy, MH not described.

References: Cunliffe M, Burrows FA (1985). Anaesthetic implications of nemaline rod myopathy. *Canadian Anaesthesia Society Journal*, 32, 543–7.

Stackhouse R (1994). Anesthetic complications in a pregnant patient with nemaline myopathy. *Anesthesia and Analgesia*, 79, 1195–7.

Nesidioblastosis

Characteristics: Autonomous insulin secretion unaffected by blood glucose. Neonatal/infantile apnoea, hypoglycaemia, hypotonia, seizures.

Key points: Total pancreatectomy needed, monitor perioperative blood glucose.

Reference: Bellwoar C *et al.* (1996). Anaesthetic management of a neonate with nesidioblastosis. *Paediatric Anaesthesia*, 6, 61–3.

Neurofibromatosis

Characteristics: Café au lait spots, astrocytomas, seizures, kyphoscoliosis.

Key points: Potential difficult airway and positioning, avoid proconvulsants, occult phaeochromocytoma in 5%.

Reference: See Further reading.

New variant Creutzfeldt–Jacob disease (nvCJD) (see also p. 518)

Characteristics: Psychiatric symptoms occur early. Progressive neurological signs including ataxia, involuntary movements and cognitive impairment develop. Similar to CJD.

Reference: Weihl CC, Roos RP (1999). Creutzfeldt–Jakob disease, new variant Creutzfeldt–Jakob disease, and bovine spongiform encephalopathy. *Neurology Clinics*, 17, 835–59.

Niemann–Pick disease

Characteristics: Accumulation of sphingomyelin in reticuloendothelial macrophages of many organs (liver/spleen/bone marrow), hepatosplenomegaly, mental retardation.

Key points: Anaemia, thrombocytopenia and respiratory failure.

Noonan's syndrome

Characteristics: Short stature, mental retardation, cardiac defects (pulmonary stenosis, VSD, hypertrophic cardiomyopathy), micrognathia, short webbed neck, pectus excavatum, vertebral anomalies, renal failure, lymphoedema.

Key points: Possible difficult intubation, cardiac dysfunction, platelet and coagulation defects, check renal function.

References: Grange CS (1998). Anaesthesia in a parturient with Noonan's syndrome. *Canadian Journal of Anaesthesia*, 45, 332–6.

McLure HA, Yentis SM (1996). General anaesthesia for caesarean section in a parturient with Noonan's syndrome. *British Journal of Anaesthesia*, 77, 665–8.

Ondine's curse

See Alveolar hypoventilation.

Opitz–Frias syndrome (hypospadias dysphagia syndrome)

Key points: Recurrent pulmonary aspiration of intestinal contents, achalasia of the oesophagus, subglottic stenosis, hypertelorism, micrognathia, high arched palate.

Reference: Bolsin SN, Gillbe C (1985). Opitz–Frias syndrome. A case with potentially hazardous anaesthetic implications. *Anaesthesia*, 40, 1189–93.

Osler–Weber–Rendu syndrome

See Haemorrhagic telangiectasia.

Osteogenesis imperfecta (fragilitas ossium)

Characteristics: Inherited connective tissue disorder, bone fragility, frequent fractures and/or deformities, blue sclera.

Key points: Teeth easily damaged, excessive bleeding, tendency to hyperthermia—probably not MH.

Reference: Cho E *et al.* (1992). Anaesthesia in a parturient with osteogenesis imperfecta. *British Journal of Anaesthesia*, 68, 422–3.

Osteopetrosis (Albers–Schonberg disease)

Characteristics: Group of disorders characterized by increased bone in the skeleton associated with changes in modelling with overgrowth. Range of severity, brittle bones, nerve compression syndromes, hearing loss, mental retardation, bone marrow involvement leads to leucoerythroblastic anaemia.

Key points: Airway/ventilation problems, cervicomedullary stenosis (cord trauma during intubation), thrombocytopenia, hepatosplenomegaly (reduced FRC), reduced myocardial contractility (hypocalcaemia). Careful moving and positioning—risk of fractures, head and mandibular involvement may complicate intubation.

Reference: Burt N *et al.* (1999). Patients with malignant osteopetrosis are at high risk of anesthetic morbidity and mortality. *Anesthesia and Analgesia*, 88, 1292–7.

Paramyotonia congenita (Eulenberg's disease)

Characteristics: Variant of Hyperkalaemic periodic paralysis, cold induced myotonia, flaccid paralysis, worsened by exercise.

Key points: Assess sensitivity to cold and frequency of myotonic episodes. Warm theatre/fluids/patient. Normal response to non-depolarizing muscle relaxants. Avoid suxamethonium. Central neural blocks safe. No MH tendancy.

Reference: Grace RF, Roach VJ (1999). Caesarean section in a patient with paramyotonia congenita. *Anaesthesia and Intensive Care*, 27, 534–7.

Patau's syndrome (trisomy 13)

Characteristics: Multiple craniofacial, cardiac, neurological, and renal anomalies. 'Rockerbottom feet'.

Key points: Difficult airway, thoracic kyphoscoliosis, ineffective cough, post-operative respiratory problems, apnoeic episodes, full cardiac assessment (80% have severe malformations), impaired renal function, polycythaemia and platelet dysfunction.

References: Martlew RA, Sharples A (1995). Anaesthesia in a child with Patau's syndrome. *Anaesthesia*, **50**, 980–2.

Pollard RC, Beasley JM (1996). Anaesthesia for patients with trisomy 13 (Patau's syndrome). *Paediatric Anaesthesia*, **6**, 151–3.

Pemphigus vulgaris

Characteristics: Autoimmune disease causing impaired cell adhesion within the epidermis. Bullous eruptions of skin and mucous membranes.

Key points: Avoid friction (monitors, lines, airway manipulation, positioning, etc.). Possible ulceration/bullae/oedema of glottis after intubation (lubricate everything well), careful fluid/electrolyte balance (include losses from bullae). Perioperative steroids to reduce exacerbation, regional/general anaesthetic acceptable.

References: Mahalingham TG *et al.* (2000). Anaesthetic management of a patient with pemphigus vulgaris for emergency laparotomy. *Anaesthesia*, **55**, 160–2.

Vatashsky E, Aronson HB (1982). Pemphigus vulgaris: anaesthesia in the traumatised patient. *Anaesthesia*, **37**, 1195–7.

Pendred's syndrome

Characteristics: Genetic defect in thyroid hormone synthesis, hypo-thyroidism, goitre, deafness.

Key points: As for Hypothyroidism.

Reference: Reardon W (1999). Prevalence, age of onset, and natural history of thyroid disease in Pendred syndrome. *Journal of Medical Genetics*, **36**, 595–8.

Pfeiffer's syndrome (acrocephalosyndactyly type V)

Characteristics: Growth and developmental retardation, sagittal cranio-synostosis, hypertelorism, low set ears, micrognathia with mandibular ankylosis, congenital heart defects, and genital anomalies.

Key points: Solid cartilaginous trachea lacking rings may be present.

Reference: Moore MH *et al.* (1995). Pfeiffer syndrome: a clinical review. *Cleft Palate and Craniofacial Journal*, **32**, 62–70.

Pharyngeal pouch

Characteristics: Epithelial lined diverticulum above the upper oesophageal sphincter, often asymptomatic, sometimes associated with dysphagia.

Key points: Tracheal soiling not prevented by cricoid pressure. Empty pouch manually (by patient) prior to induction or with large bore nasopharyngeal tube. Consider intubation in head down position or under local anaesthetic.

Phenylketonuria

Characteristics: Defective phenylalanine-4-hydroxylase, cerebral damage, mental retardation, epilepsy.

Key points: Sensitive to opioids/barbiturates, consider inhalation induction, monitor blood glucose.

Reference: Celiker V *et al.* (1993). Anesthetic management of a patient with hereditary fructose intolerance and phenylketonuria. *Turkish Journal of Pediatrics*, **35**, 127–30.

Pickwickian syndrome

Characteristics: Morbid obesity, episodic somnolence, hypoventilation.
Key points: Hypoxaemia, polycythaemia, pulmonary hypertension, cardiac failure, difficult access/positioning, prone to wound infection, DVT/PE risk. Sensitive to respiratory depressants, regional anaesthesia ideal for peripheral surgery. Alert ICU following major surgery, CPAP beneficial. (See p. 67.)
Reference: Neuman GG *et al.* (1986). Perioperative management of a 430-kilogram (946-pound) patient with Pickwickian syndrome. *Anesthesia and Analgesia*, **65**, 985–7.

Pierre–Robin syndrome

Characteristics: Cleft palate, micrognathia, mandibular hypoplasia, congenital heart disease.
Key points: Difficult airway, receding mandible fails to hold tongue forward in normal position—falls against posterior pharyngeal wall, assess for heart anomalies.
Reference: Rasch DK *et al.* (1986). Anaesthesia for Treacher–Collins and Pierre–Robin syndromes: a report of three cases. *Canadian Anaesthesia Society Journal*, **33**, 364–70.

Plott's syndrome

Characteristics: Laryngeal-abductor paralysis, psychomotor retardation and sixth nerve palsy.
Key points: Stridor at rest, cyanosis during crying/exertion, postoperative upper airway control.
Reference: McDonald D (1998). Anaesthetic management of a patient with Plott's syndrome. *Paediatric Anaesthesia*, **8**, 155–7.

Plummer–Vinson syndrome (Patterson–Brown–Kelly syndrome)

Characteristics: Upper oesophageal web, dysphagia, iron-deficiency anaemia, glossitis, angular stomatitis, increased risk of postcricoid carcinoma.
Key points: Regurgitation risk, anaemia.
Reference: Hoffman RM, Jaffe PE (1995). Plummer–Vinson syndrome. A case report and literature review. *Archives of Internal Medicine*, **155**, 2008–11.

Pneumatosis cystoides intestinalis

Characteristics: Multiple intramural gas-filled cysts in the gastrointestinal tract, disturbed bowel function, may be associated with systemic sclerosis.
Key points: Avoid nitrous oxide.
Reference: Sutton DN, Poskitt KR (1984). Pneumatosis cystoides intestinalis. Nitrous oxide anaesthesia and the rapid effect of oxygen therapy. *Anaesthesia*, **39**, 776–80.

Pompe's disease

See Glycogenoses type II.

Post-poliomyelitis syndrome

Characteristics: New neuromuscular symptoms occurring > 15 years after clinical stability has been attained in patients with a prior history of symptomatic poliomyelitis. Limb atrophy, slow progression with periods of stabilization.
Key points: Respiratory muscle involvement, bulbar dysfunction.

Potter's syndrome (bilateral renal agenesis)

Characteristics: Incompatible with life, bilateral renal agenesis, pulmonary hypoplasia, characteristic facial features.

Key points: Ventilation may be impossible despite intubation.

Reference: Van der Weyden (1982). Potter's syndrome [letter]. *Anaesthesia and Intensive Care*, **10**, 90.

Prader–Willi syndrome

Characteristics: Mental retardation, severe obesity, polyphagia, dental caries, short stature, congenital muscle hypotonia, hypogonadism, cardiovascular anomalies.

Key points: Obesity may be extreme, hypotonia, difficult venous access, altered thermoregulation, arrythmias, convulsions, blood glucose should be maintained intravenously during starving, perioperative respiratory problems may occur.

Reference: Dearlove OR *et al.* (1998). Anaesthesia and Prader–Willi syndrome. *Paediatric Anaesthesia*, **8**, 267–71.

Progeria (premature ageing)

Characteristics: Feature of many syndromes.

Key points: IHD/hypertension/cardiomyopathy at young chronological age. Plan technique around 'physiological age'.

Reference: Nguyen NH *et al.* (2001). Anaesthesia for a child with progeria. *Paediatric Anaesthesia*, **11**, 370–1.

Progressive external ophthalmoplegia (PEO)

Key points: Sensitive to all induction agents.

Reference: James RH (1986). Induction agent sensitivity and ophthalmoplegia plus [letter]. *Anaesthesia*, **41**, 216.

Proteus syndrome

Characteristics: Congenital progressive hamartomatous disorder, partial bilateral gigantism, hemihypertrophy (often one whole side of the body), macrocephaly, scoliosis, cystic lung changes. (probably explains 'the Elephant Man'). (See Klippel–Trenaunay syndrome.)

Key points: Difficult airway (See Bullous cystic lung disease.)

Reference: Pennant JH, Harris MF (1991). Anaesthesia for Proteus syndrome. *Anaesthesia*, **46**, 126–8.

Prune-belly syndrome (Eagle–Barrett syndrome)

Characteristics: Almost exclusively male, abdominal muscle deficiency, complex genitourinary malformations and bilateral undescended testes. May die in neonatal period from pulmonary hypoplasia, also associated with congenital heart disease, skeletal anomalies and imperforate anus.

Key points: Optimize pulmonary function, poor cough due to muscle weakness, beware postoperative respiratory distress, careful fluid balance. Renal failure may coexist.

References: Heisler DB *et al.* (1994). Pectus excavatum repair in a patient with prune belly syndrome. *Paediatric Anaesthesia*, **4**, 267–9.

Henderson AM *et al.* (1987). Anaesthesia in the prune belly syndrome. *Anaesthesia*, **42**, 54–60.

Pseudoxanthoma elasticum (Groenbald–Strandberg disease)

Characteristics: Hereditary disorder of elastic tissue, four types with variable features including fragile connective tissue, vascular complications (slow progressive occlusive arterial disease), retinal changes with early blindness and myopia, high arched palate, blue sclera. Lungs unaffected.

Key points: Fragile tissue—haemorrhage with minor trauma (including airway). High incidence of hypertension, IHD, valvular disease, dysrythmias. Care in fixing IV lines.

References: Krechel SL *et al.* (1981). Anesthetic considerations in pseudoxanthoma elasticum. *Anesthesia and Analgesia*, **60**, 344–7.

Levitt MW, Collison JM (1982). Difficult endotracheal intubation in a patient with pseudoxanthoma elasticum. *Anaesthesia in Intensive Care*, **10**, 62–4.

Pulmonary cysts

Key points: Can increase in size and rupture during anaesthesia (especially with nitrous oxide).

Refsum's disease

Characteristics: Defective metabolism of phytanic acid, sensorimotor polyneuropathy, ataxia, retinal damage, deafness.

Key points: Document pre-existing neurology before performing regional blocks.

Rett syndrome

Characteristics: Devastating disabling female neurological disease, abnormal respiratory control (hyperventilation/apnoea) when awake, scoliosis, long QT, sudden death.

Key points: Full respiratory assessment ideal but may be technically difficult, respiratory pattern normal under general anaesthetic, prolonged weaning, high pain threshold (abnormal processing).

Reference: Dearlove OR, Walker RW (1996). Anaesthesia for Rett syndrome. *Paediatric Anaesthesia*, **6**, 155–8.

Rigid spine syndrome

Characteristics: Very limited spinal flexion, generalized proximal limb weakness, limb contractures, progressive scoliosis, restrictive ventilatory defect, pulmonary hypertension, RV failure.

Key points: Difficult intubation, flexible ETT provides better fit in hyperextended trachea. Avoid suxamethonium (K+). Cardiomyopathy, check ECG (conduction defects), low MH risk, care with muscle relaxants, careful positioning/padding, consider HDU/ICU postoperatively.

Reference: Jorgensen BG *et al.* (1999). Anaesthetic implications of rigid spine syndrome. *Paediatric Anaesthesia*, **9**, 352–5.

Riley–Day syndrome

See Familial dysautonomia.

Romano–Ward syndrome

Characteristics: Congenital delay of cardiac depolarisation, prolonged Q-T interval.

Key points: Sudden death at any age during induction of anaesthesia, ?consider pacing preoperatively.

Reference: Ponte J, Lund J (1981). Prolongation of the Q-T interval (Romano–Ward syndrome): anaesthetic management. *British Journal of Anaesthesia*, **53**, 1347–50.

Rubinstein–Taybi syndrome

Characteristics: Microcephaly, mental retardation, broad thumbs and toes, craniofacial abnormalities, recurrent respiratory infections, congenital heart disease (33%).

Key points: Difficult airway, search for CVS disease (arrhythmias occur), chronic lung disease.

References: Critchley LA et al. (1995). Anaesthesia in an infant with Rubinstei–Taybi syndrome. *Anaesthesia*, **50**, 37–8.

Stirt JA (1981). Anesthetic problems in Rubinstein–Taybi syndrome. *Anesthesia and Analgesia*, **60**, 534–6.

Russell–Silver syndrome

Characteristics: Short stature, facial and limb assymetry, mandibular hypoplasia, micrognathia, macroglossia, sweating. Fasting hypoglycaemia, mental retardation, congenital heart disease may coexist.

Key points: Difficult airway (including mask fit), intra-operative glucose monitoring, temperature control (minimal body fat). Monitor neuromuscular block (normal doses may relatively underdose).

Reference: Dinner M et al. (1994). Russell–Silver syndrome: anesthetic implications. *Anesthesia and Analgesia*, **78**, 1197–9.

Saethre–Chotzen syndrome

Characteristics: Craniosynostosis, micrognathia, renal failure.

Key points: Difficult intubation.

Scheie syndrome (mucopolysaccharidosis V)

Characteristics: Metabolic disease characterized by abnormal accumulation and excretion of mucopolysaccharides.

Key points: Ischaemic heart disease, valvular insufficiency, difficult intubation, joint stiffness, and mental retardation.

Reference: Nakayama H et al. (1994). Anesthesia in a patient with Scheie syndrome. *Masui*, **43**, 1385–8. (See also Further reading.)

Scimitar syndrome

Key points: Anomalous venous drainage of the right lung into the inferior vena cava, right lung hypoplasia, scimitar-shaped radiographic shadow of the anomalous vein gives the syndrome its name.

Seckel syndrome

Characteristics: Rare syndrome of chromosome aberration, bird-headed dwarfism, microcephalus, other minor deformities.

Key points: Preoperative laryngeal and renal assessments.

Reference: Shiraishi N et al. (1995). Anesthetic management of Seckel syndrome: a case report. *Masui*, **44**, 735–8.

Shprintzen syndrome (velocardiofacial syndrome)

Characteristics: Facial dysmorphism, cleft palate, cardiovascular malformations, mild/moderate mental retardation/learning difficulties.

Reference: Meinecke P *et al*. (1986). The velo-cardio-facial (Shprintzen) syndrome. Clinical variability in eight patients. *European Journal of Pediatrics*, **145**, 539–44.

Shy–Drager syndrome (central nervous and autonomic degeneration)

Characteristics: Progressive neurovegetative disorder with primary autonomic failure, severe orthostatic hypotension with syncope, anhydrosis, disordered thermoregulation, impotence/urinary incontinence, respiratory obstruction/sleep apnoea.

Key points: Increased aspiration risk (gut motility disorder plus laryngeal weakness), IPPV may cause CVS instability (reduced venous return), ensure normovolaemia. Regional blocks used successfully, consider fludrocortisone to sustain plasma volume.

References: Dewhurst A, Sidebottom P (1999). Anaesthetic management of a patient with multiple system atrophy (Shy–Drager syndrome) for urgent hip surgery. *Hospital Medicine*, **60**, 611.

Niquille M *et al*. (1998). Continuous spinal anesthesia for hip surgery in a patient with Shy–Drager syndrome. *Anesthesia and Analgesia*, **87**, 396–9.

Simmond's syndrome and Sheehan's syndrome (postpartum pituitary necrosis)

Characteristics: Pituitary infarction following postpartum haemorrhage, variable degree of pituitary insufficiency.

Key points: Assess endocrine derangement.

Sipple syndrome (multiple endocrine adenomatosis type IIa)

Characteristics: Phaeochromocytoma, medullary carcinoma of thyroid with or without parathyroid hyperplasia.

Key points: Assess degree of endocrine dysfunction, treat as for Phaeochromocytoma.

Sjogren's syndrome (keratoconjunctivitis sicca)

Characteristics: Dry eyes without rheumatoid arthritis, may also have dysphagia/abnormal oesophageal motility, other autoimmune disease, renal tubular defects, pulmonary hypertension, peripheral neuropathy, vasculitis.

Key points: Assess for other systemic conditions. Worsened by anticholinergic drugs, improved by humidification.

Reference: Takahashi S *et al*. (1990). Anesthetic management of a patient with Sjogren's syndrome and pulmonary fibrosis. *Masui*, **39**, 1393–6.

Smith–Lemli–Opitz syndrome

Characteristics: Micrognathia, mentally defective, thymic hypoplasia.

Key points: Difficult intubation, intrinsic lung disease, possibly susceptible to infection.

Reference: Choi PT, Nowaczyk MJ (2000). Anesthetic considerations in Smith–Lemli–Opitz syndrome. *Canadian Journal of Anaesthesia*, **47**, 556–61.

Spinal muscular atrophy

Characteristics: Peripheral motor neurons affected, upper motor neurons spared. Types I–IV increase in rate of progression, muscular wasting. (See also Amyotrophic lateral sclerosis.)

Key points: Weak respiratory muscles (IPPV advisable), abnormal reaction to muscle relaxants. If relaxants are essential monitor blockade and ensure full reversal. Avoid suxamethonium (K^+ and myotonic contractures). Post-operative respiratory support may be indicated, aspiration risk with bulbar involvement.

Reference: Shime N *et al.* (1990). Anesthetic management of a patient with progressive spinal muscular atrophy. *Masui*, **39**, 918–20.

Strumpell's disease

Characteristics: Progressive spastic paresis predominantly affecting lower extremities.

Key points: Avoid suxamethonium, sensitive to non-depolarizing muscle relaxants, regional anaesthesia probably acceptable, poor respiratory function/reserve.

Reference: McTiernan C, Haagenvik B (1999). Strumpell's disease in a patient presenting for Cesarean section. *Canadian Journal of Anaesthesia*, **46**, 679–82.

Sturge–Weber syndrome

Characteristics: Unilateral angiomatous lesions of the leptomeninges/ upper face, contralateral hemiparesis, seizures, mental retardation.

Key points: Full evaluation for associated abnormalities, careful intubation/ extubation (angiomas of mouth/upper airway), prevent rise in ICP/IOP.

Reference: Batra RK *et al.* (1994). Anaesthesia and the Sturge–Weber syndrome. *Canadian Journal of Anaesthesia*, **41**, 133–6. (See also Further reading.)

Takayasu's disease (pulseless disease, occlusive thromboaortopathy, or aortic arch syndrome)

Characteristics: Chronic autoimmune inflammatory disease, elastic tissue replaced by fibrous tissue leading to blood vessel narrowing/ occlusion/ aneurysms (preferentially large arteries—aorta and branches) and hence its alternative names. Often self-limiting.

Key points: Hypertension, IHD, cerebrovascular disease. Control cerebral perfusion (BP, CO_2 etc.). If on steroids may require supplement, non-invasive blood pressure measurements may be inaccurate. Many have postoperative CVS complications from poorly controlled hypertension.

References: Henderson K, Fludder P (1999). Epidural anaesthesia for caesarean section in a patient with severe Takayasu's disease. *British Journal of Anaesthesia*, **83**, 956–9.

Kawaguchi M *et al.* (1993). Intraoperative monitoring of cerebral haemodynamics in a patient with Takayasu's arteritis. *Anaesthesia*, **48**, 496–8.

Tangier disease (familial alpha-lipoprotein deficiency)

Characteristics: Deficient HDL apoprotein, accumulation of cholesterol in reticuloendothelial tissue, enlarged orange tonsils, hepatosplenomegaly, corneal opacities, polyneuropathy.

Key points: Sensitivity to muscle relaxants, IHD, anaemia, thrombocytopenia.

TAR syndrome (thrombocytopenia, absent radius)

Key points: May also have Fallot's tetralogy.

Tay–Sachs disease (familial amaurotic idiocy)

Characteristics: Accumulation of GM2 gangliosides in the CNS and periph-eral nerves, progressive cerebral degeneration, seizures, dementia, blindness,

death before 2 years, characteristic macular cherry spot appearance.
Key points: No documented problems, progressive neurology leads to respiratory complications.

Thrombotic thrombocytopenic purpura

Characteristics: Rare severe disease composing triad of haemolytic anaemia, consumptive thrombocytopenia, CNS dysfunction. Often scheduled for therapeutic splenectomy.
Key points: Preferably postpone elective surgery until period of remission. Check coagulation, renal, liver function. Consider prophylactic antiplatelet drugs, corticosteroids. platelet transfusion contraindicated (may worsen disease). Use packed cells and FFP, strict asepsis (often immunocompromised), avoid IM route, avoid nasal intubation, control BP (renal and cerebral perfusion), care with positioning.
Reference: Pivalizza EG (1994). Anesthetic management of a patient with thrombotic thrombocytopenic purpura. *Anesthesia and Analgesia*, **79**, 1203–5.

Tourette syndrome

Characteristics: Profane vocalizations, repetitive speech, muscle jerking.
Key points: Do not confuse tic like behaviour with seizure activity on induction/emergence. Sedating premedication beneficial, continue normal medication, pimozide may cause prolonged Q-T.
Reference: Morrison JE, Lockhart CH (1986). Tourette syndrome: anaesthetic implications. *Anesthesia and Analgesia*, **65**, 200–2.

Toxic epidermal necrolysis ('scalded skin syndrome')

Characteristics: Split at level of stratum granulosum, epidermal erythema/blistering/necrosis, worsened by lateral shearing forces. Can be drug related.
Key points: Prevention of friction (monitors, lines, airway manipulation, positioning, etc.), consider fluid losses from blisters/exposed areas of dermis.

Treacher–Collins syndrome

See Mandibulofacial dysostosis.

Trisomy 13

See Patau's syndrome.

Trisomy 18

See Edward's syndrome.

Trisomy 21 (Down's syndrome)

See p. 212.

Tuberous sclerosis (Bourneville's disease)

Characteristics: Neurocutaneous syndrome, facial angiofibromas, epilepsy, mental retardation, CVS/CNS/renal hamartomas.
Key points: Hamartomas may affect airway/lungs/CVS with spontaneous rupture/bleeding. Spontaneous pneumothoraces, careful positioning and padding, avoid proconvulsants, consider full preoperative CVS assessment (cardiac rhabdomyoma).
Reference: Schweiger JW et al. (1994). The anaesthetic management of the patient with tuberous sclerosis complex. *Paediatric Anaesthesia*, **4**, 339–42. (See also Further reading.)

Turner's syndrome

Characteristics: XO chromosome, micrognathia, short webbed neck, coarctation/dissecting aortic aneuryms/pulmonary stenosis, renal anomaly (50%).
Key points: Possible difficult intubation, assess CVS/renal function, care with renally excreted drugs.

Urbach–Wiethe disease

Characteristics: Type of histiocytosis (see Hand–Schuller–Christian disease), hyaline deposits in larynx and pharynx—hoarseness/ aphonia.
Key points: Cautious intubation, laryngeal opening may be small.

Urine drinking in psychiatric patients

Characteristics: Produces moderate to severe hyponatraemia.
Key points: Correct electrolyte abnormality, consider other aspects of psychiatric condition.

Von Recklinghausen's disease

See Neurofibromatosis.

Von Willebrand's disease (pseudohaemophilia)

See p. 140.

WAGR syndrome

Characteristics: Wilms tumour, anirida, genitourinary abnormalities, retardation.

Weaver's syndrome

Characteristics: Unusual craniofacial appearance, micrognathia.
Key points: Airway/intubation problems, may have large stature in adulthood.

Weber–Christian disease

Characteristics: Global fat necrosis (including retroperitoneal, pericardial, peritoneal, meningeal).
Key points: Associated organ dysfunction (e.g. adrenals, constrictive pericarditis). Avoid trauma to superficial fat during movement, positioning during surgery (cold, heat, pressure).

Wegener's granuloma

Characteristics: Necrotizing granulomas in inflamed vessels of multiple organ systems (CNS/CVS/renal/RS).
Key points: Consider laryngeal stenosis, pneumonia, bronchial destruction, CVS valvular dysfunction, abnormal cardiac conduction, arteritis (cerebral aneurysms, arterial line difficulty), IHD, renal failure, peripheral neuropathy.

Welander's muscular atrophy

Characteristics: Peripheral muscular atrophy, good prognosis.
Key points: Sensitive to thiopental, muscle relaxants and opioids.

Werdnig–Hoffman disease (spinal muscular atrophy type I acute, and type II chronic)

See Spinal muscular atrophy.

Wermer syndrome (type 1 endocrine adenomatosis)

Characteristics: Parathyroid, pituitary, adrenal, thyroid adenomas and pancreas islet cell tumours—can all coexist.
Key points: Assess degree of different endocrine dysfunctions.

Werner syndrome (premature aging syndrome)

See Progeria.

Wiedemann–Rautenstrauch syndrome (premature aging syndrome)

See Progeria.

William's syndrome

Characteristics: Congenital stenosis of aortic/pulmonary valves, hypocalcaemia in infancy (20%), stellate blue eyes.

Wilson's disease

Characteristics: Inborn error of copper metabolism, basal ganglia degeneration, neurological symptoms, hepatic and renal failure.
Key points: Respiratory complications, difficulty reversing muscle relaxants.
Reference: el Dawlatly AA *et al.* (1992). Anesthetic management for cesarean section in a patient with Wilson's disease. *Middle East Journal of Anesthesiology*, **11**, 391–7.

Wiskott–Aldrich disease

Characteristics: Faulty presentation of antigen to macrophages, thrombocytopenia.
Key points: Immunodeficiency, recurrent infections, anaemia, coagulopathy.

Wolf–Hirschorn syndrome

Characteristics: Rare chromosomal abnormality, severe psychomotor retardation, seizures, VSD/ASD, characteristic facies, midline fusion abnormalities, many die by age 2 (cardiac failure or bronchopneumonia).
Key points: Assess for system dysfunction, MH risk unproven.
Reference: Ginsburg R, Purcell-Jones G (1988). Malignant hyperthermia in the Wolf–Hirschorn syndrome. *Anaesthesia*, **43**, 386–8.

Wolfram syndrome

Characteristics: Diabetes insipidus, diabetes mellitus, optic atrophy, deafness.
Key points: Fluid and electrolyte problems.

Wolman's syndrome

Characteristics: Familial xanthomatosis, adrenal calcification, hepatosplenomegaly, hypersplenism.
Key points: Anaemia, thrombocytopenia, platelet transfusion may only be successful after splenectomy.

Zellweger syndrome (cerebrohepatorenal syndrome)

Characteristics: Poor suck, failure to thrive, flat/round face, micrognathia, cleft palate, polycystic kidneys, apnoeas, congenital heart defects, hypotonia, areflexia, seizures, hepatomegaly, biliary dysgenesis.

Key points: Difficult intubation, assess CVS, care with muscle relaxants.
Reference: Govaerts L *et al.* (1982). Cerebro-hepato-renal syndrome of Zellweger: clinical symptoms and relevant laboratory findings in 16 patients. *European Journal of Pediatrics*, **139**, 125–8.

Further reading

Baines D, Keneally J (1983). Anaesthetic implications of the mucopolysaccharidoses: a fifteen-year experience in a children's hospital. *Anaesthesia and Intensive Care*, **11**, 198–202.

Diaz JH (2000). Perioperative management of children with congenital phakomatoses. *Paediatric Anaesthesia*, **10**, 121–8.

Katz J, Benumof JL, Kadis LB (1990). *Anesthesia and uncommon diseases.* WB Saunders, Philadelphia.

Rushman GB, Davies NJH, Cashman JN (ed.) (1999). Dictionary of key points about rare diseases. In: *Lee's synopsis of anaesthesia*, pp. 353–81. Butterworth-Heinemann, Oxford.

Russell SH, Hirsch NP (1994). Anaesthesia and myotonia *British Journal of Anaesthesia*, **72**, 210–16.

Smith GB, Shribman AJ (1984). Anaesthesia and severe skin disease. *Anaesthesia*, **39**, 443–55.

Walker RWM *et al.* (1994). Anaesthesia and the mucopolysaccharidoses. A review of the airway problems in children. *Anaesthesia*, **49**, 1078–88.

For detailed information about rare conditions try: Online Mendelian Inheritance in Man, OMIM (TM). McKusick-Nathans Institute for Genetic Medicine, Johns Hopkins University (Baltimore, MD) and National Center for Biotechnology Information, National Library of Medicine (Bethesda, MD), 2000. World Wide Web URL: http://www.ncbi.nlm.nih.gov/omim/. (Click on 'Search the OMIM Database' and enter the name of the condition in the search field).

Section II
Anaesthesia for surgical specialties

Chapter 13
Day case surgery

Peter Davies

General principles

A surgical day case is a patient who is admitted for investigation or operation on a planned non-resident basis and who nonetheless requires facilities for recovery.

Royal College of Surgeons Guidelines 1992

Organization

Organization is the key to efficient good-quality day surgery and requires close cooperation between all agencies involved, including surgeons, anaesthetists, day case unit staff, general practitioners, and patients themselves.

Facilities

An efficient organization requires 'ring fenced' theatres and ward space. Day cases on inpatient wards or theatres will suffer cancellation when there are bed shortages and emergency operations. Self-contained units with their own facilities, within an acute hospital, probably offer the best option.

Staff

Senior staff should perform day case anaesthesia and surgery. Much of the surgery and anaesthesia may be viewed as routine or simple, but it must be performed to a high standard for day units to operate efficiently.

Patient selection

In theory all patients should follow a sequential pathway. All patients should be preassessed by specially trained nurses, according to set day case criteria. However, preassessment should be approached flexibly as different methods work for different patient groups.

- With short waiting times, patients can be reviewed at the hospital on the day of their surgical outpatient appointment.
- Some patient groups can be telephone assessed; in particular those who have direct access surgery (not seeing a surgeon until the day of surgery).
- Older patients need earlier preassessment at the hospital so that tests can be performed and the results reviewed prior to surgery.
- In some hospitals surgeons book day cases after reviewing them and instructions are sent out by clerical staff. This can work well as long as the surgeon is senior and is fully conversant with the requirements of day surgery.

Patient agreement:

I confirm that a responsible adult will remain with me overnight following my discharge from hospital after my operation. I agree not to drive, cycle, operate machinery, or take alcohol for a minimum of 24 hours after my anaesthetic. If in any doubt after this time, please seek medical advice.

Driving under the influence of anaesthetic drugs might be considered a criminal offence and could affect insurance cover.

Patient:..Date:............

Day case selection criteria

Health status: Generally fit and healthy (ASA 1 and 2). Patients with significant cardiovascular or respiratory disease, insulin-dependent diabetics, or those with gross obesity are not suitable.

Age: Patients should be older than 6 months. There is no upper age limit; physiological fitness should be considered rather than chronological age.

Complexity of surgery: Operations lasting more than 60 min and those associated with a risk of significant postoperative pain, haemorrhage, or prolonged immobility should not be performed.

Transport: All patients must be escorted home by a responsible, informed adult and be adequately supervised during their recovery at home for a minimum of 24 h.

Social support: Patients must have suitable home conditions with adequate toilet facilities and a telephone should be readily available for advice in an emergency.

Geography: The patient should live within 1 hour's travelling distance from the hospital.

Preassessment nurses will discuss with the patients their health, details concerning their admission, and give written instructions about the day of surgery. It is important that patients read the advice and sign a patient agreement.

Some patients who fall outside the guidelines need to be discussed on an individual basis and may include:

- Some ASA 3 patients who would do better in a day case environment rather than as an inpatient, e.g. chemotherapy patients, stable diabetics.

- Many paediatric anaesthetists will anaesthetize babies as young as 6 weeks on a day case basis (provided infant was not premature).

- Moderate obesity in itself does not preclude day stay surgery, but does cause unpredictable problems in terms of length of surgery and anaesthesia. BMI is not the ideal tool for assessing fitness for day surgery, but provides preassessment nurses with guidance. Obese patients should be scheduled mid morning to allow preoperative antacid therapy time to work and still allow time for recovery. Remember that obesity may cause as many problems to the surgeon as to the anaesthetist. In general a BMI >35 is not suitable (BMI = weight (kg)/height^2 (m)).

Common coexisting disease

- Stable asthmatics are suitable for day surgery. Regular hospitalization, oral steroid therapy, and poor control of symptoms would suggest unsuitability.

- Stable epileptics on medication are suitable for day surgery. Avoid propofol if they have a driving licence (see p. 171).

- Well-motivated, well-controlled diabetics having operations with a low incidence of postoperative nausea can be managed as day cases, with either general or local anaesthesia.

Cancellations and DNAs (did not attend)

Most cancellations on the day of surgery can be avoided by careful patient selection by experienced staff. It is often unavoidable to cancel patients who have an acute illness, i.e. a heavy cold, or an exacerbation of previously well controlled asthma. However, diseases such as undiagnosed hypertensive disease or uncontrolled atrial fibrillation should be discovered by preassessment at the day surgery unit.

Starvation instructions

- Morning lists: no solid food after midnight and free clear fluids up to 0630 h.
- Afternoon lists: no solid food after 0630h and free clear fluids up 1130h.

Preoperative verbal and written instructions are important so that milky drinks are avoided. In practice, accept drinks with 1 to 2 teaspoons of milk but treat any more as solid food and require a 6 h fast.

Driving

Patients should not drive for at least 24 h postoperatively because of residual effects of the anaesthetic. Remember that some operations themselves will preclude driving for longer because of pain and limited movement, e.g. arthroscopy and inguinal hernia repair. This advice must be contained in the preoperative verbal and written instructions given to the patient.

Preoperative investigation

The following tests should be performed when appropriate:

- FBC only in patients with the possibility of anaemia, e.g. menorrhagia.
- Sickle cell test in patients of Afro-Caribbean origin.
- Electrolytes and creatinine in patients on diuretics.
- Blood sugar in patients who are diabetic or have a urinalysis positive for glucose.
- ECG in all patients over the age of 55 and younger patients if they have a cardiac history or signs (hypertension, dysrhythmias, diabetics).
- Chest radiograph only for patients with COAD, breathlessness, severe chest or cardiac history. Also patients with unexplained or unexpected chest problems or signs. Very few day surgery patients should need a preoperative chest radiograph.

Conduct of anaesthesia

Use local anaesthetic, or short-acting general anaesthetic drugs which have few residual psychomotor effects and a low incidence of postoperative nausea or vomiting (PONV).

Preoperative

- Nurses, surgeon, and anaesthetist will need to undertake an adequate history and examination as a full medical clerking is not usually performed by junior medical staff. This should include blood pressure measurement and cardiorespiratory examination. Consent should be performed by the operating surgeon either in the outpatient department or on the day of surgery.

- Avoid premedication if at all possible. If necessary use oral midazolam (up to 0.5 mg/kg) in a little undiluted sweet fruit cordial (as it tastes awful) for children, or temazepam (10–20 mg) in adults.

- There is no evidence for any increase in regurgitation/aspiration in day case patients so the routine use of antacid drugs is probably unnecessary. However, in those with a history of regurgitation ranitidine (300 mg PO) or omeprazole (40 mg PO) is appropriate.

- NSAIDs, e.g. diclofenac 50–100 mg, given orally or rectally, reach peak effect after 1–2 h and are a useful adjunct to anaesthesia, with very few side-effects. Remember that slow release oral preparations do not reach steady state concentrations until after several doses, and are thus not useful for early analgesia.

Perioperative

- Total intravenous anaesthesia with propofol is widely used. Inhalation of oxygen-enriched air will also allow omission of nitrous oxide. Propofol induction with isoflurane/sevoflurane maintenance is an alternative.

- Incremental fentanyl, often 2–4 μg/kg in divided doses.

- Diclofenac (PO/PR) and local anaesthetic for every suitable patient/operation.

- Whenever possible use a laryngeal mask airway, avoiding intubation, muscle relaxants, and reversal agents where possible. Laryngeal masks for gynaecological laparoscopy and armoured laryngeal masks for wisdom tooth extraction, and many nasal operations can be used safely in most circumstances.

- Antiemetics are not indicated routinely but should be reserved for treatment of any PONV or prophylaxis in those with a history of PONV.

Postoperative

- The inclusion of opioids, NSAIDs, and local anaesthetics should provide early analgesia. If more analgesia is needed it is imperative to treat it early. 50–75 μg fentanyl provides good, fast-onset analgesia.

- Give morphine if stronger analgesia is required. Remember that pain worsens nausea.

- Simple oral analgesics may be of help, as may physical therapies such as hot-water bottles, particularly for the cramping lower abdominal pain following gynaecological surgery.

Postoperative nausea and vomiting

A multifactorial approach to the prevention of PONV should be used. Early ambulation is a risk factor for PONV, so all day case patients should be treated as high risk. PONV must be fully controlled before discharge home.

TIVA propofol, omitting nitrous oxide, mutimodal analgesic therapy, good hydration, and minimal (2 h) fluid fast are appropriate. This is a recipe approach which works well and leaves a small number of patients requiring treatment, which can then be cost effectively done with a 5-HT3 antagonist such as ondansetron.

Regional anaesthesia

Regional anaesthesia is widely used in Europe and North America for day case anaesthesia. PONV is reduced. Timing and planning are important as blocks take a longer time to set up or wear off compared with general anaesthesia. Perform spinal anaesthetics early on the list, to allow maximum time for recovery. Spinals must have worn off completely before discharge to allow safe ambulation. However, it is reasonable to discharge patients with working plexus blocks thus allowing the benefit of prolonged postoperative analgesia. Remember that patients need special instructions on care of the anaesthetized part so as to avoid inadvertent damage. This would include a sling for patients with brachial plexus blocks.

Local anaesthesia and sedation

With increased use of local anaesthetics, short-acting sedative drugs will inevitably be used to increase tolerability. It must be noted that sedation is a poor adjunct to an imperfect local anaesthetic block. However, judicious use of intermittent midazolam or propofol infusions (TCI 1–1.5 μg/ml) can provide good amnesia with few postoperative effects. If sedation is to be used it must be provided and monitored by someone other than the operating surgeon.

Specific blocks

- Field block: excellent for LA hernia repair as provides postoperative analgesia and obviates the need for general anaesthesia.
- Spinals: use 25/26 gauge pencil point needles and 0.25% heavy bupivacaine (1:1 diluted 0.5% heavy bupivacaine and sterile saline). This gives a similar onset of anaesthesia with a shorter discharge time (4 versus 6 h).
- Epidurals are less suitable due to the time factor in achieving block.
- Caudals: use dilute solutions (0.125% bupivacaine) add preservative free ketamine 0.5 mg/kg or clonidine 1 μg/kg to prolong the block for up to 24 h. Warn the patients about ambulation difficulties.
- Brachial plexus blocks: use axillary approach (low incidence of pneumothorax). If used with GA use dilute local anaesthetic (0.25% bupivacaine) to minimize motor block. If without GA, take onset time into account when planning the list.
- The use of femoral nerve blocks is controversial as mobilization is difficult.

Specific discharge criteria

Spinals

Full recovery of motor power and proprioception.

Passed urine.

Brachial plexus blocks

Some regression of motor block.

Understanding of protection of partially blocked limb.

Lower limb blocks

Some regression of motor block.

Adequate mobility demonstrated on crutches.

Understanding of protection of partially blocked limb.

Discharge drugs

All patients should have a supply of suitable oral postoperative analgesics at home or be given it to take home. Inguinal hernia repair, laparoscopic surgery, wisdom tooth extraction, etc. should be given at least 2 days' supply of analgesics (diclofenac 50 mg three times a day, Cocodamol—a combination of codeine/paracetamol 30 mg/500 mg 2 tablets four times a day or similar).

Discharge criteria

Stable vital signs.

Fully awake and orientated.

Able to eat and drink.

Passed urine (urological surgery) and after spinal/caudal.

Ambulant.

Pain and nausea well controlled.

At least a 1 h wait postoperatively is a sensible condition of discharge.

Discharge organization

Intravenous cannula removed and wound checked.

Written and verbal discharge information.

Discharge drugs.

Suture removal organized if required.

GP letter.

Contact telephone number.

Collected by responsible adult.

Postoperative admission

Reasons for overnight admission:

- Do not fulfil discharge criteria before unit closes.
- Observation after surgical or anaesthetic complications.
- Unexpectedly more extensive surgery.
- Inadequate social circumstances.
- Uncontrolled pain or PONV.

Overall unanticipated admission occurs in between 0.5 and 2.0% of cases, depending on the mix of surgery.

Gynaecology and urology have the highest admission rates. Surgical causes of hospital admission are three to five times greater than anaesthetic causes. Common anaesthetic reasons for hospital admission are inadequate recovery, nausea and vomiting, and pain. Anaesthesia-related complications are more frequent with general anaesthesia than with local anaesthesia plus sedation or regional anaesthesia. Surgical reasons include bleeding, extensive surgery, perforated viscus, and further treatment. Admissions still occur when social circumstances have changed, i.e. patient has no one for 24 h supervision.

Further reading

Chung F, Mezei G (1999). Adverse outcomes in ambulatory anesthesia. *Canadian Journal of Anesthesia*, **46**, R18-R26.

Liu S S (1997). Optimizing spinal anesthesia for ambulatory surgery. *Regional Anesthesia*, **22**, 500–10.

Peng PWH, Chan VWS, Chung FFT (1997). Regional anaesthesia in ambulatory surgery. *Ambulatory Surgery*, **5**, 133–43.

Rowe WL (1998). Economics and anaesthesia. *Anaesthesia*, **53**, 782–8.

Website of the British Association of Day Surgery: www.bads.co.uk (for updates and new day surgery links).

Website of the Society of Ambulatory Anesthesia: www.sambahq.org (use 'search' for 'core curriculum').

Chapter 14
General surgery

Peter MacIntyre

General principles of anaesthesia for laparotomy

Laparotomy is a major physiological insult. Perioperative complications are common and often unpredictable. Even after ensuring that the patient's physiological status is optimized, fluid replacement and analgesia are adequate, and appropriate monitoring is carried over into the postoperative period, complications may still occur. High dependency or intensive care is often appropriate.

General considerations

Anaesthesia is usually straightforward in the young patient having simple bowel resection. However, abdominal surgery is more common in elderly people compromised by underlying disease, undergoing prolonged procedures associated with major fluid shifts and cardiorespiratory stress. Recent studies on optimization have shown that close attention to anaesthetic detail, particularly ensuring an adequate circulating volume and cardiac output, is associated with an improved outcome. In some hospitals a proportion of these patients are admitted to HDU/ICU prior to surgery, although this is not routine in the United Kingdom.

Preoperative

- Ischaemic heart disease and cardiac failure increases the risk of surgery and should be optimally controlled.
- Respiratory function should be optimized and physiotherapy commenced before surgery. Examine the chest radiograph if available.
- Consider overnight IV fluids prior to operation if creatinine is high, patient is jaundiced or dehydrated, or if fluid intake inadequate. Bowel preparation can result in significant hidden dehydration.
- Exclude contraindications to regional anaesthesia, e.g. patient refusal, infection around proposed site of epidural, coagulation disorders.
- Discuss analgesia options and obtain at least verbal consent if a central neuraxial block considered.
- Check the thromboprophylaxis regimen (ensure low molecular weight heparins are given at least 12 h in advance of neuraxial block).
- Discuss rapid sequence induction, if this is required. Consider ranitidine or omeprazole premedication.
- Consider whether HDU/ICU care is indicated perioperatively and book bed if appropriate.

Perioperative

- Large bore IV access. Gaining extra IV access during surgery may be difficult especially if the patient is in the lithotomy position.
- Start IV infusion as soon as the patient arrives in the anaesthetic room/ theatre if it has not been started preoperatively. Long extension sets may be required.
- Hypotension is common following induction (relative dehydration) and may require the use of vasopressors.

- Check if a nasogastric tube is required—ask the surgeon to check the position during surgery.
- Prophylactic antibiotics (p. 896).
- Establish appropriate invasive monitoring.
- Establish active patient warming, e.g. fluid warmer, hot air blanket, insulation.
- Postoperative nausea and vomiting are common, consider an antiemetic in theatre, and prescribe postoperatively.
- Keep one arm out on an arm support to allow vascular access and neuromuscular monitoring.
- Be prepared for the lithotomy position and head down tilt—may need PEEP to maintain oxygenation.
- Muscle relaxation is essential until the abdomen is closed (this helps the surgeon).
- Empty stomach if appropriate by aspirating the nasogastric tube before waking up and extubating.

Postoperative

- Continue active patient warming.
- Prescribe postoperative supplemental oxygen for up to 72 h.
- Arrange a check chest radiograph if a CVP line sited intra-operatively.
- Continue close monitoring of fluid status. Frequent monitoring of pulse, blood pressure, urine output, CVP (if appropriate), fluid loss (urine, drains, ileostomy, blood, etc.), and conscious level. In high-risk patients and following major surgery measure urine output hourly for at least 48 h.
- Consider daily FBC and U+E until normal bowel function returns. Correct electrolyte abnormalities and anaemia.
- Monitor and treat pain.

Perioperative mortality and morbidity

Surgery and anaesthesia for intra-abdominal procedures carries a high risk of complications. Upper abdominal procedures have an increased risk compared with lower gastrointestinal procedures. Significant complications primarily affect the respiratory, cardiovascular, and renal systems. Mortality rates associated with intra-abdominal procedures may be as high as 5%, with upper abdominal surgery twice as likely to result in death than lower abdominal procedures. In studies on postoperative mortality, deaths following cardiac, vascular, and abdominal surgery represent 60–80% of all deaths reported. Predictors of severe adverse perioperative outcome (including death) include a history of CCF/MI less than 1 year ago, ASA 3 or 4 and age >50 years.

Intra-operative invasive monitoring

When to use invasive monitoring is controversial. Consider the extra information it will provide against the possible risks involved.

Postoperative paralytic ileus

Bowel function begins to return 24–36 h postoperatively, but does not return to normal until 48–72 h. Prolonged ileus leads to collection of fluid and gas in

Suggested indications for invasive monitoring	
Central venous pressure	large fluid shifts, major blood loss, CVS or renal compromise, inotropes, prolonged surgery
Arterial line	Major blood loss, unstable patient, arrhythmias, CVS compromise, blood gas sampling
Oesophageal Doppler	Monitors beat by beat pulse waveform and can indicate inadequate filling, pump performance, and afterload. Will determine whether fluids, inotropes, vasodilators, or vasoconstictors are needed
Pulmonary artery catheter	Where difference is expected with performance between left and right side of heart, cardiac failure

the bowel resulting in distension, increased pain, nausea, vomiting, and delayed discharge. The aetiology of ileus is multifactorial and includes:

• manipulation of the bowel
• hormonal stress response
• increased sympathetic activity
• postoperative pain
• immobility
• opioids
• hypokalaemia.

Analgesia

Abdominal incisions are extremely painful for several days following the operation and can be associated with changes in FRC and ability to cough. In general three levels of analgesia are used:

• Simple IM/SC opioids for less invasive procedures, e.g. appendicectomy, reversal of colostomy.
• Opioids by continuous intravenous infusion or PCA can be used, particularly for lower abdominal procedures. Continuous infusion techniques can be particularly effective in the elderly population who may be confused postoperatively and unable to utilize a PCA (ensure additional oxygen therapy and hourly sedation/pain scoring).
• Epidural techniques, which may be particularly beneficial for upper abdominal surgery, prolonged procedures, and high-risk patients

Regular paracetamol (PO/PR) and NSAIDS when appropriate should also be prescribed.

Epidural analgesia

This is commonly used for patients undergoing laparotomy. Advantages include:

• Improved pain relief. Thoracic epidurals using local anaesthetic and/or epidural opioids provide superior analgesia compared with systemic opioid analgesia. Epidural opioids improve analgesia compared with local anaesthetic alone. Effectiveness relies on appropriate placement. The catheter should be placed at a level corresponding to the dermatome innervating the middle of the abdominal incision. The range for abdominal incisions is usually T6–T12. Failure of analgesia is common if the catheter is placed too low.

- Improved postoperative gastrointestinal motility. Improved recovery of bowel motility is seen with appropriately used epidural catheters due to reduced inhibitory gastrointestinal tone and increased intestinal blood flow. Low-dose epidural opioids do not seem to decrease intestinal motility.
- Improved postoperative patient mobilization.
- Improved postoperative respiratory function resulting in a reduced incidence of pneumonia, respiratory failure, and radiological markers of pulmonary complications, e.g. atelectasis.
- Potentially improved myocardial oxygenation. Pain, activation of the sympathetic nervous system, and the stress response can increase heart rate, coronary vasoconstriction, and myocardial workload, increasing the risks of myocardial ischaemia and infarction.
- Reduction in thromboembolism.
- Reduced sedation and postoperative nausea/vomiting.
- Possible reduction in overall mortality.[1]

Disadvantages associated with the use of epidurals include:
- Risks related to placement of the epidural catheter.
- Epidural failure (can be as high as 30% for postoperative analgesia).
- Perioperative hypotension. This should be treated aggressively depending on the aetiology.
- Postoperative motor blockade impeding patient mobilization.
- Itching associated with epidural opioids.

Practical considerations for epidural analgesia

- The catheter should be sited at an appropriate level to provide analgesia to the site of the skin incision (T10–T11 for lower abdominal procedures, T8–T9 for upper abdominal procedures). Siting the epidural awake is probably safer—patient feedback during insertion can be useful in alerting the anaesthetist to potential problems.
- Intra-operatively. Epidural loading dose 50–100 μg fentanyl in 8–10 ml 0.5% bupivacaine (divide into 4–5 ml boluses) and assess response. Top up with 3 ml 0.25% bupivacaine as needed. Bupivacaine takes 15–20 min to achieve its maximum spread and top ups should be performed cautiously. Intravenous supplementation with a short-acting opioid or an increase in the volatile agent may be required until the block is sufficient. An extensive sympathetic block may develop with relatively low volumes of local anaesthetic.

1   Rodges A *et al.* (2000). Reduction of postoperative mortality and morbidity with epidural or spinal anaesthesia: results from overview of randomised trial. *British Medical Journal*, **321**, 1493.

- Where extensive bleeding is expected, or in patients who are cardiovascularly unstable, it is often wise not to use epidural local anaesthetic until postoperatively. Epidural opioids alone are often a safer option.
- The effectiveness of epidurals varies during surgery. Surgeons manipulating organs or pulling on mesentery may cause stimulation, even with a good block. AP resection (which requires analgesia and anaesthesia across thoracic, lumbar, and sacral dermatomes) can prove problematic. Effectiveness of the epidural can be improved with the use of epidural opioids and larger volumes of weak anaesthetic solution, e.g. 0.125% bupivacaine. Despite this it can be difficult to effectively anaesthetize sacral dermatomes and it may be necessary to supplement with systemic analgesia/anaesthesia. Use short-acting opiates, e.g. remifentanil, alfentanil, fentanyl, to reduce postoperative complications. The epidural catheter should still be sited in the low thoracic region as the major source of pain relates to the abdominal incision.
- Treat hypotension with fluids and vasopressors. Ensure renal perfusion is maintained and avoid prolonged periods of relative hypotension.
- Postoperatively an appropriate regime consists of a mixture of local anaesthetic and opioid, e.g. bupivacaine 0.167% + diamorphine 0.1 mg/ml (2–8 ml/h), bupivacaine 0.125% + fentanyl 4 μg/ml (2–8 ml/h).
- Epidural analgesia may not be appropriate in very sick/septic patients undergoing emergency laparotomy for intra-abdominal obstruction/catastrophe. Problems with persistent hypotension may limit the analgesic effect and compromise renal blood flow, plus increased risks of epidural haematoma/infection.
- If an epidural is contraindicated use IV morphine in theatre and recovery and then PCA or a morphine infusion postoperatively.

Temperature control

Patients undergoing general anaesthesia become hypothermic due to:

- anaesthetic-induced impairment of thermoregulatory control
- a cool operating environment
- surgical factors promoting heat loss.

Hypothermia develops with a characteristic three-phase pattern.

- Phase 1: redistribution of body heat as the tonic vasoconstriction that normally maintains the core to periphery temperature gradient is inhibited. Occurs during the first hour and results in a reduction in core temperature of 1–1.5 °C.
- Phase 2: core temperature then decreases linearly at a rate determined by the difference between heat production and heat loss. Patients undergoing an operation under general anaesthesia not only have increased losses (radiation, conduction, convection, evaporation) but also have a reduced metabolic rate and therefore reduced heat production. Lasts 2–3 h.
- Phase 3: when core temperature drops to a sufficiently low value vasoconstriction is triggered and the temperature reaches a plateau phase of about 3–4 °C below normal.

Efforts to reduce operative hypothermia are aimed at preventing the linear decrease in phase 2 and increasing the total body heat to minimize the drop in core temperature seen with redistribution. This involves:

- An HME filter which humidifies and warms inhaled gases reducing losses from the respiratory tract.

- A fluid warmer to prevent conductive heat loss associated with the administration of cold fluids.
- A hot air warming blanket reducing radiation loss and increasing total body heat.
- Insulation to exposed areas, e.g. the wrapping the head reduces heat loss.

Patients undergoing laparotomy have large increases in heat loss compared to those normally associated with anaesthesia. If a thoracic epidural is used, the compensatory vasoconstriction responsible for phase 3 is lost and severe hypothermia can occur. Every effort must be made to avoid hypothermia and its complications. In recovery the residual effects of general anaesthesia, continued epidural vasodilatation, inhibition of shivering, and continuing fluid administration can result in further hypothermia. The above techniques should be carried over into recovery.

Fluid management

Fluid loss occurs pre-, intra-, and postoperatively in patients undergoing laparotomy. Causes of fluid loss include:

- Preoperative: reduced fluid intake secondary to the underlying disease process, increased fluid losses, e.g. ileostomy, vomiting, laxative use for bowel preparation, preoperative starvation.
- Intra-operative: large evaporative losses from the peritoneal cavity through the abdominal incision, sequestration of fluid into the omentum and bowel lumen (third space loss), blood loss, evaporative loss from the respiratory tract, urine production, nasogastric losses.
- Postoperative: ongoing sequestration of fluid into the omentum and bowel (paralytic ileus), ongoing losses from the nasogastric tube, urine production, ongoing blood loss.

These losses must be replaced with an individualized fluid regime. Those with large preoperative fluid deficits should have IV fluids preoperatively on the ward or HDU. Losses should be carefully charted on a regular basis particularly nasogastric drainage, blood loss, and urine output. During surgery, crystalloid maintenance rates are between 10 and 30 ml/kg/h. For prolonged procedures, requiring large volumes of crystalloid, Hartmann's solution is preferable.

Nasogastric tubes

When deciding on which nasogastric tube to use consider:

- duration of use
- the indication
- diameter.

Duration

With prolonged use, complications such as local tissue irritation/ necrosis/ perforation (nares, nasopharynx, oesophagus, stomach), and degradation of the nasogastric tube become more pertinent. The most important consideration in preventing these complications is the material that the nasogastric tube is made from. The maximum recommended durations of use for the various materials used in the manufacture of nasogastric tubes are:

- PVC 1 week
- polyurethane 2–4 weeks
- silicone >4 weeks.

Indication

There are four basic types of nasogastric tube:

* Gastric tube: approximately 100 cm long with an open-ended, non-weighted tip. This is the most basic type of tube. The open-ended tip allows easier aspiration and wash out of the stomach but at the expense of increased risk of trauma to the stomach wall, i.e. 'tissue grab' during the process of aspiration.

* Leven gastro-duodenal tube: approximately 125 cm long with closed non-weighted tip. Reduces the risk of tissue grab and is long enough to pass into the duodenum/jejunum if nasogastric feeding is likely.

* Ryles tube: approximately 125 cm long with the same characteristics as the Leven tube except that the tip is weighted using tungsten. The tungsten weight makes passage of the tube into the stomach easier and aids peristalsis in moving the tube tip out of the stomach and into the small intestine.

* Salem sump tube: approximately 100 cm long with a closed non-weighted tip. At the proximal end there is a sump tube, which if left open to air reduces tissue grab even when negative pressure is applied to the nasogastric tube. These tubes are designed for active decompression of the GIT using continuous gentle aspiration.

Diameter

Nasogastric tubes come in a range of diameters from 8–18 FG. The bigger the gauge the easier it is to drain and decompress the stomach but the greater the risk of tissue grab and patient discomfort. One of the main complaints of patients following laparotomy is discomfort and pain related to the nasogastric tube.

For most laparotomies a PVC/polyurethane 16 FG Ryles or Salem tube is adequate. For procedures such as a laparoscopic cholecystectomy, where decompression of the stomach aids surgical access or where active decompression of the GIT is anticipated postoperatively, then the Salem tube is preferable.

Operation	Description	Time (h)	Pain	Position	Blood loss (litres)	Notes
Hemicolectomy	Resection of right or left hemicolon	1–3	++++	Supine	0.5	Low thoracic epidural or opioid infusion/PCA
Sigmoid colectomy	Resection of sigmoid colon with bowel anastomosis	1–3	++++	Supine. Head down. May need Lloyd-Davies	0.5–1.0	Low thoracic epidural or opioid infusion/PCA
Hartmann's procedure	Resection of sigmoid colon with colostomy	1–3	++++	Supine. Head down. May need Lloyd Davies	0.5–1.0	Low thoracic epidural or opioid infusion/PCA
Anterior resection	Resection of rectum	2–3	++++	Head down. Lloyd Davies	0.5–1.5	Low thoracic epidural
AP resection	Resection of rectum and anus	2–4	+++++	Head down. Lloyd Davies	0.5–2.0	Low thoracic epidural. Can be difficult to block sacral nerve roots. CVP line
Gastrectomy	Resection of stomach	2–3	+++++	Supine	0.5–1.0	High thoracic epidural, Consider CVP/art line
Cholecystectomy	Resection of gall bladder	1	+++ /++++	Supine	0.5	Right upper quadrant incision. PCA
Closure of loop colostomy or loop ileostomy	Local closure of colostomy or loop ileostomy	0.5–1	++	Supine	ns	Still requires muscle relaxation. May need PCA. If difficulties arise can proceed to more extensive procedure
Reversal of Hartmann's	Laparotomy. Bowel ends re-anastomosed	1–2.0	++++	Supine. Head down. May need Lloyd Davies	0.5–1.5	Low thoracic epidural

The sick laparotomy

(See also 'Anaesthesia for the Septic Patient' p. 682.)

Patients for emergency intra-abdominal surgery are at a much greater risk of perioperative complications than those presenting electively. The time available for preparation varies from only a few minutes to 12 h or more. The key is to strike the correct balance between the benefits of preoperative resuscitation and those of timely surgery. The principles described earlier regarding the care of the patient undergoing a laparotomy apply equally in the emergency situation.

Preoperative assessment

- Discuss the probable diagnosis with the surgical team. The emergency laparotomy can be broadly divided into a bleeding problem (e.g. AAA, splenic laceration, avulsed vessel), intestinal perforation (e.g. perforated duodenal ulcer, intestinal ischaemia), or acute intestinal obstruction.
- Bleeding problems present with hypovolaemic shock. Treat appropriately, but these cases need immediate treatment and resuscitation can occur during transfer to theatre and immediately prior to induction. Consider anaesthetizing the patient on the operating table with the surgeon scrubbed and the patient prepared for surgery.
- Intestinal perforation/obstruction produces a greater metabolic derangement. Time spent on a detailed assessment and adequate resuscitation pays dividends perioperatively.
- Careful examination of cardiorespiratory status is important and can reveal subtle clues regarding the severity of illness. Pulse oximetry is useful in those who are dyspnoeic.
- Investigations should include FBC, electrolytes (include magnesium if possible), LFTs, clotting, ECG, chest radiograph, and cross-match.
- ABGs are used to assess the degree of acidosis and oxygenation and may yield important information regarding the severity of illness, resuscitation, and the appropriate environment for perioperative care.

Preoperative preparation

- A careful balance must be struck between preoperative optimization and surgical urgency. Patients presenting with an intra-abdominal catastrophe (acute obstruction/perforation) are often extremely unwell, with marked hypovolaemia, hypoperfusion, acidosis, severe renal impairment, and sepsis.
- Optimize the patient's cardiorespiratory status as far as possible in the time available. This may require admission to ICU/HDU, invasive monitoring of CVP and arterial pressure, aggressive rehydration, and possibly inotropic support. If ICU/HDU is not available, theatre recovery may be an option. Aggressive preoperative optimization in this group of patients is often beneficial in the perioperative period.
- Oxygen should be administered to most emergency laparotomies in the preoperative period especially if hypotensive or with an oxygen saturation of less than 95% on pulse oximetry or arterial blood gas measurement.
- Aggressive fluid management is essential. The first priority is to restore intravascular volume and perfusion. Initial resuscitation should be with

colloid or blood depending on the haemoglobin. Once an adequate circulating volume is achieved, prescribe crystalloid and/or colloid to maintain hydration and perfusion. Fluid resuscitation should be guided by CVP measurement, or at least hourly urine output.

- Urinary catheter: start hourly measurement of urine output and use to guide fluid therapy.
- A nasogastric tube should be inserted in patients presenting with intestinal obstruction to relieve gastric distension and reduce the risk of aspiration.
- Electrolytes should be corrected as far as possible. Hypokalaemia and hypomagnesaemia provoke cardiac arrhythmias. Control diabetes with an insulin/dextrose infusion.
- Metabolic acidosis should improve with aggressive fluid and cardiovascular manipulation. If the pH does not respond and remains low (<7.2) the patient is at high risk. Consider whether there may be an underlying metabolic problem (e.g. diabetic ketoacidosis) or pathology (e.g. bowel ischaemia). If surgery is indicated and the pH unresponsive, 100–200 ml of 8.4% sodium bicarbonate IV should be considered.
- Problems with clotting should be addressed and treated appropriately.
- Analgesia is not contraindicated in the acute abdomen. Use IV morphine. Avoid NSAIDs in the critically ill (renal damage, decreased platelet function, etc.).
- Give antibiotics where appropriate.

Perioperative care

- Aspirate the nasogastric tube prior to induction.
- Pre-oxygenate.
- Rapid sequence induction.
- Have a large-bore IVI connected to pressurized fluids (gelofusine) and infusing rapidly.
- Choice of induction agent depends on cardiovascular stability. A single dose of etomidate is unlikely to have major effects on the adrenocortical axis. Propofol or thiopental are more likely to cause hypotension in this group. Give any induction agent slowly allowing for the delay in onset.
- Relaxants. Following suxamethonium use atracurium/cis-atracurium (metabolism not dependent on renal function). In the acidotic patient the duration of action of these drugs is prolonged.
- Analgesia. Regional analgesia is often a poor choice in this group due to persisting hypotension and the risks of unmasking hypovolaemia. Fentanyl or morphine are good options. Give with induction and supplement as needed. TIVA using ketamine is sometimes useful.
- Vasopressors and vagolytics should be drawn up before induction (atropine, glycopyrrolate, ephedrine, and metaraminol). If hypotension persists prepare an adrenaline or noradrenaline infusion and start preoperatively.
- Monitoring. Invasive arterial and central venous pressure monitoring are extremely useful in this group and should be inserted preoperatively. Continue in recovery and postoperatively as required.
- Patient warming should be as for any laparotomy.

Postoperative

- ICU/HDU care is often necessary for early and aggressive treatment of hypothermia, cardiorespiratory compromise, sepsis, coagulopathy, borderline urine output, etc. Consider postoperative ventilation for 24 h if the patient is particularly hypothermic or cardiovascularly unstable perioperatively.
- Frequent review of postoperative fluids should be undertaken, guided preferably by CVP measurement.
- Urine output should be measured hourly intra- and postoperatively. If <0.5 ml/kg/h urgent review is necessary.
- Postoperative chest radiograph to check the position of the CVP line.
- Oxygen should be administered for a minimum of 72 h postoperatively.
- Pain—consider continuous morphine infusion. PCA is often not practical due to postoperative confusion.

General principles for laparoscopic surgery

Laparoscopic techniques have been developed for many operations including cholecystectomy, fundoplication, vagotomy, hemicolectomy, hernia repair, appendicectomy, and oesophagectomy.

Compared with laparotomy the major advantages are:

- Reduced tissue trauma required for surgical exposure.
- Reduced wound size and postoperative pain.
- Improved postoperative respiratory function: Following open cholecystectomy FVC is reduced by approximately 50% and changes are still evident up to 72 h postoperatively. Following laparoscopic cholecystectomy FVC is reduced by approximately 30% and is normal at 24 h postoperatively.
- Reduced postoperative ileus.
- Earlier mobilization.
- Shorter hospital stay.

Surgical requirements

- Gravitational displacement of abdominal viscera from the operative site.
- Decompression of abdominal viscera, especially the stomach (nasogastric tube) and bladder (urinary catheter). Prevents injury on trocar insertion.
- Pneumoperitoneum. This separates the abdominal wall from the viscera. An intra-abdominal pressure of 15 mmHg is adequate for most procedures. Modern equipment has an automatic limit on abdominal pressure. Beware older equipment which may not have an automatic limit, as can deliver gas flows producing an intra-abdominal pressure greater than 40 mmHg.
- Carbon dioxide can be used to create the pneumoperitoneum. This has the advantage of being non-combustible allowing the use of diathermy or laser. Disadvantages include systemic absorption and peritoneal irritation producing pain.

Intra-operative effects of laparoscopic surgery

- Pneumoperitoneum raises intra-abdominal pressure. Physiological changes are minimized if the intra-abdominal pressure <15 mmHg. This value should be monitored on the insufflation equipment. Physiological effects include:

Respiratory	Diaphragmatic displacement, reduced lung volumes and compliance, increased airway resistance, increased V/Q mismatch, hypoxia/hypercapnia from hypoventilation, increased risk of regurgitation
CVS	Increased systemic vascular resistance, raised mean arterial pressure, compression of IVC, reduced venous return, reduced cardiac output
Renal	Reduced renal blood flow, reduced glomerular filtration rate, reduced urine output

- Patient positioning. With upper abdominal procedures the patient is placed head up (reverse Trendelenberg position). For lower abdominal procedures the patient is placed head down (Trendelenberg position). The usual tilt is 15–20 degrees. Some left tilt is usual with cholecystectomy. These postures may further stress CVS and respiratory function.
- Systemic carbon dioxide absorption may produce hypercarbia and acidosis.
- Extraperitoneal gas insufflation occurs through a misplaced trocar or when gas under pressure dissects through tissue defects. It may cause subcutaneous emphysema, pneumomediastinum, pneumopericardium, or pneumothorax.
- Venous gas embolism may occur when the trocar is inadvertently positioned in a vessel. Presents as acute right heart failure, reduced $ETCO_2$, arrhythmias, myocardial ischaemia, hypotension, elevated CVP.
- Unintentional injuries to intra-abdominal structures—major vessels, viscera, liver, and spleen. May not be detected during surgery. Presents postoperatively with pain, hypotension, hypovolaemia, peritonitis, septicaemia.

Anaesthetic management

Preoperative

- Contraindications to laparoscopic surgery are relative. Successful laparoscopic procedures have been carried out on patients who were anticoagulated, markedly obese, or pregnant.
- Fit and young patients tolerate the physiological changes well.
- Elderly patients and those with cardiac or pulmonary disease have more marked and varied responses.
- NCEPOD 1996/1997 recommended caution in patients who were ASA >3, age >69 years, those who had a history of cardiac failure, and those with widespread ischaemic heart disease.
- Patients with marked respiratory or cardiac disease must be thoroughly reviewed and optimized preoperatively and have a surgeon experienced in the procedure as the operator. Beware of patients being admitted on the day of surgery without the appropriate preoperative preparation.
- Prescribe paracetamol 1 g PO and an NSAID, e.g. diclofenac 50–100 mg PO, 2 h preoperatively.
- Be prepared to convert to an open procedure (1–7%).

Perioperative

- General anaesthesia with endotracheal intubation to protect against pulmonary aspiration, aids ventilation and allows IPPV. Use IPPV to overcome the respiratory effects of pneumonperitoneum and hypercarbia. Good muscle relaxation reduces the intra-abdominal pressure needed for adequate surgical exposure. Monitor relaxants.
- Induction: avoid excess stomach inflation from mask ventilation.
- Nasogastric tube: insert and aspirate. This deflates the stomach reducing the risk of gastric injury during trocar insertion and improves surgical exposure.
- Use a urinary catheter for lower abdominal procedures. This decompresses the bladder and reduces the risk of injury.
- Ventilate to normocarbia. Raised intra-abdominal pressure and systemic absorption of carbon dioxide will require increased minute volume and raised airway pressures.

- Watch for inadvertent endobronchial intubation if the patient is positioned head down with pnuemoperitoneum.
- Opioids: short acting opioids, e.g. fentanyl, alfentanil, can be used intra-operatively to cover what can be an intense but short-lived stimulus.
- Nitrous oxide: concerns regarding problems with bowel distension and postoperative nausea and vomiting have not been substantiated.
- Volatiles: avoid halothane—sensitized myocardium in the presence of hypercarbia—because of a risk of arrhythmias.
- Fluids: avoid hypovolaemia as this exaggerates the deleterious CVS effects of the procedure.
- Gas insufflation into the peritoneal cavity with stretching of the peritoneum, raised intra-abdominal pressure and altered patient positioning can cause a range of clinical responses:
  - Sympathetic response: hypertensive, tachycardia, increased cardiac output is the most common response. Treatment: increase volatiles, short-acting opioid, e.g. alfentanil, remifentanil, vasodilator, and/or beta-blocker.
  - CVS depression with a fall in cardiac output: hypotension, tachycardia, or bradycardia. Treatment: fluids, vasodilators, inotropes.
  - Vagal response: asystole, sinus bradycardia, nodal rhythm, hypotension. Treatment: vagolytics.
- If there is intra-operative hypoxia consider:
  - Hypoventilation—pneumoperitoneum, position, inadequate ventilation.
  - V/Q mismatch—reduced FRC, atelectasis, endobronchial intubation, extraperitoneal gas insufflation, bowel distension, pulmonary aspiration, and rarely pneumothorax.
  - Reduced cardiac output—IVC compression, arrhythmias, haemorrhage, myocardial depression, venous gas embolism, extraperitoneal gas.
- Subcutaneous emphysema during the procedure spells DANGER—stop gas insufflation and check for extraperitoneal gas insufflation.
- At end of operation encourage the surgeon to expel as much CO_2 as possible to reduce pain. Local anaesthetic to wound sites.
- For laparoscopic cholecystectomy remove the nasogastric tube before taking the patient to recovery. For other procedures check with the surgeon.

Postoperatively

- Pain varies significantly and is worst in the first few hours postoperatively. It ranges from shoulder tip pain (diaphragmatic irritation) to deep-seated pain from the surgery. Significant pain extending beyond the first day raises the possibility of intra-abdominal problems.
- Prescribe regular paracetamol and NSAIDs with opioid PRN.
- Nausea and vomiting: over 50% of patients require antiemetics. Give intra-operatively and prescribe postoperatively.

Special considerations

- Intra-operative monitoring: standard monitoring including nerve stimulator. Respiratory monitoring is essential including $ETCO_2$ and airway pressure. In patients with severe cardiopulmonary compromise use intra-arterial blood pressure and CVP monitoring.

- LMA: some anaesthetists use an LMA for laparoscopic procedures. This is an individual choice. Potential contraindications to its use are an inexperienced surgeon, an anticipated difficult procedure, obesity, history of reflux, and pre-existing severe cardiopulmonary compromise.

- Some short procedures (e.g. laparoscopic sterilization) can be performed without muscle relaxation provided that the operator is experienced.

- Regional anaesthesia is not generally used as the sole anaesthetic technique because of the level of block required, pneumoperitoneum, patient positioning and shoulder tip pain.

- Mortality/morbidity: the incidence of adverse events is approximately 5%. The most common complication is superficial infection at the site of the umbilical trocar. There are a number of case reports describing acute hypotension, hypoxia, and cardiovascular collapse with laparoscopic surgery. The cause is probably multifactorial. Be prepared to convert to an open procedure if the patient is too unstable.

- Open versus laparoscopic procedures: in the case of cholecystectomy the laparoscopic technique, unless surgically impossible, is the technique of choice even in high-risk patients because of postoperative advantages. Mortality following open cholecystectomy overall is less than 1% but in the elderly population can be up to 10%. The adverse event rate following open cholecystectomy is approximately 20%. For other procedures little good evidence exists.

- Laparoscopic appendicectomy: not recommended if perforated appendix is suspected. It has the advantage of allowing diagnosis and preventing unnecessary laparotomy in 20% of cases. Potential advantages are a better cosmetic result, reduced wound pain, and a more rapid return to normal activities, but these are not proven. Risks of laparoscopic appendicectomy are pneumoperitoneum and prolonged surgery; it is also more expensive.

- Laproscopic inguinal hernia: more applicable for indirect hernias. Direct hernias are more challenging. High-risk cases are best done open under local anaesthetic. There are no clear postoperative advantages, with the total length of incisions essentially the same for the two procedures. The laparoscopic technique has disadvantages associated with a GA and pneumoperitonuem.

Laparoscopic cholecystectomy

Procedure	Laparoscopic removal of gall bladder
Time	1–2 h
Pain	++/++++
Position	Supine, 15–20 degree head up, table tilted towards surgeon
Blood loss	Not significant
Practical technique	GA, ETT, IPPV

Preoperative

* Patients typically 'fair, fat, female, forty'.
* The procedure is potentially painful.

Perioperative

* The stomach may need deflating, hence insert a larger bore nasogastric tube—remove it at end of surgery.
* 16 gauge IV access—blood loss may become significant.
* Combination of pneumoperitoneum and obesity may make ventilation difficult.
* Head up/sideways tilt.
* Surgical time is very variable and operator dependent.
* Ask the surgeon to infiltrate port sites with local anaesthetic at the end.
* Conversion to open procedure 1–7%. This is usually due to difficulty identifying the cystic duct, suspected common bile duct injury, uncontrolled bleeding from the cystic artery, stones present in the common bile duct, or acute inflammatory changes.

Postoperative

* High incidence of PONV.
* Pain can be severe and may require opioids.

Special considerations

* This can be a very stimulating and painful procedure, particularly during diathermy around the liver.
* Analgesic requirements can be reduced by asking the surgeon to spray local anaesthetic onto the gall bladder bed before starting dissection (20 ml bupivacaine 0.25%).

Appendicectomy

Procedure	Resection of appendix
Time	20–40 min
Pain	++/+++
Position	Supine
Blood loss	Not significant
Practical technique	Rapid sequence induction, ETT, IPPV, ilio-inguinal block

Preoperative

- Patients are usually aged 5–20 years and are fit.
- Can present in the elderly. May be the presenting condition of caecal adenocarcinoma requiring right hemicolectomy.
- Consent required for suppositories.
- Check fluid status.
- If considering ilio-inguinal block, warn of possible associated femoral nerve blockade.

Perioperative

- Rapid sequence induction.
- Muscle relaxation required for surgery.
- Replace fluid deficit.
- Give PR diclofenac and PR paracetamol.
- Right ilio-inguinal nerve block gives useful postoperative analgesia, or ask the surgeon to infiltrate locally.
- Extubate awake and in left lateral.

Postoperative

- Prescribe paracetamol, NSAIDs, morphine, and antiemetic until tolerating oral fluids.
- Maintenance fluids.

Special consideration

- Regional anaesthesia is an option in adults if GA contraindicated.

Inguinal hernia repair

Procedure	Repair of inguinal muscular canal defect through which bowel protrudes
Time	30–60 min
Pain	++/+++
Position	Supine
Blood loss	Not significant
Practical techniques	GA, SV LMA, inguinal field block
	Spinal
	Local infiltration and/or sedation

Preoperative

• Patients are usually adult males or young children.

Perioperative

• Will need opioid if not using a local technique.
• If using an inguinal field block the surgeon may need to inject a local anaesthetic into the spermatic cord. More likely if the genitofemoral nerve is not blocked preoperatively.

Postoperative

• Significant co-morbidity associated with age—give supplemental oxygen for 24 h.

Special considerations

• May be booked as a day case procedure.
• If day case, prescribe opioid analgesia to take home, e.g. tramadol 50–100 mg four times a day.
• Laparoscopic hernia repair (see earlier).
• Some surgeons do all inguinal hernias under local anaesthetic, some none. In a high-risk patient repair under local anaesthetic is best.
• Mesh insertion usually requires administration of prophylactic antibiotics.

Haemorrhoidectomy

Procedure	Excision of haemorrhoids
Time	20 min
Pain	++/+++
Position	Supine, lithotomy, head down
Blood loss	Not significant
Practical technique	GA, SV LMA and/or caudal
	Spinal ("saddle block")

Preoperative

- Assess suitability for LMA + lithotomy + head down position. Consider ETT if the patient is obese.

Perioperative

- Opioid analgesia—short but intensely painful stimulus. Fentanyl and/or alfentanil is a good option.
- Ensure sufficient depth of anaesthesia—beware laryngospasm/airway difficulties if the depth of anaesthesia is insufficient.
- Caudal anaesthesia is useful for postoperative analgesia (bupivacaine 0.25% 20 ml), but beware the risk of urinary retention. Infiltration by the surgeon during the procedure is probably as effective.
- Potential for bradycardia/asystole as surgery starts. Have atropine available.

Postoperative

- Best to avoid the PR route of drug administration.

Special considerations

- Beware spinal followed by an immediate head down tilt.
- Anal stretch is an intense stimulus. Before the surgeon performs this manoeuvre deepen the anaesthetic, e.g. increase volatile and give a bolus of alfentanil (500 μg). The anal stretch can also produce an increase in vagal tone. Be prepared for this.
- If the patient has a murmur remember to give SBE prophylaxis.
- A sacral only spinal block ("saddle block") using heavy bupivacaine is a useful alternative with little effect on cardiovascular dynamics.

Testicular surgery

Procedure	Removal/biopsy of testis, marsupulization of hydrocele, vasectomy, testicular torsion
Time	30 min–1 h
Pain	++/+++
Position	Supine
Blood loss	Not significant
Practical techniques	GA, LMA and/or spermatic cord block
	Spinal
	LA infiltration

Preoperative

• May be suitable for day case surgery.

Perioperative

• Beware vagal responses—have atropine ready.

Special considerations

• Innervation of testes and scrotum: somatic innervation is via ilioinguinal, genitofemoral, pudendal, and posterior scrotal nerves (branches of posterior cutaneous nerve of the thigh) with nerve root contributions from L1–S3. Autonomic innervation is from the sympathetic chain T10–L4 and the parasympathetic plexus S1–S3. Local techniques therefore need to cover T10–S3.

• A spermatic cord block can be used as an adjunct to a GA or as part of an LA technique for scrotal surgery. The block covers all nerves except the pudendal and posterior scrotal branches. If used as part of a local anaesthetic technique supplemental infiltration of the scrotal skin is therefore required.

• Spermatic cord is best blocked under direct vision by the surgeon. However, if a local technique is planned:
  • Identify the pubic tubercle.
  • Insert the needle 1 cm below and medial to the pubic tubercle.
  • Insert the needle until bone is contacted.
  • Withdraw the needle slightly and, if aspiration is negative, inject a total of 15–20 ml of local anaesthetic in three to four passes at different angles.
  • Alternatively, feel for the spermatic cord as it enters the top of the scrotum and infiltrate 5 ml local anaesthetic around the cord.

Further reading

Chui PT, Gin T, Oh TE (1993). Anaesthesia for laparoscopic general surgery. *Anaesthesia and Intensive Care*, **21**, 163–71.

Cunningham AJ (1998). Anaesthetic implications of laparoscopic surgery. *Yale Journal of Biology and Medicine*, **71**, 551–78.

Ruskis AF (1982). Effects of narcotics on gastrointestinal tract, liver, kidneys. In: Kitahata LM, Collins JG (ed.), *Narcotic analgesic in anesthesiology*, pp. 143–156. Williams & Wilkins, Baltimore.

Sessler DI (2000). Perioperative heat balance. *Anaesthesiology*, **92**, 578–96.

Van Aken H, Rolf N (1999). Clinical Anaesthesiology: thoracic epidural anaesthesia. *Bailliere's Best Practice and Research*, **13** (1), 9–109.

Chapter 15
Endocrine surgery

Paul Marshall

Thyroidectomy

Procedure	Removal of all or part of the thyroid gland.
Time	1–2 h depending on complexity
Pain	+/++
Position	Bolster between shoulders with head ring. Head up tilt
Blood loss	Usually minimal. Potentially major if retrosternal extension
Practical techniques	IPPV + ETT

General considerations (see also p. 80)

* Complexity can vary from removal of a thyroid nodule to removal of long-standing retrosternal goitre to relieve tracheal compression.
* Retrosternal goitre is usually excised through a standard incision, but occasionally a sternal split is required.
* Recurrent laryngeal nerves and four parathyroid glands should be preserved.
* Straightforward unilateral surgery can be performed under superficial and deep cervical plexus block but general anaesthesia is usual.

Preoperative

* Assess the resting pulse rate and ensure that the patient is as near euthyroid as possible.
* Ask about duration of goitre. Longstanding compression of the trachea may be associated with tracheomalacia. A rapid increase in size suggests the possibility of malignancy.
* Check for complications associated with hyperthyroidism: AF, tachycardia, proptosis.
* Ask about positional breathlessness. Make a routine assessment of the airway (p. 866).
* Examine the neck. How big is the goitre? Note the consistency of the gland (hard suggests malignancy). Can you feel below the gland (retrosternal spread)? Is there evidence of tracheal deviation (check radiograph)?
* Look for signs of SVC obstruction.
* Listen for stridor.
* Check the range of neck movements preoperatively and do not extend them outside of their normal range during surgery.

Investigations

* FBC, electrolytes, Ca^{2+}, and thyroid function tests are routine.
* Chest radiograph. Check for tracheal deviation and narrowing. In suspicious or complex cases lateral thoracic inlet views are necessary to exclude retrosternal extension and to detect tracheal compression in the anterior–posterior plane (retrosternal enlargement may be asymptomatic).

◆ CT scan accurately delineates the site and degree of airway encroachment and may also indicate tracheal invasion by carcinoma. It is advisable if there are symptoms of narrowing (e.g. stridor, positional breathlessness), more than 50% narrowing on the radiograph or suspicion of malignancy. Plain radiographs overestimate diameters due to magnification effects and cannot be relied on when predicting endotracheal tube diameter and length.

◆ ENT consultation for nasendoscopy to document cord function. This is mandatory for medicolegal purposes. Preoperative cord dysfunction may be asymptomatic. Possible causes of dysfunction are previous surgery and malignancy. Fibreoptic examination also defines any possible laryngeal displacement (useful in airway planning).

◆ Benzodiazepine premedication is usual. Give an antisialogogue if planning fibreoptic or inhalation induction. Preoperative paracetamol/NSAIDs (oral or rectal) helps postoperative pain control.

Airway planning

The majority of cases are straightforward even when there is some tracheal deviation or compression. Preoxygenation should be followed by intravenous induction and a neuromuscular blocking drug (after checking that the lungs can be inflated manually).

The following features should lead to a more considered approach and may require discussion with the surgeon and radiologist:

◆ Malignancy. Cord palsies are likely. Distortion and rigidity of surrounding structures mean that lumen of trachea may not allow a standard ET tube to pass. There is the possibility of intraluminal spread. The larynx may be displaced. Also the tumour may produce glottic or supraglottic obstruction and/or lower tracheal/bronchial obstruction as well as midtracheal obstruction.

◆ Significant respiratory symptoms or > 50% narrowing on chest radiograph or lateral thoracic inlet view. CT will help determine management. If a 7 mm tube can be accommodated and if the site of obstruction is sufficiently above the carina to accommodate a cuff and bevel then a conventional approach is possible.

◆ Coexisting predictors of difficult intubation.

Options to secure the airway for complicated thyroid surgery

◆ Inhalation induction with sevoflurane (p. 879) in patients with stridor and suspected difficult upper airway. This should be preceded by antisialogogue premedication. Sevoflurane in Heliox may be useful in cases of marked airway narrowing. Stridor and decreased minute ventilation delay the onset of sufficiently deep anaesthesia for intubation. Topical local anaesthetic may be useful. Be prepared for rapid lightening of consciousness whilst attempting intubation.

◆ Fibreoptic intubation. (p. 882). Attempts to pass a fibreoptic bronchoscope in an awake patient with stridor are difficult as the narrowed airway may become obstructed by the instrument. May be useful where there is marked displacement of the larynx or coexisting difficulties with intubation, e.g. ankylosing spondylitis.

◆ Tracheostomy under local anaesthetic. This will only be possible if the tracheostomy can be easily performed below the level of obstruction.

- Ventilation through a rigid bronchoscope is a backup option when attempts to pass an ETT down the trachea fail. The surgeon and necessary equipment should be immediately available for complex cases, particularly involving significant mid-lower tracheal narrowing.

Perioperative

- Eye padding and tape are important, especially if exophthalmos.
- Full relaxation is required to accommodate tube movements. Local anaesthetic spray on the ETT reduces the stimulation produced by tracheal manipulation during the surgery.
- Fix the ETT with tape, avoiding ties around the neck. Armoured ETTs are preferred by most anaesthetists and should probably be used in cases with significant tracheal compression.
- Head and neck extension with slight head up tilt.
- Consider a superficial cervical plexus block for postoperative analgesia. Some surgeons infiltrate subcutaneously with local anaesthetic and adrenaline before starting.
- Arms to sides, IV extension.
- Communicate with the surgeon if there are excessive airway pressures during manipulation of the trachea. Obstruction may be due to airway manipulation distal to the tube or the bevel of the tube abutting on the trachea.
- Monitor muscle relaxants on the leg.
- In cases of longstanding goitre some surgeons like to feel the trachea before closing to assess tracheomalacia. They may ask for partial withdrawal of the endotracheal tube so that the tip is just proximal to the site of the goitre.
- At end of surgery reverse muscle relaxant and extubate. Any respiratory difficulty should lead to immediate reintubation. The traditional practice of inspecting the cords immediately following extubation is difficult and unreliable. Possible cord dysfunction and postoperative tracheomalacia is better assessed with the patient awake and sitting up in the recovery room.

Postoperative

- Intermittent opioids with oral/rectal paracetamol and NSAIDs.
- The opioid requirement is reduced with subcutaneous infiltration or superficial cervical plexus blocks.
- Use fibreoptic nasendoscopy if there is doubt about recurrent laryngeal nerve injury.

Postoperative stridor

- Haemorrhage with tense swelling of the neck. Remove clips from skin, and sutures from platysma/strap muscles to remove the clot. In extremis this should be done at the bedside. Otherwise return to theatre without delay.
- Tracheomalacia. Longstanding goitre may cause tracheal collapse after surgery. Immediate reintubation followed by tracheostomy may be necessary. Tracheal reconstruction may be needed at a later date.
- Bilateral recurrent laryngeal nerve palsies. This may present with respiratory difficulty immediately postoperatively or after a variable period. Stridor may only be obvious when the patient becomes agitated. Assess by

fibreoptic nasendoscopy. May require tracheostomy. Laryngeal surgery may be possible at a later stage to allow decannulation of the tracheostomy.

• Laryngeal oedema. This is unusual but may occur if there has been a traumatic intubation or with more extensive neck surgery (e.g. radical neck dissection). May require corticosteroids and humidification.

Other postoperative complications

Hypocalcaemia

Hypocalcaemia from parathyroid removal is rare. Serum calcium should be checked at 24 h and again daily if low.

• Presentation: may present with signs of neuromuscular excitability, tingling around the mouth, or tetany. May progress to fits or ventricular arrhythmias.

• Diagnosis: carpopedal spasm (flexed wrists, fingers drawn together) may be precipitated by cuff inflation (Trousseau's sign). Tapping over the facial nerve at the parotid may cause facial twitching (Chvostek's sign). Prolonged QT interval on ECG.

• Treatment: serum calcium below 2 mmol/litre should be treated urgently with 10 ml 10% calcium gluconate over 3 min plus oral alfacalcidol or dihydroxycholecalciferol 1–5 μg orally. Check level after 4 h and consider calcium infusion if still low. If hypocalcaemic but level above 2 mmol/litre treat with oral calcium supplements.

Thyroid crisis

This is rare as hyperthyroidism is usually controlled beforehand with anti-thyroid drugs and beta-blockers. May be triggered in uncontrolled or undiagnosed cases by surgery or infection.

• Diagnosis: tachycardia and rising temperature. May be difficult to distinguish from MH. Higher mixed venous $PvCO_2$ and higher CPK in MH.

• Treatment: see p. 80.

Pneumothorax

Pneumothorax is possible if there has been dissection behind the sternum.

Further reading

Farling PA (2000). Thyroid disease. *British Journal of Anaesthesia*, **85**, 15–28.

Parathyroidectomy

Procedure.	Removal of solitary adenoma or four-gland hyperplasia
Time	1–3 h
Pain	+/++
Position	Bolster between shoulders with head ring. Head up tilt
Blood Loss	Usually minimal
Techniques	IPPV + ETT

General considerations (see also p. 83)

- Usual indication for operation is primary hyperparathyroidism from parathyroid adenoma.
- With preoperative localization, removal of simple adenoma has been described using sedation and local anaesthesia. General anaesthesia is more usual.
- Carcinoma may require en bloc dissection.
- Total parathyroidectomy may also be performed in secondary hyperparathyroidism associated with chronic renal failure.

Preoperative (see also p. 83)

- Hypercalcaemia is usual. With moderate elevation ensure adequate hydration with 0.9% normal saline. Levels over 3 mmol/litre should be corrected before surgery as follows:
  - urinary catheter
  - normal saline 1 litre in first hour then 4–6 litres over 24 h
  - Pamidronate 60 mg in 500 ml saline over 4 h
  - watch for fluid overload. CVP measurement may be necessary in some patients. Monitor electrolytes including magnesium, phosphate, and potassium.
- Preoperative imaging and unilateral exploration are usual for adenoma. Some surgeons request intravenous methylthioninium chloride (methylene blue) 5 mg/kg in 500 ml dextrose saline given over 1 h immediately preoperatively to show up adenoma during the operation. Transient falls in the SpO_2 reading may occur if this drug is infused too rapidly in theatre.
- Secondary hyperparathryoidism occurs secondary to low serum calcium in chronic renal failure. In this situation:
  - Total parathyroidectomy may be required. Control afterwards is easier if no functioning parathyroid tissue is left.
  - Dialysis will be required preoperatively.
  - The risk of bleeding is increased.
  - Alfacalcidol is usually started preoperatively.

• Hypertension is more common in primary hyperparathyroidism. Raised parathyroid hormone appears to be a good clinical predictor of left ventricular hypertrophy in haemodialysis patients.

Perioperative

• Similar anaesthetic considerations as for thyroid surgery.
• Airway encroachment is not usually a problem.
• Operation times may be unpredictable, especially if frozen section or parathyroid assays are performed.
• Consider active heat conservation.

Postoperative

• Serum calcium checked at 6 and 24 h. Hypocalcaemia may occur (for diagnosis and treatment see above under Thyroidectomy). Persisting hypercalcaemia is unusual.
• Continuation of alfacalcidol in secondary hyperparathyroidism lessens the chance of hypocalcaemia postoperatively.
• Perform fibreoptic nasendoscopy if recurrent laryngeal nerve damage is suspected.
• Pain not usually severe, especially with local anaesthetic infiltration or superficial cervical plexus blocks. Rectal paracetamol is useful. Avoid NSAIDs in patients with poor renal function.

Further reading

Mihai R, Farndon JR (2000). Parathyroid disease and calcium metabolism. *British Journal of Anaesthesia*, **85**, 29–43.

Phaeochromocytoma

- Phaeochromocytomas are tumours of chromaffin cells which secrete nor-adrenaline, adrenaline, or dopamine in decreasing incidence. Some tumours secrete more than one catecholamine.
- 90% occur in the adrenals, 10% are bilateral, but tumours may be located anywhere along the sympathetic chain from the base of the skull to the pelvis.
- Most are benign, a few are malignant.
- They occur in all age groups, less commonly in children.
- Can occur in association with multiple endocrine neoplasia (MEN) 2A where medullary thyroid carcinoma and parathyroid adenomas coexist, or MEN2B with medullary thyroid carcinoma and marfanoid features. Both of these have abnormalities of the ret oncogene, an abnormality on chromosome 10.
- Also found in patients with neurofibromatosis and Von Hippel–Lindau syndrome.

Presentation

- Hypertension can be constant, intermittent, or insignificant.
- The association of palpitations, sweating, and headache with hypertension has a high predictive value.
- Anxiety, nausea and vomiting, and weakness and lethargy are also common features.
- Acute presentations include pulmonary oedema, myocardial infarction, and cerebrovascular episodes.
- Can present perioperatively, and unless the diagnosis is considered and appropriate treatment instituted the mortality is high—up to 50%.

Diagnosis

- Clinical suspicion.
- Once the diagnosis has been considered then urinary catecholamines or their metabolites are measured either over 24 h or more conveniently overnight.
- When diagnosis is confirmed then localization is the next stage.
- Traditionally the use of CT radiocontrast was thought capable of provoking phaeo crises and its use has been avoided in unblocked patients. Modern contrast agents may be used.
- MIBG (meta-iodobenzylguanidine) scan—a radio-labelled isotope of iodine which is taken up by chromaffin tissue.
- MRI.
- It is usual to search in the abdomen first and widen the search in the unusual situation that the tumour is extra-adrenal. Extra-abdominal. MIBG is particularly helpful in revealing phaeochromocytomas in unusual sites.

Investigations relevant to anaesthesia

* Pay particular attention to the CVS including cardiac echo (patients with persistent hypertension, those with any history of ischaemia or evidence of heart failure). Patients can present with a catecholamine cardiomyopathy.
* Blood glucose—excess catecholamines result in glycogenolysis and insulin resistance and some patients become frankly diabetic.

Preoperative

* Unless there are pressing reasons refer the patient to a team with experience in the management of this condition. In the author's opinion it is not acceptable to manage an occasional patient with this condition; respected opinion and clinical governance would support this view.
* The usual management is sympathetic blockade with first alpha- and then beta-blockers (phenoxybenzamine and atenolol). The advantages to the patient of preoperative blockade are resolution of symptoms and prevention of the effects of surges in BP. Preoperative blockade allows the safe conduct of anaesthesia for the removal of the tumour by preventing hypertensive responses to induction of anaesthesia, and limits the surges in blood pressure seen during tumour handling. Avoid unopposed beta-blockade because of the theoretical risk of increasing vasoconstriction and precipitating a crisis. Although this has been reported, many patients will already have received beta-blockers for hypertension before presentation without adverse effects. Some patients report stopping them because of intolerance or feeling unwell. In patients with asthma in whom beta-blockade may be inadvisable it is usually possible to use only alpha-blockade.
* Prazosin and doxazosin have been used. As these are competitive selective alpha 1 blockers they do not inhibit presynaptic NA re-uptake and thus avoid the tachycardia seen with non-selective alpha blockade. However, competitive block may be overcome by very large amounts of secreted hormone (phenoxybenzamine is a non-competitive alpha blocker). The literature contains reports both in favour and against the use of selective blockade.
* Calcium channel blockers, particularly nicardipine, have been used and probably work via inhibiting noradrenaline mediated calcium influx in smooth muscle. They do not affect catecholamine secretion by the tumour. Evidence in the literature is varied and control of BP during surgical removal has not always been good.
* Metyrosine is an inhibitor of catecholamine synthesis. It is toxic and it is not widely used.
* The use of magnesium has been reported. It blocks catecholamine release, blocks receptors, is a direct vasodilator, and is possibly myocardial protective. The use of magnesium has not gained widespread support.
* It has been suggested that modern cardiovascular drugs, along with invasive monitoring and better understanding of the physiology, should allow safe removal of the tumours without preoperative preparation.
* Patients with phaeochromocytoma are very varied as are their tumours; patients with severe hypertension and troublesome symptoms may have a smooth intra-operative course and others with minimal symptoms may

develop acute pulmonary oedema, heart failure, and die. Any study on patients with phaeochromocytoma inevitably has small numbers of patients and may not cover the entire spectrum of activity. With increased genetic testing more patients are being diagnosed before they become symptomatic—the behaviour of these patients may not be the same. Until further experience has been gained, the author recommends caution in changing what is a safe, tried, and tested regime of alpha- and beta-blockade.

Assessment of sympathetic blockade

* 24-h ambulatory blood pressure monitoring. Aim for BP less than 140/90 throughout the 24-h period, with heart rate <100 beats/min.
* Lying and standing BP and heart rate. Should exhibit a marked postural drop with compensatory tachycardia.
* The duration of blockade is determined by the practicalities of tumour localization and scheduling of surgery. Some authors have recommended hours and others weeks, usually in small series with good results.
* Blockade is started to treat symptoms as well as to prepare for surgery.

Perioperative

* Perform open or laparoscopic adrenalectomy either through a midline, transverse, or flank incision (introduction of gas for laparoscopic resection can result in hypertension in normal subjects and may be exaggerated in patients with phaeochromocytomas).
* Blockade should be continued until the evening before the procedure.
* Premedication as required (e.g. temazepam 20–30 mg).
* Monitoring to include direct BP and CVP (triple lumen to allow drug infusions). Consider a PA catheter in patients with CVS disease or catecholamine cardiomyopathy.
* Large-bore intravenous access.
* Consider an epidural for a laparotomy. Remember that the sympathetic blockade of epidurals is proximal to the site of catecholamine action and will not oppose catecholamine-induced vasoconstriction.
* Monitor and maintain temperature, particularly during laparoscopic resection which can be prolonged.
* Induction: avoid agents which release histamine and thus catecholamines (use etomidate or propofol, alfentanil, and vecuronium).
* Hypotension is unlikely, but may be treated with judicious use of adrenaline.
* Maintenance: isoflurane with nitrous oxide or air and oxygen. Give an epidural with opioid and local anaesthetic if that is appropriate to the surgical approach, otherwise fentanyl/alfentanil/remifentanil until tumour removal when, if necessary, morphine can be substituted for postoperative analgesia.
* Fluctuations in BP tend to be transient and medication needs to be able to respond in a similar fashion. SNP is effective and is preferred to phentolamine, nicardepine, or magnesium because it provides rapid control with no prolonged effects. The doses required are unlikely to lead to toxicity.
* Control heart rate at <100 beats/min with propranolol.

- Once the tumour is resected the BP will take several minutes to decline. Prevent hypotension after tumour removal by ensuring an adequate pre-load. Maintain a high CVP of 10–15 mmHg. Several litres of crystalloid may be needed.
- Hypotension after resection can be due to a low cardiac output or a low SVR. Treat the first with adrenaline and the latter with noradrenaline.
- It is unusual to still require inotropic support by the time the patient is ready to leave theatre unless there are coexisting medical problems.

Postoperative

- The patient should be nursed in an HDU or ICU for 12 h.
- Monitor blood glucose. Catecholamines cause an increase in glucose levels: in the acute absence of catecholamines blood glucose may drop sufficiently to produce unconsciousness. Residual beta-blockade may limit response to this and patients commonly require intravenous glucose maintenance for 12–24 h postoperatively.
- If both adrenals are resected the patient will require steroid support immediately.
- Even when only one adrenal is removed patients may occasionally be relatively hypoadrenal and require support. If this is suspected (e.g. un-expectedly low BP) a small dose (50 mg) of hydrocortisone will do no harm whilst the result of a cortisol estimation is awaited.

Special situations

- Pregnancy. There are many reports of the combination of a newly diag-nosed phaeochromocytoma and pregnancy. Overall mortality is up to 17%.
- Phenoxybenzamine and propranolol are safe.
- If phaeochromocytoma is diagnosed before midtrimester it should be resected at this stage.
- There is a high mortality associated with normal delivery; consider LSCS with or without resection of the phaeochromocytoma at the same procedure.

Management of an unexpected phaeochromocytoma

- Any patient who has unexplained pulmonary oedema, hypertension, or severe unexpected hypotension should prompt consideration of the diag-nosis; however, it can be very difficult. There is no quick available test to support the diagnosis in the acute situation.
- Once the diagnosis has been considered, if possible, surgery should be dis-continued to allow acute treatment, investigation, and blockade prior to definitive surgery. Attempts to remove the tumour during a crisis may result in significant morbidity or even mortality.
- Treatment acutely should consist of vasodilators and intravenous fluid; this may be counterintuitive in a patient with severe pulmonary oedema. The circulating volume in patients with phaeochromocytoma may be markedly reduced and vasodilatation will result in a profound drop in blood pressure. Glyceryl trinitrate can usually be successfully titrated in this situation.
- Patients who present with hypotension have an acutely failing heart due to profound vasoconstriction. These are the most difficult ones in whom to

make the diagnosis and to treat. Additional catecholamines in this situation merely fuel the fire but are difficult to resist. The mortality rate is very high.

Further reading

Hull CJ (1986). Phaeochromocytoma—diagnosis, preoperative preparation and anaesthetic management. *British Journal of Anaesthesia*, **58**, 1453–68.

O'Riordan JA (1997). Pheochromocytomas and anesthesia. *International Anesthesiology Clinics*, **35**, 99–127.

Prys-Roberts C (2000). Phaeochromocytoma—recent progress in its management. *British Journal of Anaesthesia*, **85**, 44–57.

Chapter 16
Vascular surgery

Mark Stoneham

General principles

Most vascular surgery involves operating on arterial vessels diseased or damaged by atherosclerosis, which causes poor peripheral blood flow (ischaemia) or embolic phenomena. The mortality of elective aortic surgery is 7%[1], and following emergency aortic surgery at least 50%. Mortality and morbidity are markedly increased in the presence of uncontrolled cardiovascular disease. Operations may be long, and involve blood transfusion, marked fluid shifts, and significant impairment of lung function.

- Vascular patients are often elderly, arteriopathic, and have significant associated disease. Hypertension (66% of patients), ischaemic heart disease (angina, MI), heart failure, diabetes mellitus, and COPD (at least 50% are current or ex-smokers) are common. Many patients are taking aspirin, beta-blockers, diuretics, heart failure medications, and, perhaps, insulin or oral hypoglycaemics.
- Some patients will already be receiving anticoagulants, many others will receive anticoagulants perioperatively, so consider the pros and cons of regional techniques carefully. However, regional techniques may reduce morbidity and mortality (see below).
- Many patients have serial operations, e.g. AAA followed by aortobifemoral bypass followed by femorodistal bypass, followed by amputation. There may be several previous anaesthetic records to review.
- 30–40% of vascular operations are semiurgent or emergency, often occurring out of hours, which has implications therefore for the grade of anaesthetist involved.
- All patients receiving vascular grafts (usually Gortex® or Dacron®) require prophylactic antibiotic cover.
- Measure NIBP in both arms—there may be significant differences due to arteriopathy (use the higher of the two values clinically).
- Develop a working relationship with your vascular surgeon—you will have a better chance of being warned of untoward events (e.g. aortic clamping/unclamping, sudden massive blood loss etc.).

Preoperative assessment

The preoperative assessment should quantify the extent of any cardio-respiratory disease, both in terms of the planned surgical procedure and the postoperative period. Carefully consider (and document) whether regional anaesthesia is appropriate—it may have advantages, but may be contra-indicated in an anticoagulated patient.

Take a careful history and examine the patient. Include direct questions about exercise tolerance (distance on the flat and ability to climb stairs) and ability to lie supine.

- Investigations: routinely FBC, electrolytes and creatinine, ECG, chest radiograph.

---

1 Bayly PJ *et al.* (2001). In-hospital mortality from abdominal aortic surgery in Great Britain and Ireland. *British Journal of Surgery*, **88**, 687–92.

• For elective aortic surgery and for patients with symptomatic or new cardiac disease, a dynamic assessment of cardiac function is required. This should involve at least an echocardiogram, which will also give the left ventricular ejection fraction (EF). In patients with underlying ECG abnormalities or symptomatic heart disease an exercise ECG or stress echocardiography are recommended. Alternatives include radionucleide thallium scan or multigated acquisition scan (MUGA). Patients with critical ischaemic heart disease should be referred for cardiological opinion for angiography and possible coronary revascularization before aortic surgery. Patients undergoing urgent vascular procedures may have to undergo surgery before dynamic investigations can be performed. However, elective surgery can wait until such an assessment is available.

• Lung function tests should be performed in patients with significant respiratory disease presenting for AAA repair.

Premedication

• Some patients may require anxiolysis.

• There is some evidence that beta-blockers such as atenolol or bisoprolol given preoperatively may reduce cardiovascular mortality following major vascular surgery.[2] This may even hold true for a single dose. However, this is controversial and not routinely done.

2 Poldermans D *et al.* (1999). The effect of bisoprolol on perioperative mortality and myocardial infarction in high-risk patients undergoing vascular surgery. *New England Journal of Medicine*, **341**, 1789–94.

Regional anaesthesia and analgesia in vascular surgical patients

Regional anaesthesia may be used alone for distal vascular surgery and is also increasingly used for carotid surgery with supplemental sedation. Epidural analgesia is commonly used to supplement general anaesthesia for AAA. The advantage of regional techniques include:

- Improved patient monitoring (carotid endarterectomy with awake patient)
- Improved blood flow in legs, reduced DVT incidence, reduced reoperation rate (peripheral revascularization).[3]
- Postoperative pain relief (AAA, distal revascularization, amputation).
- Reduced pulmonary complications (AAA surgery).
- Pre-emptive analgesia for amputations with possible reduction in phantom limb pain.
- Treatment of proximal hypertension during aortic cross-clamp

Epidural catheters and anticoagulation[4] (see p. 998)

The small but finite risk of epidural haematoma should be weighed up against the benefits of regional anaesthesia for each individual patient. As a general guide, epidural insertion/removal should not be performed:

- in patients taking anticoagulants with INR >1.5
- in patients with other demonstrable coagulopathy, e.g. platelets $<100 \times 10^9$/litre
- in patients who have received thrombolysis in the last 24 h (urokinase/streptokinase)
- within 4 h of Minihep administration
- within 12 h of LMWH administration
- within 2 h of systemic heparinization.

  Epidurals should probably be avoided if cardiac-type heparin doses (e.g. 20 000 units) are to be used.

3 Perioperative Ischemia Randomized Anesthesia Trial Study Group (1993). *Anesthesiology*, **79**, 422–34.

4 Horlocker TT Wedel DJ (2000). Regional anesthesia and pain. *Medicine*, **25**, 83–98.

Aortic aneurysm repair

Procedure	Excision of aortic aneurysmal sac and replacement with synthetic graft (may be tube graft or trouser graft if the anastomosis is to the iliac or femoral vessels)
Time	2–4 h
Pain	++++
Position	Supine, arms out (crucifix)
Blood loss	500–2000+ ml (cross-match six units). Suitable for autotransfusion
Practical technique	ETT + IPPV, arterial + CVP lines. Epidural if possible

Preoperative

- Elderly, often multiple coexisting disease.
- Mortality for elective surgery is 5–10%; causes are predominantly myocardial infarction and multiorgan failure.
- Careful preoperative assessment is essential. Scrutinize ECG for signs of ischaemia and check for any renal impairment. Needs dynamic cardiac assessment preoperatively (see above). Check access sites for CVP and arterial line.
- Depending on local practice, arrange HDU/ICU for postoperative care. Alert the patient to this plan especially if a period of postoperative IPPV is planned. Preoptimization is performed in some units—patients are admitted to the HDU/ICU a few hours preoperatively to have lines etc. inserted and to have haemodynamic status 'optimized'. This is controversial.
- Continue the usual cardiac medications. Consider adding a beta-blocker (e.g. atenolol 25 mg) to the premedication.

Perioperative

- Draw up vasoconstrictors (ephedrine and metaraminol) and have vasodilators (GTN) and beta-blockers (labetalol) available.
- Two 14G or greater intravenous access. A hot air warmer and IVI warmer are essential. Intra-operative temperature should be monitored.
- A Level-1® fluid warmer or equivalent is very useful for complex case/redo/suprarenal clamp as these cases may bleed very rapidly due to surgical problems/acidosis/hypothermia. Cell savers are indicated in cases where blood loss is greater than 1000 ml.
- Arterial line and thoracic epidural (T6–T11) preinduction. Take a baseline blood gas sometime before cross-clamping.
- Have at least two syringe drivers present—inotropes, vasodilators, and eventually the epidural will all need them.

- Use a five-lead ECG (leads II and V5)—this increases the sensitivity for detection of myocardial ischaemia.
- Triple lumen CVP after induction. Consider inserting a PA introducer in complex cases as this will allow rapid fluid administration and facilitates PA catheter insertion if necessary (use right internal jugular or left subclavian vein to facilitate easier insertion of pulmonary catheter if required).
- Consider PA catheter if severe CVS/RS disease, e.g. ejection fraction <25%, FVC <2 litres.
- Consider isovolaemic haemodilution preinduction (see p. 917). AAA is ideal for this as you can return the patient's blood (with platelets and clotting factors) as the aortic cross-clamp is coming off. As a rough guide: Hb 10–12 g/dl take one unit, Hb 12–14 g/dl take two units, Hb 14–16 g/dl take three units.
- Careful induction with monitoring of invasive arterial blood pressure. Use moderate-/high-dose opioid, e.g. remifentanil (must have epidural) or high-dose fentanyl (5–10 μg/kg). Treat hypotension with fluids at first and then cautious vasoconstriction.
- Rebound hypertension may occur during endotracheal intubation (place the nasogastric tube at the same time).
- Hypothermia is likely unless energetic efforts are made to maintain temperature during induction, line insertion, and perioperatively. Warming blankets should not be placed on the lower limbs whilst the aortic cross-clamp is in place as this may worsen lower limb ischaemia.
- Insert a urinary catheter for hourly measurement of urine output.
- Heparin will need to be given just before cross-clamp—3000–5000 units is usual. This may be reversed after unclamping with protamine 0.5–1 mg/100 units heparin IV slowly—causes hypotension if given too fast.
- Proximal hypertension may follow aortic cross-clamping and is due to a sudden increase in SVR, increased SVC flow, and sympathoadrenal response. It may be treated by deepening the anaesthetic and/or a bolus of beta-blocker (labetalol 5–10 mg) and/or GTN infusion and epidural local anaesthetic.
- Whilst the aorta is clamped, metabolic acidosis will develop due to ischaemic lower limbs. Maintaining minute ventilation will cause a respiratory alkalosis to develop which will minimize the effects of this metabolic acidosis on pH when the aorta is unclamped. Check arterial blood gases to assess haematocrit, metabolic acidosis, respiratory compensation, and ionized calcium.
- Cross-clamp time is usually 30–60 min. During this time, start giving fluid, aiming for a moderately increased CVP, e.g. 5 mmHg greater than at the start of the case by the time unclamping occurs. This helps with cardiovascular stability, reduces sudden hypotension following cross-clamp removal, and may help preserve renal function. Release of the cross-clamp one limb at a time also helps with haemodynamic stability.
- Hypotension following aortic unclamping is caused by a decrease in SVR, relative hypovolaemia, and myocardial 'stunning' due to return of cold metabolic waste products from the legs, etc. Treat with IV fluids and/or lighten anaesthetic depth and/or small doses of inotropes, e.g. adrenaline 10 μg aliquots (1 ml of 1:100 000) and/or a bolus of calcium gluconate (up to 10 ml 10%). You may need inotropes for a while postoperatively.

◆ For fluid replacement, give isotonic crystalloid or colloid to replace insensible losses, third space losses, and initial blood loss. Give blood products when a deficiency is identified, i.e. if the haematocrit is <25% give blood, or known thrombocytopenia (<100 × 10^9/litre) give platelets. Check an activated clotting time (normal <140 s) if you suspect coagulopathy. Thromboelastography (if you have access to it) will give you the whole coagulation picture.

Postoperative

◆ ICU or HDU is essential postoperatively. HDU may be appropriate for otherwise fit patients who can be extubated at the end of the case. Extubate if warm, haemodynamically stable, and with a working epidural. Otherwise wake up and extubate slowly on the ICU.

◆ Opioid infusion and/or PCA if no epidural. Routine observations including invasive arterial and central venous pressure monitoring and urine output should be continued postoperatively to assess haemodynamic stability. There is a potential for large fluid shifts which need replacement. Also assess distal pulses.

◆ Hypothermia should be treated aggressively.

Special considerations

◆ Management of epidural. A bolus of epidural diamorphine 2.5–5 mg at induction will last for at least 12 h. This is much more effective than epidural fentanyl. Use epidural LA sparingly until the aorta is closed. It is easier to treat the hypotension of aortic unclamping with a functioning sympathetic nervous system.

◆ Renal failure occurs in 1–2% and is multifactorial in origin. It is much more likely if the cross-clamp is suprarenal. There is no evidence that dopamine prevents renal failure, merely acting as an inotrope. Mannitol is used routinely by some (0.5 g/kg during cross-clamp time) as it is a free-radical scavenger and an osmotic diuretic. Avoid hypovolaemia and monitor urine output hourly.

Emergency repair of abdominal aortic aneurysm

A true anaesthetic and surgical emergency. An aortic aneurysm may rupture acutely—in which case cardiovascular collapse is the commonest presentation. Death is likely unless the rupture is contained in the retroperitoneal space. Alternatively, the aneurysm can dissect along the arterial intima or can expand rapidly. In these cases, back pain with or without abdominal pain is the usual presentation. Prehospital mortality for ruptured AAA is 50% and 50% of those reaching hospital also do not survive. Management is as for elective AAA, with the following additional considerations:

- Where doubt exists, diagnosis is confirmed by ultrasound or CT scan if time is available. Get IV lines in early.

- If hypovolaemic shock is present, resuscitate to a systolic pressure of 90–100 mmHg until the aortic cross-clamp is applied. Avoid hypertension, coughing, and straining at all costs as this may precipitate a further bleed. Titrate intravenous morphine against patient's pain.

- Minimum lines preinduction are two 14G peripheral cannulas and (ideally) an arterial line. Use of the brachial artery may be necessary and sometimes an arterial 'cut down' indicated. Central venous access can wait until after the cross-clamp is applied. Where venous access is difficult insert a PA catheter sheath into the right internal jugular vein.

- Epidural analgesia is rarely appropriate because of time constraints preoperatively and coagulopathy postoperatively.

- A urinary catheter can be placed before or after induction.

- Induction must be in the operating theatre, with the surgeons scrubbed, surgical preparation completed, drapes on, and blood available in theatre and checked. Rapid sequence induction is appropriate using preoxygenation and suxamethonium. Suitable induction agents include etomidate/ fentanyl or ketamine. As soon as the endotracheal tube is confirmed as being in the trachea ($ETCO_2$) the surgeons can start. Treat hypotension with rapid infusion of intravenous fluids and small doses of vasopressors/ inotropic agents.

- Hot air warming and at least one warmed IVI are essential (a Level-1® blood warmer is invaluable).

- Have both intravenous lines running maximally at induction. One assistant should be dedicated to managing the intravenous fluid and ensuring an uninterrupted supply.

- Hypothermia, renal impairment, blood loss, and coagulopathy are common perioperative problems. Hypothermia is a particular hazard, as even if surgery goes well, the patient will continue to bleed on the ICU. Platelet function is markedly reduced below 35 °C. Whilst there is no place for routine administration of platelets and FFP, consider early use when they are needed.

- Do not attempt to extubate at the conclusion of surgery—a postoperative period of ventilation on the ICU is essential to allow correction of biochemical and haematological abnormalities.

Thoracoabdominal aortic aneurysm repair

Procedure	Excision of aortic aneurysmal sac extending above the origin of the renal arteries and replacement with a synthetic graft. May involve thoracotomy and the need for one-lung ventilation
Time	3–6 h
Pain	+++++
Position	Supine, arms out (crucifix), may be R lateral if thoracotomy
Blood loss	1000–? ml (cross-match eight units, plus platelets and FFP)
Practical technique	DLT + IPPV, arterial + CVP lines. Thoracic epidural

Thoracic aneurysms of the ascending aorta require median sternotomy and cardiopulmonary bypass. Transverse aortic arch repairs often require hypothermic circulatory arrest as well.

Special considerations

As for infrarenal aortic aneurysm repair, with the following considerations:

- The aneurysm can compress the trachea and distort the anatomy of the upper vasculature.
- Intensive care is essential postoperatively for a period of ventilation and stabilization.
- The aortic cross-clamp will be much higher than for a simple AAA. This means that the kidneys, liver, and splanchnic circulation will be ischaemic for the duration of the cross-clamp.
- Access to the thoracic aorta may require one-lung ventilation—thus a left-sided double lumen tube (DLT) may be required. A Univent® tube is a possible alternative, which consists of a normal ET tube with a bronchial blocker within. The blocker may be advanced into either lung, and then used for suction and oxygenation of the collapsed lung. It may be withdrawn postoperatively so the Univent® tube does not need changing at the end of surgery. Check the position of the DLT after turning to the lateral position.
- Proximal hypertension following aortic cross-clamping is more pronounced. Use aggressive vasodilatation with GTN (infusion of 50 mg/50ml run at 0–5 ml/h) or esmolol (2.5 g/50 ml at 3–15 ml/h).
- Hypotension following aortic unclamping is often severe, requiring inotropic support postoperatively—use adrenaline 1:10 000 starting at 5 ml/h.
- Acidosis may be a particular problem due to the metabolic acidosis that develops during cross-clamping and an additional respiratory acidosis due to prolonged one-lung ventilation.

- Renal failure occurs in up to 25% of cases—principally related to the duration of cross-clamp. Monitor urine output, give mannitol 25 g before cross-clamping, and maintain the circulating volume during the case.

- Spinal cord ischaemia leading to paralysis may develop. This is related to the duration of cross-clamping and occurs because a branch of the thoracic aorta (artery of Adamkiewicz) reinforces the blood supply of the cord. Techniques used for prevention (none are infallible) include: CSF pressure measurement and drainage through a spinal drain, spinal cord cooling through an epidural catheter, intrathecal magnesium, distal perfusion techniques, cardiopulmonary bypass, and deep hypothermic circulatory arrest. Surgeons performing this surgery have their own preferred techniques.

- Fluid balance is as for infrarenal AAA, although blood loss will be more extreme, blood transfusion will almost certainly be required, and platelets and FFP are more commonly required.

- Patients require ventilation postoperatively until acidosis and hypothermia are corrected and the lungs are fully re-expanded.

Carotid endarterectomy

Procedure	Removal of an atheromatous plaque in the internal carotid artery (ICA). The ICA is clamped, opened, the plaque stripped off, and then the artery closed either directly or with a Gortex or vein patch
Time	1–3 h
Pain	++
Position	Supine, head up. Contralateral arm board
Blood loss	Minimal (cross-match two units)
Practical techniques	Cervical plexus block + sedation, arterial line. ETT + IPPV, arterial line

An operation to reduce the incidence of stroke in symptomatic (TIA or CVA) patients with a 70% or greater carotid stenosis. Unfortunately it has a combined mortality and major stroke incidence of 2–5%. Patients are usually elderly arteriopaths similar to those presenting for aortic surgery (see above). Dynamic cardiac assessment is not usually required.

Monitoring cerebral perfusion during carotid cross-clamping is an important, but controversial, area. Advocates of regional anaesthesia cite the advantages of having a conscious patient in whom neurological deficits are immediately detectable and treatable by the insertion of a carotid shunt or pharmacological augmentation of blood pressure. Under general anaesthesia, other techniques may be used for monitoring cerebral perfusion, including: measurement of carotid artery stump pressure, electroencephalograph (EEG) processing, monitoring somatosensory evoked potentials, transcranial Doppler of the middle cerebral artery, and, more recently, near-infrared spectroscopy. Individuals units will have their own protocols.

Preoperative

- Elderly patients, often with severe cardiovascular disease, most are hypertensive. At least 50% of deaths following carotid endarterectomy (CEA) are cardiovascular in origin, thus hypertension must be controlled preoperatively. Aim for 160/90.
- Determine the normal range of blood pressure from ward charts. Measure BP in both arms.
- Document pre-existing neurological deficits so that new deficits may be more easily assessed.
- Draw up vasoconstrictors (e.g. ephedrine and metaraminol) and have vasodilators available (e.g. GTN, labetalol).
- Consider cerebral monitoring techniques—there will be protocols in your particular unit.
- Premedication: sedative/anxiolytic, particularly if using GA.

Perioperative

* 20G and 14G IV access plus an arterial line for measurement of invasive arterial blood pressure. All these need to be in the contralateral arm, which may be out on an arm board.
* Monitoring: five-lead ECG, arterial line, NIBP, SpO_2, $ETCO_2$.
* Maintain blood pressure within 20% of the baseline value. During carotid cross-clamping, maintain BP at or above baseline. If necessary use vaso-constrictors, e.g. metaraminol (10 mg diluted up to 20 ml, give 0.5 ml at a time) to achieve this.

General anaesthesia for CEA

* Careful IV induction. Blood pressure may be very labile during induction and intubation. Give generous doses of short-acting opioids at induction. Consider spraying the cords with lidocaine (lignocaine). Most anaesthetists use an endotracheal tube although the LMA has been used (the LMA cuff has been shown to reduce carotid blood flow but this is of unknown significance). Secure the tube and check connections very carefully (the head is inaccessible during surgery).
* Remifentanil infusion combined with superficial cervical plexus block gives ideal conditions, with rapid awakening. Otherwise isoflurane/opioid technique. Maintain normocapnia.
* Extubate before excessive coughing develops. Close neurological monitoring in the recovery until fully awake.

The 'awake carotid'

* Cervical dermatomes C2–C4 may be blocked by deep and/or superficial cervical plexus block or cervical epidural (very rarely used in the United Kingdom).
* Patient preparation and communication are vital. A thorough explanation of the benefits of the awake technique is invaluable and avoids the need for heavy sedative premedication.
* For the deep block use three 5 ml injections of 0.5% bupivacaine at C2, 3, and 4 or a single injection of 10–15 ml 0.5% bupivacaine at C3. Reinforce this with 10 ml 0.5% bupivacaine injected along the posterior border of the sternocleidomastoid (superficial block). Avoid the deep block altogether in patients with respiratory impairment as they may not tolerate the unilateral diaphragmatic paralysis which can ensue. Infiltration along the jawline helps to reduce pain from the submandibular retractor.
* Ensure the patient's bladder is emptied preoperatively. Give IV fluids only to replace blood loss—a full bladder developing whilst the carotid is cross-clamped is a potential disaster.
* Sedation (e.g. propofol target controlled infusion 0.5–1 µg/ml) may be carefully employed during block placement and dissection. Once dissection is complete, patient discomfort is much reduced. No sedation during carotid cross-clamping will allow continuous neurological assessment. Administer oxygen throughout.
* An L-bar angled over the patient's neck allows good access for both surgeon and anaesthetist.

- Despite an apparently perfect regional block, around 50% or so of patients will require LA supplementation by the surgeon, particularly around the carotid sheath and if the carotid bifurcation is very high.
- Monitor the patient's speech, contralateral motor power, and cerebration. Neurological deficit presents in three ways:
  - profound unconsciousness on cross-clamping
  - subtle but immediate deficit, e.g. confusion, slurred speech, delay in answering questions
  - deficit after a variable period of time which may be related to relative hypotension.
- Attentive monitoring of the patient is vital, particularly during cross-clamping. If neurological deficit develops, a shunt should be inserted immediately, although you may have to use considerable tact/skill to re-assure the patient, maintaining the airway whilst the shunt is being inserted. Recovery should be rapid once the shunt is in place—if it is not, convert to general anaesthesia. Pharmacological augmentation of blood pressure may improve cerebration by increasing the pressure gradient of collateral circulation across the circle of Willis. Approximately 2.5% of patients will require conversion to general anaesthesia (use of an LMA is probably easiest).
- For patients who do not tolerate regional anaesthesia, GA is the best option.

Postoperative

- Careful observation in a well-staffed recovery for 2–4 h is mandatory. HDU is optimal if available, particularly for those patients who develop a neurological deficit.
- Airway oedema is common—in both GA and regional cases—presumably due to dissection so close to the airway. Cervical haematoma additionally occurs in 5–10% of cases. These cases need very careful observation in recovery. Immediate re-exploration is required for developing airway obstruction due to haematoma (the regional block should still be working). Remove skin sutures in recovery as soon as you have made the diagnosis to allow drainage of the haematoma.
- Haemodynamic instability is common postoperatively. Hyperperfusion syndrome, consisting of headaches and ultimately haemorrhagic CVA, is caused by areas of brain previously 'protected' by a tight carotid stenosis being suddenly exposed to hypertensive blood pressures. Thus blood pressure must be controlled. Careful written instructions should be given to ward staff about haemodynamic management. An example is:
  - If systolic BP >160 mmHg, call house officer and consider giving labetalol 5–10 mg boluses IV or a hydralazine infusion.
  - If systolic BP <100 mmHg, give colloid 250 ml stat. and call house officer.
- New neurological symptoms and signs require immediate surgical consultation.

Peripheral revascularization operations

Procedures	Bypass operations performed for patients with occlusive arterial disease of the legs. The long saphenous vein or a Gortex graft is used to bypass the occluded artery.
	Femoropopliteal bypass—femoral to above-knee popliteal artery
	Femorodistal bypass—femoral to anterior or posterior tibial artery
	Femorofemoral crossover graft—from one femoral artery to another
Time	1–6 h
Pain	+++
Position	Supine
Blood loss	Usually 500–1000 ml (cross-match two units)
Practical techniques	Combined spinal/epidural with sedation, ?arterial line.
	ETT/IPPV ?LMA

Preoperative

- These procedures constitute a large proportion of elective vascular surgery. The duration of surgery is unpredictable—overruns are not uncommon.

- The usual attention should be paid to preoperative assessment of the cardiovascular system. However, this surgery is better tolerated than aortic surgery. A dynamic assessment of cardiac function is not usually necessary unless there have been new developments, e.g. unstable angina.

- The choice between general and regional anaesthesia is up to the individual. There is some evidence that regional anaesthesia is associated with lower reoperation rates.[5] Long operations (>3 h) may make pure regional techniques impractical, but they are is still possible.

Perioperative

- IV access: ensure at least one large (14 or 16G) IV cannula with an infusion which runs freely.

- Use invasive arterial pressure monitoring for long cases (over 2 h), if haemodynamic instability is expected or in sicker patients. Otherwise use standard monitoring with five-lead ECG if available. CVP monitoring is rarely required.

- General anaesthetic techniques include ETT with IPPV or LMA/SV. The surgeon should be able to perform femoral nerve block perioperatively, which will give good analgesia, including the saphenous vein harvesting incision.

---

5 Perioperative Ischemia Randomized Anesthesia Trial Study Group (1993). *Anesthesiology*, **79**, 422–34.

- Regional anaesthesia is an alternative to GA offering good operating conditions with excellent postoperative pain relief. Spinal anaesthesia alone may not give enough time for some procedures. The combination of spinal and epidural anaesthesia is ideal. If the patient can lie affected side down, hyperbaric bupivacaine (2–2.5 ml 0.5%) can be used to produce a very dense spinal block on that side. Consider giving epidural diamorphine 2–3 mg initially, then start an epidural infusion of 0.25% bupivacaine at 5–10 ml/h after 1 h. Always give supplemental oxygen. If the patient wants to be sedated, use the CO_2 sampling tubing within the oxygen face mask so that respiratory rate can be monitored as well. Propofol TCI is ideal.
- Heparin, e.g. 3000–5000 units, will need to be given before clamping—reverse with protamine 0.5–1 mg/100 units heparin slowly after unclamping.

Postoperative

- Epidural infusion.
- Oxygen overnight if you have given epidural diamorphine.
- PCA if no epidural. Pain may even be less than the preoperative, ischaemic pain.

Axillobifemoral bypass

Procedure	Extraperitoneal bypass (trouser graft) from axillary artery to femoral arteries
Time	2–4 h
Pain	++++
Position	Supine
Blood loss	<1000 ml
Practical technique	GA—ETT, IPPV, arterial line, ?CVP

This is often a last-chance operation for patients with completely occluded aortic or iliac arteries. Some will already have had aortic surgery and have infected grafts. It is an extraperitoneal operation, so patients with severe cardiorespiratory disease who might be excluded from aortic surgery may tolerate it better. However, do not be misled—it is still a long operation, which can involve significant blood loss, morbidity, and even mortality.

Preoperative

♦ The usual comments about preoperative assessment of vascular patients apply. Try to obtain recent information about cardiac function. An echo-cardiograph can easily be done at the bedside.

♦ Some of these patients will be very sick either from their pre-existing cardiorespiratory disease or from having infected aortic grafts. Surgery may be their only hope of life although equally it can also be a rapid road to their demise. Provided the patient understands this, the operation may be appropriate despite high risk. These are not cases for inexperienced trainees to do alone.

Postoperative

♦ General anaesthesia with ETT and IPPV is appropriate. An arterial line and a large-gauge cannula is mandatory, CVP monitoring is optional.

♦ Heparin/protamine will be required at clamping/unclamping.

Postoperative

♦ Extubation at the end of surgery is usually possible, but a period of time on the HDU is recommended if at all possible.

♦ PCA for postoperative analgesia.

Amputations

(Below knee, through knee, above knee, Symes, digits, etc.)

Procedures	Removal of necrotic or infected tissue due to vascular ischaemia.
Time	30–120 min
Pain	++++
Position	Supine
Blood loss	Usually 200–500 ml
Practical technique	Spinal or epidural with sedation
	GA + sciatic/femoral blocks

Preoperative

- Patients are often very sick, bed-bound, or diabetic with significant cardiovascular disease who have had repeated revascularization attempts previously.
- Many will be in considerable discomfort preoperatively (less so the diabetics) and may be on large doses of enteral or parenteral opioids. Regional analgesia may therefore give more predictable results than parenteral opioids postoperatively.

Perioperative

- Spinal anaesthesia with hyperbaric bupivacaine and sedation offers excellent anaesthesia, which can be directed affected side down. The duration of block (and postoperative pain relief) can be extended with intrathecal diamorphine (0.25–0.5 mg). Clonidine 15 μg intrathecally has also been used.
- Epidural analgesia offers better postoperative analgesia and can be sited preoperatively if required (pre-emptive analgesia).
- General anaesthesia with LMA/SV or ETT/IPPV is also an option, but additional regional blockade is advisable (combined sciatic and femoral blocks will ensure analgesia for up to 24 h).
- Occasionally these patients are septic due to the necrotic tissue. The only way they will get better is to have the affected part amputated thus the operation should not be cancelled for this reason.

Postoperative

- Regional analgesia is the best option, otherwise PCA.
- Phantom limb pain is a real problem for amputees—it occurs in 60–70% at some time. It is important to distinguish it from pain in the residual stump that can be treated by conventional analgesic techniques. Phantom limb pain is highly resistant to treatment and these patients often require chronic pain management.

- Pre-emptive analgesia (i.e. siting and using the epidural preoperatively) is believed by some to reduce the incidence and severity of chronic pain.[6] This is controversial.

6 Bach S, Noreng MF, Tjellden NU (1988). Phantom limb pain in amputees during the first 12 months following limb amputation after preoperative lumbar epidural blockade. *Pain*, **33**, 297.

Thoracoscopic sympathectomy

Procedures	For patients with sweaty palms/axillae. The sympathetic trunk is divided via a thoracoscope inserted through a small axillary incision
Time	30–60 min
Pain	++
Position	Supine, affected arm on arm board
Blood loss	Minimal
Practical technique	IPPV via double lumen tube
	SV via LMA

- Patients are usually young, fit people with hyperhidrosis (sweaty palms and axillae).
- The surgical technique involves cutting the thoracic sympathetic trunk at T2 or T3 thoracoscopically.
- Traditionally this is done using one-lung anaesthesia (double lumen tube), with the patient in the reverse Trendelenburg position.
- A simpler technique involves the patient breathing spontaneously through an LMA. When the surgeon insufflates CO_2 into the pleural cavity, the lung is pushed away passively, allowing surgery to take place. The degree of shunt produced is less dramatic than with one-lung ventilation. Assisted ventilation must be avoided, except to re-inflate the lung manually at the end. The CO_2 insufflator machine regulates intrapleural pressures.
- With either technique, at the conclusion of the procedure, the lung must be re-expanded (under the surgeon's direct vision) to prevent pneumothorax.
- Local anaesthetic can be deposited by the surgeon directly onto the sympathetic trunk and into the pleural cavity.
- A postoperative chest radiograph is required to confirm that the lung is reinflated.
- Some surgeons like to perform bilateral sympathectomies in the same operation. This is a much more challenging operation. It can lead to very profound hypoxia when the second lung is collapsed due to persistent atelectasis in the first lung. It is certainly inappropriate for all but the very fittest patients.

First rib resection

Procedures	Resection of the first/cervical rib in patients with thoracic outlet syndrome
Time	1–2 h
Pain	++
Position	Supine, affected arm on arm board
Blood loss	Minimal
Practical technique	IPPV via COETT, avoid relaxants if possible

- Patients are usually young and fit.
- The position is similar to that for thoracoscopic sympathectomy.
- Muscle relaxants should be avoided, as the surgeon needs to be able to identify the brachial plexus perioperatively. Intubate under opioid/induction agent alone or use mivacurium/opioid and then hyperventilate with isoflurane/opioid or similar.
- At the conclusion of surgery, the wound is filled with saline and manual ventilation performed with sustained inflation pressures >40 cmH$_2$O. This is to check for a lung leak and exclude a pleural injury.
- A superficial cervical plexus block provides good analgesia postoperatively.
- A postoperative chest radiograph is required in recovery.

Varicose vein surgery

Procedures	Removal of tortuous veins of the lower extremities: High tie and strip — long saphenous vein removal (sometimes bilateral) Short saphenous vein surgery — tied off in popliteal fossa
Time	30 min to 3 h
Pain	++
Position	Supine or prone for short saphenous surgery
Blood loss	Up to 1000 ml
Practical technique	LMA/SV for most, ETT/IPPV for prone

- Patients are usually young and fit.
- The main operation is usually combined with multiple avulsions to remove varicosities. These are minute scars, which can, however, bleed profusely.
- Blood loss can be minimized by elevating the legs.
- Patients may need combined long and short saphenous surgery (i.e. two operative incisions on the same leg) and may require turning during the operation. In selected slim patients without risks of aspiration, this can be done with the patients breathing spontaneously through an LMA.
- A combination of NSAIDs and local anaesthetic into the groin wound gives good postoperative analgesia. Caudal anaesthesia is possible for prolonged re-explorations.
- Bilateral surgery is common and takes 30–60 min per incision.
- Redo surgery is also common and can be very prolonged.

Other vascular procedures

Operation	Description	Time (min)	Pain	Position	Blood loss	Notes
Femoral or brachial embolectomy	Removal of clot from artery	60	+/++	Supine	minimal	LA ± sedation commonest
Aortic stent insertion	Radiological insertion of stent to aortic aneurysm	90 or more	+	Supine	Potentially massive	In X-ray under sedation/light GA but needs lines/monitoring as for AAA
Popliteal aneurysm repair	Bypass of aneurysmal peripheral artery	60–120	++/+++	Supine or prone	<500 ml	As for fem-pop bypass

Further reading

Caldicott L, Lumb A, McCoy D (1999). *Vascular anaesthesia, a practical handbook.* Butterworth Heinemann, Oxford.

O'Connor CJ, Rothenburg DM (1995). Anesthetic considerations for descending thoracic aortic surgery: Parts 1 and 2. *Journal of Cardiothoracic and Vascular Anesthesia*, **9**, 581–8, 734–47.

Paul SD, Eagle KA (1995). A stepwise strategy for coronary risk assessment for non-cardiac surgery. *Medical Clinics of North America*, **79**, 1241–61.

Stoneham MD, Knighton JD (1999). Regional anaesthesia for carotid endarterectomy. *British Journal of Anaesthesia*, **82**, 910–19.

Wilke HJ, Ellis JE, McKinsey JF (1996). Carotid endarterectomy: perioperative and anesthetic considerations. *Journal of Cardiothoracic and Vascular Anesthesia*, **10**, 928–49.

Chapter 17
Cardiac surgery

Bruce Martin and Michael Sinclair

Coronary blood flow

- Right and left coronary arteries originate from the anterior and left aortic sinuses respectively, just above the aortic valve leaflets.
- The right coronary artery descends in the right atrioventricular (AV) groove, continues around the inferior border of the heart, and joins with the circumflex branch of the left coronary artery in the posterior atrioventricular groove. It gives rise to acute marginal branches at the inferior border of the heart, supplying the right ventricle. In approximately 85% of individuals it terminates as the posterior descending artery, supplying the posteroinferior aspect of the left ventricle and intraventricular septum, this is described as a right dominant system.
- The left coronary artery leaves the left aortic sinus as the left main stem, posterior to the pulmonary trunk, and after a short distance divides into the left anterior descending and circumflex arteries. The left anterior descending artery passes down the anterior interventricular groove and around the apex, giving rise to septal and diagonal branches, which supply the septum and the free wall of the left ventricle respectively. These branches are important landmarks when describing lesions of the left anterior descending artery. The circumflex artery passes along the left AV groove, supplying the lateral free wall of the left ventricle via obtuse marginal branches, numbered one to three and in 15% of cases gives rise to the posterior descending artery, a left dominant system. Crucially this means that the left coronary artery supplies the entire left ventricle, the intraventricular septum and the AV node.
- 75% of myocardial venous return drains into the right atrium via the coronary sinus in the posterior AV groove, 20% returns via the anterior cardiac vein.
- 5% of myocardial venous return drains directly into the left ventricle via the thebesian, anterior sinusoidal and anterior luminal veins. These constitute a fixed shunt and contribute to the dilution of oxygenated blood.
- Coronary blood flow at rest is 250 ml/min or 5% of cardiac output, with near maximal oxygen extraction.
- Flow can increase up to five times with exertion, predominantly under the control of metabolic autoregulation. Adenosine, from the breakdown of ATP, and hypoxia are the major vasodilators.
- Coronary blood flow to the left ventricle only occurs during diastole.
- A right ventricular pressure of 25 mmHg minimally affects blood flow in the right coronary artery; whereas flow in the left coronary artery may stop and possibly reverse with a left ventricular pressure of 120 mmHg.
- Tachycardia shortens the time for diastole and will eventually reduce coronary blood flow. A heart rate of 90–100 beats/min will normally optimize coronary flow and therefore cardiac output.

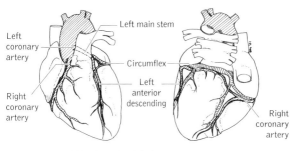

Fig 17.1 Arterial blood supply of the heart.

Cardiopulmonary bypass

Cardiopulmonary bypass (CPB) replaces the work of heart and lungs whilst the heart is arrested, allowing for a bloodless and stable surgical field. The bypass machine consists of an integrated, disposable unit made up of reservoir, oxygenator, and heat exchanger connected via a series of roller pumps on the permanent part of the machine. Membrane oxygenators are most commonly used. These contain minute hollow fibres, similar to those used for haemofiltration, giving a large surface area for gas exchange (2–2.5 m^2). Gas exchange occurs down concentration gradients; increasing the gas flow removes more CO_2 and increasing FiO_2 increases oxygenation.

Prior to CPB, full anticoagulation of the patient is required with an activated clotting time (ACT) recorded at greater than 400 s. Blood is siphoned from the inferior vena cava (IVC) and superior vena cava (SVC) into the reservoir, where it is filtered/defoamed. It is pumped through a heat exchanger, to alter the temperature as required, and then through the oxygenator, before being returned to the patient via a narrow arterial cannula placed in the aortic root. The bypass circuit is primed with 1000 ml of crystalloid (Hartmann's solution), heparin 5000 units, and occasionally mannitol (0.5 g/kg). The bypass machine normally delivers non-pulsatile flow with a cardiac index of 2.4 litres/min/m^2.

The perfusionist can control mean arterial pressure (MAP) by adjusting flow from the pump and by the use of vasoconstrictors/ vasodilators. MAP is normally maintained between 50 and 70 mmHg. Volume, as colloid/blood, can be added to the reservoir or removed by ultrafiltration, to maintain a haematocrit of 20–30%. Drugs may also be added to the circuit.

Cardiopulmonary bypass causes haemolysis, platelet damage, and consumption of coagulation factors. This is usually minimal for the first 2 h. Suction from the surgical field drains directly into the reservoir and powerful suction can exacerbate haemolysis. Other potential problems involve poor venous drainage, aortic dissection, and gas embolization. The risk of a cerebrovascular episode (CVE) ranges from 1–5% and is associated with several risk factors:

- age
- aortic atheroma
- previous CVE
- diabetes mellitus
- type of surgery (aortic arch replacement >valve replacement >coronary artery surgery).

Cognitive changes are common (up to 80% of all patients) in the perioperative period and persist in 30% of patients. These are caused by particulate matter (platelets, atheroma etc).

Instituting cardiopulmonary bypass

- Before cannulation, systolic blood pressure should be decreased (to 80–100 mmHg) to reduce the risk of aortic dissection.
- Prior to instituting bypass, the patient should be anticoagulated with heparin 300 IU/kg (usual dose 20 000–25 000units). ACT must be confirmed at >400 s.

- Prepare and pressurize cardioplegia to 300 mmHg, ensuring a bubble-free circuit if cold cardioplegia is being used.
- Once on bypass the ventilator is turned off and an intravenous anaesthetic (propofol 6 mg/kg/h) started. A bolus of midazolam or a vaporizer mounted on the bypass machine are alternatives.
- The perfusionist maintains a perfusion pressure of 50–70 mmHg by modifying flow/filling and the use of alpha agonists such as metaraminol.
- Blood gases and ACT are checked every 30 min.
- The patient's temperature is actively lowered, or allowed to drift, to 28–34 °C, depending on the type of surgery and surgical preference.

Coming off bypass

- This is a team effort between surgeon, anaesthetist, and perfusionist. The aim is to wean the patient from the bypass machine allowing the heart and lungs to re-establish normal physiological function.
- Before coming off bypass:
  - the temperature should have returned to 37 °C
  - potassium should be 4–5 mmol/litre
  - haematocrit should be >24%.
- Have protamine drawn up (1 mg/100 IU heparin—usually 3 mg/kg).
- The venous line is progressively clamped and the heart gradually allowed to fill/eject. It is usual practice to come off bypass with the patient relatively 'underfilled'. This avoids over-distension of the ventricles, which may not yet function normally.
- The perfusionist will transfuse 100 ml boluses as required. Be vigilant, watch the heart performance and filling carefully. If the ventricle is performing poorly, start a small amount of adrenaline.
- Heart rate should be 70–100 beats/min and sinus rhythm (if possible). Defibrillate and use atropine/isoprenaline/adrenaline as necessary.
- Ventilate with 100% oxygen and ensure the lung bases are expanded.
- When the surgeon requests protamine, clearly inform the perfusionist to turn off the suction and administer slowly IV. The systemic arterial pressure will decrease due to vasodilation and volume should be administered via the aortic cannula. Severe pulmonary hypertension can occur.

Post-bypass management

- Ensure adequate anaesthesia and analgesia with a volatile agent (i.e. halothane/isoflurane) and an opioid.
- Systolic blood pressure should be controlled between 80 and 140 mmHg by careful filling and adjustments of GTN/adrenaline infusions, as necessary.
- If the patient is persistently hypotensive or bleeding, inform the surgeon before the chest is closed.

Cardioplegia

This is either crystalloid or blood based. It contains potassium (20 mmol/litre) magnesium, and procaine and when rapidly infused renders the heart asystolic. Further doses are repeated every 20 min or when electrical activity returns. The advantages of blood cardioplegia are largely theoretical and based on the assumption that haemoglobin will carry oxygen and thus help reduce myocardial damage. Reperfusion (warm blood) cardioplegia is sometimes used towards the end of bypass to wash out products of metabolism and give an oxygen 'boost' to the myocardium. Cardioplegia is usually administered anterograde (via the coronary arteries), but retrograde cardioplegia may be delivered via the coronary sinus.

Temperature management

During bypass, the patient's temperature may be allowed to 'drift' down to 34 °C, or the patient can be actively cooled to a lower temperature (28–34 °C). Generally, a cooler temperature allows better cerebral protection, but a warmer temperature is preferred for the heart. Different centres vary in approach, and the technique of hypothermia often reserved for more complex cases.

Intermittent cross-clamping and fibrillation

When performing coronary arterial grafts, the surgeon can use either cardioplegia (conventional) or intermittent cross-clamping with fibrillation. With intermittent cross-clamping the aorta is cross-clamped and a fibrillator pad placed underneath the heart. When the heart fibrillates oxygen demand is reduced, and the lower end of a graft can be sutured. After each graft the cross-clamp is removed and the heart cardioverted into sinus rhythm. The top end will then be sutured onto the aorta. Advantages are that no cardioplegia is used (hence a lower incidence of complete heart block) and after each graft is attached, the ECG can be inspected for any ischaemia. However, as the heart is not protected by cardioplegia, surgical time needs to be kept to a minimum to avoid myocardial damage.

Potassium management

For myocardial stability following CPB it is important to maintain serum potassium levels between 4 and 5 mmol/litre. Hypokalaemia usually develops and should be treated with aliquots of 20 mmol KCl. This is preferably administered whilst on CPB, thus avoiding the need to administer via a central line, directly onto an unstable myocardium.

'Alpha-stat' versus 'pH-stat' arterial gas interpretation

The pH-stat and alpha-stat regimes differ in terms of whether $PaCO_2$ and pH are maintained within normal values when measured at the temperature of the patient or when measured at 37 °C.

- pH-stat: $PaCO_2$ and pH are maintained near 5.0 kPa and 7.4 respectively, when measured at actual body temperature, a process called 'temperature correction'. Thus, during hypothermia, CO_2 is added to the bypass machine. When measured in a blood-gas machine at 37 °C, this will suggest a high $PaCO_2$ and a low pH (similar to a respiratory acidosis).

- alpha-stat: attempts to duplicate the normal response of poikilothermic animals, in which $PaCO_2$ during hypothermia decreases when corrected for body temperature. Using the alpha-stat regime, $PaCO_2$ values are not corrected for temperature and are kept in the normal range when measured at 37 °C by the blood gas analyser.

When the two methods are compared for hypothermic CPB at 28 °C, a 3 kPa difference in $PaCO_2$ levels exists. This $PaCO_2$ gradient has been shown to significantly alter cerebral blood flow since cerebrovascular carbon dioxide responsiveness is maintained.

Potentially harmful effects of pH-stat management include:

- Increased cerebral blood flow, possibly increasing the embolic load to the brain (i.e. air/debris).
- Increased cerebral blood flow to non-ischaemic areas may cause a steal phenomenon.
- 'Respiratory acidosis' (increased CO_2) may disrupt normal cellular function.

Theoretical advantages of pH-stat management include:

- Acidosis counteracts the leftward shift of the oxygen dissociation curve associated with hypothermia, so that release of oxygen from haemoglobin is enhanced.
- Depressed enzymatic activity associated with acidosis may potentiate the total amount of metabolic depression caused by hypothermia.

The potentially harmful effects of pH-stat management would seem to outweigh any advantages. The alpha-stat technique is now more commonly used.

Volatile agents and CPB

Halothane, isoflurane, enflurane, and sevoflurane have all been used successfully during cardiac anaesthesia. They all cause vasodilatation, cardiac depression, and bradycardia in a dose-dependent manner. Isoflurane has been shown in the animal model to cause a 'steal' phenomenon, but this has not been convincingly demonstrated in man. A large study in the 1990s compared all different anaesthetic techniques then in use for cardiac surgery and concluded that there was no difference between the anaesthetic used in terms of either morbidity or mortality. Halothane is the volatile agent that has been used the longest and the more recently introduced volatile agents (enflurane, isoflurane, or sevoflurane) would not appear to have any advantages over it. However, there is evidence that for repeat anaesthesia, the incidence of hepatitis following halothane administration may be higher than that with the other agents.

Risk scoring

The Parsonnet risk stratification scheme can be used to score the risk and predict the mortality rate in cardiac surgical patients. However, it should only be used as a guide to surgical outcome.

Parsonnet risk stratification scheme

Risk factor		Score
Female gender		1
Age	70–74	7
	>75	12
Ejection fraction	Good	0
	Fair (30–49%)	2
	Poor (<30%)	4
Obesity	>1.5 times ideal weight	3
Diabetes		3
Hypertension	Systolic >140 mmHg	3
Reoperation	First reoperation	5
	Second or subsequent operation	10
Preop. intra-aortic balloon pump	Present for surgery	2
LV aneurysm		5
Valve surgery: mitral	PA pressure <60 mmHg	5
	PA pressure >60 mmHg	8
Valve surgery: aortic	Gradient <120 mmHg	5
	Gradient >120 mmHg	7
Valve and CABG		2
Emergency surgery following cardiac catheter		10
Dialysis dependent		10
Catastrophic states		10–50
Other circumstances (asthma etc.)		2–10

Score	Risk	Predicted mortality
0–4	Good	1%
5–9	Fair	5%
10–14	Poor	9%
15–19	High	17%
>20	Very high	31%

Coronary arterial bypass grafting

Procedure	Bypassing a coronary artery stenosis with an arterial or venous graft
Time	3 h
Pain	+++/++++
Position	Supine +/– crucifix
Blood loss	Moderate (cross-match four units)
Practical technique	ETT, IPPV, arterial/CVP, urinary catheter, usually on CPB

Preoperative

- Commonly associated medical problems include hypertension, COPD, diabetes, cerebrovascular disease, and renal dysfunction.
- History of angina, recent MI, or CVE.
- Investigations: recent FBC, U&Es, chest radiograph, ECG, and angiogram. Respiratory function tests and echocardiography may be necessary.
- Careful assessment of left ventricular function:
  - orthopnoea and paroxysmal dyspnoea are important symptoms of LV failure
  - exercise ECG
  - coronary angiography within past 12 months
  - echocardiography assessment (transthoracic or transoesophageal):
    - >50% LV ejection fraction = good LV
    - 30–50% LV ejection fraction = moderate LV
    - <30% LV ejection fraction = poor LV
  - most useful assessment of left ventricular function is exercise tolerance.
- Parsonnet's scoring system (see p. 342).
- Premedication with intramuscular opioid and anticholinergic (e.g. papaveretum/hyoscine 15 mg/0.3 mg for an adult male, very amnesic and soporific). Prescribe oxygen supplementation from time of premedication.
- Continue all cardiac medication preoperatively (some centres stop aspirin/ACE inhibitors).

Perioperative

- Peripheral venous and arterial lines awake, preoxygenate and induce with fentanyl 10–15 µg/kg and etomidate 5–10 mg. Paralyse with pancuronium 0.1 mg/kg and maintain anaesthesia with halothane 0.5–1.5% in an oxygen and air mixture. Insert internal jugular lines and urinary catheter.
- Five-lead ECG with ST segment monitoring is advised (lead II for rhythm and V5 for ischaemia).
- Use a nasopharyngeal temperature probe.
- Indications for a pulmonary arterial flotation catheter include:

- all ventricles with an ejection fraction <30%
- all mitral valves, as filling and PA pressures are important postoperatively
- all patients with raised preoperative creatinine
- a perioperative alternative is to insert a left atrial line or a transoesophageal echo probe can be used to assess filling and ventricular function.

- Avoid hypertension and tachycardia. Aim for cardiovascular stability with volume, GTN infusion, and careful boluses of metaraminol 0.5–1 mg.
- Prophylactic antibiotics timed to coincide with skin incision:
  - flucloxacillin 2 g (vanconycin 1 g IV with premed if penicillin allergy or MRSA risk)
  - gentamicin 1.5 mg/kg
- Anticipate blood pressure surge with sternotomy, cover with fentanyl/halothane increase and/or GTN.
- Give heparin 300 IU/kg and ensure ACT >400 s pre-bypass.
- Maintain systolic blood pressure in range 80–100 mmHg for aortic cannulation.
- Continue as for bypass.
- Once the chest is closed and the patient stable, transfer intubated to recovery.
- Patients usually require plenty of filling postoperatively, particularly if bleeding, diuresing well, and vasodilating as they warm up. If cardioplegia has been used, temporary pacing wires will be inserted and pacing may be needed in the short term.

Postoperative

- Check FBC, clotting, arterial blood gases, and ensure blood loss is less than 200 ml/h.
- Once warm, awake, weaned, and not bleeding (i.e. a stable patient) extubate. Administer morphine (0.02 mg/kg/h) with GTN to keep systolic BP <140 mmHg to protect the graft 'top-ends' and reduce bleeding.

Special considerations

- For severe left main stem disease, maintain arterial pressure at preoperative values, as this is crucial to myocardial perfusion.
- Unstable angina with poor ventricles: consider PAFC and insertion of an intra-aortic balloon pump (IABP) in the anaesthetic room.
- Thoracic epidurals are used in some centres, claiming improved haemodynamic stability and excellent postoperative pain relief, but this is controversial due to the perceived risk of epidural haematoma and tetraplegia following anticoagulation for CPB.
- Arterial grafts (internal mammary/radial artery) are prone to spasm, therefore maintain GTN infusion postoperatively.

Redo coronary arterial bypass graft

Preoperative

* There is often poor LV function.
* Venous/arterial access as for CABG but often more difficult.
* Cross-match six units.

Perioperative

* A pulmonary arterial flotation catheter introducer is useful if rapid infusion is necessary.
* Have external defibrillator pads in situ on the patient, as VF is a risk at sternotomy and dissection of adhesions. This can be a problem with the use of diathermy as it obscures the ECG and with VF all you may see is a flat arterial trace (be vigilant)!
* Have blood available in theatre.
* There is a risk of torrential bleeding as the right ventricle may be stuck by adhesions to the underside of the sternum.
* Consider using a fibrinolytic inhibitor such as aprotonin during the procedure. Test dose of 1 ml, then 2 million units (200 ml) loading dose, 2 million units into the prime and then 500 000 units (50 ml) per hour peroperatively.

Postoperative

* There is increased risk of postoperative bleeding.
* There may be problems related to poor LV function.

Emergency coronary arterial bypass graft (failed angioplasty)

Preoperative
* The patient will be collapsed in periarrest with the need for urgent surgery to correct ischaemia.
* Should have good femoral venous and arterial access from the 'cath lab'.
* Patient will probably need inotropes, if not already started. Must attain some degree of stability or an arrest will follow induction.
* An IABP can help poor coronary perfusion by increasing diastolic pressure, plus ventricular function by off-loading the heart.

Perioperative
* May need a pulmonary arterial flotation catheter, but do not waste time if speed is important. It can be done later during the case.
* Cautious induction with a reduced dose of fentanyl (250–500 μg) and etomidate (4–6 mg). Cardiovascular stability is essential.
* Adrenaline should be prepared to be given as a bolus, 10 or 100 μg/ml as necessary.
* Institute CPB as soon as possible.

Postoperative
* Inotropes should be maintained post-CPB and/or IABP.
* There is no urgency to extubate the patient. A period of stability is required.
* There are likely to be many infusions running.
* There is a high risk of renal failure.

Mitral stenosis

Procedure	Replacement of mitral valve
Time	3–4 h
Pain	+++/++++
Position	Supine
Blood loss'	1000–1500 ml (cross-match four units)
Practical techniques	On CPB

The anatomical problems and consequences of particular valve lesions should be understood to appreciate the physiological requirements necessary for forward flow of blood before and after valve replacement.

Mechanical valves tend to be used in younger patients, as they should last forever. However, anticoagulation (warfarin) is needed to prevent clot formation around the valve. In elderly patients, porcine (homograft) valves can be used, as long-term anticoagulation is not needed. These valves probably only last for about 15 years.

Preoperative

- Frail, flushed, in atrial fibrillation with a fixed cardiac output and possible pulmonary hypertension.
- Almost always due to rheumatic heart disease, normally asymptomatic for 20 years.
- Surgery required if dyspnoea on mild exertion/at rest.
- Normal valve surface area = 4–6 cm^2
  - symptom free until 1.5–2.5 cm^2
  - moderate stenosis = 1–1.5 cm^2
  - critical stenosis <1 cm^2.
- Continue antiarrhythmic therapy and convert those on warfarin to heparin preoperatively.
- Echocardiography and angiography to assess pulmonary arterial pressure, ventricular function, and coronary arteries.
- Opioid/anticholinergic premedication with oxygen supplementation.

Perioperative

- Heart rate: mitral flow is relatively fixed, keep below 100 beats/min and in sinus rhythm if possible to maximize the time for diastole and coronary blood flow.
- Preload: does not normally need augmenting pre-bypass.
- SVR: because of fixed cardiac output the SVR is often raised, avoid reducing it, as the diastolic pressure will fall and with it coronary blood flow.

Venodilation will also reduce cardiac return and cardiac output for which the heart cannot compensate.

* Contraction: severe mitral stenosis leads to pulmonary hypertension and with it right ventricular failure. The left ventricle is normally unaffected until end-stage disease. Check ABGs regularly to avoid hypoxia/hypercarbia and exacerbation of pulmonary hypertension. Adrenaline may be required if the right ventricle is very dilated and failing.
* Heart rate: disruption of conducting pathways from surgery can cause arrhythmias, requiring atropine or isoprenaline.

Post-bypass

* Preload: keep well filled, as obstruction to flow has been removed (PAWP 13–16 mmHg).
* SVR: a reduction will now also encourage forward flow.
* Contraction: adrenaline may be required if the right ventricle is struggling and may help a stiff left ventricle.

Special considerations

* Use a pulmonary arterial flotation catheter to assess filling and requirement for ionotropy.
* Pulmonary arterial pressures take several days/weeks to reduce. Nitric oxide may help.
* Catastrophic atrioventricular (AV) disruption, where the heart bursts, in the first few days is rare and fatal.

Aortic stenosis

Procedure	Replacement of aortic valve
Time	3 h
Pain	+++/++++
Position	Supine
Blood loss	1000–1500 ml (cross-match four units)
Practical techniques	On CPB

Preoperative

- As a result of a congenital bicuspid valve (found in 1–2% of the population) or rheumatic heart disease. Bicuspid valves are often asymptomatic for 60 years and rheumatics for 40 years.
- A gradient exceeding 50 mmHg or an aortic orifice of <0.75 cm² in an average size adult is generally considered to represent critical obstruction to left ventricular outflow.
- Surgery indicated if the gradient is >70 mmHg with a good LV, and >50 mmHg with a poor LV.
- If a known gradient is decreasing, this is a sign of LV failure.
- The triad of symptoms of angina, syncope, or CCF indicates a life expectancy of <5 years.
- A sudden change in heart rhythm (e.g. atrial fibrillation) can cause rapid LV failure.
- Perform echocardiography and angiography to assess LV function and coronary blood flow.
- Aortic stenosis causes LV hypertrophy, with no increase in LV volume and a stiff non-compliant ventricle with poor diastolic function (relaxation). This increases oxygen demand. If long-standing the LV fails, LVEDP increases (causing mitral regurgitation and a high PAP) and ultimately RV failure.

Perioperative

- Heart rate: 'aortic stenosis—always slow'. Tachycardia is not well tolerated as it shortens diastole, hence the time for coronary blood flow, and increases oxygen demand. Atrial kick of the sinus rhythm improves filling of a stiff LV.
- Preload: should be increased to aid filling of stiff LV, beware of GTN reducing preload and cardiac output.
- SVR: must be aggressively maintained with alpha agonists. A reduction in diastolic pressure may critically reduce coronary blood flow to a hypertrophied LV.
- Contraction: the stiff and thickened LV may require adrenaline.

Post-bypass

- Preload: volume is still very important for adequate filling and perfusion of a stiff LV.
- SVR: an infusion of noradrenaline may be required once well filled.
- Contraction: adrenaline may be required to improve LV performance.

Special considerations

- Consider a pulmonary artery flotation catheter as filling is crucial, particularly in the postoperative period. Pre-bypass, the high pulmonary arterial pressure in long-standing aortic stenosis may underestimate LV filling.
- Good myocardial protection for a hypertrophied ventricle is the key to a good outcome.

Mitral regurgitation

Procedure	Replacement of mitral valve
Time	3 h
Pain	+++/++++
Position	Supine
Blood loss	1000–1500 ml (cross-match four units)
Practical techniques	On CPB

Preoperative

- Acute: rupture of a papillary muscle due to MI or endocarditis, causing pulmonary oedema.
- Chronic: rheumatic in origin, usually some stenosis as well and asymptomatic for up to 40 years.
- 75% have atrial fibrillation. Continue antiarrhythmic therapy and change warfarin to heparin.
- Symptoms of tiredness and dyspnoea reduce life expectancy to <5 years.
- The LV is essentially volume overloaded, which increases pulmonary arterial pressure and may cause RV failure.
- Once symptoms of failure cannot be controlled medically, surgery is indicated.

Perioperative

- 'Full, fast, and forward for a regurgitant lesion.'
- Heart rate: relative tachycardia reduces the time for regurgitation and increases forward flow.
- Preload: keep the patient well filled, again to encourage forward flow.
- SVR: an increase in SVR increases the regurgitant fraction. Alpha agonists should be avoided if there is a drop in blood pressure—volume is usually the answer. Avoid bradycardia.
- Contraction: inotropes are rarely needed pre-bypass, with acute mitral regurgitation an intra-aortic balloon pump may help.

Post-bypass

- LV function is often over estimated in mitral regurgitation, as the pulmonary circulation provides a low-pressure release system for a poor ventricle. On replacing the valve the LV has to work harder, which may precipitate failure and the need for adrenaline.
- Preload: filling is still very important.
- SVR: a reduction will benefit forward flow.
- Contraction: adrenaline may be required for a tiring LV.

Special considerations

- Consider a pulmonary arterial flotation catheter as LV contractility and correct filling are essential.
- An IABP may also be of use in the short term for a struggling LV.

Aortic regurgitation

Procedure	Replacement of aortic valve
Time	3 h
Pain	+++/++++
Position	Supine
Blood loss	1000–1500 ml (cross-match four units)
Practical techniques	On CPB

Preoperative

- There are many causes of aortic regurgitation: rheumatic or non-rheumatic valve disease or in association with aortic root dilation or dissection.
- Chronic aortic regurgitation may be asymptomatic for 20 years. Angina is a late symptom indicating end-stage disease.
- The LV is essentially volume overloaded which increases sympathetic drive, causing tachycardia, increased contractility, peripheral vasodilatation, and fluid retention to increase preload. LV hypertrophy occurs with LV dilation and an increased LV volume.
- Surgery is indicated once symptomatic.

Perioperative

- 'Full, fast, and forward for a regurgitant lesion.'
- Heart rate: cardiac output is rate dependent, increasing the rate reduces diastole and forward flow is encouraged. Avoid bradycardia and aim for a rate of 90 beats/min.
- Preload: LV is stiff with increased volume, so keep well filled. Sinus rhythm is of benefit but patients are usually in atrial fibrillation.
- SVR: anaesthesia causes a reduction in SVR, reducing the regurgitant fraction and encouraging forward flow. A vasodilator may improve this, but may also reduce venous return/preload.
- Contraction: if LV function is poor an inotrope may be required.

Post-bypass

- Preload: because of LV dilatation, filling is essential and must be maintained.
- SVR: a reduction will encourage forward flow, particularly if the LV is impaired.
- Contraction: an inotrope may be required. An inodilator (milrinone or enoximone) will reduce the SVR and improve LV function at the same time.

Special considerations

- An intra-aortic balloon pump is contraindicated in aortic regurgitation, but may be useful post-bypass.

- Careful control of blood pressure is needed pre-bypass in patients with aortic root dilatation or dissection. Try to keep systolic blood pressure <120 mmHg with GTN.
- With mixed lesions go with the dominant lesion.

Thoracic aortic surgery

Procedure	Replacement of ascending aorta/aortic arch with a tubular graft
Time	3–4 h
Pain	+++/++++
Position	Supine
Blood loss'	1000– >2500 ml (cross-match eight units)
Practical techniques	On CPB ± deep hypothermic circulatory arrest

General points

Thoracic aortic aneurysms and dissection are usually due to atherosclerosis. They can be divided into two groups, those with hypertension and those with hereditary conditions such as Marfan's syndrome. More than 66% have co-existing ischaemic heart disease, and dilatation of the aortic root with aortic regurgitation is common. They are classified as type A, involving the ascending aorta to the brachiocephalic artery, and type B, the arch/descending aorta. Type A and those involving the arch are treated surgically, the remainder of type B (descending lesions) are treated medically. Arch involvement, although rare, is treated surgically, under deep hypothermic circulatory arrest. They may present as elective or emergency procedures.

Preoperative

- For emergency dissections, control of blood pressure, bleeding, and fluid resuscitation are the main problems. An arterial line and good venous access are essential; a CVP line can be inserted later.
- 10 units of blood need urgent cross-matching and once in theatre, warn the laboratory regarding the need for clotting factors, platelets, and more blood later.
- GTN/labetalol infusion may be required to keep the systolic pressure <120 mmHg.

Perioperative

- Once stable they should be treated as patients with aortic regurgitation, by avoiding bradycardia, reducing afterload, and keeping well filled.
- Inotropes should be avoided as any dissection can increase.
- Aprotinin, 2 million units, is administered to the patient, 2 million units added to the bypass prime, and then continued IV at 500 000 units/h peroperatively to reduce clot breakdown.
- Femoral artery cannulation is usually required as the ascending aorta is to be resected.
- If the aortic root is involved the aortic valve may need replacement and coronary arteries reimplanting.
- Regular ABGs and monitoring of acid–base for indices of organ perfusion.

- Administer standard heparin (300 IU/kg) and maintain ACT >600 s. Aprotinin does require a longer clotting time.
- Adrenaline may be required before coming off bypass.

Post-bypass

- Bleeding and control of the arterial pressure are major problems.
- Continue aprotinin infusion and administer FFP and platelets as needed.
- Careful control of systolic pressure at <120 mmHg.
- Renal and gut perfusion are also potential problems, so keep the patient warm and well filled.

Special considerations

Circulatory arrest

Protection of the central nervous system by deep hypothermia during prolonged periods of circulatory arrest is necessary if the arch of the aorta is to be operated on, as it is not possible to perfuse the cerebral vessels easily on bypass. Hypothermia depresses the metabolic rate and oxygen consumption in the brain and also seems to protect cerebral integrity during reperfusion. The maximum safe duration of deep hypothermic circulatory arrest (DHCA) is thought to be approximately 45 min at 18 °C. This value comes from experimental evidence in animals as well as from clinical experience. In neonates, this can be extended to 60 min. Most centres do not rely solely on hypothermia to protect the brain; the head can be packed in ice and thiopental (7 mg/kg) added to the pump prime, in an effort to decrease cerebral metabolic demand further. The shorter the period of DHCA the better. Incidence of postoperative neurological problems is directly proportional to the time of DHCA.

- To aid rapid cooling, and to ensure that the brain is cooled, a vasodilator (GTN) is given. This prevents localized vasoconstriction due to hypothermia.
- Once the circulation has been arrested, all infusions and pumps are stopped.
- It is essential to measure both core and skin temperature and to make sure the core temperature reaches <20 °C.
- On rewarming, start propofol infusion (3–6 mg/kg/h as tolerated), order 4 units FFP and 1 large unit platelets, as these patients frequently encounter bleeding problems.
- Mannitol 0.5 g/kg may also be given to encourage a diuresis.
- When core temperature reaches 35 °C start adrenaline (0.05–0.1 μg/kg/min) to improve cardiac function and GTN (3–5 mg/h), if tolerated, to maintain vasodilatation to help rewarming.
- A steep head down tilt is used to allow air out of the aortic graft.

Keeping the patient warm is difficult as it takes a considerable time to warm thoroughly. Skin temperature must be >33 °C with a core temperature of >37 °C, before attempting to come off bypass. Do not be rushed as rebound cooling occurs in recovery, which will exacerbate poor myocardial function and any coagulopathy.

Pulmonary thromboembolectomy

Procedure	Removal of clot/tumour from pulmonary artery
Time	2–3 h
Pain	++/+++
Position	Supine
Blood loss	1000–1500 ml (cross-match four units)
Practical techniques	On CPB

Preoperative

- The patient is usually collapsed—'Airways, Breathing, Circulation'.
- There are usually emboli from pelvic or leg veins.
- Presentation with tachycardia, tachypnoea, hypoxia, cyanosis with distended neck veins and signs of RV failure.
- A healthy heart requires 60–80% of the pulmonary trunk to be obstructed before RV failure.
- Urgent cardiopulmonary bypass to re-establish oxygenation is the priority, so rapid decision-making is essential.

Perioperative

- Once the decision is taken to operate speed is the key—allow no delays. Heparin is easily forgotten.
- Intubate and ventilate with 100% oxygen, maintaining perfusion with inotropes as necessary and institute CPB as soon as possible.
- The surgeons should consider placing an IVC filter postembolectomy.

Post-bypass

- Inotropes are likely to be needed, keep well filled and reduce SVR with vasodilators if tolerated.
- Nitric oxide may help reduce a raised pulmonary arterial pressure. Delay heparinization (following CPB) for 24 h to reduce surgical bleeding.

Special considerations

- Very high right-sided pressures may open the foramen ovale and cause right to left shunting. This will worsen hypoxia and may allow paradoxical emboli, causing a CVE.
- With significant pulmonary emboli the capnograph will detect very little or no CO_2. Following embolectomy, if successful, this should show dramatic improvement, as the pulmonary circulation is re-established.

Cardioversion

Procedure	d.c. shock to convert an arrhythmia back to sinus rhythm
Time	5–10 min
Pain	–
Position	Supine
Blood loss	Nil
Practical techniques	Propofol ± LMA
	COETT if full stomach

Preoperative

• Atrial fibrillation is the commonest arrhythmia and may be acute or chronic.

• Often a remote site, with patients who are cardiovascularly unstable and have a full stomach.

• Requires an experienced anaesthetist with full anaesthetic equipment, monitoring, and trained help.

• If possible transfer to an anaesthetic room in theatre with help nearby.

• Treat as for any surgical procedure, premed with antacid prophylaxis if possible and have a physician ready to cardiovert the patient.

• Potassium should be in the normal range, as the myocardium may become unstable.

• If in AF >48 h and not anticoagulated the left atrium should be checked for clot with a transoesophageal echo before cardioversion. This can be done under propofol sedation. If clot is present anticoagulation for 4 weeks is required and then check again. If clear, continue with propofol and secure the airway as appropriate.

Perioperative

• Full monitoring, with ECG leads connected through the defibrillator and synchronized to R wave.

• Preoxygenate, induce slowly with a minimal dose of propofol and maintain the airway using a facemask, LMA, or COETT if there is a risk of aspiration.

• Consider etomidate if cardiovascularly unstable.

• Opioids are not usually necessary—except if intubating, when alfentanil may be appropriate.

• Safety during defibrillation—follow the ALS protocol.

• If there is atrial fibrillation, start with a shock of at least 200 J.

• If there is atrial flutter, start with a shock of 50 J, and if that fails increase by increments of 50 J.

Postoperative

* Aim to maintain spontaneous ventilation throughout the procedure.
* Turn the patient into the recovery position with supplemental oxygen and recover with full monitoring as for any anaesthetic.

Special considerations

* Patients in chronic AF may have atrial thrombus, which can embolize (see above).
* Digoxin increases the risk of postcardioversion arrhythmia and should be omitted on the day.
* Amiodarone improves the success of cardioversion to sinus rhythm.
* Defibrillation paddles should be kept at least 12.5 cm away from a pacemaker.

Anaesthesia for implantable defibrillators

Procedure	Implanting pacemaker/defibrillator
Time	1–3 h
Pain	+
Position	Supine
Blood loss	Nil
Practical technique	LA + sedation
	GA: ET/IPPV or LMA/SR

- Implantable defibrillators are placed in patients who are at risk of sudden death due to malignant cardiac arrhythmias. Patients range from young and otherwise fit adults with normal cardiac contractility, to extremely compromised cardiac patients.
- The procedure may be straightforward, when two venous wires (sensing and shocking) are positioned transvenously, or complex when pacemakers are replaced or the coronary sinus is catheterized to gain access to the LV muscle.
- The procedure is expensive (£20 000 for the electronic box). In some units cardiologists provide their own sedation service.
- During the procedure VF is induced on a number of occasions to test the device. The patient needs to be sedated during this phase.
- Invasive monitoring (arterial line) is advisable for any patients with impaired contractility.
- The cardiologist usually gains access via the left cephalic vein and uses fluoroscopy to guide the position of the leads.
- Careful asepsis is important to avoid infection of the prosthesis. IV antibiotics are usually given.
- Watch the total doses of local anaesthetic used by the cardiologist!

Preoperative

- Careful assessment is required to assess the functional cardiac reserve. Use local anaesthesia and sedation for anyone who is compromised.
- Ensure resuscitation drugs and equipment are available, as well as an external defibrillator (usually applied via stick-on pads).
- Draw up vasopressors and vagolytic drugs ready for use (ephedrine/metaraminol/glycopyrrolate). Have dedicated, skilled assistance.
- Insert an arterial line and large venous cannula under light sedation.

Perioperative

- If sedation is chosen give small doses of midazolam and fentanyl until comfortable, cooperative, but sleepy, then connect TCI propofol. Set to run at 0.5–1 μg/ml. Aim for light sleep during which the patient maintains their own airway. Administer additional oxygen. Just before defibrillator testing deepen the sedation.

- If GA is planned ensure recovery is planned preoperatively. Light anaesthesia only is required and care is needed on induction as many of these patients have limited cardiac reserve. An X-ray table may not tip and induction may be safer on a tilting trolley.
- ECG is recorded by the cardiologist.

Special considerations

- During VF testing, if the device does not work, do not allow the heart to be stopped for long!
- After VF and shocking the BP may remain low for a short period. Vasopressors may be required.
- If the patient has an existing pacemaker which is to be changed and the cardiologist is using diathermy, complete loss of pacemaker function can occur.
- Do not allow yourself to be distracted by the range of other activities taking place.
- A large plastic sheet (similar to an awake carotid set-up) allows the anaesthetist access to the patient's airway without compromising sterility.

Further reading

Hwang NC, Sinclair M (ed.) (1997). *Cardiac anaesthesia: a practical handbook.* Oxford University Press, Oxford.

Kaplan J (ed.) (1998). *Cardiac anesthesia.* Grune & Stratton, New York.

Patel RL, Turtle MRJ, Chambers DJ *et al.* (1993). Hyperfusion and cerebral dysfunction: effect of differing acid-base management during cardiopulmonary bypass. *European Journal of Cardiothoracic Surgery*, 7, 457–64.

Reeves JG (1999). Towards the goal of optimal cardiac anesthesia.Editorial. *Journal of Thoracic and Cardiovascular Anesthesia*, **13**, 1–2.

Slogoff S, Keats AS (1989). Randomised trial of primary anesthetic agents on outcome of coronary artery bypass operations. *Anesthesiology*, **70**,179–88.

Tuman KJ, McCarthy RJ, Spiess BD *et al.* (1989). Does choice of anesthetic agent significantly affect outcome after coronary artery surgery. *Anesthesiology*, **70**, 189–98.

Chapter 18
Thoracic surgery

David Sanders

General principles

Successful thoracic anaesthesia requires the ability to control ventilation of the patient's two lungs independently, skilful management of the shared lung and airway, and a clear understanding of the planned surgery. Good communication between surgeon and anaesthetist is essential.

Patients undergoing thoracic surgery are commonly older and less fit than other patients (30% are aged over 70 years, 50% are ASA grade 3 or above). Long-term smoking, bronchial carcinoma, pleural effusion, empyema, oesophageal obstruction, and cachexia are all common and can significantly reduce cardiorespiratory physiological reserve.

Anaesthesia—general points

- Discuss the planned procedure and any potential problems with the surgeon.
- Optimize lung function before elective surgery—try to stop patients smoking, arrange preoperative physiotherapy and incentive spirometry.
- The lateral decubitus position with the operating table 'broken' to separate the ribs is used for many operations.
- Use the ability to isolate and ventilate each lung independently when it is appropriate.
- Mechanical ventilation after pulmonary surgery stresses suture lines and increases air leaks and the risk of chest infection so avoid postoperative IPPV if possible.
- Minimize postoperative respiratory dysfunction by providing good analgesia and physiotherapy.
- Prescribe postoperative oxygen therapy routinely to compensate for increased V/Q mismatch. Warmed humidified 40% oxygen via a facemask is recommended after pulmonary surgery. Nasal cannulae delivering oxygen at 3 litre/min are better tolerated and satisfactory for most other patients.

Important clinical scenarios, which may be encountered by the thoracic anaesthetist, are:

- Subglottic obstruction of the trachea or carina either from extrinsic compression (retrosternal thyroid, lymph node masses, etc.) or invasion of the lumen, usually by a bronchial or oesophageal carcinoma.
- Dynamic hyperinflation of the lungs following positive pressure ventilation in patients with severe emphysema, bullae, lung cysts, or in the presence of an airway obstruction which acts as a 'flap valve' and results in gas trapping. Progressive lung distension creates the mechanical equivalent of a tension pneumothorax. This increase in intrathoracic pressure and pulmonary vascular resistance compromises venous return and right ventricular function and dramatically reduces cardiac output. If undiagnosed the situation can rapidly degenerate into an 'EMD arrest'. Emergency treatment is to disconnect the patient from the ventilator and open the tracheal tube to the

atmosphere, relieve any airway obstruction, and support right ventricular function. Remember—'if in doubt let it [the trapped gas] out'![1]

- Mediastinal shifts can occur due to large pleural effusions, tension pneumothorax and lateral positioning. Significant shifts cause unilateral lung compression and a severe reduction in cardiac output. Prompt recognition and correction of the underlying cause is vital

1 Conacher I (1998). Dynamic hyperinflation—the anaesthetist applying a tourniquet to the right heart. *British Journal of Anaesthesia*, **81**, 116–17.

Preanaesthetic assessment

* Patients require a standard assessment with particular emphasis on their cardiorespiratory reserve.
* Examine the chest radiograph and CT scans. Check for airway obstruction and tracheal or carinal distortion or compression because this can cause difficulties with placement of double lumen tubes.
* Patients with significant cardiac disease are clearly a high-risk group.

Preoperative assessment of patients for lung resection

Based on history, examination and simple pulmonary function tests, patients may be classified as:

* Clinically fit with good exercise tolerance and normal spirometry—accept for surgery.
* Having major medical problems, minimal exercise capacity, and grossly impaired pulmonary function tests—reject for surgery.
* Having reduced exercise capacity (short of breath on climbing two flights of stairs) and abnormal spirometry with or without moderate coexisting disease—require assessment as follows and careful evaluation of risks and benefits of surgery.

Pulmonary function tests are often used to determine suitability for lung resection surgery by estimating postoperative lung function. Always consider the results in the context of patient's general health and proposed resection.

* Generally accepted minimum preoperative values for FEV_1 for the following procedures are: pneumonectomy >55%, lobectomy >40%, wedge resection >35% of predicted value.
* Estimated postoperative FEV_1 <800 ml or postoperative FVC <15 ml/kg suggest a need for postoperative ventilation and increased mortality (it is difficult to generate an effective cough with an FVC <1 litre).[2]
* Exercise pulse oximetry can provide a useful clinical assessment in difficult cases. Failure to cover at least 300 m or a fall in SpO_2 of more than 4% in a 'six minute walk test' indicate a poor prognosis.
* The predicted postoperative value for pulmonary function tests is:
  preoperative value × (5 – number of lobes resected)/5.

  The goal is for a postoperative FEV_1 >35% of predicted normal for the patient (0.8–1.0 litre for an average man).

2 Gass GD, Olsen GN (1986). Preoperative pulmonary function testing to predict postoperative morbidity and mortality. *Chest*, **89**, 127–35.

Analgesia

A thoracotomy incision is extremely painful. Inadequate pain relief increases the neurohumoral stress response, impairs mobilization and respiration leading to an increase in respiratory complications, and may, in some patients, result in a post-thoracotomy chronic pain syndrome. Good analgesia is crucial and a technique combining NSAIDs, a regional block, intra-operative opioids, and regular postoperative oral analgesia is recommended.

Perioperative intercostal nerve blocks or percutaneous paravertebral blocks are useful for thoracoscopic procedures and can be combined with postoperative patient-controlled opioid analgesia. Unless specifically contraindicated, patients undergoing thoracotomy or thoracoabdominal incisions should receive continuous thoracic epidural or paravertebral regional analgesia. It is important to match the level of the block to that of the incision – usually T5/6 or T6/7. Perioperative epidural blockade should be established cautiously (3–4 ml of 0.25% bupivacaine) as an extensive thoracic sympathetic block can cause a major reduction in cardiac output and severe hypotension. Preincision percutaneous paravertebral injection of 0.5% bupivacaine (0.3 ml/kg) followed by a continuous postoperative infusion of bupivacaine (0.5% for 24 h and then 0.25% for 3–4 days) at 0.1 ml/kg/h via a surgically placed paravertebral catheter provides excellent post-thoracotomy analgesia.[3]

3   Richardson J, Lönnqvist PA (1998). Thoracic paravertebral block. *British Journal of Anaesthesia*, **81**, 230–8.

Isolation of the lungs

- Achieving independent ventilation of the lungs is not always straight-forward.
- One-lung ventilation (OLV) is associated with a number of complications and should be used only when the benefits outweigh the risks.
- 'Any anaesthetist using this technique should ensure that they have appropriate training and experience to use this technique safely' (NCEPOD Report 1996–97).

Advantages of OLV
- Protects the dependent lung from blood and secretions.
- Allows independent control of ventilation to each lung.
- Improves surgical access and reduces lung trauma.

Disadvantages of OLV
- One-lung ventilation inevitably creates a shunt and may cause hypoxia.
- The correct choice and positioning of endobronchial tubes is crucial.
- Increases technical and physiological challenge.

Indications for isolation and separation of the two lungs
- To avoid contamination of a lung in cases of infection, massive pulmonary haemorrhage, or bronchopulmonary lavage.
- To control the distribution of ventilation in massive air leaks or severe unilateral lung disease (e.g. giant bullae or lung cysts).
- Improving access for surgery is a relative indication for OLV. If isolation of the lung proves difficult the need to pursue OLV should be discussed with the surgeon since satisfactory access can often be achieved by careful lung retraction.

Techniques
- Double lumen endobronchial tubes (DLTs) are the commonest and most versatile approach.
- Bronchial blockers (Univent tube or Arndt endobronchial blocker) are occasionally useful, especially in patients who are difficult to intubate or have distorted tracheobronchial anatomy or a tracheostomy.
- Single lumen endobronchial tubes are of mainly historical interest.

Double lumen endobronchial tubes
- The commonest method of achieving OLV.
- Traditional reusable red rubber DLTs are still used in some specialist centres but disposable plastic (polyvinylchloride (PVC)) tubes are probably in wider general use.
- Described as 'right' or 'left' according to the main bronchus they are designed to intubate.
- Right-sided tubes have a hole or slit in the wall of the endobronchial section to facilitate ventilation of the right upper lobe.

- Sizes of plastic DLTs are given in Charriere (Ch) gauge (equivalent to French gauge), which is the external circumference of the tube in millimetres. Thus a 39 Ch tube has an external diameter of about 13 mm.
- The lumens of DLTs are small compared to standard single-lumen tubes used in adults. The internal diameters of the lumens of the 39 and 35 Ch 'Broncho-Cath' DLTs are only 6.0 and 5.0 mm respectively.
- Bronchoscopic placement and checking requires a narrow scope (less than 4 mm diameter), ideally with an integral battery light source for ease of manipulation.
- A major contraindication to use of a DLT is very distorted tracheobronchial anatomy or an intraluminal lesion—placement is likely to be difficult and possibly dangerous.

Types of DLT

- Carlens (left-sided): has a carinal 'hook' to aid correct placement.
- Whites (right-sided): has a carinal hook and a slit in the tube wall for the right upper lobe.
- Robertshaw (right- and left-sided): D-shaped lumens; traditionally a red rubber reusable tube, now available as a single-use version and in small, medium, and large sizes.
- Single-use PVC (right- and left-sided): high-volume, low-pressure cuffs; bronchial cuff and pilot tube coloured blue; radiopaque marker stripe running to tip of bronchial lumen; available in sizes 28–41 Ch, e.g. 'Broncho-Cath' (Mallinckrodt) or 'Sheribronch' (Sheridan).

Selection of a DLT

- Use the largest DLT which will pass easily through the glottis. 41 Ch or 39 Ch gauge PVC tube (large or medium Robertshaw) for males, 37 Ch gauge PVC tube (medium Robertshaw) for females. Small individuals may need a 35 Ch gauge or small Robertshaw tube.
- Use a left-sided tube unless the surgery involves a left pulmonary resection or abnormal bronchial anatomy is likely to obstruct intubation of the left main bronchus. A left-sided tube is less likely to block a lobar bronchus and gives a greater tolerance to shifts in tube position which inevitably occur when the patient is moved.

Placement of the DLT

- Assess the risks/benefits of using a DLT. Examine the radiographs, CT scans, and any previous bronchoscopy reports for tracheobronchial anatomy and lung pathology—is there distortion or narrowing which will interfere with bronchial intubation?
- Check the Y connector and that the 15 mm connectors are inserted into the proximal ends of the DLT lumens. (Broncho-Caths come with these connectors in a separate packet.)
- Most plastic DLTs are supplied with a malleable stylet which can be used to adjust the curve of the tube to facilitate intubation.
- Commence intubation with the concavity of the endobronchial section of the DLT facing anteriorly—once the tip is past the glottis partially withdraw the stylet and rotate the tube by 90° to bring the oropharyngeal curve into the sagittal plane. Turn the patient's head to the side opposite to the

bronchus to be intubated (i.e. to the right for a left-sided DLT) and gently slide the tube down the trachea until resistance is felt to further advancement.

- At this stage treat DLT as an ordinary ETT—inflate only the tracheal cuff to achieve a seal and confirm ventilation of both lungs.
- It is easy to push plastic DLTs in too far. The patient's height is the main determinant of correct insertion depth—the usual insertion depth to the teeth corner of the mouth in a patient 170 cm (5 ft 7 in) tall is 29 cm (depth changes by 1 cm for every 10 cm (4 in) change in the patient's height).[4]

Clinical confirmation of DLT position

- The next step is to check the tube position and establish isolation of the lungs. Beware of pathology affecting clinical signs—compare with preoperative clinical examination findings and radiology.
- Be systematic—it is easy to get confused!
- Start by checking ventilation through the bronchial lumen. Clamp off the gas flow to the tracheal lumen at the Y-connector and open the sealing cap on the tracheal lumen to air.
- Look for movement of the chest—is there appropriate unilateral expansion?
- Listen—auscultate gas entry to both lungs and listen at the proximal end of the open lumen for leaks around the bronchial cuff. Inflate the bronchial cuff 1 ml at a time (use a 5 ml syringe) until the leak stops. If a reasonable seal cannot be obtained with <4 ml of air the tube is either incorrectly placed or too small for the patient. Check specifically that all lobes are ventilated, especially the right upper if using a right-sided DLT.
- Feel—assess compliance by 'bagging' right, left, and both lungs. Very poor compliance (high inflation pressures) which is not explained by the patient's pathology suggests malposition—peak pressure on OLV should be <35 cmH$_2$O.
- Close the sealing cap, remove the Y-connector clamp, and then confirm it is possible to isolate and achieve OLV of the opposite lung via the tracheal lumen.
- Endobronchial tubes often move when the patient is placed in the lateral position. Recheck isolation and OLV once the patient is in position and before surgery starts.

Fibreoptic bronchoscope

- Ideally the position of every DLT should be checked bronchoscopically. At the very least a suitable bronchoscope must be immediately available to assess DLT placement if there are clinical problems with the tube or with OLV.
- This is invaluable where bronchial intubation is difficult and can be used to 'railroad' the tube into the correct main bronchus. Insert the bronchoscope via the bronchial lumen, partially withdraw the DLT so its tip lies in the trachea, locate the carina with the scope, and advance into the appropriate main bronchus, then slide the tube into position.

4 Brodsky JB, Benumof JL, Ehrenwerth J, Ozaki GT (1991). Depth of placement of left double-lumen endobronchial tubes. *Anesthesia and Analgesia*, 73, 570–2.

- Several bronchoscopic studies have shown that up to 80% of DLTs are mal-positioned to some extent even when the clinical signs are satisfactory. The upper surface of the bronchial cuff (blue) should lie just below the carina when visualized via the tracheal lumen.

- Always confirm positioning of a right-sided tube by bronchoscopy. The lateral 'slit' in the wall of the distal bronchial lumen should be aligned with the right upper lobe bronchus.

Management of one-lung ventilation

The physiology is complex and some aspects remain controversial.[5] One-lung ventilation inevitably creates a shunt through the unventilated lung and the crucial factor in managing OLV is to minimize the effects of this shunt. Hypoxic pulmonary vasoconstriction and the influence of anaesthetic agents upon it has little relevance to the routine clinical management of thoracic anaesthesia.

Initiating OLV

- Start with typical ventilator settings during two-lung ventilation (FiO_2 0.33, tidal volume, V_T, 10–12 ml/kg, airway pressure (P_{AW}) <25 cmH$_2$O).

- Increase FiO_2 to 0.5 and decrease V_T to 8–10 ml/kg before initiating OLV.

- Clamp the Y-connection to the non-dependent lung and open the sealing cap on that lumen of the DLT to allow the gas to escape.

- Observe the airway pressure closely. It will normally increase, often by 30–40%.

- If P_{AW} is excessive (>35 cmH$_2$O), or rises very abruptly with each inspiration, exclude mechanical causes (e.g. a kinked connector, clamp incorrectly placed) and DLT malposition or obstruction (e.g. ventilating lobe rather than lung, sputum plugs, opening of tracheal lumen against wall of trachea).

- Adjust V_T and ventilation profile to limit P_{AW}, ideally to <30 cmH$_2$O.

- Observe SpO_2 and ETCO$_2$ closely. If necessary increase the ventilatory rate to maintain the original minute volume and carbon dioxide clearance.

- Check with the surgeon that the lung is collapsing (this may take a few minutes in patients with obstructive airway disease) and that mediastinum has not 'sunk' into dependent hemithorax.

Hypoxia on OLV

- Hypoxia is a frequent complication of OLV, and is more common when the right lung is collapsed.

- It usually occurs after a few minutes of OLV (as oxygen in the non-ventilated lung is absorbed).

- SpO_2 dips but then often rises again a few minutes later as the non-ventilated lung collapses more completely and blood flow through it decreases.

- Increase FiO_2 and try to ensure an adequate cardiac output.

- Confirm the correct positioning of the DLT—are all lobes ventilated? Check with a fibreoptic bronchoscope if unsure.

5 Benumof JL, Alfrey DD (1994). Physiology of one-lung ventilation. In: Miller RD (ed.) *Anesthesia*, 4th edn, Ch 52. Churchill Livingstone,

- If partial collapse of the ventilated (dependent) lung is suspected ('sinking' mediastinum) try 5–10 cmH$_2$O PEEP on that lung—this may help, but the effect is unpredictable.
- If still hypoxic warn the surgeon, partially reinflate the non-dependent lung and then apply 5–10 cmH$_2$O CPAP via a simple reservoir bag/APL valve arrangement (CPAP System, Mallinckrodt®) supplied with 100% oxygen from an auxiliary oxygen flow-meter or cylinder. This will reliably improve saturations—simply insufflating oxygen into the collapsed non-dependent lung will not.
- If hypoxia persists use intermittent inflation of the non-dependent lung with oxygen breaths from the CPAP circuit—this needs to be coordinated with surgical activity.
- If these manoeuvres are not successful return to two-lung ventilation.
- Persisting with OLV in the face of continuing hypoxia (SpO$_2$ <92%) is dangerous and can rarely be justified.

Returning to two-lung ventilation

- Gently suction the non-ventilated lung to clear any blood or pus—use the long suction catheter supplied with the DLT.
- Close the sealing cap on the lumen to the non-ventilated lung and release the clamp on the Y-connector.
- Switch to manual ventilation and reinflate the collapsed lung under direct vision using sustained inflations. Inflation pressures up to 35–40 cmH$_2$O can be required to fully re-expand all areas of the lung.
- Return the patient to mechanical ventilation and, unless significant volumes of lung have been resected, return to original two-lung ventilator settings and FiO$_2$.
- Adjust the respiratory rate to maintain normocapnia.
- Always be prepared to return to OLV immediately should problems occur, e.g. a large air leak from the operated lung.

Bronchial blocker technique

- A balloon-tipped catheter ('blocker') is manipulated through a single lumen tracheal tube into the appropriate main (or lobar) bronchus with the aid of a narrow fibreoptic bronchoscope.
- Good lubrication of both bronchoscope and blocker is essential.
- The position of the blocker should be rechecked after the patient has been positioned for surgery.
- The lung or lobe is isolated from ventilation by inflating the balloon or cuff within the bronchus. The isolated lung slowly collapses as the trapped gas is absorbed or escapes via the blocker's narrow central lumen.
- Collapse can be accelerated by ventilating with 100% oxygen for a few minutes and then inflating the blocker at the end of expiration when the lung volume is at its minimum.
- Reinflation of the collapsed lung usually requires deflation of the blocker and consequently loss of isolation of the lungs. (A correctly positioned DLT will maintain separation of the airways to each lung until extubation.)

- During pneumonectomy or sleeve resection (bronchial reanastomosis) the blocker has to be withdrawn to allow surgical access to the bronchus.

There are two modern forms of bronchial blocker—both more costly than a standard disposable DLT:

- The Univent tube: a single lumen tube with an internal channel in its wall containing an adjustable blocker bearing a high-volume, low-pressure cuff.
- The Arndt wire-guided endobronchial blocker (COOK™): a stiff catheter with a cylindrical cuff and an adjustable 'wire' loop at its tip which guides the blocker along the outside of a fibreoptic bronchoscope into the required bronchus. Supplied with a special adapter which allows it to be deployed through a conventional single lumen or cuffed tracheostomy tube.

Indications for using a bronchial blocker

- On the rare occasions when isolation of a lobar bronchus is required (localized bronchiectasis or haemorrhage, lung abscess, or bronchopleural fistula).
- In patients who are difficult to intubate or have a permanent tracheostomy.
- To avoid the reintubation required to change to or from a DLT in patients receiving pre- or postoperative IPPV.

Rigid bronchoscopy and stent insertion

Procedure	Endoscopic inspection of the tracheobronchial tree—may include biopsy, insertion of airway stents or removal of foreign body
Time	5–20 min
Pain	+
Position	Supine with head and neck extended
Blood loss	Usually minimal
Practical techniques	TIVA with propofol boluses or infusion, alfentanil and intermittent suxamethonium. IPPV through bronchoscope with oxygen via Venturi needle and Sanders injector

Preoperative

- Check for airway obstruction—stridor, tracheal tumour on CT scan, or foreign body.
- Suitable as a day case procedure in appropriate patients.
- Warn about postoperative coughing, haemoptysis, and suxamethonium myalgia.
- Often combined with mediastinoscopy to assess suitability for lung resection.

Perioperative

- Give full preoxygenation.
- Confirm the surgeon is in the theatre before inducing the patient.
- Boluses of midazolam (2–3 mg) and alfentanil (500–1000 μg) facilitate induction and may reduce the risk of awareness.
- A preinduction 'taming' dose of non-depolarizing relaxant (e.g. vecuronium 0.5 mg) can reduce suxamethonium pains.
- Normally induce in the anaesthetic room, transfer to the theatre with a face mask, and give suxamethonium just prior to bronchoscopy.
- If there is potential airway obstruction (foreign body or tracheal compression) inhalation induction in the theatre with sevoflurane in oxygen is recommended until the airway is secure.
- Coordinate ventilation with surgical activity.
- Observe or palpate the abdomen to detect recovery of muscle tone.
- Suction the upper airway and confirm adequate muscle power before removing the scope.

Postoperative

- Turn the patient biopsied side down to avoid bleeding into the normal lung.
- Sit fully upright as soon as awake.

• Blood clot can cause severe lower airway obstruction requiring immediate intubation , suction, and repeat bronchoscopy.

Special considerations

• The airway is unprotected so patients at risk of regurgitation should be pretreated to reduce the volume and acidity of gastric secretions (oral omeprazole 40 mg the night before and 40 mg 2–6 h before the procedure).

• The procedure is very stimulating generating a marked hypertensive response.

• There is a need to obtund extreme cardiovascular responses and provide profound relaxation but with prompt return of laryngeal reflexes and spontaneous respiration.

• Vocal cords can be sprayed with local anaesthetic (4% topical lidocaine (lignocaine)) but this will not prevent carinal reflexes and may impair post-operative coughing.

• Rarely biopsy can precipitate a life-threatening airway bleed.

• Stent insertion can be technically difficult and may involve periodic loss of airway control.

• A short acting non-depolarizing muscle relaxant can be employed but it is difficult to achieve the profound paralysis required using mivacurium.

• Bradycardias caused by repeat doses of suxamethonium are seldom seen during rigid bronchoscopy in adults. Atropine should be drawn up but routine administration is not recommended since this will exacerbate any tachycardia.

Mediastinoscopy/mediastinotomy

Procedure	Inspection of structures in superior and anterior mediastinum via small suprasternal or anterior intercostal incision
Time	20–30 min
Pain	+
Position	Supine or slightly head up, arms by sides and head ring with bolster under shoulders
Blood loss	Usually minimal but potential for massive haemorrhage, G&S
Practical techniques	IPPV via single lumen tube

Preoperative

- Suitable as a day case procedure in appropriate patients.
- Check for superior vena cava obstruction and tracheal deviation or compression due to large mediastinal masses.
- Often preceded by a rigid bronchoscopy ('Bronch and Med').

Perioperative

- Tape eyes and check tracheal tube connectors; the head will be obscured by drapes.
- Boluses of IV fentanyl during surgery.
- Insert a 14 or 16G cannula in lower leg vein after induction (see below).
- Watch for surgical compression of the trachea—monitor tidal volume and airway pressures
- Monitor BP in the left arm and put the pulse oximeter on the right hand (see below).

Postoperative

- NSAIDs and PRN paracetamol and codeine phosphate.

Special considerations

- There is the potential for massive haemorrhage from the great vessels—the risk is increased in patients with SVC obstruction (hence the cannula in the leg): may require immediate median sternotomy.
- The brachiocephalic artery can be compressed by the mediastinoscope restricting blood flow to the right arm and carotid artery leading to a risk of cerebral ischaemia, hence the pulse oximeter on the right hand to monitor perfusion.
- Mediastinotomy can cause a pneumothorax.

Lung surgery: wedge resection, lobectomy, and pneumonectomy

Procedure	Excision of pulmonary tissue either selectively (wedge resection or lobectomy) or a whole lung (pneumonectomy)
Time	2–4 h
Pain	+++++
Position	Lateral decubitus with table 'broken', elbows flexed to bring forearms parallel to face with upper arm in gutter support
Blood loss	200–800ml—occasionally significantly more; G&S, cross-match two units for lobectomy/pneumonectomy
Practical techniques	IPPV via DLT using OLV during resection phase. Epidural or paravertebral regional anaesthesia with catheter for postoperative analgesia, arterial line for pneumonectomy and less fit patients

Preoperative

- Cancer is the commonest indication for lung resection—others include benign tumours, bronchiectasis, and TB.
- Assess the cardiorespiratory reserve and estimate post-resection lung function (see p. 366).
- Assess the airway with respect to placement of a DLT.
- Plan the postoperative analgesia regime.

Perioperative

- Select an appropriate DLT and check lung isolation carefully after intubation.
- Use a left-sided tube unless the surgery involves a left lobectomy or pneumonectomy or abnormal bronchial anatomy is likely to obstruct intubation of the left main bronchus.
- Intravenous infusion in upper arm—14 or 16G cannula.
- Radial arterial lines function better in the dependent arm as that wrist is usually extended.
- CVP monitoring can be unreliable in the lateral position with an open chest. Central lines are not recommended for routine use but may be indicated for access purposes or postoperative monitoring.
- OLV facilitates surgery and prevents soiling of the dependent lung.
- Continuous display of the airway pressure/volume loop is a valuable adjunct to monitoring and managing OLV.

- Surgical manipulation often causes cardiac and venous compression which reduces cardiac output and blood pressure and may cause arrhythmias.
- Suction the airway to the collapsed lung prior to reinflation.
- The bronchial suture line is 'leak tested' under saline by manual inflation to 40 cmH$_2$O.
- Titrate IV fluids to losses and duration of surgery. Avoid excessive fluid replacement especially in pneumonectomy.
- Preoperative epidural or paravertebral block with a surgically inserted catheter. Epidural can be used peroperatively but cautious incremental boluses are recommended (3 ml of 0.25% bupivacaine).

Postoperative

- Aim to extubate the patient awake at the end of the procedure and sit them upright in theatre.
- Prescribe continuous supplementary oxygen—humidified is preferable but nasal cannulae are more likely to stay on the patient in the ward.
- Ensure good analgesia is achieved.
- A chest radiograph is usually required in the recovery room.

Special considerations

- Occasionally patients with bronchial carcinoma may have 'non-metastatic' manifestations (Eaton–Lambert myasthenic syndrome or ectopic hormone production).
- Unilateral pulmonary oedema has been reported on re-expansion of the collapsed lung.
- Perioperative mortality from pneumonectomy is 5%. Increased pulmonary vascular pressures predispose to postpneumonectomy pulmonary oedema which occurs in 4% of patients and has an 80% mortality.
- Arrhythmias, especially atrial fibrillation, are quite common after pneumonectomy and many advocate prophylactic digitalization (digoxin 500 µg IV over 30 min perioperatively followed by 250 µg/day orally for 4–5 days).

Thoracoscopy and video-assisted thoracoscopic surgery procedures

Procedure	Inspection of the thoracic cavity via a telescope passed through an intercostal incision. Used for drainage of effusions, lung and pleural biopsy, pleurectomy, pericardial biopsy and window
Time	45 min–2 h
Pain	+++/++++
Position	Lateral decubitus with table 'broken', elbows flexed to bring forearms parallel to face with upper arm in gutter support
Blood loss	Minimal to 200 ml, G&S
Practical techniques	IPPV and OLV via left-sided DLT. Percutaneous paravertebral block/catheter or intercostal blocks, ± arterial line

Preoperative

- Assess as for a thoracotomy.
- Much less invasive than thoracotomy with less postoperative deterioration of lung function.
- Discuss regional analgesia and where appropriate PCA.

Perioperative

- Consider invasive arterial pressure monitoring for high-risk or compromised patients.
- Intravenous infusion in the upper arm; arterial line in the radial artery of the dependent arm.
- Boluses of fentanyl (50–100 µg) provide satisfactory intra-operative analgesia.
- Commence OLV before insertion of the trocar to reduce the risk of lung injury.
- Good collapse of the lung in the operative hemithorax is required for surgical access.
- Intercostal or paravertebral blocks. A paravertebral catheter can be inserted under thoracoscopic guidance for more extensive procedures.

Postoperative

- Extubate, sit up, and start supplementary oxygen in theatre before transfer to recovery.
- A chest radiograph is required in recovery to confirm full lung re-expansion.

- Although a thoracotomy is avoided patients still need balanced analgesia as for lung resection. PCA morphine may be required for 24–48 h for more painful procedures such as pleurectomy, pleurodesis, or wedge resections.
- Encourage early mobilization.

Special considerations

- This is not a minor procedure—there is always the possibility of conversion to an open thoracotomy.
- An epidural not usually necessary but is worth considering for bilateral procedures.

Lung volume reduction surgery and bullectomy

Procedure	Non-anatomical resection of regions of hyperinflated and poorly functioning pulmonary tissue
Time	2–5 h
Pain	+++/+++++
Position	Median sternotomy (bilateral surgery)—supine with arms to sides. Thoracotomy—lateral decubitus (as for lung resection)
Blood loss	200–800 ml, cross-match two units
Practical techniques	Effective thoracic epidural preinduction. GA with TIVA, relaxant, DLT—extreme care with IPPV and OLV

Lung volume reduction surgery is a developing surgical treatment for severe respiratory failure secondary to emphysema. The aim is to reduce the total lung volume to more physiological levels by resecting most diseased areas thereby improving respiratory function. Most of these patients belong to a group in which general anaesthesia would normally be avoided at all costs!

Preoperative

* Patients require intensive assessment, careful selection, and optimization prior to surgery.
* Cardiac assessment for lung volume reduction surgery should include coronary angiography and right heart catheterization to evaluate IHD, ventricular function, and pulmonary artery pressures.
* Patients are often on corticosteroids—perioperative supplementation is required.
* A clear understanding of pathophysiology and adequate thoracic experience is essential for safe anaesthetic management.[6]

Perioperative

* Surgery may be performed via sternotomy, thoracotomy, or by video-assisted thoracoscopic surgery.
* There is a serious risk of rupturing emphysematous bullae with IPPV causing leaks and tension pneumothorax.
* Nitrous oxide is contraindicated.
* Continuous spirometry, invasive arterial, and CVP monitoring are essential.

6 Conacher ID (1997). Anaesthesia for the surgery of emphysema. *British Journal of Anaesthesia*, **79**, 530–8.

- Clinical assessment of DLT placement is difficult—verify the position bronchoscopically.
- Limit the risk of 'gas trapping' and dynamic pulmonary hyperinflation by deliberate hypoventilation and permissive hypercapnia ($PaCO_2$ up to 8.5 kPa). Recommend V_T 6–8 ml/kg, 10–12 breaths/min , I:E ratio 1:4 and peak airway pressure <30 cmH_2O.
- Disconnect from the ventilator intermittently to allow the lungs to 'empty'.
- Bronchospasm and sputum retention with mucus plugging can be a problem.
- Use colloids for fluid replacement to minimize the risk of pulmonary oedema.

Postoperative

- HDU or ICU care will be required—extubate as soon as possible.
- Anticipate and accept raised $PaCO_2$ (7–9 kPa) and adjust FiO_2 to maintain SpO_2 in the range 90–92%.
- Watch closely for air leaks—use a maximum of 10 cmH_2O suction on intercostal drains.
- Requires excellent pain relief, skilled physiotherapy, and a pulmonary rehabilitation programme.

Special considerations

- The commonest complication is prolonged air leak—more than 7 days in 50% of patients.
- Mortality from a recent series is 5–10%.
- A large-scale randomized trial currently in progress in the United States.
- Patients with an isolated congenital bulla or 'lung cyst' require the same careful intra-operative anaesthetic management but are usually much fitter and do not normally require invasive cardiological assessment.

Drainage of empyema and decortication

Procedure	Surgical removal of pus (empyema) and organized thick fibrinous pleural membrane (decortication)
Time	Drainage 20–40 min
	Decortication 2–3 h
Pain	+++/+++++
Position	Lateral decubitus for thoracotomy
Blood loss	Simple drainage: minimal
	Decortication: 500–2000 ml, cross-match three units
Practical techniques	GA with cautious IV induction, relaxant, intubation, and IPPV
	DLT advised for decortication (risk of air leaks); single lumen tube adequate for drainage procedures, arterial line/CVP

Preoperative

- Interpleural infection is usually secondary to pneumonia, intercostal drains, or chest surgery.
- Patients are often debilitated by chronic infection and may be frankly septic. Confirm the patient is on appropriate antibiotic therapy.
- Respiratory function is often already compromised by pneumonia or prior lung resection.
- Check for the presence of a bronchopleural fistula created by erosion into the lung.

Perioperative

- Empyema is usually drained by rib resection and insertion of a large-bore intercostal drain.
- Thoracoscopy may be used to break down loculated effusion or empyema and free pleural adhesions.
- Decortication requires a standard thoracotomy anaesthetic and epidural analgesia since pleural changes often preclude a paravertebral catheter.
- Decortication frequently causes significant haemorrhage, and air leaks are common.
- Invasive arterial and CVP monitoring are advised for all but the fittest patients.

Postoperative

* Balanced analgesia with regular paracetamol, NSAIDs (check renal function), regional block (intercostal blocks useful for drainage procedures) and supplementary opioids.
* High-dependency care is recommended after decortication.

Special considerations

* The surgical principle is to remove infected tissue including pleural 'peel', fully re-expand the lung, and obliterate infected pleural space.
* Decortication is a major procedure which requires careful evaluation of risks and benefits in elderly, frail, and sick patients.
* Lobectomy may occasionally be required during decortication if a massive air leak or severe parenchymal lung damage occurs.

Repair of bronchopleural fistula

Procedure	Closure of communication between the pleural cavity and trachea or bronchi
Time	2–3 h (for thoracotomy approach)
Pain	++++/+++++
Position	Keep sitting upright with the affected side tilted down until the good lung is isolated, then lateral decubitus for thoracotomy
Blood loss	300–800 ml, G&S, cross-match two units if anaemic
Practical techniques	Rapid IV induction and fibreoptic guided endobronchial intubation with DLT
	Awake fibreoptic guided intubation with DLT
	Intubation with DLT under deep inhalation anaesthesia with spontaneous ventilation

Preoperative

- Features are productive cough, haemoptysis, fever, dyspnoea, subcutaneous emphysema, and a falling fluid level in the postpneumonectomy space on the chest radiograph.
- The severity of symptoms is proportional to the size of the fistula—big fistulae with large air leaks cause severe dyspnoea and may necessitate urgent respiratory support.
- Patients are often debilitated with respiratory function compromised by infection and prior lung resection.
- Check previous anaesthetic charts for ease of intubation and type of DLT used.
- Check the anatomy of the lower airway carefully on the chest radiograph—it is often distorted by previous surgery.
- Require supplementary oxygen, a functioning chest drain, and IV antibiotics and fluids.

Perioperative

- Key principles are to protect the 'good' lung from contamination and to control the distribution of ventilation.
- Small or moderate fistulae are usually assessed by bronchoscopy and may be amenable to sealing with tissue glue.
- Commence invasive arterial pressure monitoring before induction.
- Awake intubation with local anaesthesia is considered to be the safest option but ultimately the choice of technique depends upon individual circumstances. However, failure to adequately isolate the lungs after induction will put the patient at grave risk.

- IPPV increases gas leakage, causing loss of tidal volume and the risk of tension pneumothorax.
- Endobronchial intubation must be under direct vision with a fibreoptic bronchoscope to ensure correct placement in the bronchus contralateral to the fistula—the potential exists to enlarge the fistula by inappropriate placement.
- TIVA is recommended—delivery of volatile agents may be unreliable with large gas leaks. Ketamine may be useful in high-risk patients.

Postoperative

- Plan HDU/ICU care for all but the most straightforward cases.
- Minimize airway pressures during ventilation and extubate as soon as possible.
- Use the standard post-thoracotomy analgesic regimen but watch renal function with NSAIDs.

Special considerations

- Most fistulae are postoperative complications of pneumonectomy or lobectomy but some are secondary to pneumonia, lung abscesses, or empyema.
- Anaesthesia for repair of bronchopleural fistula is challenging and is not recommended for an 'occasional' thoracic anaesthetist!

Tips for controlling a massive air leak (i.e. unable to ventilate effectively)

If a DLT cannot be positioned satisfactorily the following are worth attempting:

- Intubate with an uncut cuffed 6 mm diameter single lumen tube—pass a fibreoptic bronchoscope through the tube into the intact main bronchus and 'railroad' the tube into the bronchus to isolate and ventilate the good lung.
- Ask the surgeon to pass a rigid bronchoscope into the intact main bronchus and slide a long flexible bougie or COOK™ airway exchange catheter (which allows jet ventilation) into the bronchus—remove the bronchoscope and railroad a single lumen tube.
- If all else fails an Arndt endobronchial blocker or a large Fogarty embolectomy catheter passed into the fistula via a rigid bronchoscope may control the leak temporarily.

Pleurectomy/pleurodesis

Procedure	Stripping of parietal pleura from the inside of the chest wall (pleurectomy)
	Production of adhesions between parietal and visceral pleura either chemically (talc, tetracycline) or by physical abrasion (pleurodesis)
Time	Pleurectomy 1–2 h
	Pleurodesis 20–40 min
Pain	+++/++++
Position	Lateral decubitus for open thoracotomy or VATS. May be supine for pleurodesis
Blood loss	Minimal if thoracoscopic; up to 500 ml for thoracotomy, G&S
Practical techniques	IPPV, DLT, and OLV advised for open/VATS procedures. A single lumen tube is usually adequate for pleurodesis

Preoperative

- Patients fall into two groups: young and fit with recurrent pneumothoraces (check for asthma) and older patients compromised by COPD or recurrent pleural effusions (check respiratory reserve).
- Check a recent chest radiograph for pneumothorax and/or effusion.
- A preoperative intercostal drain is advised if pneumothorax is present.
- Check the planned surgical approach.
- Discuss postoperative analgesia and regional technique.

Perioperative

- Keep airway pressures as low as possible in patients with a history of pneumothorax.
- Be alert for pneumothoraces—they can tension rapidly on IPPV even with a drain in situ and can be on the 'healthy' side; avoid nitrous oxide in this group of patients.
- Collapse the lung during instillation of irritant to facilitate pleural coating—if using a single lumen tube preoxygenate and then briefly disconnect the lungs from the ventilator.
- Aim for full expansion of the lung at the end of the procedure to appose parietal and visceral pleura.

Postoperative

- Extubate and sit the patient upright before transfer to the recovery room.

- A chest radiograph is needed in the recovery room to check full lung expansion—suction on intercostal drains may be prescribed by the surgeon to assist expansion.
- Pleural inflammation can cause severe pain.
- A balanced analgesic regimen with regular paracetamol, NSAIDs, and either a thoracic epidural (bilateral procedures) or a combination of morphine PCA with intercostal blocks or, if feasible, a paravertebral catheter.

Special considerations

- Pleurectomy is usually performed for recurrent pneumothorax—combined with stapling of lung tissue responsible for recurrent air leaks (usually apical 'blebs' or small bullae).
- Pleurodesis is often used to manage malignant pleural effusions (mesothelioma, metastatic carcinoma)—there can be large volumes of fluid causing significant respiratory compromise.
- Patients with very large pleural effusions (over halfway up the hemithorax on chest radiograph or >1500 ml) are at risk of circulatory collapse when turned 'effusion side up' for surgery. The mechanism is probably a combination of mediastinal shift and high intrathoracic pressure on IPPV reducing venous return and cardiac output. Drain the effusion with the patient supine before turning to the lateral position.

Oesophagectomy

Procedure	Total or partial excision of oesophagus with mobilization of stomach (occasionally colon) into chest with anastomosis to proximal oesophagus to restore continuity
Time	3–6 h
Pain	+++++
Position	Supine with arms by sides and/or lateral decubitus for thoracotomy
Blood loss	500–1500 ml; cross-match two units
Practical techniques	IPPV, DLT useful if thoracotomy. Art/CVP lines, urinary catheter, thoracic epidural or paravertebral catheter for thoracoabdominal incision

Preoperative

- Establish indication for surgery—usually oesophageal cancer but occasionally for non-malignant disease (benign stricture, achalasia).
- The anaesthetic plan requires understanding of the surgical approach:
  - transhiatal: laparotomy and cervical anastomosis
  - Ivor–Lewis: laparotomy and right thoracotomy
  - thoracoabdominal: left thoracotomy crossing costal margin and diaphragm
  - McKewan three-stage: laparotomy, right thoracotomy, and cervical anastomosis.
- Preoperative malnutrition or cachexia is common and is associated with a higher risk of postoperative morbidity and mortality.
- Requires careful cardiorespiratory assessment.
- Plan for the duration of surgery and the need to reposition the patient during the procedure.
- Preoperative adjuvant chemotherapy may leave residual immunosupression.
- Book HDU or ICU according to the patient's fitness and local protocols.

Perioperative

- Consider all patients with oesophageal disease to be at risk of regurgitation so rapid sequence induction with cricoid pressure is advised.
- If thoracotomy is planned use a DLT and OLV to facilitate surgical access and reduce trauma to the lung.
- Plan regional anaesthesia according to the surgical approach—paravertebral LA infusion with morphine PCA for thoracoabdominal approach or for laparotomy/thoracotomy a mid-thoracic epidural (using 3 ml boluses

of 0.25% bupivacaine perioperatively and postoperative infusion of 5 mg diamorphine in 50 ml 0.167% bupivacaine at 2–8 ml/h).

- A nasogastric tube will be required initially. It is removed for resection and reinserted under surgical guidance following anastomosis.
- Do not put an internal jugular line on the side required for cervical anastomosis.
- Monitor core temperature and be obsessional about keeping the patient warm (efficient fluid warmer and forced air warming blanket).
- Stay ahead with fluid replacement—aim for 10 ml/kg/h of crystalloid plus colloid or red cells to replace blood loss.
- Check Hb (Haemacue® ideal) and blood gases intra-operatively—watch for metabolic acidosis suggesting inadequate tissue perfusion.
- Arrhythmias and reduced cardiac output causing hypotension frequently occur during intrathoracic oesophageal mobilization.
- Change DLT to a single lumen tube to improve surgical access prior to cervical anastomosis (if performed).

Postoperative

- Require intensive and experienced nursing care in a specialist ward, high-dependency unit or intensive care.
- If cold (<35.5 °C) or haemodynamically unstable ventilate until the condition improves.
- Aim for a minimum urine output of 1 ml/kg/h.
- Use a jejunostomy or nasoduodenal tube for early enteral feeding.

Special considerations

- Oesophagectomy has one of the highest perioperative mortality rates of all elective procedures (up to 5% even in specialist centres).
- 66% of deaths are from systemic sepsis secondary to respiratory complications or anastomotic breakdown.
- Over 30% of patients suffer a major complication.
- Occasional practice in anaesthesia (or surgery) for oesophagectomy is not recommended.

Chest injury

The emergency diagnosis and initial treatment of major thoracic trauma is described on p. 440. This section deals with the anaesthetic management for definitive repair of ruptures of the diaphragm, oesophagus, and tracheo-bronchial tree.

General considerations

- Serious chest injuries are frequently associated with major head, abdominal, or skeletal injuries and appropriate attention and priority must be given to their management (cervical spine immobilization, laparotomy to arrest bleeding, splintage of limb fractures).

- Fewer than 30% of patients with thoracic trauma require a thoracotomy but persistent bleeding from intercostal drains exceeding 200 ml/h is an indication for urgent surgery.

- Most deaths from thoracic trauma are due to exsanguination. Good IV access with two large-bore cannulas will allow rapid infusion.

- Emergency thoracotomy in the resuscitation room is seldom indicated and is rarely associated with a favourable outcome.

- Standard principles of emergency anaesthesia should be applied.

- Maintain a high index of suspicion for tension pneumothorax during IPPV—an intercostal drain does not guarantee protection.

- Massive air leaks usually indicate significant tracheobronchial injury (see below).

- Patients with major thoracic trauma are at high risk of multiple organ failure and require postoperative management in an intensive care unit.

Repair of a ruptured diaphragm

- Clinical features and diagnosis are described on p. 441.
- May present as a chronic condition or as an intestinal obstruction of herniated bowel—check preoperative fluid and electrolyte status.
- The defect should be closed promptly but seldom needs to be done as an emergency.
- The surgical approach is via a standard lateral thoracotomy or thoraco-abdominal incision.
- Intra-operative management is as for fundoplication.
- Avoid nitrous oxide—it distends the bowel and may make reduction of hernia more difficult.
- DLT and OLV facilitate surgical access for repair.
- A nasogastric tube should be used to decompress the stomach.

Repair of a ruptured oesophagus

- Clinical features and diagnosis are described on p. 442—surgical emphysema and pleural effusions are frequently present.
- Other causes of oesophageal rupture include excessive abdominal straining and uncoordinated vomiting (Boerhaave's syndrome). Oesophageal per-

foration can be caused by foreign bodies but is often iatrogenic (during endoscopic procedures).

- Mediastinitis is followed rapidly by sepsis and systemic inflammatory response syndrome with associated problems of circulatory shock, renal failure, and ARDS.
- The principles of surgical management are initially drainage and prevention of further contamination.
- Initial careful endoscopic assessment will determine the extent of oesophageal disruption.
- Small tears in unfit frail patients may be managed conservatively with chest drainage and nasogastric suction but normally urgent surgery is required.
- Patients should be stabilized preoperatively in ICU with chest drainage, IV fluid replacement, analgesia, invasive monitoring, and inotropic support.
- Intra-operative management is as for oesophagectomy.
- Upper and lower oesophageal injuries require right and left thoracotomy respectively.
- Primary closure is possible if the oesophagus is healthy, if not oesophagectomy will be required.
- Arrhythmias, particularly atrial fibrillation, are common due to mediastinitis.
- Change the DLT for a single lumen tube before transfer to intensive care for postoperative ventilation.
- Even patients who are stable at the end of the repair procedure remain at high risk of major complications for several days.
- Early postoperative feeding—either parenteral or via feeding jejunostomy.
- There is a significant incidence of dehiscence resulting in oesophagopleurocutaneous fistula and high mortality.

Repair of tracheobronchial injury

- Most patients with significant tracheal or bronchial disruption do not reach hospital alive.
- Clinical features of laryngeal and tracheobronchial injuries are described on p. 442.
- The priority is 100% oxygen and relief of tension pneumothorax which may require two large-bore intercostal drains with independent underwater seals.
- If ventilation and oxygenation are acceptable call for thoracic surgical assistance and try to assess and identify the site of airway injury by fibreoptic bronchoscopy before intubation.
- Airway management and anaesthetic principles apply as for a large bronchopleural fistula (p. 385).
- Adequate positive pressure ventilation may be impossible with a single lumen tube.
- A torn bronchus can be isolated by fibreoptic guided intubation of the contralateral intact main bronchus with an appropriate DLT.
- An uncut single lumen tube can be bronchoscopically guided past an upper tracheal tear so its cuff lies distal to the injury.

- Once the airway is secure and ventilation is stabilized proceed to urgent thoracotomy for repair.
- Carinal disruption may require cardiopulmonary bypass to maintain oxygenation during repair.
- Inappropriate management can lead to later stenosis and long-term airway problems.

Other thoracic procedures

Operation	Description	Time	Pain	Position/ approach	Blood loss/ X-match	Notes
Fibreoptic bronchoscopy	Visual inspection of tracheobronchial tree ± biopsy and bronchial brushings/lavage	5–10 min	+	Supine	None	GA rarely used. Single lumen tube (SLT) (8–9 mm) with bronchoscopy diaphragm on angle piece. IPPV with relaxant appropriate to duration. Expect high airway pressures while scope in ETT. Suction can empty breathing system
Lung biopsy	Diagnostic sampling of lung tissue for localized or diffuse abnormality	30–60 min	+++/++++	Lateral/VATS or minithoracotomy	Minor/G&S: X-match if anaemic	DLT and OLV facilitates VATS procedures. Patients with diffuse disease can have very poor lung function—risk of ventilator dependence and significant mortality
Oesophagoscopy and dilatation (O&D)	Visual inspection of oesophagus via rigid or fibreoptic scope ± dilatation of stricture with flexible bougies	5–20 min	+	Supine	None	Regurgitation risk so rapid sequence induction advised. SLT on left side of mouth—watch for airway obstruction and ETT displacement during procedure. Flexible oesophagoscopy often done under IV sedation

Operation	Description	Time	Pain	Position/approach	Blood loss/X-match	Notes
Oesophageal stent insertion	Endoscopic placement of tubular stent through oesophageal stricture	10–30 min	+/++	Supine	None	Often emaciated, may be anaemic. Preop. IV fluids to correct dehydration. Rapid sequence induction, SLT, and awake extubation in lateral position. Small risk of oesophageal rupture
Fundoplication	'Antireflux' procedure for hiatus hernia — fundus of stomach wrapped round lower oesophagus	2–3 h	++++/+++++	Supine/laparotomy. Lateral/left thoracotomy. Laparoscopic procedure also	Moderate/G&S: if Hb <12 X-match 2 units	Often obese — check respiratory function. Rapid sequence induction or awake fibreoptic intubation mandatory. Nasogastric tube required. DLT helpful for thoracic approach. Epidural or paravertebral and PCA recommended
Pectus excavatum repair	Correction of 'funnel chest' deformity of sternum	3–5 h	+++/+++++	Supine — arms to sides/midline sternal incision or subcostal	Moderate to severe: X-match 3 units	Primarily cosmetic unless deformity severe. Usually young fit adults. GA, IPPV via SLT and midthoracic epidural recommended. Risk of pneumothoraces

Operation	Description	Time	Pain	Position/ approach	Blood loss/ X-match	Notes
Thymectomy	Excision of residual thymic tissue and/or thymoma from superior and anterior mediastinum	2–3 h	++/+++	Supine – arms to sides/median sternotomy	Moderate: X-match 2 units	Usually for myasthenia gravis. Check for airway compression, other autoimmune diseases, thyroid function and steroid therapy. GA, IPPV via SLT, minimal or no relaxant and monitoring of neuromuscular transmission. May need postop. ventilatory support (see p. 186)

Chapter 19
Neurosurgery
Tracey Clayton and Alex Manara

Intracranial pressure (ICP)

Normal ICP is between 5 and 12 mmHg. Changes in ICP reflect changes in the volume of the intracranial contents held within the confines of the rigid skull (brain substance 1200–1600 ml, blood 100–150 ml, CSF 100–150 ml, ECF <75 ml). Compensatory mechanisms initially reduce the effect of an intracranial space-occupying lesion on ICP. These mechanisms involve displacement of CSF into the spinal subarachnoid space, increased absorption of CSF, and a reduction in intracranial blood volume. However, a critical point is reached when these compensatory mechanisms are overwhelmed and a further small increase in intracranial volume results in a steep rise in intracranial pressure (Fig. 19.1). If a lesion develops slowly it may reach a relatively large volume before causing a significant rise in ICP. In contrast, a lesion that appears relatively small on a CT scan may have developed quickly allowing little time for compensation.

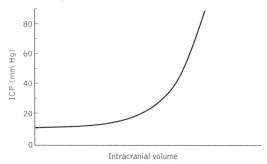

Fig 19.1 Compliance curve for the intracranial contents.

Causes of raised ICP

- Increased brain substance: tumour, abscess, and haematoma.
- Increased CSF volume: hydrocephalus, benign intracranial hypertension.
- Increased blood volume:
  - increased cerebral blood flow: hypoxia, hypercarbia, volatile anaesthetic agents
  - increased cerebral venous volume: increased thoracic pressure, venous obstruction in the neck, head down tilt, coughing.
- Increased extracellular fluid: cerebral oedema.

Cerebral perfusion pressure (CPP)

CPP is the effective pressure that results in blood flow to the brain:

$$CPP = MAP - (ICP + VP).$$

Venous pressure (VP) at the jugular bulb is usually zero or less and therefore CPP is related to ICP and mean arterial pressure (MAP) alone.

Cerebral blood flow (CBF)

Cerebral blood flow is normally autoregulated. This maintains a constant blood flow between mean arterial pressures (MAP) of 50–140 mmHg. Outside these limits of autoregulation cerebral blood flow varies passively with perfusion pressure. In patients with chronic hypertension the lower and upper limits of autoregulation are higher than normal so that a blood pressure that may be adequate in a normal patient may lead to cerebral ischaemia in the hypertensive patient. Autoregulation is also impaired or abolished acutely in the presence of a brain tissue acidosis as may occur with hypoxia, hypercarbia, acute intracranial disease, and following head injury.

Cerebral blood flow varies with:

- Metabolism. CBF is primarily determined by the metabolic demands of the brain. CBF is therefore increased during epileptic seizures and in association with pain and anxiety. Conversely CBF is reduced in coma, hypothermia, and following the administration of anaesthetic agent such as propofol or barbiturates.

- Carbon dioxide tension. Hypocapnea results in cerebral vasoconstriction and a reduction in CBF. The greatest effect is at normal $PaCO_2$ where a change of 1 kPa results in a 30% change in blood flow. Arterial pressure modifies the response of the cerebral circulation to hyperventilation. High perfusion pressures are associated with an increased responsiveness to hyperventilation, whereas hypotension of 50 mmHg abolishes the effect of increased or decreased $PaCO_2$ on CBF.

- Oxygen tension. PaO_2 is not a particularly important determinant of CBF, a value of less than 7 kPa being required before cerebral vasodilatation occurs.

- Temperature. Hypothermia reduces cerebral metabolism thereby reducing CBF. Metabolism falls by approximately 5% for every degree centigrade reduction in body temperature.

- Viscosity. There is no effect on CBF when the haemotocrit is between 30 and 50%. CBF will increase with reduced viscosity outside this range.

- Anaesthetic agents (see p. 402).

Measuring intracranial pressure (ICP)

Ventricular

A catheter inserted into a lateral ventricle via a burr hole is the gold standard for the measurement of ICP. The catheter is connected to either a pressure transducer or fibreoptic pressure measuring device This method allows the drainage of CSF as a treatment option to reduce ICP. Disadvantages of the technique are risk of haemorrhage at insertion and the risk of ventriculitis if the catheter is left in position for a prolonged period. This technique may be difficult in patients with cerebral oedema and small ventricles.

Subdural

A hollow bolt is inserted into the skull via a burr hole. The dura is incised and a pressure transducer or fibreoptic device is passed into the subdural space. Haemorrhage and infection are possible complications. Subdural ICP monitoring tends to underestimate ICP.

Intraparenchymal

Microminiature silicone strain gauge monitors can be inserted into the brain parenchyma to monitor ICP. These are becoming increasingly popular because of their ease of insertion and accuracy, particularly in intensive care when they can be inserted by non-neurosurgical staff.

Extradural

Catheters in the extradural space are not a reliable method of monitoring ICP and have been largely abandoned.

General principles of anaesthesia in the presence of raised ICP

Identify those patients with a raised ICP preoperatively. Symptoms and signs include:

- Early:
  - headache and vomiting
  - seizures, focal neurology, papilloedema.
- Late:
  - increasing blood pressure and bradycardia
  - agitation, drowsiness, coma
  - Cheyne–Stokes breathing, apnoea
  - ipsilateral then bilateral pupillary dilatation
  - decorticate then decerebrate posturing.
- Investigations: evaluate CT/MRI scans for the presence of generalized oedema, midline shift, acute hydrocephalus, and the size of any lesion and associated oedema.

Management aims

Do not increase ICP further:

- Avoid increasing cerebral blood flow by avoiding hypercarbia, hypoxia, hypertension, and hyperthermia. Always use controlled ventilation to manipulate $PaCO_2$ and ensure good oxygenation. In situations where autoregulation is lost there may be unpredictable effects on CBF with even modest increases in blood pressure. Ensure adequate analgesia and depth of anaesthesia.
- Avoid increasing venous pressure. Avoid coughing and straining, the head down position, and obstructing the neck veins with ETT ties.
- Avoid further cerebral oedema. While patients are generally fluid restricted, it is important to maintain intravascular volume and CPP. Do not use hypotonic solutions such as Hartmann's solution or dextrose-containing solutions. Fluid flux across the blood–brain barrier is determined mainly by the plasma osmolality not oncotic pressure. Maintenance of a high normal plasma osmolality is essential.
- Maintain CPP: hypotension will result in a decreased cerebral perfusion pressure in the presence of a raised ICP. To preserve CPP, normotension is maintained prior to opening the dura using fluids as well as catecholamines if necessary.
- Avoid anaesthetic agents that increase ICP (see below).

Specific measures to decrease ICP:

- Reduce cerebral oedema using osmotic or loop diuretics, or the two combined. Give mannitol 0.25–1 g/kg as an infusion over 15 min or furosemide (frusemide) 0.25–1 mg/kg. Insert a urinary catheter in all patients receiving diuretics.

- Modest hyperventilation to $PaCO_2$ of 4.0–4.5 kPa has a transient effect in reducing ICP for 24 h. Excessive hyperventilation will result in cerebral ischaemia, and may result in a loss of autoregulation. However, remember that $ETCO_2$ is lower than $PaCO_2$.
- Corticosteroids are useful in reducing oedema associated with tumours and abscesses but their use is controversial in head injury. They take several hours to work. Dexamethasone 4 mg 6-hourly is often given electively pre-operatively.
- Cerebrospinal fluid may be drained via an external ventricular drain or ventriculoperitoneal shunt.
- Position the patient with a head up tilt of 30 degrees to reduce central venous pressure. Ensure that the MAP is not significantly reduced as the overall result could be a reduction in CPP.

Anaesthetic agents and ICP

Volatile agents

Volatile agents reduce cerebral metabolism and oxygen demand. However, they also increase cerebral blood flow and ICP and abolish autoregulation in sufficient doses. Halothane causes the greatest increase in ICP and isoflurane the least. ICP is unaffected by concentrations of less than 1 MAC of isoflurane. Sevoflurane and desflurane appear to have similar CNS and CVS effects to isoflurane. Enflurane may cause seizures, particularly in association with hypocapnoea, and has no place in neuroanaesthesia. Nitrous oxide is a weak cerebral vasodilator causing an increase in CBF and therefore ICP. In addition it has been shown to increase cerebral metabolic rate.

Intravenous anaesthetic agents

All IV anaesthetic agents decrease cerebral metabolism, CBF, and ICP with the exception of ketamine, which increases ICP and should be avoided in neuroanaesthesia. Carbon dioxide reactivity and autoregulation of the cerebral circulation are well maintained during propofol and thiopental anaesthesia. Both offer a degree of neuroprotection as a result of reduced cerebral metabolism and therefore oxygen demand.

Other drugs

- Suxamethonium causes a rise in ICP through muscle fasciculation increasing venous pressure. However, this effect is moderate, short-lived, and of little clinical relevance. Suxamethonium should still be used in acute situations such as head injury when rapid intubation is required in the presence of a potentially full stomach. In elective cases intubation and muscle relaxation can be achieved following a non-depolarizing relaxant.
- Narcotic analgesics have little effect on CBF and ICP if respiratory depression with a consequent increase in $PaCO_2$ is avoided. Carbon dioxide reactivity is maintained. Although there were concerns initially that alfentanil may increase ICP this was shown to be secondary to hypotension resulting in cerebral vasodilation and a consequent increase in cerebral blood volume. This has not proven to be significant if the drug is administered slowly or infused, and serves to re-emphasize the importance of maintaining MAP.

Craniotomy

Procedure	Craniotomy for excision or debulking of tumours, e.g. meningiomas, astrocytomas. Burr hole biopsy to establish a tissue diagnosis. Drainage of cerebral abscess
Time	1–12 h
Pain	+/+++
Position	Supine, head up tilt or lateral decubitus
Blood loss	0–2000 ml, G&S or cross-match two units
Practical techniques	ETT, IPPV, arterial line, CVP

Preoperative

* Assess the patient for symptoms and signs of raised intracranial pressure. Document any neurological deficits.

* Intracranial tumours may be metastatic, the primary sites including the lung, breast, thyroid, and bowel.

* Assess the gag and cough reflexes.

* Check the CT/MRI scans for the site and size of tumour and features of a raised ICP. Meningiomas may reach a large size before producing clinical signs and if very vascular may result in significant intra-operative blood loss. The duration and complexity of the procedure are determined by the size, site, and vascularity of lesions being excised or debulked.

* Patients receiving diuretic therapy or who have been vomiting may have disordered electrolytes. Patients receiving preoperative dexamethasone may be hyperglycaemic.

* Restrict IV fluids to 30 ml/kg/day of normal saline if cerebral oedema is present. Avoid glucose-containing solutions—they may cause hyper-glycaemia which is associated with a worse outcome after brain injury, and also reduce osmolality resulting in increased cerebral oedema.

* Sedative premedication should be avoided in patients with raised ICP.

* Ensure graduated compression stockings are fitted for thromboembolic prophylaxis. Anticoagulation increases the risk of serious haemorrhage and is best avoided.

* Prophylactic or therapeutic phenytoin may be required (a loading dose of 15 mg/kg followed by a single daily dose of 3–4 mg/kg).

* Discuss with the surgeon the anticipated duration of the procedure since this is very variable (multiply the estimate by two!).

Perioperative

* Patients undergoing a burr hole biopsy require standard monitoring. Those scheduled for craniotomy also need invasive blood pressure and CVP measurement, neuromuscular monitoring, and core temperature. Urine output should be measured in long cases and in those who receive diuretics or mannitol.

- Anaesthesia can be induced with thiopental 3–5 mg/kg or propofol 1–3 mg/kg, followed by an opioid such as fentanyl 5 µg/kg and a non-depolarizing relaxant like vecuronium 0.15 mg/kg. Give IV induction agents slowly to avoid reducing blood pressure and CPP. Additional agents such as alfentanil 10 µg/kg, lidocaine (lignocaine) 1.5 mg/kg or a beta-blocker (labetalol 5 mg increments) may be required to attenuate the hypertensive response to intubation. Lidocaine spray to the larynx and vocal cords may reduce coughing. Use an armoured ETT to prevent kinking and secure in place with tapes as ties may cause venous obstruction. Cover and protect the eyes.

- Patients may be placed in the supine or lateral position depending on the surgical approach. Avoid extreme neck flexion or rotation, which may impair cerebral venous return, and maintain a head up tilt. If the head is turned to the left or the right for surgery, support the shoulder to reduce the effect of rotation on the neck veins. The head is often secured in place using a Mayfield three-point fixator. The application of the pins can cause a marked hypertensive response which should be prevented by infiltration of the pin sites with local anaesthetic. Alternatively give a further dose of fentanyl (1–2 µg/kg), alfentanil (10 µg/kg), or propofol (0.5–1 mg/kg).

- Anaesthesia is maintained using either isoflurane (<1 MAC) or a propofol infusion. Avoid N_2O if the ICP is raised. Ensure adequate analgesia using top-up doses of fentanyl. Alternatively use an infusion of alfentanil (25–50 µg/kg/h) or of remifentanil (0.5 µg/kg/min until craniotomy, reduced to 0.25 µg/kg/min for the rest of the procedure). Maintain neuro-muscular relaxation throughout with a non-depolarizing muscle relaxant such as atracurium or vecuronium.

- Aim for normotension for most procedures. Modest hypotension is required infrequently to improve the surgical field for the removal of very vascular tumours. Mild hypocapnoea is used in tumour surgery. Aim for a $PaCO_2$ of 4–4.5 kPa (30–35 mmHg). Use normal saline as maintenance fluid, replacing blood loss with colloid or blood.

- Maintain normothermia using a hot air warmer, particularly during pro-longed procedures. Hypothermia is only indicated for procedures where the cerebral blood supply is at risk (see vascular lesions).

- Use an intermittent pneumatic compression device to the calves or feet throughout the procedure for thromboprophylaxis.

- Following the completion of the intracranial surgery, closure of the dura and scalp takes at least half an hour. Sudden hypertension on awakening may be treated with small boluses of propofol, lidocaine (lignocaine), or labetalol. Avoid coughing on the endotracheal tube if possible.

Postoperative

- Many routine craniotomies can be managed postoperatively on an ade-quately staffed neurosurgical ward. Continued monitoring of the patient's conscious level and neurological state is essential. Consider postoperative sedation and ventilation if there is continuing cerebral oedema or if the patient was severely obtunded preoperatively.

- The majority of patients (>90%) will experience pain in the mild to moderate range after craniotomy. Codeine phosphate (60–90 mg) com-bined with regular paracetamol is usually sufficient for postoperative analgesia. If not patient-controlled analgesia with morphine may be used.

Special considerations

- NSAIDs should only be used for postoperative analgesia after careful consideration. While they reduce opioid requirements and enhance opioid analgesia, they certainly increase the bleeding time and a postoperative intracranial haematoma is potentially disastrous. Many patients will also have received diuretics and are potentially hypovolaemic. This may exacerbate the renal toxicity of NSAIDs.

- A central line is indicated for the majority of craniotomies to allow measurement of CVP, infusion of vasoactive drugs, and the aspiration of air in the case of venous air embolism. This is most commonly inserted in the antecubital fossa using a long line. However, in experienced hands the insertion of an internal jugular line does not worsen raised ICP.

Ventriculoperitoneal shunt

Procedure	CSF drainage for treatment of hydrocephalus
Time	45–120 min
Pain	++
Position	Supine, head up tilt
Blood loss	Not significant
Practical techniques	ETT, IPPV

Shunts are inserted for hydrocephalus. The CSF is diverted from the cerebral ventricles to other body cavities from where it is absorbed. Most commonly a ventriculoperitoneal shunt is created. On rare occasions ventriculoatrial or ventriculopleural shunts are inserted. An occipital burr hole enables a tube to be placed into the lateral ventricle and it is then tunnelled subcutaneously down the neck and trunk and inserted into the peritoneal cavity through a small abdominal incision. A flushing device can be placed in the burr hole to keep the system clear, and a valve system is incorporated to prevent CSF draining too rapidly with changes in posture.

Preoperative
- As for craniotomy (p. 403).
- Many patients requiring shunts are children and the usual paediatric considerations need to be remembered.
- Patients often have raised intracranial pressure.
- Emergency cases may have a full stomach requiring a rapid sequence induction.

Perioperative
- Shunt procedures are shorter and simpler than craniotomies. Use routine monitoring. Arterial and central venous lines are not required.
- Antibiotic treatment or prophylaxis is required and strict antisepsis protocols are normally followed to reduce the incidence of shunt infection.
- Advancing the trocar to allow tunnelling of the shunt is particularly stimulating. Additional analgesia and/or muscle relaxation is often required at this stage.

Postoperative
- Any deterioration in the patient's conscious level is an indication for a CT scan to exclude shunt malfunction or subdural haematoma.

Special considerations
- Patients are at risk of intracranial haemorrhage if CSF is drained too rapidly.
- Shunts often block or become infected, requiring revision.
- Watch for signs of pneumothorax as the trocar is placed subcutaneously.

Evacuation of intracranial haematoma

Procedure	Evacuation of extradural or subdural haematoma
Time	1.5–3 h
Pain	+/+++
Position	Supine, head up
Blood loss	200–2000 ml, cross-match two units
Practical techniques	ETT, IPPV, arterial line, CVP

Intracranial haematoma may be extradural, subdural, or intracerebral:

Extradural
Urgent evacuation is required and certainly within an hour of pupillary dilation. The haematoma is usually the result of a tear in the middle meningeal artery. It is virtually always associated with a skull fracture, except in children when a fracture may be absent.

Subdural
Subdural haematomas result from bleeding from the bridging veins between the cortex and dura. Early evacuation of acute subdural haematomas improves outcome. Chronic subdural haematomas occur in the elderly, usually after trivial injury. They present insidiously with headaches and confusion and may be evacuated via burr holes under local anaesthesia.

Intracerebral
Intracerebral haematomas occur secondary to a head injury, a bleed from an intracranial aneurysm, or in hypertensive individuals. It may also occur as a complication of treatment with warfarin.

Preoperative
* As for head injury (p. 420).
* Most patients will have a reduced and possibly deteriorating GCS.
* Intracranial pressure will be raised in most patients.
* Patients may have associated injuries to the chest, pelvis, or abdomen requiring resuscitation and treatment in their own right. Protect the cervical spine if necessary.
* Patients may have a full stomach requiring rapid sequence induction.
* Check blood clotting profile and the availability of blood products prior to surgery.

Perioperative
* As for craniotomy (p. 403).
* Patients require standard monitoring including invasive blood pressure monitoring. CVP monitoring should be instituted in trauma patients.

- Ensure smooth induction and normotension to maintain CPP using catecholamines if necessary. Assume that the ICP is 20 mmHg and that the minimum acceptable MAP is therefore 90 mmHg to achieve a CPP of 70 mmHg.
- Ensure head up tilt; avoid nitrous oxide, ventilate to an $ETCO_2$ of 4 kPa and give mannitol (0.5–1 g/kg) and furosemide (fusemide) (0.25–1 mg/kg) as required.
- Once decompression has occurred there may be a decrease in systemic blood pressure which can usually be treated with volume replacement.

Postoperative

- Ventilate those patients in coma preoperatively, or with a 'tight' brain at craniotomy, on ITU for 12–24 h postoperatively. Management can be guided by a protocol that aims to maintain CPP and prevent secondary insults to the brain (see p. 424).

Special considerations

- It is essential for various teams to communicate and set priorities in the management of patients with multiple injuries. The priorities will vary from patient to patient with evacuation of an intracranial haematoma being paramount in one patient, while in another control of intra-abdominal haemorrhage and cardiovascular stabilization may be required before evacuation of the intracranial haematoma.

Posterior fossa surgery

Procedure	Excision of posterior fossa tumour
Time	3–14 h
Pain	+/+++
Position	See below
Blood loss	100–2000 ml, G&S
Practical techniques	ETT, IPPV, art line, CVP, ?monitoring for venous air embolism

The posterior fossa lies below the tentorium cerebelli and contains the pons, medulla, and cerebellum. Within the brainstem lie the main motor and sensory pathways, the lower cranial nerve nuclei, and the centres that control respiration and cardiovascular function. An increase in pressure in this area results in decreased consciousness, hypertension, bradycardia, respiratory depression, and loss of protective airway reflexes. The exit pathways for CSF from the ventricular system are also located here and if obstructed result in hydrocephalus. Space-occupying lesions and surgical disturbance in this area can therefore have a profound physiological impact.

Preoperative

- Patients with posterior fossa lesions may have a reduced level of consciousness and impaired airway reflexes. Bulbar palsy may lead to silent aspiration. Pulmonary function must be assessed.

- Assess intracranial pressure—it may be raised. If hydrocephalus is present, ventricular drainage may be required before the definitive procedure.

- Assess fluid status—the patient may be dehydrated if vomiting. A reduced intravascular volume will result in hypotension on induction or if placed in the sitting position.

- Check electrolytes and glucose, particularly if taking diuretics or steroids.

- Assess cardiovascular function, particularly the presence of untreated hypertension, postural hypotension, and septal defects.

Perioperative

- As for craniotomy (p. 403).

- Insert a nasogastric tube if the patient has, or is at risk of, postoperative bulbar dysfunction.

- Further specialized monitoring is required for posterior fossa surgery including monitoring for venous air embolism (p. 418) and nerve tract injury. The appropriate electrophysiological monitor used to detect nerve tract injury depends upon the neural pathway at risk during the procedure. Spontaneous or evoked electromyographic activity, somatosensory evoked potentials, or brainstem auditory evoked potentials are frequently monitored.

- Lumbar CSF drainage is occasionally requested to improve surgical conditions and to reduce the incidence of postoperative CSF leaks.
- Some centres advocate the avoidance of N_2O. In addition to increasing cerebral metabolic rate and CBF, it may also worsen the outcome of air embolism. Finally, there is a risk that if N_2O is used once the skull is closed, any residual intracranial air will increase in volume and cause pneumocephalus.
- While some still recommend spontaneous respiration for posterior fossa surgery, the consensus is to use muscle relaxation and IPPV.
- Surgical interference with the vital centres may result in sudden and dramatic cardiovascular changes. Warn the surgeon since more gentle retraction or dissection usually resolves the problem. Only use drugs such as atropine and beta-blockers if absolutely necessary as they make the interpretation of further changes difficult.

Patient positioning

Surgical access to the posterior fossa requires the patient to be in the sitting, prone, or lateral position. Careful attention is required in positioning the patient as the procedures are often prolonged.

Sitting position

The use of this position is declining. It should only be employed where specifically indicated and by experienced practitioners. This position provides optimum access to midline lesions, improves cerebral venous drainage, and lowers intracranial pressure. However, significant complications include haemodynamic instability, venous air embolism, and the possibility of paradoxical air embolism, pneumocephalus, and quadriplegia. Absolute contraindications to the use of this position include cerebral ischaemia when upright and awake, and the presence of a patent ventriculoatrial shunt or patent foramen ovale (should be screened preoperatively). Relative contraindications are uncontrolled hypertension, extremes of age, and COPD. To achieve this position the head and shoulders are gradually elevated with the neck partially flexed and the forehead resting on a horseshoe ring mounted on a frame. Avoid excessive head flexion since this can cause jugular compression, swelling of the tongue and face, and cervical cord ischaemia.

Prone position

This position allows good surgical access without the risks specifically associated with the sitting position. Abdominal compression should be avoided as it results in an increased cerebral venous pressure. This is achieved by adequately supporting the chest and pelvis.

Lateral position

The lateral or 'park bench' position is particularly suitable for lateral lesions such as acoustic neuroma or operations on a cerebellar hemisphere. The neck is flexed and the head rotated towards the floor ensuring that the jugular veins are not obstructed. Pressure points over the shoulder, greater trochanter, and peroneal nerves should be protected.

Postoperative

- Most patients can be safely extubated and managed on a properly staffed neurosurgical ward postoperatively.

- Postoperative airway obstruction can occur after posterior fossa surgery due to macroglossia, partial damage to the vagus, or excessive flexion of the cervical spine.
- Surgery on medullary or high cervical lesions carries a significant risk of postoperative impairment of respiratory drive.
- The patient should be admitted to ICU for ventilation if the preoperative state was poor, the surgical resection was extensive, if there is significant cerebral oedema, or there are intra-operative complications.

Special considerations

- Acoustic neuroma. The facial nerve is particularly vulnerable and is monitored using electromyographic needles placed over the face. This allows the surgeon to identify the nerve and when it is at risk during dissection. In this situation neuromuscular blockade should not be used. Often eighth nerve function is also monitored to preserve any hearing the patient still has. This requires a constant level of anaesthesia so that neurophysiological changes can be attributed to the surgery rather than variations in anaesthetic depth. These requirements are best met using an opioid infusion (alfentanil or remifentanil) combined with a constant level of anaesthesia using a low concentration of an inhalation agent or a propofol infusion.
- Venous air embolism (see p. 418).
- Postoperative analgesia is managed as after craniotomy. Posterior fossa surgery is reputed to cause more postoperative pain than supratentorial surgery, although this is questionable.

Posterior fossa lesions

Tumour	Notes
Gliomas	Cerebellar astrocytomas, ependymomas, particularly arising from the fourth ventricle
Medulloblastoma	Often arising from the vermis of the cerebellum, usually in children
Acoustic neuroma	Arising from the eighth nerve in the cerebellopontine angle, usually benign
Haemangioblastoma	Young adults
Meningiomas	Less common in the posterior fossa
Metastatic tumours	
Abscesses and haematoma	
Vascular lesions	Aneurysms of the superior cerebellar, posterior inferior cerebellar, and vertebral arteries
Developmental lesions	Arnold–Chiari malformation

Vascular lesions

Vascular lesions presenting for surgical management are usually either intracranial aneurysms or arteriovenous malformations.

Intracranial aneurysms

- Berry aneurysms occur at vessel junctions, cerebral arteries having a weaker, less elastic muscle layer than systemic vessels. They may occur in association with atherosclerosis, polycystic kidneys, hereditary haemorrhagic telangectasia, coarctation of the aorta, and Marfan's, Ehlers–Danlos, and Kleinfelter's syndromes. Mycotic aneurysms may occur in rheumatic fever.
- The most common sites are the internal carotid system (41%), the anterior cerebral artery (34%), and the middle cerebral artery (20%).
- They are more common in females, occur mainly in 40–60 year-old age group and in 25% of cases they are multiple. In the United Kingdom the incidence is 10–28 per 100 000 of the population per year. The prevalence of aneurysm is 6% of the population in prospective angiographic studies.
- Aneurysms do not usually rupture until they are greater than 5 mm in diameter. They then present as a subarachnoid or intracerebral haemorrhage. The classic symptoms of a subarachnoid haemorrhage are sudden onset of severe headache with loss of consciousness that may be transient in mild cases. Occasionally a patient presents with a focal neurological deficit due to the pressure of an enlarging aneurysm on surrounding structures.
- Grading of subarachnoid haemorrhage (World Federation of Neurosurgeons): the grade of the subarachnoid haemorrhage influences morbidity and mortality. It is also of value in deciding whether to operate or coil early (grades 1–3) or to wait (grades 4 and 5):

Grade	GCS*	Motor deficit
1	15	–
2	13–14	–
3	13–14	+
4	7–12	+/–
5	3–6	+/–

*See p. 421.

Arteriovenous malformations

- These are dilated arteries and veins with no intervening capillaries.
- They may present clinically with subarachnoid haemorrhage or seizures.
- High blood flows through such lesions may 'steal' blood from surrounding tissue leading to ischaemia.

Complications of aneurysmal subarachnoid haemorrhage

Neurological complications

Rebleeding

- The initial bleed and subsequent bleeds are the main cause of mortality. The highest risk period is in the first 24 h during which there is a risk of rebleeding of 4%. After that there is a further risk of 1.5% per day for the next 4 weeks.

- There is a 60% risk of death with each episode of rebleeding. The main aim of management is to prevent rebleeding by controlling the aneurysm surgically by clipping it or angiographically by obliterating it endoluminally.

- Surgery was previously delayed for up to 10 days, as early surgery is more difficult, and to wait for the peak of vasospasm to pass.

- The introduction of nimodipine has resulted in earlier surgery, ideally within 72 h of the subarachnoid haemorrhage. Grade 1 or 2 patients may be operated upon immediately.

Delayed neurological deficit

- Delayed neurological deficit may present as focal or diffuse deficits and is a major cause of morbidity following subarachnoid haemorrhage, and is secondary only to rebleeding as the main cause of mortality.

- It is associated with vasospasm which is caused by substances released as the subarachnoid blood undergoes haemolysis. The most likely spasmogenic agent is oxyhaemoglobin.

- Although angiographic vasospasm occurs in up to 75% of studied patients who have had a subarachnoid haemorrhage, only half of these patients develop delayed neurological deficit. Up to 20% of symptomatic patients will develop a stroke or die of vasospasm despite optimal management.

- Delayed neurological deficit peaks 3–12 days and 2 weeks after the initial bleed. With increasingly early surgery for aneurysms, it is now commonly seen postoperatively.

- Treatment is as follows:

  - Calcium channel blockers. Nimodipine is a relatively selective calcium channel antagonist with effective penetration of the blood–brain barrier. It is started at the time of diagnosis and continued for 3 weeks using a dose of 60 mg nasogastrically or orally 4-hourly. Alternatively it can be administered intravenously (1 mg/h increasing to 2 mg/h) either centrally or through a peripheral vein together with a fast flow of fluids. Nimodipine may cause systemic hypotension which should be aggressively treated with fluids and, if necessary, catecholamines.

  - Hypertensive, hypervolaemic therapy with or without haemodilution ('triple H therapy'). This treatment is based on the theory that vasospasm can be prevented or reversed by optimizing cerebral blood flow. Goals are to increase cardiac output and blood pressure using volume expansion and then vasoactive drugs. The resulting haemodilution may improve cerebral blood flow by reducing viscosity. Disagreement exists as to the fluids and drugs that should be used and as to which haemodynamic goals to aim for. Suggested values are normal MAP + 15%, CVP >12 mmHg, haematocrit 30–35%. Some centres advocate the use of PA catheters to monitor therapy. Noradrenaline (0.025–0.3 μg/kg/min) or dobutamine (2–15 μg/kg/min) are used to increase MAP.

- In some centres balloon angioplasty or intra-arterial papaverine are also used.

Hydrocephalus

Blood in the subarachnoid space may obstruct drainage of CSF and result in hydrocephalus and a raised ICP. Sudden reduction in pressure with the insertion of a ventricular drain may increase the risk of rebleeding by reducing the transmural pressure across the aneurysm. Hydrocephalus must be ruled out by CT scan before attributing neurological deterioration to delayed neurological deficit/vasospasm.

Other neurological complications

These include seizures and cerebral oedema.

Medical complications

Life-threatening associated medical problems occur in nearly 40% of patients, and account for about 23% of deaths after subarachnoid haemorrhage. Many of the cardiorespiratory complications following subarachnoid haemorrhage are related to the massive sympathetic surge and catecholamine release following the subarachnoid haemorrhage.

- Severe LV dysfunction and cardiogenic shock can both occur after subarachnoid haemorrhage, and despite their severity can be reversible with the use of dobutamine. Nearly 45% of patients with subarachnoid haemorrhage who undergo echocardiography will have an ejection fraction of <50% or regional wall motion abnormalities.
- ECG abnormalities. Up to 27% of patients will have ECG changes following a subarachnoid haemorrhage, T-wave inversion being the most common. Other changes include ST segment abnormalities and Q-wave inversion. They are strongly associated with a poor neurological grade but are not predictive of all-cause mortality.
- Neurogenic pulmonary oedema. This is initially a hydrostatic pulmonary oedema resulting from a catecholamine-induced increase in pulmonary artery pressure, followed by damage to the pulmonary microvasculature and an increase in pulmonary capillary permeability.
- Hyponatraemia. Many patients with subarachnoid haemorrhage are hypovolaemic and hyponatraemic as a result of a natriuresis secondary to excessive atrial natriuretic peptide release. Fluid restriction is therefore an inappropriate way to correct the hyponatraemia, which should be managed with sodium repletion.
- Other complications include deep vein thrombosis, pneumonia, and hepatic, renal, and GI dysfunction.

Outcome following subarachnoid haemorrhage

Approximately 20% of patients will die from subarachnoid haemorrhage at the time of the initial bleed. Of those who survive to reach hospital a further 15% will die within 24 h, and 40% will make a good recovery.

Anaesthesia for vascular lesions

Procedure	Clipping of intracranial aneurysm
Time	3–6 h
Pain	+/+++
Position	Supine, head up, lateral or prone
Blood loss	200–2000 ml, cross-match two units
Practical techniques	ETT, IPPV, art line, CVP

Clipping an aneurysm involves the use of microsurgery to apply a spring clip across the neck of the aneurysm. Aneurysms arising from branches of the vertebral or basilar arteries require a posterior fossa craniotomy, whilst others may be reached from a frontal or frontoparietal approach. There is often a need to control the aneurysm prior to clipping. Applying a temporary clip to a vessel proximal to the aneurysm usually does this.

Preoperative

* Assess the effects of the haemorrhage and any pre-existing arterial disease on the brain and other organs.
* Ensure adequate fluid intake, and that fluid is not being unnecessarily restricted.
* Nimodipine treatment should be instituted.
* Patients are initially treated with bed rest and analgesia and are therefore prone to DVT and chest infections. Heparin is contraindicated. Ensure graduated compression stockings are fitted.
* Phenytoin (a loading dose of 15 mg/kg followed by a single daily dose of 3–4 mg/kg) should be prescribed prophylactically for the majority of patients.
* Note the site of the intracranial aneurysm and discuss with the surgeon the surgical approach planned and the anticipated difficulty. Predictable difficulties will influence the decision to use induced hypothermia, barbiturates, and other forms of cerebral protection.

Perioperative

* As for craniotomy (p. 403) but note the following:
* Standard monitoring including invasive blood pressure monitoring should be instituted prior to induction. A CVP line can be inserted after induction. It will be useful not only intra-operatively but also in the postoperative period to help guide triple H therapy.
* Ensure adequate venous access with a large-bore cannula.
* Aim to avoid increases in arterial pressure that may result in aneurysm rupture, but maintain sufficient cerebral blood flow to ensure adequate cerebral perfusion pressure and help counteract vasospasm. Aim for the preinduction BP ± 10%.

- Hypocapnoea can result in cerebral ischaemia after subarachnoid haemorrhage and must be avoided. Ventilation should be adjusted to maintain a normal $PaCO_2$.
- Monitor the core temperature. Allow the temperature to drift down until the aneurysm is secured, then rewarm the patient.
- Modern neurosurgical practice is to use temporary spring clips rather than induced hypotension. The latter may still be required in difficult cases or if rupture occurs. In this situation aim for a systolic blood pressure of 60–80 mmHg. Moderate hypotension may be achieved using isoflurane (up to 1.5 MAC). Further hypotension is achieved using labetalol (5–10 mg increments). Sodium nitroprusside is rarely used. Hypotension must not be induced in the presence of vasospasm.
- If rupture occurs:
  - call for help
  - increase IV infusions and start blood transfusion
  - inducing hypotension helps to reduce bleeding
  - ipsilateral carotid compression.
- Other cerebral protection measures should be considered electively if temporary clipping of a major cerebral vessel is planned or in case of aneurysm rupture. These include inducing hypothermia to a temperature of 32 °C and the administration of thiopental (3–5 mg/kg bolus intravenously followed by 3–5 mg/kg/h afterwards). Ideally EEG monitoring should be used when infusing thiopental. This allows the titration of the dose to burst suppression.

Postoperative

- ICU/HDU care is required postoperatively for patients with a poor grade preoperatively, those who had a stormy perioperative course, and those requiring treatment for vasospasm.
- Codeine phosphate and regular paracetamol may be prescribed for analgesia.
- A decrease in the Glasgow coma score (see later) may indicate vasospasm, an intracranial haematoma, or hydrocephalus.

Special considerations

It is becoming increasingly common to control intracranial aneurysm by the insertion of platinum Guglielmi detachable coils (GDC) via catheters inserted in the femoral artery.

- The procedure is undertaken in the angiography suite by neuroradiologists. Ensure skilled anaesthetic assistance and the same anaesthetic and monitoring facilities that would be available in theatre for a clipping procedure.
- Patients require general anaesthesia using techniques similar to that described for clipping aneurysms except that a CVP line is not commonly used.
- It is important to maintain MAP and a normal $PaCO_2$.
- Rupture of the aneurysm during the procedure occurs in approximately 1 in 300 cases and is almost invariably fatal.
- The overall mortality of the procedure is 5.1% at 6 months.

Arteriovenous malformations (AVM)

- Surgery is not urgent unless the AVM or a resulting haematoma is causing pressure effects.
- The procedure may be associated with significant blood loss. Check that blood is available in theatre and ensure adequate IV access.
- Blood may be shunted through the AVM resulting in relative ischaemia to the surrounding tissue. When the lesion is excised, a relative hyper-perfusion of surrounding tissue may occur resulting in cerebral oedema and increased ICP.
- There is no risk of vasospasm and when indicated hypotension may be induced with relative safety. This is achieved using isoflurane and/or labetalol as outlined above.
- In children AVMs can cause high output failure due to intracerebral shunt. CCF may be precipitated by excision of the lesion.

Venous air embolism

- Venous air embolism (VAE) can occur during any operation in which the operative site is higher than the right atrium. Its incidence is particularly high during craniotomy in the sitting position, and when the surgeon is dissecting tissues that do not allow veins to collapse despite a negative pressure within them (e.g. the emissary veins in the posterior fossa).
- VAE causes pulmonary microvascular occlusion resulting in increased physiological dead space. Bronchoconstriction may also develop. A large volume of air causes frothing within the right atrium leading to obstruction of the right outflow tract and a reduction in cardiac output.
- Signs of VAE include hypotension, arrhythmias, increased PA pressure, decreased $ETCO_2$, and hypoxia.
- N_2O may worsen the outcome from VAE although its use does not increase the risk of VAE.

Detection of VAE

- $ETCO_2$ is generally the most useful monitor as it is widely available and sensitive. Air embolism results in a sudden reduction in $ETCO_2$. Hyperventilation, low cardiac output, and other types of embolism will also result in reduction in $ETCO_2$.
- Doppler ultrasound is the most sensitive non-invasive monitor. It uses ultra high-frequency sound waves to detect changes in blood flow velocity and density. Unfortunately, it is not quantitative and does not differentiate between a massive air embolism and a physiologically insignificant air embolism. Positioning the probe and diathermy interference can prove problematic.
- Transoesophageal echo allows determination of the amount of air aspirated but is more invasive, difficult to place, and needs expertise to interpret.
- Pulmonary artery catheters are invasive but sensitive monitors for VAE. However, an increase in PA pressure is not specific for air.
- The least sensitive monitor is a precordial or oesophageal stethoscope to detect a 'millwheel' murmur. This is only apparent after massive VAE, which is usually clinically obvious.

Prevention

- Avoid the sitting position unless essential.
- Elevate the head only as much as necessary.
- Ensure adequate volaemia to reduce the risk of hypotension on sitting and to raise the CVP.
- Small amounts of PEEP (5–10 cmH_2O) may reduce the risk of air entrainment.
- A 'G-suit' or medical antishock trousers may be used to increase venous pressure and reduce hypotensive episodes in patients in the sitting position.

Treatment

- Treatment is supportive.

- Inform the surgeon, who should flood the operative field with fluid. This stops further entrainment of air and allows the identification of open veins that can be cauterized or waxed if within bone.
- Stop N_2O if in use and increase the FiO_2 to 1.0.
- If possible position the operative site below the level of the heart to increase venous pressure.
- Aspirate air from the CVP line. The tip should be placed close to the junction of the SVC and the right atrium.
- Support the blood pressure with fluid and vasopressors.
- If a large volume of air has been entrained, and surgical conditions permit, turn the patient into the left lateral position to attempt to keep the air in the right atrium.
- Commence CPR if necessary.

Paradoxical air embolism

- Air emboli may enter the systemic circulation via Thebesian veins in the heart and bronchial vessels. It is also a possibility if the patient has a patent foramen ovale. Such defects may be small and not picked up preoperatively.
- Small volumes of air in the systemic circulation can have disastrous consequences.
- Intracardiac septal defects are an absolute contraindication to surgery in the sitting position.

Perioperative management of severe head injury

The aims of managing patients with severe head injury are to identify and treat promptly life-threatening injuries (such as intracranial haematoma) and to reduce the incidence of secondary brain damage. Approximately 30% of patients with a severe head injury will also have significant extracranial injuries. Most head injury morbidity results from a delay in diagnosing and evacuating an intracranial haematoma or the failure to correct hypoxia and hypotension. Assessment and resuscitation proceed according to the principles taught in the advanced trauma life support system (ATLS). (See also p. 437).

Airway/breathing
The airway must always be managed with cervical spine control.
* Secure, maintain, and protect a clear airway. Intubate if:
  * the airway is compromised
  * there is ventilatory failure
  * GCS <9
  * the patient has seizures
  * it is required to facilitate CT scan
  * it is necessary for the management of other injuries.
* Management of intubation:
  * A rapid sequence induction is required with cricoid pressure and manual in-line stabilization of the head and neck.
  * Use thiopental 3–5 mg/kg or propofol 1–3 mg/kg with suxamethonium 1–2 mg/kg and fentanyl 2–5 µg/kg.
  * Ventilate to a $PaCO_2$ of 4.5–5.3 kPa (35–40 mmHg).
  * Maintain oxygenation (SaO_2 >95%).
  * Maintain sedation with a propofol infusion (1–3 mg/kg/h).
  * Insert an orogastric tube; nasogastric tubes are contraindicated until a fractured base of skull has been excluded.
  * Consider vasopressors if the patient is hypotensive and providing hypovolaemia has been corrected/excluded.

Circulation
Ensure control of haemorrhage and maintenance of BP. A single episode of hypotension is associated with a doubling of mortality. Hypotension in a head injured patient is a medical emergency and must be corrected immediately:
* Secure IV access.
* Give 0.9% saline as maintenance fluid.
* Maintain systolic BP >120 mmHg. Use colloid and blood if required.
* If in doubt insert a CVP line to guide fluid management.
* If the patient is still hypotensive use vasopressors (noradrenaline or other alpha-agonist).

- Aim for Hb >10 g/dl.
- Do not assume that the head injury or scalp wounds cause persistent hypotension or tachycardia. Extracranial injuries must be excluded and considered in devising a definitive treatment plan and priorities.

Paediatric considerations

- Maintain BP >90 mmHg.
- Consider intraosseous access if venous access is difficult.
- Note that blood loss from a scalp wound may be significant.
- For children weighing <15 kg, use 4% glucose/0.18% saline as maintenance fluid.
- Beware of hypothermia.

Disability

- Perform a rapid assessment of Glasgow coma score (see Table) and pupillary responses on arrival and repeat regularly.
- Document any limb weakness, abnormal eye movements, obvious cranial nerve injury, or signs of a fractured base of skull.

Exposure

- Perform a complete secondary survey and treat injuries as required. Log roll patient at all times.

The Glasgow coma scale and score (normal score is 15)

Response	Score
Eye opening response	
Spontaneously	4
To speech	3
To pain	2
None	1
Best motor response (in arms)	
Obeys commands	6
Localization of painful stimuli	5
Normal flexion to painful stimuli	4
Spastic flexion to painful stimuli	3
Extension to painful stimuli	2
None	1
Best verbal response	
Orientated	5
Confused	4
Inappropriate words	3
Incomprehensible sounds	2
None	1

Best motor response (upper limbs)	Best verbal response (to pain)
Obeys commands 6 (>2 years)	Orientated 5 (>5 years)
Localizes to pain 5 (<2 years)	Words 4 (>1 year)
Normal flexion to pain 4 (>6 months)	Vocal sounds 3 (>6 months)
Spastic flexion to pain 3 (<6 months)	Cries 2 (<6 months)
Extension to pain 2	None 1
None 1	

Modification of GCS for children under 5. Using this scoring system the maximum GCS is 9 at 0–6 months, 11 at 6–12 months, 13 at 1–2 years, and 14 at 2–5 years. The eye opening response is the same as for adults, the motor and verbal responses modified for age as shown in the Table.

- Perform radiography of the cervical spine, chest, and pelvis.
- Persistent hypotension indicates extracranial injury.

Management of seizures
- Give diazemuls 0.1–0.2 mg/kg IV.
- Phenytoin 15 mg/kg over 15 min.
- Thiopental 3 mg/kg if required.
- Recheck ABC.

Management of increased ICP
- Give mannitol 0.5 g/kg (wt [kg] x 2.5 = ml of 20% mannitol).
- Manually hyperventilate for 30 s and reassess pupillary response.

Decision to consult neurosurgical unit

Condition	Action
Critical: Not obeying commands plus deteriorating GCS and/or progressive focal signs (motor or pupillary)	Immediate neurosurgical consultation. Transfer/scan as agreed. Do not delay
Severe: Not obeying commands but GCS stable. Systemically stable	Arrange urgent CT scan. Neurosurgical consultation with CT. Image link and transfer as appropriate
Moderate: Obeying commands but impaired consciousness. GCS stable	If CT scan is normal and GCS is stable or improving, observe. If CT scan is abnormal, and clinical progress is unsatisfactory consult with neurosurgeons

What the neurosurgical unit needs to know at time of referral
- Patient's age and previous medical history if known.
- History of injury—time, cause, and mechanism.
- Neurological state:
  - conscious level on arrival at hospital

- trend in GCS
- pupil responses
- best motor response.
- Cardiorespiratory status, BP, and pulse rate.
- Injuries including skull fractures and extracranial injuries.
- Management so far:
  - airway protection and ventilation status
  - circulatory status and fluid therapy
  - first aid treatment of associated injuries
  - drugs given.

CT scans (See also p. 659)

- A CT scan is indicated for:
  - high-velocity trauma
  - neurological signs and/or impaired level of consciousness
  - skull fracture or suspected base of skull fracture
  - deteriorating GCS or new neurological signs.
- The CT scanner is a dangerous place.
- Scan only after the patient has been resuscitated.
- All head injured patients requiring CT scan should be intubated and escorted by an anaesthetist.
- In some situations it is appropriate to transfer the patient to the neuro-surgical centre before scanning.

Transfer of the head injured patient (See also pp. 438, 688)

Do not transfer a patient until life-threatening extracranial injuries have been stabilized and there is no persistent hypotension.

- The patient should be intubated, sedated, and paralysed.
- Check ETT and ensure adequate IV access (×2).
- Patients must be accompanied by an anaesthetist and a nurse, both of whom have appropriate experience.
- Monitor and record SpO_2, BP (preferably via arterial line), ECG, $ETCO_2$, and pupillary responses every 15 min.
- Continue cervical spine protection.
- Treat raised ICP as previously described.

Equipment checklist:

- adequate oxygen
- airway equipment (self inflating bag, laryngoscope, ET tube, airway, mask, suction)
- CT scans
- venous cannulas
- fluids
- drugs (anaesthetics, neuromuscular blockers, vasopressors, mannitol, diazemuls, cardiac arrest drugs)
- defibrillator.

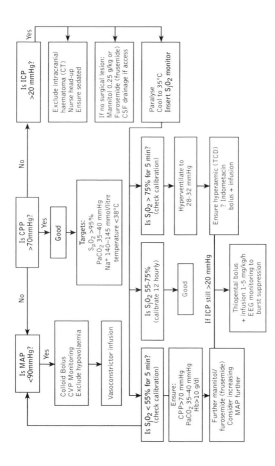

Fig 19.2 Postoperative and intensive care management of the severely head-injured adult.

Postoperative and ICU management of the head injured patient

- The management of the head injured patient on the ICU is similar for a postoperative patient and one not requiring surgery. Patients are best managed using a protocol designed primarily to maintain an adequate CPP and cerebral oxygenation and to identify and treat causes of secondary brain insults (Fig. 19.2).
- The causes of secondary insult are:
  - intracranial: haematoma, oedema, convulsions, hydrocephalus, abscess, hyperaemia
  - systemic: hypotension, hypoxia, hyponatraemia, pyrexia, anaemia, sepsis, hypercarbia.
- On current evidence, steroids should not be routinely administered to patients following severe head injury.

Brainstem death

The most common causes of brainstem death are head injury, cerebrovascular accidents (including subarachnoid haemorrhage), cerebral tumours, and hypoxic brain injury. To diagnose brainstem death the patient needs to fulfil certain preconditions and have absent brainstem reflexes.

Preconditions

- The patient is apnoeic and dependent on mechanical ventilation.
- The cause of the coma must be established to be an irreversible structural cause of brain injury in an apnoeic patient dependent on ventilatory support.
- Reversible causes for brainstem depression have been excluded: sedatives, muscle relaxants, alcohol, hypothermia, and metabolic or endocrine disturbances.

Absence of brainstem responses

- The tests of brainstem reflexes should only be performed once the pre-conditions and exclusion criteria are fulfilled.
- The pupils are fixed and do not respond to light. The direct and consensual responses should be observed. The pupils are usually dilated but this is not essential for the diagnosis.
- The corneal reflex is absent.
- There is no motor response within the cranial nerve distribution to painful stimuli applied centrally or peripherally. Spinal reflexes may persist in brainstem-dead patients, and may even return after an initial absence.
- The oculovestibular reflex is absent. There is no eye movement in response to the injection of 20 ml of ice-cold water into the external auditory meatus, direct access to the tympanic membrane should be verified using an auroscope. The eyes should be observed for at least 30 s after the injection.
- There is no gag reflex or cough reflex in response to a suction catheter passed into the pharynx or down the endotracheal tube.
- Apnoea is present on disconnection from mechanical ventilation. This test is done last, to avoid unnecessary hypercarbia should any of the other reflexes be present. The patient should be preoxygenated by ventilating with 100% oxygen for 5 min before disconnection. The patient is then disconnected and observed for any respiratory movement for 10 min. The $PaCO_2$ should be measured at the end and should be high enough to ensure an adequate stimulus to ventilation (over 6.7 kPa (50 mmHg) in a previously normal individual). Hypoxia should be avoided during apnoea. This can be achieved by passing a suction catheter down the endotracheal tube and supplying 5–10 litre/min of oxygen and monitoring the SpO_2.

Other considerations

- The diagnosis of brainstem death should be made by two medical practitioners with experience in the field, one of who must be the consultant in charge of the patient or an ICU consultant. The second must be one of the above or their deputy, have been registered for at least 5 years, and have had previous experience of the procedure.
- Both must satisfy themselves that the preconditions have been met and neither should be a member of the transplant team.

- The tests must be performed on two occasions separated by an adequate time interval to satisfy all concerned.
- The diagnosis should not normally be considered until at least 6 h after the onset of apnoeic coma or 24 h after the restoration of the circulation if the cause was cardiac arrest.
- The results are recorded on a special form and death is certified after the second set of tests.
- No additional tests are required in the United Kingdom, but other countries may require EEG, carotid angiography, or brainstem evoked potentials.
- The time of death is the completion of the first set of brainstem criteria, and this should be the time recorded in the notes and on the death certificate.
- The coroner needs to be informed of most of these patients due to the underlying diagnosis, and if organ donation is contemplated.
- Care of the relatives is essential at this time irrespective of whether the patient is to be an organ donor or not.

Further reading

Moss E (1994). Anaesthesia for cerebro vascular surgery. *Current Anaesthesia and Critical Care*, 5, 2–8.

Pickard JD, Czosnyka M (1993). Management of raised intracranial pressure *Journal of Neurology, Neurosurgery and Psychiatry*, 56, 845–58.

Joshi S, Dash HH, Ornstein E (1997). Anaesthetic considerations for posterior fossa surgery. *Current Opinions in Anesthesiology*, 10, 321–6.

Porter JM, Pidgeon C, Cuningham AJ (1999). The sitting position in neurosurgery: a critical appraisal. *British Journal of Anaesthesia*, 82, 117–28.

Cottrell JE (1996). Trends in neuroanaesthesia. *Canadian Journal of Anaesthesia*, 43, R61-R74.

Chapter 20
Trauma surgery

Jerry Nolan

Immediate trauma care

Preparation

Advance warning before the arrival of a severely injured patient in the accident department allows accident department staff to decide whether to alert the trauma team. Essential resuscitation drugs, fluid, and equipment should be prepared before the patient's arrival.

The trauma team

Trauma patient resuscitation is most efficient if undertaken by a team of appropriately trained doctors and nurses. In this way a variety of tasks can be undertaken simultaneously.

Immediate care—ATLS

The Advanced Trauma Life Support (ATLS) programme was established by the American College of Surgeons[1] and provides a framework on which the immediate management of the trauma patient is based. The initial management is considered in four phases:

- primary survey
- resuscitation
- secondary survey
- definitive care.

Although the first two phases are listed consecutively, they are performed simultaneously. The secondary survey, or head-to-toe examination of the patient, is not started until the patient has been adequately resuscitated.

Primary survey and resuscitation

The primary survey ('ABC principles') looks sequentially for immediately life-threatening injuries:

- Airway with cervical spine control.
- Breathing.
- Circulation and haemorrhage control.
- Disability—a rapid assessment of neurological function.
- Exposure—while considering the environment, and preventing hypothermia.

Airway and cervical spine

The priority during resuscitation of any severely injured patient is to ensure a clear airway and maintain adequate oxygenation. Initially, this is achieved with basic airway manoeuvres with or without adjuncts such as a Guedel or nasopharyngeal airway. Every patient with multiple injuries should receive high-concentration oxygen. In the unintubated, spontaneously breathing patient this should be given with a mask and reservoir bag ($FiO_2 = 0.85$).

---

1 The American College of Surgeons Committee on Trauma (1997). *Advanced trauma life support program for physicians: Instructor manual.* American College of Surgeons, Chicago.

Assume the presence of a spinal injury in any patient who has sustained significant blunt trauma until appropriate clearance procedures have been completed. This implies that the patient has been examined by an experienced clinician and appropriate radiological procedures have been completed. A reliable clinical examination cannot be obtained if the patient:

- has sustained a significant closed head injury
- is intoxicated
- has a reduced conscious level from any other cause
- has significant pain from an injury, which 'distracts' attention from the neck.

Tracheal intubation

Indications for immediate intubation of the severely injured patient include:

- airway obstruction unrelieved by basic airway manoeuvres
- impending airway obstruction, e.g. from facial burns and inhalation injury
- GCS <9
- haemorrhage from maxillofacial injuries compromising the airway
- respiratory failure secondary to chest or neurological injury
- the need for resuscitative surgery
- uncooperative patients requiring further investigations.

Nasal intubation is contraindicated in the presence of a basal skull fracture because of the risk of accidental intracranial placement! The most appropriate technique for emergency intubation of a patient with a potential cervical spine injury is:

- Manual in-line stabilization of the cervical spine by an assistant whose hands grasp the mastoid processes and hold the head firmly down on to the trolley. This reduces neck movement during intubation. Traction should not be applied to the neck.
- Preoxygenation.
- Intravenous induction of anaesthesia. All anaesthetic induction agents have the potential to produce or worsen hypotension and the choice of induction agent is less important than the way it is used. Extreme caution is essential in patients who may be hypovolaemic—if at all possible, some fluid resuscitation should precede anaesthetic induction.
- Paralysis with suxamethonium 1.5 mg/kg (though in experienced hands rocuronium 1 mg/kg is acceptable).
- Application of cricoid pressure—some advocate the two-handed technique, which may reduce cervical spine movement.
- Direct laryngoscopy and oral intubation.

Placing the patient's head and neck in neutral alignment will tend to make the view at laryngoscopy difficult—expect 20% of patients to have a grade 3 view of the larynx. Use of a gum-elastic bougie and McCoy levering laryngoscope is recommended. If intubation of the patient proves impossible insertion of an LMA may provide a temporary airway, but may not prevent aspiration. The intubating LMA (ILMA) may be easier to insert in the neutral position and provides the opportunity for blind intubation, but consistent success requires ongoing practice. Needle cricothyroidotomy with a 14G cannula followed by jet inflation of oxygen from a high-pressure source

(400 kPa) will provide satisfactory oxygenation but the airway is not protected and the cannula is subject to kinking and displacement. Surgical cricothyroidotomy, using a scalpel and a 6.0 mm ID tracheostomy tube, is probably a more reliable procedure if the patient cannot be intubated by conventional methods.

Breathing — immediately life-threatening chest injuries

- Tension pneumothorax. Reduced chest movement, reduced breath sounds, and a resonant percussion note on the affected side, along with respiratory distress, hypotension, and tachycardia, indicate a tension pneumothorax. Deviation of the trachea to the opposite side is a late sign, and neck veins may not be distended in the presence of hypovolaemia. Treatment is immediate decompression with a large cannula placed in the second intercostal space, in the mid-clavicular line on the affected side. Once intravenous access has been obtained, a large chest drain (36FG) should be placed in the fifth intercostal space in the anterior axillary line and connected to an underwater seal drain.

- Open pneumothorax. Any open pneumothorax should be covered with an occlusive dressing and sealed on three sides.

- Massive haemothorax. This is defined as > 1500 ml blood in a hemithorax and will result in reduced chest movement and a dull percussion note, in the presence of hypoxaemia and hypovolaemia. A chest drain is placed once volume resuscitation has been started.

Cardiac tamponade

Consider cardiac tamponade while examining the chest, particularly if the patient has sustained a penetrating injury to the chest or upper abdomen. Distended neck veins in the presence of hypotension are suggestive of cardiac tamponade, although after rapid volume resuscitation myocardial contusion may also present in this way. Muffled heart sounds are quite meaningless in the midst of a busy resuscitation room. Sophisticated trauma facilities will allow immediate access to ultrasound, which is the most reliable method for diagnosis. If cardiac tamponade is diagnosed or suspected after penetrating injury and the patient is deteriorating despite all resuscitative efforts, an urgent thoracotomy and pericardiotomy will be required. If there is time, this is best undertaken in an operating room; however, in extremis, resuscitative thoracotomy can be undertaken in the emergency room. In the absence of a suitably experienced surgeon, pericardiocentesis may provide temporary relief from the tamponade while awaiting definitive treatment.

Circulation — management of hypovolaemia

Major external haemorrhage is controlled with direct pressure. Hypovolaemic shock can be conveniently divided into four classes according to the percentage of the total blood volume lost, and the associated symptoms and signs. The table provides rough guidance only. Haemorrhage alone, in the absence of significant tissue injury, results in relatively less tachycardia and may be easily overlooked, particularly in young, fit people who are able to compensate to a remarkable degree. A fall in systolic pressure suggests a loss of >30% of total blood volume (approximately 1500 ml in a 70 kg adult). A deteriorating conscious level due to hypovolaemia suggests at least 40–50% loss of blood volume.

Classification of hypovolaemic shock according to blood loss (adult)

	Class I	Class II	Class III	Class IV
Blood loss (%)	<15	15–30	30–40	>40
Blood loss (ml)	750	800–1500	1500–2000	>2000
Systolic blood pressure	Unchanged	Normal	Reduced	Very low
Diastolic blood pressure	Unchanged	Raised	Reduced	Unrecordable
Pulse (beats/min)	Slight tachycardia	100–120	120 (thready)	>120 (very thready)
Capillary refill	Normal	Slow (>2 s)	Slow (>2 s)	Undetectable
Respiratory rate	Normal	Tachypnoea	Tachypnoea (>20/min)	Tachypnoea (>20/min)
Urine output (ml/h)	>30	20–30	10–20	0–10
Extremities	Normal	Pale	Pale	Pale, cold, clammy
Complexion	Normal	Pale	Pale	Ashen
Mental state	Alert	Anxious or aggressive	Anxious, aggressive or drowsy	Drowsy, confused or unconscious

- Two short, large-bore intravenous cannulas (14G or larger) should be inserted rapidly. Take blood samples for FBC, electrolytes, and cross-match from the first cannula.
- If peripheral access is difficult use the external jugular vein, femoral vein (avoid in abdominal/pelvic/leg injury), cut-down on a peripheral vein (long saphenous at the ankle), or perform central venous cannulation. If the central route is to be used for rapid fluid resuscitation a relatively short, large-bore catheter (e.g. 8.5Fr pulmonary artery introducer sheath) is essential.
- Insert an arterial cannula for blood gas sampling and invasive blood pressure monitoring. Severely injured patients will have a marked base deficit and its correction by the infusion of appropriate fluid (not bicarbonate) will help to confirm adequate resuscitation.

Fluids

Crystalloid or colloid is suitable for the initial fluid resuscitation. The volume status of the patient is best determined by observing the change in vital signs after a reasonably large fluid challenge (2 litres of Hartmann's solution or 1 litre of colloid). Failure to improve the vital signs suggests ongoing haemorrhage, and the need for immediate surgical intervention and blood transfusion. A full cross-match will take 45 min, group-confirmed blood can be issued in 10 min, and group O blood can be obtained immediately. It is nearly always possible to wait for at least group-confirmed blood; major incompatibility reactions when using group-confirmed blood are extremely rare. Until more data are available from studies on acute trauma patients, the haemoglobin concentration of the severely injured patient should probably be targeted at greater than 8–9 g/dl.

All intravenous fluids should be properly warmed. A high-capacity fluid warmer will be required to cope with the rapid infusion rates used during resuscitation of trauma patients. Hypothermia (core temperature less than 35 °C) is a serious complication of severe trauma and haemorrhage, and is an independent predictor of mortality. Hypothermia has a number of adverse effects:

- It causes a gradual decline in heart rate and cardiac output while increasing the propensity for myocardial dysrhythmias and other morbid myocardial events.
- The oxyhaemoglobin dissociation curve is shifted to the left by a decrease in temperature, thus impairing peripheral oxygen delivery in the hypovolaemic patient at a time when it is most needed.
- Shivering may increase oxygen consumption and compound the lactic acidosis that typically accompanies hypovolaemia.
- Even mild hypothermia inhibits coagulation significantly and increases the incidence of wound infection.

In the presence of uncontrolled haemorrhage:

- Aggressive fluid resuscitation may simply accelerate bleeding and increase mortality.
- Inadequate fluid resuscitation will cause hypoperfusion of vital organs and may induce life-threatening ischaemia.
- Until surgical control of haemorrhage has been achieved, fluid resuscitation should be targeted at a blood pressure that will almost produce ade-

ital organ perfusion (permissive hypotension). This target will
d on age and coexisting morbidities. In the normally fit patient aim
ressure around 80 mmHg systolic. In the elderly or those with
cant co-morbidity a systolic pressure of around 100 mmHg may be
appropriate.

cy of minimal fluid resuscitation is likely to be extremely detrimental
ents with severe head injury. Hypotension will substantially increase
rbidity and mortality following severe head injury and attempts
must be made to maintain an adequate cerebral perfusion as soon as possible. In a patient with even slightly raised intracranial pressure, this implies
the need for a mean arterial pressure of at least 90 mmHg.

Once haemorrhage control has been achieved, the goals of fluid resuscitation are to optimize oxygen delivery, improve microcirculatory perfusion, and
reverse tissue acidosis. Fluid infusion should be targeted at a blood pressure
and cardiac output that results in an acceptable urine output, and a falling
lactate and base deficit.

Goals for resuscitation of the trauma patient before haemorrhage has
been controlled

Parameter	Goal
Blood pressure	Systolic 80 mmHg. Mean 50–60 mmHg
Heart rate	<120 beats/min
Oxygenation	SpO_2 >96% (peripheral perfusion allowing oximeter to work)
Urine output	>0.5 ml/kg/h
Mentation	Following commands accurately
Lactate level	<1.6 mmol/litre
Base deficit	>−5
Haemoglobin	>9.0 g/dl

Disability—rapid neurological assessment

The pupils are checked for size and their reaction to light. The Glasgow Coma
Scale (GCS) score should be assessed rapidly.

If the patient requires urgent induction of anaesthesia and intubation,
remember to perform a quick neurological assessment first.

Exposure/environmental control

The patient should be completely undressed and then protected from
hypothermia with warm blankets.

Tubes

Insert a urinary catheter; urine output is an excellent indicator of the adequacy of resuscitation. Place a gastric tube; this will allow stomach contents to
be drained and reduce the risk of aspiration. If there is any suspicion of a basal
skull fracture the orogastric route should be used.

Radiographs

Radiographs of the chest and pelvis will be required for all patients sustaining
significant blunt trauma.

Glasgow Coma Score

	Response	**Score**
Best verbal response	Orientated	5
	Confused	4
	Inappropriate words	3
	Inarticulate words	2
	Nothing	1
Best motor response	Obeys commands	6
	Localizes pain	5
	Flexion withdrawal (stimulus to supraorbital notch)	4
	Flexion to pain (decorticate rigidity)	3
	Extension to pain (decerebrate rigidity)	2
	Nothing	1
Eye opening	Eyes open	4
	Eyes open to speech	3
	Eyes open to pain	2
	No eye opening	1

The secondary survey

A detailed head-to-toe survey of the trauma patient should not be undertaken until the vital signs are relatively stable. The patient must be continually re-evaluated so that ongoing bleeding is detected early. Patients with exsanguinating haemorrhage may need a laparotomy as part of the resuscitation phase.

Head injuries

Inspect and palpate the scalp for lacerations, haematomas, or depressed fractures. Check for signs of a basal skull fracture (racoon eyes, Battle's sign—bruising over the mastoid process, subhyaloid haemorrhage, scleral haemorrhage without a posterior margin, haemotympanium, cerebrospinal fluid rhinorrhoea, and otorrhoea).

Brain injury can be divided into primary and secondary groups. Primary injury (concussion, contusion, and laceration) occurs at the moment of impact. Secondary brain injury is compounded by hypoxia, hypercarbia, and hypotension.

These factors must be prevented or treated rapidly. Resuscitation goals include:

- Mean blood pressure of at least 90 mmHg—allows for CPP of 70 mmHg in the presence of slightly raised intracranial pressure (e.g. 20 mmHg).
- SaO_2 >95%.
- $PaCO_2$ of approximately 4.5 kPa (if mechanically ventilated).

The conscious level is assessed using the GCS, which is reliable and reproducible. The trend of change in conscious level is more important than one static reading. The pupillary response and the presence of any lateralizing signs must be recorded.

Indications for intubation and ventilation after head injury

The following are indications for intubation and ventilation:

- GCS <9.
- Loss of protective laryngeal reflexes.
- Ventilatory insufficiency (PaO_2 <13 kPa on oxygen, $PaCO_2$ >6 kPa).
- Spontaneous hyperventilation causing $PaCO_2$ <3.5 kPa.
- Respiratory arrhythmia.
- Copious bleeding into mouth (e.g. skull base fracture).
- Seizures.
- To permit CT scanning.
- Before transfer to a regional neurosurgical unit:
  - significantly deteriorating conscious level, even if not in coma
  - bilaterally fractured mandible.

Indications for an urgent CT scan

Indications for an urgent CT scan include:

- Coma after resuscitation.
- Deteriorating conscious level.
- Confusion and focal signs.

- Skull fracture and GCS <15, or neurological signs.
- Multiply injured patient not fully orientated, and requiring ventilation and/or extracranial surgery.
- any head injury with previously known intracranial pathology.

Referral to a neurosurgical unit

Referral to the regional neurosurgical unit is indicated for:

- All patients with an intracranial mass.
- Primary brain injury requiring ventilation.
- Compound depressed skull fracture.
- Persistent CSF leak.
- Penetrating skull injury.
- Patients deteriorating rapidly with signs of an intracranial mass lesion.

Transfer to a regional neurosurgical unit

The regional organization of neurosurgical services in the United Kingdom dictates the frequent need for interhospital transfer of patients with serious head injuries. Guidelines for the transfer of these patients have been published jointly by the Neuroanaesthesia Society of Great Britain and Ireland and the Association of Anaesthetists of Great Britain and Ireland.[2] The Intensive Care Society has published guidelines for the transport of any critically ill patient. A doctor with at least 2 years' experience in an appropriate specialty (usually anaesthesia) and an adequately trained assistant should accompany patients with head injuries.

The patient should receive the same standard of physiological monitoring during transfer as they would receive in an intensive care unit. All notes (or photocopies), radiographs, blood results, and cross-matched blood should accompany the patient. The transfer team should carry a mobile phone. Head-injured patients must be adequately resuscitated before transfer (determined by the goals listed above).

Essential equipment for patient transfer includes:

- Portable mechanical ventilator.
- Adequate supply of oxygen.
- Portable, battery-powered multifunction monitor:
  - ECG
  - invasive blood pressure monitoring
  - central venous pressure monitoring
  - pulse oximetry
  - capnography
  - temperature.
- Suction and defibrillator.
- Battery powered syringe pumps.

2   The Neuroanaesthesia Society of Great Britain and Ireland and The Association of Anaesthetists of Great Britain and Ireland (1996). *Recommendations for the transfer of patients with acute head injuries to neurosurgical units.* The Association of Anaesthetists of Great Britain and Ireland, London.

- Intubation equipment.
- Bag-valve-mask apparatus.
- Venous access equipment.
  Essential drugs for the transfer include:
- Hypnotics—a propofol infusion is ideal for sedating intubated patients.
- Muscle relaxants.
- Analgesics, e.g. fentanyl.
- Mannitol 20%:
  - Mannitol (0.5–1.0 g/kg) may be given after discussion with the neurosurgeon. This may reduce intracranial pressure and will buy time before surgery.
- Vasoactive drugs, e.g. adrenaline, dobutamine.
- Additional resuscitation drugs.

(see also p. 688)

Chest injuries

There are six potentially life-threatening injuries (two contusions and four 'ruptures') that may be identified during the secondary survey:
- Pulmonary contusion.
- Cardiac contusion.
- Aortic rupture.
- Ruptured diaphragm.
- Oesophageal rupture.
- Rupture of the tracheobronchial tree.

Pulmonary contusion
- Inspection of the chest may reveal signs indicating considerable decelerating forces, such as seat-belt bruising.
- Pulmonary contusion is the commonest potentially lethal chest injury.
- Young adults and children have particularly compliant ribs and considerable energy can be transmitted to the lungs in the absence of rib fractures.
- The earliest indication of pulmonary contusion is hypoxaemia (reduced PaO_2/FiO_2 ratio).
- The chest radiograph shows patchy infiltrates over the affected area but may be normal initially.
- Increasing the FiO_2 may provide sufficient oxygenation—failing that the patient may require mask CPAP or tracheal intubation and positive pressure ventilation.
- Use small tidal volumes (5–7 ml/kg) to minimize volutrauma. Try to keep the peak inspiratory pressure <35 cmH_2O.
- The patient with chest trauma requires appropriate fluid resuscitation but fluid overload will compound the lung contusion.

Myocardial contusion
- Cardiac contusion must be considered in any patient with severe blunt chest trauma, particularly those with sternal fractures.
- Cardiac arrhythmias, ST changes on the ECG, and elevated CK-MB isoenzymes may indicate contusion but these signs are very non-specific—cardiac troponins may be slightly more specific for cardiac contusion.
- An elevated CVP in the presence of hypotension is the earliest indication of myocardial dysfunction secondary to severe cardiac contusion, but cardiac tamponade must be excluded.
- Echocardiography is the best method of confirming a cardiac contusion.
- Patients with severe cardiac contusion tend to have other serious injuries that will mandate their admission to an intensive care unit—the decision to admit a patient to ICU rarely depends on the diagnosis of cardiac contusion alone.
- The severely contused myocardium will require inotropic support (e.g. dobutamine or adrenaline).

Traumatic rupture of the aorta

- The thoracic aorta is at risk in any patient sustaining a significant decelerating force (e.g. fall from a height or high-speed road traffic accident). Only 10–15% of these patients will reach hospital alive and of these survivors, without surgery two-thirds will die of delayed rupture within 2 weeks.

- The commonest site for aortic injury is at the aortic isthmus, just distal to the origin of the left subclavian artery at the level of the ligamentum arteriosum. Deceleration produces large shear forces at this site because the relatively mobile aortic arch travels forward relative to the fixed descending aorta.

- The tear in the intima and media may involve either part of or the whole circumference of the aorta, and in survivors the haematoma is contained by an intact aortic adventitia and mediastinal pleura.

- Patients sustaining traumatic aortic rupture usually have multiple injuries and may be hypotensive at presentation. However, upper extremity hypertension is present in 40% of cases as the haematoma compresses the true lumen causing a 'pseudocoarctation'.

- Supine chest radiograph will show a widened mediastinum in the vast majority of cases. Although this is a sensitive sign of aortic rupture, it is not very specific—90% of cases of widened mediastinum are due to venous bleeding. Whenever practical obtain an erect chest radiograph (providing a clearer view of the thoracic aorta).

- Signs on the chest radiograph suggesting possible rupture of the aorta are wide mediastinum, pleural capping, left haemothorax, deviation of the trachea to the right, depression of the left mainstem bronchus, loss of the aortic knob, deviation of the nasogastric tube to the right, fractures of the upper three ribs (although disputed recently), or fracture of the thoracic spine.

- If the chest radiograph is equivocal, further investigation will be required. Spiral CT scan is thought to be almost as good as arteriography for delineating aortic injury and a number of centres are now using transoesophageal echocardiography to diagnose traumatic aortic ruptures.

- If a rupture of the thoracic aorta is suspected, the patient's blood pressure should be maintained at 80–100 mmHg systolic (using a beta-blocker such as esmolol), in an effort to reduce the risk of further dissection or rupture. The use of pure vasodilators, such as SNP, increases the pulse pressure and will not reduce the shear forces on the aortic wall. The patient must be transferred immediately to the nearest cardiothoracic unit.

Rupture of the diaphragm

- Rupture of the diaphragm occurs in about 5% of patients sustaining severe blunt trauma to the trunk.

- It can be difficult to diagnose initially—the diagnosis is often made late.

- Approximately 75% of ruptures occur on the left side. The stomach or colon commonly herniates into the chest and strangulation of these organs is a significant complication.

- Signs and symptoms detected during the secondary survey may include:
  - diminished breath sounds on the ipsilateral side
  - pain in the chest and abdomen
  - respiratory distress.
- Diagnosis can be made on a plain radiograph (elevated hemidiaphragm, gas bubbles above the diaphragm, shift of the mediastinum to the opposite side, nasogastric tube in the chest). The definitive diagnosis is made by instilling contrast media through the nasogastric tube and repeating the radiograph.
- Once the patient has been stabilized, the diaphragm will require surgical repair.

Oesophageal rupture

- A severe blow to the upper abdomen may result in a torn lower oesophagus as gastric contents are forcefully ejected.
- The conscious patient will complain of severe chest and abdominal pain, and mediastinal air may be visible on the chest radiograph.
- Gastric contents may appear in the chest drain.
- The diagnosis is confirmed by contrast study of the oesophagus or endoscopy.
- Urgent surgery is essential—mediastinitis carries a high mortality.

Tracheobronchial injury

- Laryngeal fractures are rare.
- Signs of laryngeal injury include hoarseness, subcutaneous emphysema, and palpable fracture crepitus.
- Total airway obstruction or severe respiratory distress is managed by intubation or a surgical airway—tracheostomy is indicated rather than cricothyroidotomy.
- Less severe laryngeal injuries may be assessed by CT before any appropriate surgery.
- Transections of the trachea or bronchi proximal to the pleural reflection cause massive mediastinal and cervical emphysema.
- Injuries distal to the pleural sheath lead to pneumothoraces—these will not resolve after chest drainage, since the bronchopleural fistula allows a large air leak.
- Most bronchial injuries occur within 2.5 cm of the carina and the diagnosis is confirmed by bronchoscopy.
- Tracheobronchial injuries will require urgent repair through a thoracotomy.

Abdominal injuries

The priority is to quickly determine the need for laparotomy, and not to waste time trying to define precisely which viscus is injured. The abdomen is inspected for bruising, lacerations, and distension. Careful palpation may reveal tenderness. A rectal examination is performed to assess sphincter tone and to exclude the presence of pelvic fracture or a high prostate (indicative of a ruptured urethra). Diagnostic peritoneal lavage, abdominal ultra-sound, or CT is indicated whenever clinical examination is unreliable:

* in patients with a depressed level of consciousness (head injury, drugs, or alcohol)
* in the presence of lower rib or pelvic fractures
* when the examination is equivocal, particularly if prolonged general anaesthesia for other injuries will make reassessment impossible.

The relative merits of diagnostic peritoneal lavage, ultrasound, and CT for the investigation of abdominal trauma are listed on p. 444. Indications of a positive peritoneal lavage include:

* More than 5 ml free blood aspirated from the peritoneal cavity.
* Enteric contents aspirated from the peritoneal cavity.
* Lavage fluid leaking into the chest drains or urinary catheter.
* $100\,000 \times 10^9$ red blood cells/litre, bile, food, or bacteria in the lavage fluid.

In experienced hands, ultrasound has a sensitivity, specificity, and accuracy comparable to diagnostic peritoneal lavage and can be done at the bedside. Focused assessment with sonography for trauma (FAST) involves scanning four distinct regions identified as the four Ps:

* pericardial
* perihepatic
* perisplenic
* pelvic.

The use of diagnostic peritoneal lavage is on the decline generally but is still the investigation of choice in the absence of personnel trained in ultrasound and when the patient is too haemodynamically unstable to be transferred to the CT scanner.

Relative merits of diagnostic peritoneal lavage, ultrasound, and CT in blunt abdominal trauma

	Diagnostic peritoneal lavage	Ultrasound	CT scan
Indication	Diagnosis of haemoperitoneum in presence of haemodynamic instability	Screening for free fluid or solid organ injury in all blunt trauma patients	Diagnosis of organ injury in haemodynamically stable patients
Advantages	Fast, 85–98% sensitivity for intra-abdominal bleeding	Fast, sensitivity 83–87%, can detect free fluid and solid organ injury	Most specific for injury (92–98%)
Disadvantages	Invasive, falsely indicates need for laparotomy in some patients who could be managed conservatively, misses injury to diaphragm or retroperitoneum	Operator dependent, misses diaphragm, bowel, and some pancreatic injuries	Takes time to transfer to scanner, misses diaphragm, bowel, and some pancreatic injuries

Pelvic fractures

- Pelvic fractures can result in life-threatening occult haemorrhage. In the hypovolaemic, shocked patient the blood is either on the floor, in the chest, in the abdomen, or in the pelvis.
- The bleeding in pelvic fractures arises mainly from the shearing and tearing of the large veins lining the posterior pelvis. Bleeding can also arise from the raw, cancellous bony surfaces. Arterial bleeding accounts for major bleeding in less than 10% of cases.
- The two main fracture types responsible for severe haemorrhage are the open book type (or AP-compression) and the vertical shear pattern.
- Suspect pelvic fracture after motor vehicle accidents, especially where the victim has been ejected from the vehicle, pedestrian–vehicle contact, motorcycle accidents, and falls from more than 3 m.
- Clinical signs are variable and unpredictable and the diagnosis is made with AP pelvic radiograph at the end of the primary survey. Widening of the symphysis greater than 2 cm or vertical displacement of one side of the pelvis indicates severe disruption and a high likelihood of major haemorrhage.

Treatment

- A widening or diastasis of the symphysis of more than 2 cm doubles the pelvic volume. Emergency treatment aims to reduce this volume and tamponade the bleeding vessels. In the emergency room, 'closing the book' using a folded sheet wrapped around the pelvis, and binding the legs together can buy precious minutes during resuscitation.
- Providing there are no over-riding airway or breathing priorities, the next step is rapid, emergency surgical stabilization of the pelvis with an external fixator. This allows strong purchase of both wings of the pelvis by means of threaded self-drilling pins and allows the book to be closed by clamping both halves of the pelvis together, tamponading the underlying venous bleeding.
- Application of an external fixator should take precedence over laparotomy in the presence of an open book or vertical shear pelvic fracture, otherwise the loss of tamponade associated with the laparotomy incision can lead to catastrophic retroperitoneal bleeding. Once the external fixator is applied, a diagnostic peritoneal lavage can be performed (above the umbilicus to avoid the pelvic haematoma). Alternatively emergency focused ultrasound may exclude associated intraperitoneal bleeding. Laparotmy can be easily carried out with the external fixator in place.
- The external fixator can be applied in the resusitation room or the operating theatre depending on local policy. The key is to apply the fixator as rapidly as possible. A recent survey of 31 acute hospitals revealed that only 8 of them could apply an external fixator within 1 h.

Associated injuries

Bladder injury 20%, urethral injury 14%. Liver and splenic injury, spinal fracture, other limb injuries.

Pitfalls

- Open fractures of the pelvis may be difficult to diagnose due to vaginal or rectal perforation, and have a 30 to 50% mortality.

- Beware urethral injury. Do not attempt to catheterize if there is marked pelvic disruption on the radiograph or marked perineal bruising and urethral bleeding. Call a surgeon who will carry out an emergency urethrogram.

- If there is no improvement in vital signs after external fixation then look for other causes of the bleeding, i.e. intraperitoneal (laparotomy), or arterial (angiography) and embolization.

Anaesthetic considerations

- These patients are usually in Class III shock and need early blood transfusion. Fixators may be applied under LA or GA.

- Patients with a fractured pelvis need analgesia. Opioids are the easiest early treatment, but an epidural is effective if not contraindicated.

Spinal injuries (see also p. 180)

If a spinal board has been used to transfer the patient to hospital it should be removed as soon as possible and certainly within 1 h. The patient must be log rolled to enable a thorough inspection and palpation of the whole length of the spine. A safe log roll requires a total of five people:

- Three to control and turn the patient's body.
- One to maintain the cervical spine in neutral alignment with the rest of the body.
- One to palpate the spinous processes for tenderness or deformities.

The person controlling the cervical spine should command the team.

Thorough clearance of the patient's spine can be a complex process:

- In the patient who is awake, alert, sober, neurologically normal, and without distracting injuries, the spine may be cleared if there is no pain at rest and, subsequently, on flexion and extension.
- All other patients will require lateral, AP, and open-mouth radiographs of the cervical spine, and lateral and AP radiographs of the thoracolumbar spine.
- If the cervical spine cannot be seen clearly, down to the junction of the seventh cervical (C7) and first thoracic (T1) vertebrae, a swimmer's view (lateral oblique with one arm raised) will be required—if these fail to show the C7–T1 junction, a CT scan will be required.
- In the obtunded patient, apparently clear, good-quality radiological views of the entire spine do not totally rule out the presence of a significant ligamentous injury to the spine. A senior clinician will need to decide whether to accept the radiological investigations as adequate for declaring the spine clear—there is no widespread consensus on this contentious issue.

In the conscious patient, a detailed neurological examination should detect any motor or sensory deficits. Spinal cord injury can be categorized as:

- incomplete paraplegia
- complete paraplegia
- incomplete quadriplegia
- complete quadriplegia.

Any motor or sensory function below the level of injury indicates an incomplete injury. A cervical or high thoracic injury may result in loss of vasomotor tone, with hypotension and bradycardia. This requires appropriate fluid and vasopressor therapy. The principles of resuscitation for the spinal injured patient are much the same as for the head injured patient; the cord perfusion pressure should be maintained and hypoxia avoided. High-dose methylprednisolone therapy (30 mg/kg within the first 15 min, followed by 5.4 mg/kg/h for the next 23 h) may improve neurological outcome if started within 8 h of the injury.

Limb injuries

Limb injuries are rarely immediately life threatening, but should be examined to ensure an adequate circulation and absence of neurological deficit. The priority is to detect injuries that may be limb threatening. Fractures should be aligned carefully and splinted appropriately, checking for pulses after each intervention. Tibial and forearm fractures are at particularly high risk of causing a compartment syndrome. The signs and symptoms of compartment syndrome are:

- Pain greater than expected and increased by passive stretching of the muscles.
- Paraesthesiae.
- Decreased sensation or functional loss of the nerves traversing the compartment.
- Tense swelling of the involved compartment.
- Loss of pulses is a very late sign—a distal pulse is usually present in a compartment syndrome.

Definitive diagnosis of a compartment syndrome is made by measurement of intracompartmental pressures using a cannula connected to a transducer. In patients with normal blood pressure, compartment pressures in excess of 30–35 mmHg are indicative of a compartment syndrome requiring urgent surgical decompression (see p. 463).

Burns (see also p. 599)

The standard 'ABC' principles apply to managing patients with severe burns. Patients with severe burns should be stabilized and transferred to the nearest burns centre.

* The patient with a thermal injury to the respiratory tract may develop airway obstruction rapidly—all patients with thermal or smoke injury to the respiratory tract must be given humidified, high-concentration oxygen.

* Measure an arterial blood gas and a carboxyhaemoglobin level.

* Consider the need for early intubation in the presence of altered consciousness, direct burns to the face or oropharynx, hoarseness or stridor, soot in the nostrils or sputum, expiratory rhonchi, dysphagia, drooling and dribbling saliva.

* Having established intravenous access, fluid resuscitation is started.

* Cover burnt areas with cling film.

* Use the simple 'rule of nines' to produce an approximate calculation the surface area of the burn. This can be calculated more precisely later using a Lund and Browder chart.

* In line with longstanding North American practice, many burns centres are now using crystalloid-based fluid resuscitation protocols. The estimated fluid replacement using crystalloid is 2–4 ml/ kg/% burn for the first 24 h. Half of this is given in the first 8 h and half over the next 16 h.

* The exact volume of fluid given depends on vital signs, central venous pressure, and urine output. Patients with full thickness burns of >10% of the body surface area will probably require blood.

* Patients with burns will require potent analgesia—this is best given as titrated intravenous opioids.

Analgesia for the injured patient

Effective analgesia should be given to the patient as soon as practically possible. If the patient needs surgery imminently, then immediate induction of general anaesthesia is a logical and very effective solution to the patient's pain. If not, intravenous opioid (e.g. fentanyl or morphine) should be titrated to the desired effect. Head injured patients will require adequate pain relief for any other injuries. Careful titration of intravenous morphine or fentanyl will provide effective pain relief without significant respiratory depression. The popular use of intramuscular codeine in head injured patients is illogical. It is a weak opioid and, in equianalgesic doses, it is a more potent histamine releaser than morphine. It has the same side-effects as morphine, including the ability to induce respiratory depression and miosis. Non-steroidal anti-inflammatory drugs (NSAIDs) provide moderate analgesia but are relatively contraindicated in patients with hypovolaemia; these patients depend on renal prostaglandins to maintain renal blood flow.

Local anaesthetic blocks are ideal for the acute trauma patient. Unfortunately, relatively few blocks are both simple and effective. Femoral nerve blockade will provide analgesia for a fracture of the femoral shaft. Intercostal nerve blocks will provide analgesia for rib fractures but the duration is relatively short. Continuous thoracic epidural analgesia will provide excellent pain relief for patients with multiple rib fractures. This will help the patient to tolerate vigorous physiotherapy and to maintain adequate ventilation. All these factors help to reduce the requirement for intubation and mechanical ventilation.

The multiply injured patient—common problems

Clinical dilemmas presented by the patient with multiple injuries include:

- The head injured patient with an abdominal injury—which of a laparotomy or brain CT should be undertaken first? If the patient is haemodynamically unstable the laparotomy has priority. Hypotension will compound any brain injury and bleeding must be controlled rapidly. If the patient is haemodynamically stable, a CT scan of both the brain and the abdomen may be appropriate.

- The head injured patient with lower limb fractures. In general, in the haemodynamically stable patient, limb fractures should be stabilized as soon as possible. In the presence of a significant brain injury, intracranial pressure should be monitored before intramedullary nailing of limb fractures.

- The patient with pulmonary contusion and lower limb fractures. Intramedullary reaming will cause some degree of fat embolism. Whether this results in significant risk to the patient is contentious. In the presence of severe pulmonary contusion, some orthopaedic surgeons would elect to stabilize lower limb fractures temporarily with an external fixator before undertaking definitive nailing at a later date.

Relatives in the resuscitation room

It is increasingly common for a relative to remain in the resuscitation room while the patient is being resuscitated. The trauma team must be made aware of the presence of the relative and a member of the emergency department nursing staff should accompany them. Relatives should be warned before any particularly invasive procedures so that they have the option to leave if they wish.

Anaesthesia for major trauma

Patients with major trauma often present at night, are poorly prepared, and may require prolonged surgery from different surgical specialties. Injuries that influence cardiorespiratory function may be unrecognized, or present during the course of surgery.

General considerations

+ Major trauma cases often require a number of procedures. Discussion by the different surgical teams will determine the best sequence of procedures. Life-saving surgery clearly takes priority, but it may be necessary/possible to perform several procedures at once.

+ Whenever possible the patient should be reviewed fully preoperatively. Include the notes and radiographs. Check for chest, cervical spine, thoracolumbar spine, and pelvic imaging. Major injuries are easily missed in A&E.

+ When the anaesthetist is unable to see the patient prior to theatre a full hand-over from the trauma team is essential—details of mechanism of injury, current injuries, investigations, resuscitation and treatment already performed, prior health problems, and medications. Blood results and cross-matched blood should be checked.

+ In theatre every patient should have a minimum of a rapid assessment along ATLS primary survey lines (airway, breathing, circulation, and disability) prior to undertaking surgery. This should not delay life-saving surgery.

+ A high index of suspicion should exist for injuries that may not have been apparent at the initial assessment, but may cause cardiorespiratory compromise—pneumothorax, spinal cord injury, cardiac tamponade, fat embolism, and occult haemorrhage.

+ Hypothermia causes significant morbidity and should be rigorously avoided/treated.

Management of anaesthesia

Team work

It is important to use all the members of the medical staff in as efficient a way as possible. Thus, one should identify the members of the anaesthetic team and brief each one clearly as to their responsibilities. Adequate, organized assistance is essential.

Circulatory access

+ Continue resuscitation during transfer to theatre. Do not delay life-saving surgery with attempts to fully resuscitate hypovolaemia from surgical bleeding.

+ Warmed venous access—preferably 14–16G cannulas or a 7Fr catheter in adults. In patients with possible subclavian injury, place lines in the lower limbs. If venous access is difficult consider a cut down/femoral line/external jugular line, or intraosseus access in children.

+ Attach one IV line to a high-performance warming system, preferably with an automatic pressurization system. One line should be dedicated for fluid resuscitation unless haemorrhage is massive: this ensures adequate heating of infused fluid. One person should be solely responsible for checking and dealing with all fluid on this line.

- An arterial line should be inserted when practical. They are not normally required immediately and should not delay surgery. Leave a limb accessible to perform cannulation during surgery. If the subclavian vessels have been injured, avoid the upper limb.
- Central venous access is not usually a priority and may be difficult due to injuries to the vasculature and hypovolaemia. It is best carried out after fluid resuscitation. A femoral line may be the most practical (and quickest) option if infusions of vasopressors/ inotropes are required.

Airway

- Endotracheal intubation is usual. In view of the higher incidence of difficult intubation in trauma patients, all the usual equipment should be available before starting induction of anaesthesia.
- Always assume a full stomach. Place a gastric tube during surgery to attempt gastric decompression. The tube should be placed orally if there are associated nasal/mid-face or base-of-skull fractures.

Ventilation

Ventilator settings may have to be adjusted from 'normal' values to take into account problems that are particular to trauma patients. Patients with actual or potentially raised ICP should have their $PaCO_2$ kept at a value of 4.5–5 kPa, to prevent rises in ICP. Patients with chest trauma may require the use of special ventilator settings, such as pressure control, reversed I:E ratio, or permissive hypercapnia. It may be necessary to use an ICU ventilator in these circumstances, especially if surgery is prolonged.

Temperature

- An oesophageal/rectal temperature probe and peripheral nerve stimulator should be placed before surgery commences.
- Try to maintain body temperature.

Blood loss

Blood loss is dependent on the type(s) of surgery undertaken, and may be massive in thoracic, hepatic, splenic, and pelvic injuries. Cross-matched blood may be unavailable—use type specific when necessary. A cell salvage system should be considered.

General and regional anaesthesia

- Regional anaesthesia may be considered as an adjunct, although preoperative urgency, haemodynamic instability, coagulopathy, and the possibility of compartment syndrome often make it impractical.
- The choice of induction agent depends on the situation. In shocked patients without head injury, IV ketamine provides the best cardiovascular stability. Induce with 1–1.5 mg/kg slowly and then add increments of 25 mg as required for maintenance.

Problems

- Unexplained hypotension and tachycardia: consider hypovolaemia, pneumothorax, pericardial tamponade, fat/air embolism.

- Unexplained hypoxia is often associated with a rise in inflation pressure: consider fat embolism and tension pneumothorax.
- Unexplained hypertension: consider pain, raised ICP (search for associated neurological signs, obtain brain CT scan), or rarely traumatic disruption of thoracic aorta. Look for different BP between left and right arms, and upper and lower limbs. Obtain either CT scan of chest, or transoesophageal echo in blunt trauma, especially in patients with rib fractures/sternal fractures/severe blunt trauma.

Changing anaesthetic teams

Major trauma cases often involve prolonged surgery, by multiple teams, and it is quite likely that the anaesthetist(s) will need to hand over the patient to different anaesthetist(s). This hand-over should be detailed and convey the following information:

- Nature of patient's injuries, including state of cervical spine and thoracolumbar spine clearance.
- Any actual or anticipated airway problems, including plan for airway (extubation?) at the end of the procedure.
- Circulatory status, and volume of cross-matched blood products available and ordered.
- Preoperative neurological status.
- Use of regional blocks, with reference to possible compartment syndrome.
- Proposed/completed surgery.
- Further investigations planned after end of surgery.
- Disposal of patient, e.g. ICU, transfer, extubation in recovery unit.
- Discussion with family.

The anaesthetist should document/sign the time and details of the hand-over on the anaesthesia record. The use of a problem list in the patient's notes is recommended for trauma patients, with an adjacent column to indicate resolution/treatment of each problem. This will reduce the chance of 'minor' problems being missed during subsequent care.

Anaesthetic considerations for cervical spine fracture

Surgery for cervical spine fracture may comprise application of stabilizing devices (Halo traction, skull tongs, plaster jacket) or definitive fixation of the bony column. Bony fixation is usually performed as a semi-elective procedure.

General considerations

- Patients will usually have suffered major trauma, although fractures can occur following minor injury in patients with pre-existing cervical spine disease.

- Controversy exists as to the best method of securing the airway for surgery in such patients. Awake intubation is safer, in that there is less risk of failed intubation. However, it may result in coughing, and can be difficult and unpleasant for the patient. Direct laryngoscopy under general anaesthesia with manual in-line neck stabilization (MILNS) has the disadvantage that it may be associated with more neck movement. The anatomical features of the patient as regards intubation and the skill of the anaesthetist are two additional factors in the management of these patients.

Anaesthesia

- Patients for halo traction, skull tong application, or other stabilizing procedures will usually be in full neck immobilization. This is removed following application of the stabilizing device. General anaesthesia is uncommon for such procedures, which are usually performed using local anaesthetic. Sedation may be required, and caution should be exercised given the likelihood of associated injuries. General anaesthesia is occasionally required for more complex stabilization or in confused/agitated/uncooperative patients. It should be performed along the lines of anterior cervical stabilization.

- Patients for open cervical spine stabilization require either an anterior or posterior approach and, in a few patients, both.

- The anaesthetist should perform a full neurological examination before induction of anaesthesia, to assess the level and extent of any spinal cord injury. This is particularly important for patients who are to be turned prone.

- Anterior approaches are usually performed in the supine head-up position, through an oblique incision across the anterior aspect of the neck. The posterior approach is performed in the prone position, using a longitudinal incision. Occasionally, fractures to C1/C2 may require an approach through the mouth.

- All types of cervical stabilization involve prolonged surgery. Endotracheal intubation is performed either with the cervical immobilization device in place, or in the case of a hard collar, with manual in-line stabilization to minimize risks of worsening any neurological injury. Awake fibreoptic intubation is the technique of choice, but may not be practical in some patients. Use of remifentanil sedation (up to 0.25 µg/kg/min) may help suppress the cough reflex in these patients, but care is needed to prevent bradypnoea and hypoxia. Young patients, or those that are confused, may require an IV induction followed by direct laryngoscopy. A range of tubes and laryngoscopes should be available, and the use of a tube stylet or gum elastic bougie is recommended.

- Arterial and venous lines should be placed in the non-dominant or non-injured arm, and must be well secured to prevent kinking. A forced air warming system should be used and urinary catheterization is required. Nasogastric decompression is usual for prolonged surgery, or for patients with pre-existing spinal cord injury.

- For prone positioning extreme care is needed during turning (involve the surgeon). It is suggested that the surgeon controls the head, while three people perform the turn into the prone position. The anaesthetist should hold the ET tube in situ, and should be in charge of timing the turn. Some centres suggest awake intubation, followed by awake positioning prior to induction of anaesthesia.

- Blood loss is rarely significant for these procedures, and so deliberate arterial hypotension is not usually required.

Anaesthesia for repair of cervical spine fracture

Procedure	Anterior/ posterior repair of cervical fracture
Time	2–6 h
Pain	++/+++
Position	Supine head up or prone for posterior approach
Blood loss	250–1000 ml, ensure cross-match four units
Practical technique	Usually awake intubation, with oral/nasal ETT, then IPPV

Preoperative

• Mostly trauma patients, often with other injuries. Sometimes older patients with fractures in a previously diseased cervical spine. Check for other manifestations of the underlying disease (e.g. rheumatoid).

• Check presence/degree of cervical spine injury, level of lesion, and likely approach.

• Check the need for postoperative ventilation and HDU care. Commoner with high lesions, which may need aggressive chest physiotherapy.

• Consider the technique of intubation. The patient may be in skull traction, which does not limit mouth opening but does limit neck movement. Full neck immobilization (with a hard cervical collar and sandbags/tape) limits both neck movement and mouth opening.

Perioperative

• Insert arterial and venous lines, preferably in the same arm.

• Intubation: awake nasal intubation is commonest,[3] but a smaller tube size results. Awake oral intubation is harder to perform, but gives a larger tube size. If the surgeon is planning an intraoral approach, check on whether an oral or nasal ETT is preferred.

• Suxamethonium is contraindicated in patients with spinal cord lesions that are more than 72 h old. In practice, it is rare to need suxamethonium, given the range of rapid onset non-depolarizing drugs that are available.

• Positioning should be in combination with the surgeon. Some request check of residual neurological function following awake intubation and after turning prone.

• Check all pressure areas before draping. Procedures are prolonged.

• Bone graft may be required, and is usually taken from the iliac crest.

3 Sidhu VS, Whitehead EM, Ainsworth QP, Smith M, Calder I (1993). A technique of awake fibreoptic intubation. Experience in patients with cervical spine disease. *Anaesthesia*, **48**, 910–13.

Postoperative

• PCA morphine is usually satisfactory.

• NSAIDs are useful.

Special considerations

• Patients with acute spinal cord lesions may demonstrate signs of neurogenic shock, with bradycardia and hypotension (see p. 180). This is best treated with judicious use of fluids and pressor agents, aided by CVP monitoring. Cervical spine surgery is rarely performed in the first few hours after injury, which makes these problems uncommon. However, spinal hyper-reflexia may occur in patients with longer-standing lesions, and these should be treated symptomatically.

• Tracheostomy is not advisable in patients scheduled for anterior fusion. Discuss with the surgeon if this is a likely option.

• CVP lines in this group of patients should avoid the jugular veins.

Anaesthetic considerations for limb fractures

Limb fractures occur in a wide range of patients, and may be solitary or occur as part of multiple trauma. The urgency of fracture reduction depends upon:

- The severity and site of the fracture, e.g. femoral fractures are treated before humerus, because of the higher risk of fat embolism syndrome.
- The age of the patient (children >adults).
- The presence of distal ischaemia (emergency).
- The presence of an open fracture (emergency).
- The presence of compartment syndrome (emergency).
- Other associated injuries (including head injury).
- The requirement for other surgery.

General considerations

- Although it is difficult to generalize, there are three main methods of limb fracture repair:
  - closed reduction, followed by stabilization with plaster/traction/sling
  - open reduction followed by plating/nail insertion/bone grafting
  - external fixation.
- Fat embolism may occur a few hours after injury or up to several days later and is commonest following tibial/femoral fractures. Look for the cardinal symptoms of: dyspnoea, confusion, anxiety, restlessness, or unexplained coma. Signs include: crepitations in the lungs, petechiae in the upper body/conjunctiva, and fluffy white exudates on fundoscopy. Investigations reveal hypoxia in severe cases, and pulmonary oedema on the chest radiograph. Lipuria is not a reliable sign. Treatment involves correction of shock from right ventricular failure, correction of hypoxia, and urgent stabilization of the fracture. The role of steroids is controversial.

Anaesthesia

- The patient should be questioned about the presence of associated injuries, including head injury. Generally, patients with recent (<24 h) moderate or severe head injury require careful consideration before proceeding to non-life-saving surgery (see below). The timing and content of the most recent meal is important, as gastric emptying may be markedly delayed after severe injury. This will influence the type of anaesthetic, and may demand precautions for the potentially full stomach.
- Blood loss is very variable, and depends on the length and complexity of the repair and the type and age of the fracture. Proximal limb fractures (femur, humerus) and use of bone grafting tend to be associated with considerably larger blood loss. The use of a tourniquet will reduce bleeding, but may be contraindicated because of the fracture type/site.
- Patients with recent head injury will need careful consideration, if the planned surgery is likely to be prolonged (>1 h). General anaesthesia can obscure the signs of deterioration in conscious level, and anaesthesia may also contribute to a rise in ICP. Therefore, consideration must be given to

either delaying surgery, or performing a cranial CT scan prior to induction of anaesthesia. Patients with actual or potentially raised ICP will benefit from the placement of an ICP monitor, ventilation to normocarbia, and a neurosurgical directed technique (see p. 420).

• Postoperative analgesia requirements depend on the duration, site, and nature of surgery to repair the fracture. Closed reductions can often be managed with a combination of perioperative opioid together with NSAIDs/paracetamol/opioid orally. More complex repairs, including external fixation, may require the use of a PCA.

Anaesthesia for limb fractures

Procedure	Closed/open reduction of limb fractures
Time	5 min to 3 h
Pain	Variable, much less for closed reductions
Position	Usually supine, may be lateral for some ankle fractures
Blood loss	Minimal for closed reductions, up to 2000 ml for open femoral nailing/wiring
Practical technique	Regional block alone
	GA ± regional block ± local infiltration according to the site/nature of reduction

Preoperative

- Discuss with the surgeon the nature and duration of the likely repair (MUA may become ORIF).
- Check that no other types of surgery are likely or required.
- Ensure the absence of other significant chest/abdominal/head injuries.
- Check the state of cervical spine clearance where relevant.
- Check the state of hydration of the patient, and the time of the last food/drink in relation to the time of injury. In practice, the stomach may never empty in some patients, particularly children, and so hard guidelines are not useful. It is better to be flexible, and if in doubt consider the patient at risk of a full stomach.
- Ensure a chest radiograph for all major trauma patients.
- Discuss with the patient/surgeon use of regional block with regard to compartment syndrome (p. 463).

Perioperative

- Ensure large-gauge infusion/IVI warmer for all open reductions involving proximal limb fractures, i.e. tibia, femur, and humerus. Do not site IV on an injured limb.
- Antibiotic prophylaxis prior to commencement of surgery/application of tourniquet.
- Ensure direct arterial monitoring and capnography for patients at high risk of fat embolism.
- Patients with pre-existing head injury may require ICP monitoring, and postoperative ventilation.

Postoperative

Analgesia should be discussed with the patient and surgeon. IV morphine via PCA/continuous infusion is often combined with NSAIDs and other simple analgesics.

Special considerations

Regional anaesthesia can be a useful addition for the provision of analgesia, and may also be used as the sole anaesthetic for some fracture reductions (e.g. Biers block for wrist fracture reductions). However, the issue of a local anaesthetic block obscuring the neurological signs of a developing compartment syndrome must be considered (p. 463). Such signs occur relatively late in the natural history of compartment syndrome, and it can be argued that the syndrome should be predicted earlier. This can often be done on clinical grounds of a high-risk injury, or by direct repeated measurement of compartment pressure. Despite this, many surgeons prefer the anaesthetist to avoid the use of local anaesthetics in patients at risk. The best strategy is to discus the problem with the surgeon beforehand.

Fat embolism may rarely occur during operative manipulation of a fracture, especially femoral, tibial, and humeral fractures. Two stages of pulmonary injury are initial RV failure, followed by an ARDS type picture. Increase inspired oxygen, treat RV failure if present, and allow rapid stabilization of fracture if possible. Steroids are of dubious value.

Compartment syndrome

Compartment syndrome is a serious limb-threatening condition that may develop in trauma or intensive care patients. Tight, unyielding fascial envelopes surround limb muscles, nerves, and vessels. When pressures within these compartments rise above capillary bed pressure, perfusion falls leading to local ischaemia of muscles and nerves. If the pressure is not relieved within a few hours of onset, irreversible changes will occur with muscle necrosis and contracture, plus nerve and vessel damage. Signs and symptoms of compartment syndrome include:

- Pain mainly over the affected compartment, worsened by passive stretching of the muscles.
- Tense swelling over the compartment, with drum-tight fascia and overlying skin.
- Paraesthesia in the distribution of nerves traversing the compartment.
- Weakness or paralysis of the limb is a late sign.
- Distal pulses are usually present.

Compartment syndrome should be anticipated in any limb injury, with or without a fracture, in crush situations or accidents with prolonged extrication times. The increase in pressure may be due to haemorrhage or oedema. Compartment syndrome can also occur with open fractures, as the compartment may not be able to decompress through the open wound. In unconscious or obtunded patients where clinical signs may be masked, or in the presence of spinal cord injuries, diagnosis is difficult. In these situations measurement of the compartmental pressure may be indicated. This can be undertaken using a pressure transducer (as in an arterial line) attached to a needle placed into the suspect compartment.

- If the compartmental pressure is within 30 mmHg of the diastolic pressure, diagnosis is confirmed.
- Release all constricting bandages, dressings or casts encircling the limb. If this does not rapidly relieve symptoms, urgent surgical fasciotomy will be required to save the limb.

Special considerations

- Keep the limb at the level of the heart. Avoid elevation as this may decrease perfusion below critical levels.
- After fasciotomy the limb should be splinted to prevent contractures and the fracture stabilized to prevent further bleeding.

Local blocks and compartment syndrome

Avoid local blocks or epidurals if the patient is at risk of developing compartment syndrome as the analgesia will mask early signs of the syndrome. The cardinal symptom is pain and this occurs early in the syndrome. The risk is especially high in tibial and forearm fractures so avoid blocks in these situations. If there is no alternative to using blocks, i.e. high anaesthetic risk patients, then compartment syndrome needs to be excluded by intra-operative monitoring of compartment pressure using indwelling catheters.

Anaesthesia for femoral neck fracture

Procedure	Cannulated screws, dynamic hip screw (DHS), cemented/uncemented hemi-arthroplasty
Time	30–120 min
Pain	+/+++
Position	Supine (?on hip table), occasionally lateral
Blood loss	250–750 ml
Practical technique	SV LMA and regional block
	Spinal ± sedation
	ET + IPPV

A fractured neck of the femur occurs predominantly in the older population, usually as a result of osteoporosis followed by a fall. Thus, patients are often frail, old, and female. An estimated 1.7 million hip fractures occurred worldwide in 1990 and this number is increasing every year. Three-month mortality is approximately 12% increasing to 21% at 1 year and there may be little difference between operative and non-operative outcomes.[4]

Preoperative

- Preoperative clerking is often short on detail in this group!
- The patient will usually be bed bound on skin traction, and may have been in hospital or unnoticed at home for some days. All medical illnesses that occur in the older population apply, plus pain, confusion, and chest infections as a direct consequence of the immobility that conservative stabilization requires. Dehydrated patients will require IV rehydration.
- Surgical treatment can be either fracture fixation or femoral head replacement and depends upon the nature of the fracture, surgical preference, previous mobility, and life expectancy of the patient. Conservative (non-operative) management is always one option for the grossly unfit.
- Determine which procedure is to be performed. Cannulated hip screws are quick, largely non-invasive procedures with a small incision and little blood loss. Cemented/uncemented hemiarthroplasty is a longer procedure, similar to a primary hip replacement. Dynamic hip screw/Richard's screw and plate are intermediate procedures (see Table).
- A decision to delay surgery should be based on a realistic attempt to improve the patient's medical condition, rather than a fruitless pursuit of 'normal' values. A mild chest infection is unlikely to improve in a bedbound elderly patient, whereas frank pneumonia with sepsis and dyspnoea may respond to rehydration, antibiotics, and chest physiotherapy. Similarly,

---

4 Parker MJ, Handoll HH (1999). Conservative versus operative treatment for extracapsular hip fractures. *Cochrane Collaboration. Cochrane Library*, issue 2.

Procedures for fractured neck of femur

Operation	Description	Time (min)	Pain (+ to +++++)	Position	Blood loss/XM	Notes
Cannulated screws	Screws across femoral neck (previously 'Garden Screws')	20	+	Supine, hip table	–	Minimally invasive, small thigh incision. Can be done with local/nerve block and sedation if necessary. X-ray guided
Richards screw and plate (RSP)	Plate along femur with compression screw into femoral head	30–45	++	Supine, hip table	<400 ml	Somewhat larger thigh incision/blood loss. X-ray guided
Dynamic hip screw (DHS)	As RSP	30–45	++	Supine, hip table	<400 ml	As RSP
Dynamic compression screw (DCS)	As RSP	30–45	++	Supine, hip table	<400 ml	As RSP
Girdlestone osteotomy	Removal of femoral head. No prosthesis	30–45	++	Supine	<400 ml	More extensive incision, but no prosthesis, hence quicker than below. Limited mobility afterwards

Operation	Description	Time (min)	Pain (+ to +++++)	Position	Blood loss/XM	Notes
Austin Moore hemiarthroplasty	Replacement of femoral head. No cement	60–90	+++	Supine	400–600ml	Similar to total hip replacement, without acetabular component
Thompson's hemiarthroplasty	Replacement of femoral head. Cemented	60–90	+++	Supine	400–600 ml	Similar to total hip replacement, without acetabular component
Exeter bipolar	Replacement of femoral head and acetabular component. Cemented	60–90	+++	Supine	400–800 ml	Similar to total hip replacement, with acetabular component

a mild hypokalaemia is often due to diuretic therapy or laxative use, and is unlikely to precipitate arrhythmias.

- An attempt should be made to control atrial fibrillation preoperatively, to prevent severe perioperative hypotension.

- Outcome studies for this age group suggest that mortality in the healthy elderly patient is similar to younger age groups. However, the older patient with co-morbidity has a much poorer outcome.[5] Thus, efforts should be directed towards ensuring that identification and stratification of risk occurs, as a result of the patient clerking and investigations.

Perioperative

- For fracture fixation the patient is usually positioned supine on a 'hip table'. This involves placement of a prop in the groin, with the table supporting the upper body only. Feet are tied into shoe supports, and the table is then elevated to allow radiographic screening and the surgeon to work at shoulder height. The anaesthetist must be aware that the patient may slide off the lower end of the table. For hemiarthroplasty the patient is lateral or supine on an ordinary operating table.

- Blood loss is variable, and depends on operator technique, the type of repair used, and the time since fracture. Much of the blood loss that is measured is old haematoma, but significant haemorrhage may occur and necessitate blood transfusion.

- The choice of anaesthetic technique is based around patient factors and the preferences of the anaesthetist. Regional and general anaesthesia are both advocated but there is little evidence to support one technique over another.[6] The options include:

  - Regional anaesthesia. Epidural, spinal, psoas plexus, and triple nerve block have all been used for operative anaesthesia and for postoperative analgesia. Sedation may be necessary but it is inadvisable to heavily sedate patients without airway support, as they are often elevated above the view of the anaesthetist and access is limited. A confused, disorientated, elderly patient on an elevated operating table can cause many problems.

  - Spinal anaesthesia may decrease the incidence of postoperative confusion and DVT, but can be associated with perioperative hypotension. A small dose of IV ketamine or alfentanil may be useful as analgesia when turning the patient before performing the block.

  - A light general anaesthetic (combined with psoas plexus or triple nerve blockade) is often better for patients with cardiovascular disease and for confused or uncooperative patients. These unilateral blocks cause less hypotensive than centroneuraxis anaesthesia and provide a degree of postoperative analgesia.

5 Cousins MT (1982). In: *Complications of anaesthesia operative risk: Postgraduate course.* New York, Elsevier.

6 Parker MJ, Handoll HH, Griffiths R (2001). Anaesthesia for hip fracture in adults. *Cochrane Collaboration.* Cochrane Library, issue 4.

- Check pressure points after placement on the 'hip table', as patients are very prone to pressure damage.
- Use some form of passive or active warming device to prevent hypothermia. Insulate the head and secure a warming blanket/polythene sheet around the chest and lower abdomen.
- Cemented hemiarthroplasty may be associated with a marked drop in arterial pressure, ETCO$_2$, and heart rate during cement insertion. Ask the surgeon to reduce insertion pressure and administer fluid and boluses of ephedrine (occasionally adrenaline 0.5–1 ml 1:10 000 aliquots may be required). Incidence may be reduced by improved surgical technique (venting the femur prior to cement impaction), avoiding relative hypovolaemia, and preloading with IV fluid (250–500 ml) before cement insertion (see p. 472).

Postoperative

- Pain is often only due to the incision, which is small for cannulated screws and DHS, but larger for hemiarthroplasty. Fracture pain will be reduced through reduction of fracture, but is still painful on rolling and turning in bed.
- Postoperative analgesia can be provided by regular IM or SC morphine. The use of NSAIDs, and more recently tramadol, can be a useful addition/alternative to more potent opioid analgesics, but beware of the side-effects in this elderly population.

Special considerations

In poor risk patients, consider whether postoperative intensive care may be appropriate. Morbidity and mortality risks should be understood by the patient or relatives and in some patients, resuscitation status should be reviewed.

Further reading

Driscoll P, Skinner D, Earlam R (ed.) (2000). *ABC of major trauma*, 3rd edn. British Medical Journal, London.

Gupta KJ, Nolan JP (1998). Emergency general anaesthesia for hypovolaemic trauma patients. *Current Anaesthesia and Critical Care*, **9**, 66–73.

Nolan JP, Parr MJA (1997). Aspects of resuscitation in trauma. *British Journal of Anaesthesia*, 79, 226–40.

General principles

Recent advances in arthroscopic and joint replacement surgery together with the ever-increasing age of the population have led to a large increase in orthopaedic workload. Patients presenting for hip and knee replacement, in particular, are often elderly and suffer with many concomitant diseases such as diabetes and cardiovascular compromise. Arthritis, with poor flexibility of multiple joints, gives a largely sedentary patient population. Many are obese, often with a significant incidence of gastric reflux. Others are the frail elderly with long-term poor dietary intake. Surgery to the lower limbs is associated with a high incidence of venous thromboembolism.

Preoperative

- Severe arthritis will limit mobility and may mask poor exercise tolerance due to other medical causes. Assessment of cardiovascular function may be difficult. Cardiologist review should be considered for patients with serious CVS disease who are scheduled for major surgery (ECG stress testing/echocardiography/angiography, see p. 20).
- Patients are often taking multiple drugs and side-effects/cross-reactions should be identified. Anticoagulants influence the choice of anaesthetic technique and may increase the risk of perioperative haemorrhage. Steroid therapy needs to be continued perioperatively.
- If central neuraxial blockade is planned in patients on thromboembolism prophylaxis ensure that the final preoperative dose is timed appropriately (see p. 998).
- Antithromboembolism measures, e.g. heparin/warfarin/stockings/leg and foot compression devices should be prescribed and used postoperatively.
- Patients with rheumatoid arthritis are at risk of atlantoaxial instability (see p. 160).

Perioperative

- Give IV antibiotic prophylaxis as per local policy. If vancomycin is used it should be given over at least 1 h to prevent hypotension.
- During surgery access may be limited and blood loss may be significant. Use a large-bore cannula and drip extension.
- Blood loss may be increased by certain types of bone structure, e.g. in Pagett's disease.
- It is important, but difficult, to monitor intra-operative blood loss. Fluids added for lavage should be from graduated containers or infusion bags and volumes used carefully recorded. Patients should be draped using a system that allows most of this fluid to be collected in the sucker together with the blood loss. Suckers should be graduated and volumes frequently checked and recorded.
- Arterial lines are commonly used due to the patient population, difficulty in fully identifying intra-operative blood loss, and the incidence of hypotension when bone cement is used. They are not required for patients without significant CVS disease undergoing uncomplicated primary hip or knee replacement or surgery using a tourniquet.

- CVP lines are not generally required. Consider them in high-risk patients undergoing revision hip arthroplasty.
- A urinary catheter should be inserted for prolonged surgery, in patients with a strong history of prostatism, or where an epidural will be used postoperatively.
- If patients are breathing spontaneously using an ordinary oxygen mask, monitor the presence of respiration and the respiratory rate by placing a capnograph sampling line in the mask. A stethoscope taped over the trachea is useful to monitor a clear airway and adequate respiration.
- The patient's temperature should be maintained with blood warmers and warm air blankets.

Postoperative

Surgeons may prescribe regular low/medium doses of indometacin postoperatively to reduce new bone growth—avoid additional NSAIDs.

Cement hypotension[1,2]

- Hypotension when using pressurized bone cement is a significant problem in approximately 10% of patients. It is probably related to release of monomer as the cement polymerizes and also to showers of micro fat emboli caused by the pressurizing. It usually only occurs during cementing of the femoral cavity in total hip replacement and revisions.

- The incidence is thought to be reduced if the socket is absolutely dry prior to insertion of the cement. This can be achieved by a combination of good surgical technique and an anaesthetic that allows hypotension at the operative site, as with subarachnoid block. A suction catheter should be placed deep into the femoral cavity by the surgeon and gradually withdrawn as the cement is pressurized. The incidence may also have been reduced by the use of more modern cements.

- Monitor fluid balance prior to insertion of cement to ensure that the patient is adequately volume loaded.

- A fall in SpO_2 may be an early sign of impending hypotension or the presence of fat emboli.

- Hypotension usually responds to normal doses of vasopressors such as ephedrine. Increase IV fluids and inspired oxygen as necessary.

- The incident is normally short lived but if hypotension persists consider other causes of hypotension such as hypovolaemia or a perioperative MI.

- If hypoxaemia persists, consider significant fat embolism.

1 Jones RH (1975). Physiologic emboli changes observed during total hip replacement arthroplasty. A clinical prospective study. *Clinical Orthopaedics*, October (112), 192–200.

2 Pitto RP, Blunk J, Kossler M (2000). Transoesophageal echocardiography and clinical features of fat embolism during cemented total hip arthroplasty study in patients with a femoral neck fracture. *Archives of Orthopaedic and Trauma Surgery*, **120**, 53–8.

Regional anaesthesia

+ Most orthopaedic operations are amenable to regional anaesthesia, either used alone with or without sedation, or used as an adjuvant to GA. Central neuraxis blockade and major nerve blocks are commonly performed.

+ In major orthopaedic surgery, blocks may provide useful postoperative pain relief and reduce the time in recovery compared with traditional general anaesthesia.

+ Some trials show a reduction in the incidence of perioperative DVT if regional anaesthesia is used.[3,4]

+ Central neuraxis blockade can be technically difficult in the elderly arthritic spine, but success is improved with experience.

Hypotensive anaesthesia

Good fixation of cement and joint prosthesis requires a dry, preferably bloodless, surgical field at the time of insertion. Regional, particularly spinal/epidural anaesthetic reduces bleeding at the surgical site without the need for other pharmacological hypotensive anaesthetic techniques which are usually contraindicated in this patient group.

Communication

It is important to communicate well with the surgeon who may not be familiar with the difficulties faced by the anaesthetist. Communication during surgery can be limited, especially if the surgical team is using modern infection control systems involving full-face helmets and personal fans. Lastly, remember that the orthopaedic theatre is one place where anaesthetists are still expected to wear facemasks.

3 Modig J (1989). Influence of regional anaesthesia, local anaesthetics, and sympathicomimetics on the pathophysiology of deep vein thrombosis [Review]. *Acta Chirugica Scandinavia*, **550** (Suppl.), 119–24 (discussion 124–7).

4 Wille-Jorgensenp *et al.* (1989). Prevention of thromboembolism following elective hip surgery. The value of regional anaesthesia and graded stockings. *Clinical Orthopaedics*, October (247), 163–7.

Tourniquets[5]

Many orthopaedic operations require a bloodless field and tourniquets can be used to achieve this. The use of the tourniquet is essentially the responsibility of the surgeon but the anaesthetist should be aware of the requirements for safe use of a tourniquet.

• Only pneumatic tourniquets should be used as mechanical tourniquets can cause areas of unpredictably high pressure in the underlying tissues.

• Small tourniquets on fingers and toes are dangerous because they are easily forgotten. It is best to use a rubber band and artery forceps and the anaesthetist should check for their removal at the end.

• Expressive exsanguination using an Esmarch bandage is contraindicated in cases of tumour or severe infection because of the risks of dissemination. It is also contraindicated if DVT is suspected—massive fatal pulmonary embolism has been reported.[6] It also represents a potential risk of left ventricular failure from fluid overload. Compression of both legs adds 15% to the circulating volume (800 ml), therefore limit to one leg only in patients at risk.

• Peripheral arterial disease is a relative contraindication to tourniquet use.

• Avoid in severe crush injuries.

• Sickle cell disease: use of tourniquets is controversial. Sickling of red blood cells under anoxic conditions causes thrombosis, but some surgeons use limb tourniquets after *full* exsanguination. If employed, it should be for as short a time as possible.

Site of application

The upper arm and thigh have sufficient muscle bulk to distribute the cuff pressure evenly and are the recommended sites. In patients with normal circulation, the cuff can be placed more distally, particularly round the calf, but should not used beyond 1 h.

Cuff width

• The American Heart Association concluded that if a sphygmomanometer cuff has a width of 20% greater than the diameter of the upper arm or 40% of the circumference of the thigh (to a maximum of 20 cm), then the pressure in the underlying central artery will be equal to that in the cuff. This avoids the need for excessively high cuff pressures. Modern silicone cuffs tend to be smaller than this, measuring 90 mm width (bladder 70 mm) for the arm and 105 mm (bladder 75 mm) for the leg.

• The tissues immediately underlying the cuff should be protected with cotton wool. This is not necessary with a correctly applied modern silicone cuff.

5   Kam PC, Kavanaugh R, Yoong FF (2001). The arterial tourniquet: pathophysiological consequences and anaesthetic implications. *Anaethesia*, **56**, p. 534–45 (review).

6   Boogaerts JG (1999). Lower limb exsanguination and embolism. *Acta Anaesthesiologica Belgiae*, **50**, 95–8.

Pressure

- Based on the unsedated patient's blood pressure measured on the ward pre-operatively.
- Upper limb: systolic BP + 50 mmHg. Lower limb: twice systolic BP. This higher pressure is needed because there is often not enough room above the operating site for a full-sized cuff.

Tourniquet time

The minimum time possible compatible with good surgery should be the aim. Notify the surgeon at 1 h and remove as soon as possible after that. If the operation is difficult, time can be extended to 1.5 h. Two hours should be regarded as a maximum but this will not be safe for all patients.

Total hip replacement

Procedure	Prosthetic replacement of femoral head and acetabulum
Time	2 h
Pain	+++
Position	Lateral or supine
Blood loss	300–500 ml, G&S
Practical technique	Spinal, with sedation or GA/LMA
	IPPV, COETT ± spinal, nerve block, or epidural

Total hip replacement is particularly amenable to spinal anaesthesia and this can be supplemented with sedation or general anaesthesia, a decision which may be partly influenced by the patient's wishes. Post spinal puncture headache is very rare in this age group with a 25G needle.

Perioperative

- Place 16G cannula in the lower arm (if a lateral position is anticipated). With proper positioning the drip will flow freely and this leaves the upper arm free for a NIBP cuff or direct arterial pressure measurement.
- Preload with IV fluids prior to performing the spinal.
- Single-shot spinal (2–3 ml bupivacaine 0.5% plain). In 'younger' patients diamorphine (0.1–0.25 mg) may be added for more prolonged analgesia.
- TCI propofol with a target infusion of 1.5–3 µg/ml is useful sedation for the lateral position, using facemask supplemental oxygen. Most patients are easy to manage with TCI alone; however, some patients may be unsettled due to pain from arthritic shoulders and other joints. Intermittent doses of midazolam, cautious narcotics or entonox/isoflurane via the Hudson mask may be useful. On occasions induction of general anaesthesia is required using an LMA.
- For the supine position (see below), consider an LMA with light isoflurane general anaesthesia.
- The addition of intrathecal narcotic can also be used to cover the longer duration of surgery necessary for a more complex primary hip replacement, usually involving some rebuilding of the acetabulum. It is a suitable technique for up to 2.5 h of surgery. Alternatively, or for longer cases, a combined spinal/epidural technique can be used. Postoperative analgesic requirements rarely require this approach for an uncomplicated primary hip replacement.
- GA (rather than sedation) with epidural should be considered for any complex primary operation because of the prolonged surgical time.
- Using an epidural postoperatively will necessitate inserting a urinary catheter (which also helps monitor fluid balance) at some stage in the majority of patients. This is best performed at the time of surgery.

• If central neuraxis blockade is contraindicated, a femoral 3 in 1 block or a psoas lumbar plexus plus lateral cutaneous nerve of thigh block can be used to supplement general anaesthesia.

• Aim to maintain BP at an adequate level based on preoperative readings.

• Intra-operative antibiotic prophylaxis will be required.

• Ensure adequate IV fluid load prior to cementing the femoral component.

Postoperative

• The surgeon usually prefers the patients to be placed on their bed in the supine position with the legs abducted using a pillow to prevent dislocation of the prosthesis.

• A technique which leads to rapid recovery of airway control and patient cooperation is therefore an advantage.

• Patients are usually mobilized at 24 to 48 h and simple IM opioids with regular paracetamol or NSAIDs are usually sufficient for postoperative analgesia. If an epidural has been inserted, a postoperative infusion can be used but is rarely necessary and needs to cease prior to mobilization.

Special considerations

• With the posterior approach the patient will be in the lateral position with the operated side up. With other approaches the patient is supine. To some extent position dictates technique. Sedation with facemask oxygen is much simpler in the lateral position where the airway is better maintained. If supine, then sedation should either be light enough to maintain airway reflexes or deeper anaesthesia with an LMA should be considered.

• Blood loss varies with different types of bone structure and levels of inflammation. It is also affected by anaesthetic technique. The average loss is 300–500 ml. A similar amount may be lost in the drain and tissues post-operatively. Blood transfusion is relatively uncommon during surgery if patients have an adequate preoperative haemoglobin. Group and saved serum is acceptable if cross-matched blood can be provided within 30 min. Haemoglobin should be checked 24 h postoperatively and treated either with transfusion or iron supplements as indicated. Patients with an Hb of >9 g/dl postoperatively rarely require transfusion. The decision to transfuse is multifactorial and includes general fitness, continuing surgical losses, and local practice. Oxygen therapy for up to 24 h is advisable in most patients.

Revision of total hip replacement

Procedure	Revision of previous total hip replacement. Revision may include one or both components
Time	2–6 h depending on complexity
Pain	+++/++++
Position	Lateral or supine
Blood loss	1 litre, occasionally considerably more, cross-match two units
Practical technique	Sedation/GA + LMA, combined spinal/epidural, art line ± CVP
	IPPV, epidural or PCA, art line ± CVP

Essentially the same as primary hip replacement except for the length of surgery, blood loss, and postoperative pain. The complexity of the surgery is very variable. First stage revision involves removal of old cement. Infection increases blood loss. One or both components may be replaced. Major reconstruction of the acetabulum and/or femur involves bone graft and wire cages. These operations are prolonged and bloody. Discuss the anticipated operation with the surgeon beforehand, but beware, it is not an exact science.

Preoperative

General principles as for total hip replacement, except:
- Patients are more elderly and usually have more medical problems.
- The operation takes longer, at least 2–3 h, often more, i.e. too long for a single-shot spinal.
- Blood loss can be significant, with 1 litre or more commonly lost perioperatively.
- Postoperative pain can be a significant problem, perhaps because of increased surgical dissection.

Perioperative

- General set up as for primary hip replacement, including a urinary catheter.
- If significant blood loss is anticipated, or the patient's CVS status indicates it, insert an arterial line and consider a CVP line.
- Depending on the length of surgery, the operative position, and patient factors a number of techniques are suitable. TCI propofol and combined spinal/epidural, spontaneous breathing with supplemental oxygen as for total hip replacement. For supine patients, or anaesthetists less familiar with this operation, an LMA is advisable. For more complex revisions, anticipated to take longer than 3 h, an IPPV technique with epidural supplementation may be more appropriate. If central neuraxis block is contraindicated consider supplementing GA with nerve blocks (femoral 3 in 1 or psoas compartment lumbar plexus plus the lateral cutaneous nerve of the thigh).

- Perioperative blood transfusion is frequently required and blood loss can be substantial. Two units of cross-matched blood should be available in theatre with the ability to obtain more within 30 min.

Postoperative

- Mobilization varies with the complexity of the revision and the strength of the reconstruction. For pain relief an epidural infusion is useful for up to 3 days, if needed, or less if earlier mobilization is required. PCA is a suitable alternative.
- Supplemental oxygen is required, particularly in the case of significant blood loss or underlying cardiorespiratory disease.

Special considerations

Blood recovery and autologous transfusion using a Bratt device or similar is often practical.

Total knee replacement

Procedure	Prosthetic replacement of the knee joint
Time	1.5–2 h
Pain	++++/+++++
Position	Supine
Blood loss	Minimal with tourniquet, 250–300 ml without. G&S
Practical technique	LMA, combined sciatic/femoral blocks
	LMA, epidural or combined spinal/epidural or spinal/nerve blocks
	ET, IPPV with either of above or IV opioid

Similar patient population to hip surgery. Generally a shorter operation with less blood loss or cement hypotension. A tourniquet is commonly used. Postoperative pain can be extreme and must be anticipated.

Preoperative

As for hip surgery

Perioperative

- The patient is always supine and therefore airway control under sedation can be a problem.
- Combination femoral and sciatic nerve blocks give good postoperative analgesia and mobilization (see below). They are easiest to combine with light GA/LMA. An alternative is epidural/GA/LMA. If regional anaesthesia is not feasible a standard GA with postoperative PCA should be considered.
- A tourniquet is commonly used, therefore perioperative blood loss is not problematic, although expect to lose up to 500 ml (and frequently more) from the drains in the first hour postoperatively. There is a trend to reduce use of the tourniquet.
- If a tourniquet is used one may see 'breakthrough' of tourniquet pain after about 1 h causing CVS stimulation and hypertension. This is more common with leg blocks and is treated by deepening anaesthesia or adding IV narcotic. In some patients, labetalol may be useful.
- Ensure the patient is well preloaded before the tourniquet is released. A short-lived reperfusion event is common (fall in BP and SpO_2, rise in $ETCO_2$) and is usually best prevented by an infusion of fluid before and as the tourniquet is released.
- An arterial line is only necessary if CVS disease is significant.

Postoperative

- Postoperative pain is usually the most significant problem and this is the main determinant of the anaesthetic technique, as discussed below.
- When blood loss into the drains continues to be brisk after the first 500 ml the surgeon will often clamp the drains for a period of time.

Special considerations

* General anaesthesia supplemented by an epidural with postoperative epidural infusion is a common technique. Combined spinal/epidural or spinal/femoral and sciatic nerve blocks may avoid the need for GA. Spinal anaesthesia on its own is suitable for the operation but leaves the problem of postoperative pain. Epidural anaesthesia on its own may not provide adequately dense analgesia or optimal muscle relaxation for the surgery.

* Femoral and sciatic nerve blocks have the following advantages:

  * Good postoperative pain relief in the first 12–24 h. Supplement with regular NSAID and oral analgesics plus parenteral narcotic (PCA or IM).

  * Avoids the need for a urinary catheter.

  * Allows the patient more mobility in bed.

  * Avoids difficulties and complications of an epidural, including patchy block. When possible, perform blocks at least 30 min prior to surgery, to allow onset time for surgical anaesthesia. This technique usually gives very good postoperative pain relief but, even with early insertion, it is unusual for it to give adequate cover perioperatively for use with sedation alone. Usually it is combined with spinal or light GA.

* Patients undertake exercises in the operated leg at 24 h postoperatively and are mobilized out of bed at 48 h. Nerve blocks fit well with this requirement, although some surgeons believe that the epidural gives better analgesic cover for the exercises. If used, it needs to be removed prior to mobilization.

Revision of total knee replacement

Same as primary knee replacement except it takes longer, 2 h plus:

* The technique is as for primary knee replacement.

* If done without a tourniquet then two units of blood should be cross-matched.

Arthroscopic lower limb procedures

General principles

- The patient population is generally younger and fitter than those having joint replacements.
- Smaller procedures are done as day cases and therefore require a technique that allows early ambulation and discharge home. The main procedures undertaken are EUA, meniscal surgery or loose body removal, synovectomy, and ligament reconstruction.
- Virtually all are done on the knee, though arthroscopy is also performed on the shoulder (p. 495), ankle, elbow, and wrist.
- Many patients are current or ex-athletes, often football or rugby players, who can be surprisingly anxious. Anaesthesia induction may prove difficult —beware the obese, 'mature' rugby player who drinks heavily.

Arthroscopy with or without excision of cartilage

Procedure	Arthroscopy, EUA, and washout ± excision of torn cartilage, removal of loose body
Time	10–60 min
Pain	++
Position	Supine with leg over side of table
Blood loss	Nil
Practical technique	GA/LMA
	EUA ± washout can be performed under LA alone

Technique

- Premed with paracetamol and NSAIDs.
- LMA/GA, a 'standard' day case anaesthetic with IV narcotics.
- A tourniquet is often used.
- Prescribe NSAIDs and strong oral analgesics to take home.
- Many surgeons instil 10–20 ml of 0.5% bupivacaine ± morphine (10 mg) into the joint cavity for postoperative pain relief.
- Simple diagnostic/washout arthroscopies can be performed under local anaesthetic when necessary. Use 1% lidocaine (lignocaine) + adrenaline to portal sites + 20 ml bupivacaine 0.25–0.5% instilled into the joint. Wait for it to work. Tourniquets are not well tolerated for more than a few minutes. IV analgesia is occasionally required.

Synovectomy

Procedure	Arthroscopy with excision of synovial membrane
Time	1–1.5 h
Pain	+++
Position	Supine
Blood loss	Nil
Practical technique	LMA and GA with femoral block

Technique

- Takes up to 1.5 h and a tourniquet is used. There may be a 'breakthrough' of tourniquet pain after about 1 h.
- There is significant pain postoperatively.
- Spontaneous breathing GA with LMA. Add IV narcotic and NSAID and prescribe intermittent narcotics and NSAID postoperatively together with oral analgesics.
- A femoral nerve block significantly reduces postoperative pain.

Cruciate ligament repair

Procedure	Arthroscopic reconstruction of anterior cruciate ligament using patellar tendon ± hamstrings
Time	1.5–2 h
Pain	+++/++++
Position	Supine
Blood loss	Nil
Practical technique	Patellar tendon repair only: LMA + GA with femoral block
	Patellar tendon and hamstring repair: LMA + GA with combined femoral/sciatic blocks
	GA + PCA

Technique

- These operations are of two main types: using the patellar tendon only for the repair and using both the patellar tendon and hamstring ligaments.
- Usually about 12 h of fairly dense analgesia is required prior to mobilization.
- If the patellar tendon only is used postoperative pain is less of a problem and a femoral nerve block is very effective for 12–24 h.
- If the hamstrings are used, the operation takes longer and there is more postoperative pain. Consider GA + femoral and sciatic nerve blocks performed prior to induction.
- Use weaker concentrations of bupivacaine (0.125–0.25%) if considering nerve blocks, so that mobilization/discharge is not delayed.
- Alternatively, combine LMA/femoral nerve block/PCA.

Ankle surgery

General principles

- Four main types of procedure: tendon transfers, open reduction and internal fixation (ORIF) of fractures, joint arthrodesis, and prosthetic joint replacement.

- Ankle arthrodesis takes 1 to 2 h. Tendon transfer is generally shorter than this and joint replacement may be longer. ORIF is variable depending on the fracture; check with the surgeon and add 30 min to this time for cleaning/draping and for application of POP at the end.

- Joint arthrodesis and replacement involve a more elderly patient population.

- These operations are amenable to regional anaesthetic techniques, either alone or, more often, as a supplement to a GA.

- Tourniquets are often used and tourniquet pain has to be considered.

- Patients may be supine or prone or, occasionally, on their side.

- In the case of ORIF following trauma, surgery may need to be undertaken urgently if distal circulation is compromised. Beware of the risk of aspiration from a full stomach and also take time to ensure that any other significant injury has been properly considered and dealt with.

- If regional block is considered for ORIF, check that there is no concern about the development of compartment syndrome postoperatively as the symptoms will be masked by the block (see p. 463).

Technique

- Tendon transfers last up to 1 h and are not particularly painful postoperatively. Use an LMA + GA and supplement with IV narcotics and an NSAID. Ask the surgeon to infiltrate LA around the surgical site.

- ORIF can be done in the same way if the patient is starved. If not, then a rapid sequence induction and ETT is needed for a GA.

- A good alternative for the ORIF and any major tendon transfer is a spinal, usually with sedation. The addition of intrathecal narcotic (e.g. diamorphine 0.1–0.25 mg) prolongs the period of analgesia but it is best avoided in the elderly.

- Arthrodesis is more painful postoperatively which limits the value of spinal anaesthesia unless followed with PCA. A good choice of technique is a sciatic nerve block, usually with LMA + GA, though it can be performed with sedation alone if the block is adequate (perform block at least 40 min prior to incision). If undertaken without GA, combine with a femoral nerve block as the saphenous nerve (terminal branch of the femoral nerve) supplies skin down to the medial malleolus of the ankle. Using a tourniquet at the level of the calf reduces the problem of breakthrough tourniquet pain.

- Ankle joint replacement is currently carried out in only a few centres. Check with the surgeon how long they expect to be. GA with sciatic block is practical.

Procedure	Time	Pain (+ to +++++)	Position	Blood loss	Practical technique
Tendon transfer/repair	Approx. 1 h	++	Supine (ruptured tendo-achilles — prone)	Nil with tourniquet	LMA + GA with infiltration of LA by surgeon Spinal if supine
ORIF of ankle fracture	Variable, 1.5–2 h	++/+++	Supine, occasionally on side or prone	Nil with tourniquet	If starved, LMA + GA; if not RSI and ETT + GA Spinal
Arthrodesis of ankle joint	1.5–2 h	+++	Supine	Nil with tourniquet	LMA + GA with sciatic nerve block or postop. PCA Spinal
Prosthetic replacement of ankle joint	2 h plus	++/+++	Supine	Nil with tourniquet	Sciatic nerve block with LMA + GA Spinal

Foot surgery

General principles

* Most operations are on the forefoot and toes, e.g. first metatarsal osteotomy, Keller's operation for removal of bunions, excision of ingrowing toenails, and terminalization of toes. Other operations are in the midfoot, such as tendon transfers and some osteotomies.
* The patient population varies and many are elderly. Those for terminalization of toes may well have concomitant problems such as diabetes and/or CVS disease.
* Osteotomies tend to be painful postoperatively.
* Surgical time is 30 min to 1 h.
* Many are done as day cases and require early ambulation and discharge with adequate pain relief.
* Many operations are amenable to regional anaesthesia. Nerve blocks make a valuable contribution to postoperative analgesia, particularly in osteotomies or excision of the nail bed, and promote early ambulation of day cases. However, onset time is relatively long and they need to be performed a full 40 min prior to surgery if planned without supplemental GA. With experience this can be made to work well but, for the less experienced or if the logistics do not allow it, it is best to undertake them primarily for postoperative pain relief in combination with LMA and GA.
* Adrenaline must not be used for 'ring' or 'web-space' blocks and is best avoided in ankle blocks if peripheral circulation is poor.
* Breakthrough pain from the tourniquet can be a problem, especially if surgery is longer than 45 min. Place the tourniquet as distally as possible to reduce this effect.
* Excision of the nail bed is painful perioperatively and requires a relatively deep GA if not supplemented with a nerve block.

Technique

* Regional blocks useful for foot surgery include ring or web-space or ankle blocks for toe surgery, ankle block for forefoot surgery and sciatic nerve block for operations on the midfoot. Most commonly these blocks are performed for postoperative pain relief and are combined with GA.
* An alternative in all cases is spinal anaesthesia.

Site	Procedure	Time (min)	Pain (+ to +++++)	Position	Blood loss/ X-match	Technique
Toes	Excision of nail bed, terminalization	30 min	+++	Supine	Nil	Ring or toe web-block with sedation or LMA/GA
Forefoot	Tendon transfers	30–60	+/++	Supine	Nil	LMA/GA + local infiltration
						Ankle block with sedation or LMA/GA
Forefoot	First metatarsal osteotomy, Keller's op. for bunions	30–60	+++	Supine	Nil	LMA/GA with ankle block or infiltration
Midfoot	Tendon transfers	30–60	+/++	Supine	Nil	LMA/GA + local infiltration
Midfoot	Osteotomy	30–60	+++	Supine	Nil	LMA/GA ± sciatic nerve block at knee

Spinal surgery

Definition

- Surgery on the spinal column between the atlanto-occipital junction and the coccyx.
- May be performed by orthopaedic or neurosurgeons depending on expertise.
- Can be loosely divided into four categories:
  - decompression of the spinal cord and nerves
  - stabilization and correction of spinal deformity
  - excision of spinal tumours
  - trauma.

General principles

- May be performed on patients of all ages and all states of fitness. Frequently includes children for scoliosis surgery, young and middle-aged adults for decompression surgery, and older patients with degenerative bone and joint disease in need of stabilization.
- Most procedures are in the prone position although anterior and lateral approaches are used. Some procedures will involve turning the patient during the operation.
- Airway access will be limited during surgery and so must be secure prior to starting.
- Excessive abdominal or thoracic pressure due to incorrect patient positioning may compromise ventilation and circulation. This must be corrected at the outset.
- Surgical blood loss can be considerable and difficult to control due to difficult surgical access. Good vascular access, accurate monitoring of fluid balance and suitable replacement fluids must be established before surgery starts.
- Long procedures necessitate active prevention of heat loss.
- Assessment of spinal function may be required during the procedure.

The prone position

A specially designed mattress allowing unhindered movement of the abdomen and chest (e.g. a Montreal mattress) should be used to minimize complications as outlined below:

- Turning the patient from prone to supine is a team event and requires formal training. The principle of 'log rolling' is used to avoid applying twisting forces in the axial plane. This is especially important for the poorly supported cervical spine, which may be unstable due to fractures or degenerative disease. The surgeon should be present as part of the team for this manoeuvre.
- Pressure on the abdomen applies pressure to the diaphragm and increases intrathoracic pressure, which in turn decreases thoracic compliance. This can lead to basal atelectasis and the need for higher lung inflation pressures, particularly in obese patients.

- Raised intra-abdominal pressure also compresses veins and decreases venous return, which may result in hypotension or increased venous bleeding from the surgical site.

- Accurate assessment of the circulation with invasive arterial monitoring and an indwelling urinary catheter is recommended for all major procedures.

- Major spinal surgery may be relatively contraindicated in obese patients and those with severe cardiorespiratory disease.

- Peripheral pressure areas are at particular risk in the prone position. Pillows and silicone pads should be used judiciously to protect all areas. Ensure that the breasts and genitalia are not trapped. During long cases it may be necessary to move the patient's limbs and head every hour to avoid stagnation of peripheral blood and the development of pressure necrosis. Pay particular attention to the nose, chin, elbows, knees, and ankles.

- The arms are usually placed 'above the head' which puts the brachial plexus at risk of stretching or being pressed against the mattress. Ensure that the axillae are not under tension after positioning.

Anaesthesia

- Plans for the recovery period should be made in advance and will be dictated by local experience. Long cases, those involving excessive blood loss, and major paediatric cases will need postoperative care in the HDU. Few patients require postoperative ventilatory support.

- Secure venous access is vital. It may be difficult to access the cannula so an extension with a three-way tap is recommended. Insert two cannulas if access is difficult, if significant blood loss is expected, or if drug infusions are required during or after the procedure (TIVA, PCA).

- Choice of anaesthetic will be dictated by personal experience but most will choose an intravenous induction with muscle relaxation and opioid supplementation. Both low-flow volatile anaesthesia and TIVA are frequently used. Short-acting agents are preferred to enable rapid assessment of neurological function at the end of surgery.

- If spinal cord integrity is at risk during surgery, it may be necessary to use spinal cord monitoring. This is a specialist service provided by a neurophysiologist but will require that muscle relaxation is allowed to wear off. It may be necessary to deepen anaesthesia during this phase, but in reality this is rarely a problem. This technique has generally superseded the 'wake up test' when patients were woken in the middle of surgery and asked to perform simple motor functions before being reanaesthetized.

- In patients with paraplegia or other large areas of muscle denervation (2 days–8 months), suxamethonium should be avoided (p. 180).

- Airway access is likely to be limited once the procedure has started, so secure oral endotracheal intubation with a non-kinking tube. Patients with unstable necks due to trauma or rheumatoid arthritis can be intubated using awake fibreoptic intubation or with manual in-line stabilization depending on the degree of instability. The tube should be moulded around the face with no bulky joints adjacent to the skin. A throat pack may be used to decrease the flow of secretions onto the pillow and the tube then secured with adhesive tape or film. Attention to detail and the use of padding is vital to ensure no pressure areas can form.

- Some centres advocate self-positioning by awake patients in order to minimize pressure problems. Regional anaesthesia with intravenous sedation without the need for airway support is then used.

- Most patients will be paralysed and ventilated for these procedures with positional considerations noted above. Check that ventilation is adequate without excessive inflation pressures before surgery starts, as the only recourse may be to return the patient to the supine position during surgery if problems develop.Check the position of the endotracheal tube when the patient has been turned.

- Blood loss may be significant, with venous oozing proving hard to control. The use of cell salvage techniques (see p. 917) is advisable for long procedures involving instrumentation of multiple levels. All patients should have samples grouped and saved and more major procedures should have blood cross-matched even if cell salvage is employed (see below).

- Moderate hypotension may help to reduce bleeding.

- Air embolism is a potential complication if large veins are exposed in under-filled patients. It may be heralded by sudden cardiovascular collapse and loss of the $ETCO_2$ trace (see p. 418).

- Prophylactic antibiotics will be prescribed for any procedure involving instrumentation or bone grafting. This will be dictated by local policy.

- The type of analgesia required will vary depending on the magnitude of surgery. Minor procedures (e.g. microdiscectomy) may manage with NSAIDs alone in association with infiltration of the site of operation with local anaesthetic. Most procedures will necessitate opioids. PCA morphine is effective after adequate intravenous loading. The use of regional analgesia is encouraged where there is no need to assess neurological function, and the use of epidural and paravertebral analgesia is growing in popularity for major procedures such as correction of scoliosis. The catheter is usually placed by the surgeon at the end of the procedure and infusions of local anaesthetic or opiates continued for several days postoperatively.

- Effective analgesia is particularly important for surgery to the thoracic spine where postoperative respiratory function will be compromised if analgesia is inadequate. Consider using incentive spirometry and chest physiotherapy.

Summary of spinal surgery procedures

Operation	Description	Time (h)	Position	Blood loss/X-match	Pain (+ to +++++)	Notes
Discectomy or microdiscectomy	Excision of herniated intervertebral disc	1–2	Prone	Not significant	+/++	Microdiscectomy can be done as day case
Cervical discectomy	Excision of herniated cervical intervertebral disc	2	Prone/head on horseshoe or halo traction pins	Not significant	++/+++	May be an emergency with neurological deficit
Spinal fusion ± decompression	Correction of spondylolisthesis or spinal stenosis for pain or instability—often several levels	1–2 (then 1 per level)	Prone	500–2000 ml, X-match 4 units	+++/+++++	Usually elderly. May take bone graft from pelvis. Metal instrumentation
Cervical fusion ± decompression	Fusion of unstable neck (e.g. arthritis, trauma)	2–3	Supine or prone. Cervical traction in place or applied at start	300–1000 ml, G&S	++/+++	Neck can be very unstable and need awake fibreoptic intubation. Application of traction pins very stimulating
Excision of spinal tumour (e.g. vertebrectomy)	Tumours may be primary or secondary from any part of the spine	2–6+	Supine, prone or lateral tilt	Potentially massive, X-match 6 units + clotting factors available	+++/+++++	Often difficult surgery with potential for excessive blood loss and neurological damage

Operation	Description	Time (h)	Position	Blood loss/ X-match	Pain (+ to +++++)	Notes
Kyphoscoliosis surgery	Correction of major spinal deformities in patients who may have severe physical disability	3–6+	Supine and /or prone	Potentially massive, X-match 6 units + clotting factors available	+++/+++++	Often in children which severe restrictive respiratory disease and coexisting abnormalities. May involve surgery in abdominal and thoracic cavities. Spinal nerve monitoring used in some centres. Massive instrumentation sometimes used. May need postop. ICU for IPPV
Repair of vertebral fracture	Repaired for neurological deficit or instability	2–6	Supine and /or prone	500–2000 ml, X-match 4 units	++/++++	Often associated with other major injury (esp. rib fracture). May be in ICU/IPPV. Neurological deficit often not reversible. NB: suxamethonium may be contraindicated

Shoulder surgery

Shoulder surgery is performed on a range of patients from fit athletes with recurrent dislocation, to the severe rheumatoid with multiple joint replacements and severe systemic disease.

General considerations

Soft tissue operations around the shoulder are often extremely painful. This pain is not predictable and may last for several days, although it is certainly worst within the first 2 days.

Anaesthesia

- The patient is usually positioned with the head distal to the anaesthetist requiring particular attention to the security of the airway. It is often easier to intubate the patient (south-facing RAE or armoured tube) except for shorter procedures where an LMA may be suitable. Long ventilator and gas sampling tubes are required.
- Venous access should be placed in the opposite arm (with a long extension) or at the ankle/foot.
- The patient may be placed supine with head up tilt, lateral, or in a deck-chair position. Repeated measurement of the blood pressure will detect falls due to head up positioning and some patients require increments of vaso-pressors when positioning. When using steep head up tilt in patients with compromised cardiovascular function, change posture slowly and consider direct arterial pressure monitoring.
- When the patient is placed in the lateral position the BP can be measured in the lower arm or in the ankle. When using ankle pressure:
  - the cuff should be of the correct size
  - a control measurement should be taken in the anaesthetic room and compared with the arm before induction of anaesthesia
  - account should be taken of the difference in vertical height from the blood pressure cuff to the head when estimating cerebral perfusion pressure.
- Although blood loss is rarely significant, patients may be unable to take oral fluids for some hours postoperatively.
- Regional anaesthesia is a useful adjunct in shoulder anaesthesia and an interscalene block is the method of choice (p. 1012). Although procedures may be performed under regional anaesthesia alone, local anaesthetic is more commonly used to supplement general anaesthesia and to provide postoperative analgesia. When planning an interscalene block, inform the patient that their whole arm may go numb, and that they may sense that full inspiration is not possible when they wake up (phrenic nerve paralysis). Interscalene block is contraindicated in patients with contralateral phrenic nerve/diaphragmatic palsy, or recurrent laryngeal nerve damage. Inter-scalene catheters can be used for prolonged postoperative analgesia.
- When an interscalene block is impractical infiltration of local anaesthetics in reasonable quantities by the surgeon may also provide postoperative analgesia. This is particularly effective in Bankart's and capsular shift operations.

- For rotator cuff repairs an epidural catheter, placed during surgery over the repair, can be used to supplement postoperative analgesia. Regular boluses (10 ml 0.25% bupivacaine 2–4 hourly) appears to work better than a continuous infusion.
- Potent analgesia is often required for 1–2 days. The combination of PCA opioid/NSAIDs/paracetamol is usually effective. Good posture (sitting up with the elbow supported on a pillow) is also important.

Further reading

Harrop-Griffiths W and Dwyer S (1999). Anaesthesia and analgesia for shoulder arthroplasty. In *Shoulder arthroplasty* (eds. G. Walch and P. Boilean). Springer Verlag, Berlin.

Total shoulder replacement

Procedure	Prosthetic shoulder replacement
Time	2–3 h
Pain	+++/++++
Position	Supine, head up, or deckchair
Blood loss	250–500 ml
Practical technique	ET + IPPV, interscalene block

Preoperative

- Many patients are elderly, severe rheumatoid disease is common
- Ask about respiratory function/reserve if planning an interscalene block (some diaphragmatic function will be lost for several hours).
- Check the airway (particularly in rheumatoid arthritis) and range of neck movement. Some patients will need fibreoptic intubation.

Perioperative

- Consider performing an interscalene block before inducing anaesthesia (see p. 1012).
- Measure blood pressure and place intravenous infusion on the opposite arm with a long extension.
- Intubate with a preformed 'south-facing' ETT.
- Hypotension is common when changing to head up position. Ephedrine (6 mg IV) is usually effective with fluid loading.
- If interscalene block has been performed, anaesthesia is usually unremarkable. Sometimes breakthrough stimulation occurs during the glenoid phase (also receives fibres from T2 which are not always covered by the block).
- If no interscalene block, load the patient with morphine and ask the surgeon to infiltrate with local anaesthetic (20–30 ml of 0.25% bupivacaine).
- Antibiotic prophylaxis.
- Monitor neuromuscular function at the lateral peroneal nerve.

Postoperative

- Pain is worst in the first 24 h postoperatively. PCA/intermittent morphine are usually satisfactory.
- NSAIDs are useful.

Special considerations

- Air/fat embolism is a rare event.
- In poor-risk patients direct arterial monitoring is advised.

Other shoulder operations

- Most shoulder surgery may be carried out using the anaesthetic guidelines above. Arthroscopic surgery is generally less painful and patients get effective postoperative analgesia if the surgeon instils 10–20 ml bupivacaine 0.5% within the joint space at the end of surgery.

- Bankart's and capsular shift operations for recurrent dislocations are more painful for larger, muscular patients but not generally as painful as cuff repairs or open acromioplasties.

- Massive cuff repairs are often extremely painful and an interscalene block is useful. PCA should be considered and a loading dose of morphine should be administered during surgery. Consider interscalene catheter with infusion of LA.

- Pain following any operation around the shoulder is unpredictable and some patients who have had short procedures suffer severe pain for several days. A flexible approach is required for analgesia.

- Beware the pain free patient following major shoulder surgery and connected to PCA morphine. When the regional block wears off, effective analgesia may take some time to establish.

Other shoulder procedures

Operation	Description	Time (min)	Pain (+ to +++++)	Position	Blood loss	Notes
Shoulder cuff repair	Repair of supraspinatus tendon	60–120	++/+++++	Lateral, supine, or deck chair	ns	Consider catheter for LA infiltration/interscalene block
Massive shoulder cuff repair	As above but more extensive	120–180	+++/++++++	Lateral, supine, or deck chair	ns	Consider catheter for LA infiltration/interscalene block
Subacromial decompression	Resection of acromion	60	++/+++++	Lateral, supine, or deck chair	ns	
Mumford's operation	Resection of acromioclavicular joint	60	++/+++++	Lateral, supine, or deck chair	ns	
Weaver–Dunn	Re-forming acromio-clavicular joint	60	++/+++	Supine	ns	
Capsular shift	Tightening of shoulder joint capsule	120	++/+++	Supine	ns	
Bankart's procedure	Tightening of shoulder joint capsule	120	++/+++	Supine	ns	
MUA for frozen shoulder	MUA to release frozen shoulder adhesions	5	+/+++	Supine	ns	LA in shoulder joint effective
Ozaki release	Open operation to release frozen shoulder	30	+/+++	Lateral, supine	ns	
Arthroscopic surgery	Diagnostic, decompression, acromioplasty, or shoulder cuff	30–120	+/+++	Lateral, deck chair	ns	LA in shoulder joint effective

ns = not significant

Hand surgery

- Hand and wrist surgery is carried out on a wide range of patients from the child with congenital defects to the severe rheumatoid with multiple medical problems.
- The majority of hand surgery procedures are suitable for local anaesthesia day surgery as the hand and wrist are relatively easy to anaesthetize with local or regional techniques, providing intra- and postoperative analgesia. The option of general anaesthesia or additional sedation is based on personal preference and specific indications/contraindications.
- Many anaesthetists use GA and either wrist block or surgical LA infiltration very successfully.
- An upper arm tourniquet is almost always used for any type of hand surgery with the possible exception of surgery for vascular insufficiency.
- Some procedures such as carpal tunnel release or trigger finger release can be done under local infiltration alone.
- Intravenous regional anaesthesia (IVRA) is suitable for procedures below the elbow of 30 min or less. It has the disadvantage of not having any postoperative analgesia. Prilocaine is the agent of choice.
- Local anaesthetic injection into tight tissue planes such as the palm or carpal tunnel may be very painful. The pain can be reduced by warming the local anaesthetic to body temperature and slow injection through a fine needle.

Advantages of regional techniques in hand surgery

- Ability to avoid opioids and deeper levels of anaesthesia (or anaesthesia altogether) to facilitate early discharge from hospital.
- When prolonged analgesia is required for postoperative physiotherapy: axillary or infraclavicular brachial plexus catheter techniques are the easiest and most reliable for hand surgery.
- When prolonged sympathectomy is required following vascular anastamoses, e.g. finger reimplantation, free-flap recipient site, etc.
- Paediatric upper limb surgery is a relative indication because of the excellent postoperative analgesia.

Contraindications to regional anaesthesia in hand surgery

- Lack of informed consent.
- Anticoagulated or coagulopathy when the bleeding may compromise vascular or neurological structures.
- Where anaesthesia will abolish postoperative clinical signs such as compartment syndrome.
- Infection over the site of needle insertion or malignant lymph nodes in the axilla or supraclavicular area.

Tourniquet

- Positioning and duration of use will be an important determinant of whether the patient is able to tolerate regional or local anaesthesia alone.

- Patients with a good brachial plexus block will usually tolerate 60 to 90 min of arm ischaemia.
- A wrist tourniquet is said to be less painful than an arm tourniquet. If a tourniquet time of greater than 90 min is planned then simultaneous wrist and arm tourniquets can be used. When ischaemic pain becomes a problem the other tourniquet is inflated and the original one deflated.
- Blood loss is rarely a consideration because of the use of the tourniquet.

Anaesthesia for hand surgery

Procedure	Various—see table
Time	20 min–2 h
Pain	+/+++
Position	Supine, arm out on table
Blood loss	Minimal
Practical technique	Regional analgesia ± LMA and SV. Tourniquet

Preoperative

- Full assessment as for GA, both because the patient may want a GA and regional anaesthesia may fail.
- Patients are often old, frail, and with systemic disease such as rheumatoid arthritis.
- Check that patients can lie flat for the proposed duration of operation, if planned to be awake.
- Assess movement of the operative arm. Can the patient achieve the necessary position for regional block or the surgery planned?

Perioperative

- Make sure the patient's bladder is empty!
- Use full monitoring whether or not GA/sedation is to be used.
- Perform local block with the patient awake or lightly sedated.
- Provide sedation or GA depending on safety and the patient's wishes. Have equipment and drugs ready to convert to sedation or GA if necessary during the operation.

Postoperative

- Surgery involving soft tissues and skin is generally less painful than surgery to the bones and joints.
- NSAIDs and paracetamol/codeine combinations are usually adequate for the less painful procedures. Opioids or regional catheter techniques may be required for the more painful.

Special considerations

- Some patients dislike the postoperative 'dead arm' after brachial plexus block. Mid humeral blocks allow the injection of different concentrations and different types of local anaesthetics to be placed around different proximal nerves. This differential block allows for recovery of movement and sensation in the non-operative area.
- Interscalene blocks are poor for hand surgery, often missing the ulnar border if not all the hand.

- Supraclavicular blocks are reliable, fast-onset blocks for the experienced practitioner, but carry a risk of pneumothorax and are not suitable for day case patients.
- Axillary blocks are less reliable and slower in onset. The musculocutaneous nerve is missed in this approach and must be blocked separately if innervating the site of surgery. The radial nerve may also be missed, as it lies lateral to (behind) the radial artery in the axilla.
- The ability to augment plexus anaesthesia with elbow or wrist blocks is essential to improve success rates.
- Tourniquet pain can be reduced by blocking the intercostobrachial nerve subcutaneously on the medial aspect of the upper arm above the level of the tourniquet.
- Adrenaline-containing solutions should be avoided near digits.

Other hand surgical procedures

Operation	Description	Time (min)	Pain (+ to +++++)	Position	Blood loss	Notes
Trigger finger release and carpal tunnel release		5–15	+	Supine with arm abducted	Minimal	These procedures can usually be carried out under local infiltration anaesthesia
Dupuytren's contractures (simple)	Usually confined to ulnar border or ulnar and median distribution. Usually less than 30 min tourniquet time	<60	+	Supine with arm abducted	Minimal	GA with wrist block or infiltration. Brachial plexus block with upper arm tourniquet ± GA. Quick procedure: wrist block with wrist tourniquet
Dupuytren's contracture (complex)	Severe disease or redo procedure may need skin grafting	60–120	+	Supine with arm abducted	Minimal	Prolonged tourniquet time means that a brachial plexus block or a GA with local block is often required
Swanson's joint replacement	MP joint replacement usually for rheumatoid.	30 per joint	++/+++	Supine with arm abducted	Minimal	Generally frailer patients with systemic disease
Tenolysis, capsulotomies, tendon grafts	These procedures may need patient participation to assess the adequacy of the procedure	15–60	+/++	Supine with arm abducted	Minimal	If hand movement is required then any block must be distal. A wrist block with sedation is usually adequate

Operation	Description	Time (min)	Pain (+ to +++++)	Position	Blood loss	Notes
Digit reimplantation	Microvascular surgery	Hours	++	Supine with arm abducted	Minimal	Regional anaesthesia for the sympathectomy is helpful. A GA is usually required because of the prolonged procedure.
Ulnar head excision or trapeziectomy	Surgery for wrist pain in rheumatoid disease	30–60	++/+++	Supine with arm abducted	Minimal	As pain is severe a single-shot brachial block or catheter technique is ideal with or without a GA

Chapter 22
Ear, nose, and throat surgery

Fred Roberts

General principles

Airway safety dominates all other considerations in ear, nose, and throat (ENT) surgery. The surgeon and anaesthetist share the airway, with access for the anaesthetist (both visual and physical) limited by drapes and instruments. The added problems of the underlying pathology and bleeding into the airway during or after surgery may also endanger the airway.

Planning and communication are essential to ensure that the techniques and equipment used by the surgeon and anaesthetist dovetail to provide good conditions for surgery whilst maintaining a safe, secure airway for the patient. Whenever a problem with the airway is suspected intra-operatively, correcting it is the first priority and the surgery must stop to allow this to be done.

Despite the widespread introduction of sophisticated monitoring, many ENT anaesthetists still regard movement of the reservoir bag with spontaneous respiration as an invaluable sign of airway integrity and favour this anaesthetic technique accordingly. To achieve intubation for spontaneous respiration, suxamethonium produces good conditions most reliably, but its side-effects can be troublesome, particularly myalgia in a patient population where early ambulation is likely. Alternatives commonly used include mivacurium, propofol, alfentanil remifentanil bolus or deep inhalational anaesthesia.

Airway management

Airway management during anaesthesia

- Traditionally an endotracheal tube (ETT) has been used for the majority of ENT work, providing airway patency and protection from aspiration of blood or surgical debris.
- Many different tubes and connectors have been designed for this, but the most widely used now are the preformed RAE tubes, originally described by Ring, Adair, and Elwyn.
- For nasal and much oral surgery an oral (south-facing) RAE tube is used, although a nasal tube (north-facing) allows easier surgical access to the oral cavity.
- A recent trend has been the use of the laryngeal mask airway (LMA), usually of the reinforced, flexible type. It appears to offer good protection against aspiration of blood or surgical material and avoids many of the problems associated with tracheal intubation. However, surgical access is restricted to a somewhat greater degree and it is more prone to displacement during surgery, with potentially catastrophic results.

Airway management at extubation

- Many ENT procedures create bleeding into the airway. It is a sensible precaution to perform careful laryngoscopy and suctioning before extubation in all cases following intraoral or nasal surgery, to ensure that the airway is clear of blood and any throat packs removed. Care must be taken not to traumatize any surgical sites during suction.
- One particular danger site for the accumulation of blood is behind the soft palate in the nasopharynx. This area is not readily visible and blood pooling here can be aspirated following extubation, with fatal results ("Coroner's clot"). This area is best cleared either by using a soft suction catheter via the nose or by rotating a Yankauer sucker so that its angled tip is placed behind the uvula.
- Irritation of the larynx by blood or from recent instrumentation can lead to coughing or laryngospasm following extubation, particularly in children.
- The traditional method for reducing this is deep extubation, a technique particularly suited to anaesthesia using spontaneous respiration. Anaesthesia is deepened at the end of surgery by increasing the concentration of volatile agent, whilst discontinuing nitrous oxide (to increase the oxygen store in the FRC).
- After careful suction a Guedel airway is inserted, the patient turned into the left lateral/head down (tonsil) position and extubated when respiration is regular. If turning the patient leads to coughing or breath holding, wait until regular respiration has returned before extubating. The patient must be kept in this position until airway reflexes return. In small children, the use of a pillow under the chest may be easier to provide the necessary postural drainage.
- If suction of the airway is necessary during the early recovery period, this can be done using a catheter left just protruding from the Guedel airway on

continuous low suction, taking care not to advance the catheter too far, which could lead to laryngospasm from irritation of the larynx.

- The major risk of using deep extubation is that of airway complications during the recovery phase, such as obstruction, laryngospasm, aspiration of blood, or even asphyxiation from large clots. If the technique is to be used, therefore, it is essential that high-quality recovery care is available.

- The alternative to deep extubation is to extubate the patient after laryngeal reflexes have returned. This approach, light extubation, is being used increasingly and is the method of choice in patients with a difficult airway. Light extubation is better suited to an IPPV-relaxant anaesthetic rather than a spontaneous breathing technique, which often leads to a substantial period of coughing and breath holding during the emergence period before extubation.

Preoperative airway obstruction

(see also p. 870)

Assessment

- Patients with preoperative airway obstruction usually present for surgery either to establish the diagnosis or to relieve the obstruction.

- The most common level for obstruction is the larynx, producing stridor (high-pitched, inspiratory noise) and markedly reduced exercise tolerance. Laryngeal obstruction may be classified as supraglottic, glottic, or subglottic.

- In adults, tumours are the commonest cause of upper airway obstruction, though haematoma or infection (including epiglottitis) is also possible. In children, infection (croup/epiglottitis) or foreign body is more likely.

- Extreme airway obstruction will cause obvious signs of respiratory distress at rest. Exhaustion and an obtunded level of consciousness are preterminal signs and, if present, immediate action must be taken to secure the airway.

- With less severe disease patients can compensate for airway obstruction very effectively (particularly if it develops slowly) and moderately severe obstruction can develop without gross physical signs being present. Features which may help to recognize a substantial degree of upper airway obstruction include:
  - a respiratory pattern with long, slow inspirations (even at rest) and associated pauses in speech
  - worsening stridor during sleep (history from spouse/night nursing staff) or exercise
  - quiet stridor may be heard much more clearly as a transmitted sound on chest auscultation.

- Lesions of the oropharynx may produce airway difficulties during anaesthesia, but rarely present as a life-threatening airway problem and their assessment is normally straightforward during the preoperative examination. The important features are the extent of limitation of mouth opening and tongue protrusion, along with the identification of any large masses that may compromise the airway.

- Other information to help the anaesthetist assess the airway may come from radiographs (plain films or CT/MRI) or an ENT clinic flexible or indirect laryngoscopy.

Management

- For the majority of patients presenting with upper airway problems, surgery will be undertaken as a planned procedure, but emergency intervention to secure the airway may be needed for life-threatening airway obstruction.

- In emergency cases, undue delays in getting the patient to theatre must be avoided. Whilst theatre is being prepared helium can be used by facemask to improve flow past the obstruction, its low density being favourable for turbulent flow. Although medical helium is premixed with oxygen, the FiO_2 is only 0.21 and additional oxygen should be used via a Y connector. Helium should only be used if it is readily available and its use must not delay the definitive airway management in theatre.

- The main problems for the anaesthetist in securing airway access are:
  - Pre-existing airway obstruction is likely to be worsened by lying the patient flat, by instrumenting the larynx, or by the use of general anaesthesia (whichever technique is used).
  - Identifying the laryngeal inlet may be difficult because of anatomical distortion (especially with supraglottic lesions).
  - Severe stenosis may limit intubation (particularly with malignant lesions at a glottic or subglottic level).
- There is little evidence to prove the benefits of any one particular anaesthetic technique. However, the use of intravenous induction agents or muscle relaxants carries the catastrophic risk of 'can't intubate/can't ventilate' in a patient unable to breath spontaneously.
- The three main options recommended for establishing secure airway access are:
  - Tracheal intubation under deep inhalational general anaesthesia using halothane or sevoflurane and direct laryngoscopy.
  - Tracheal intubation under local anaesthesia using fibreoptic laryngoscopy.
  - Tracheostomy under local anaesthesia (or under deep inhalational general anaesthesia with face mask or LMA in less severe cases).

  Mason and Fielder[1] reviewed the merits of each technique for airway obstruction at different levels, but none provides a certain, safe, and easy way to secure the airway and each represents a major challenge to the skills of those involved.
- The final decision in each case will be strongly influenced by the particular skills and experience of the anaesthetist and surgeon concerned.
- In children, deep inhalational anaesthesia is the only realistic option. Delays in getting to theatre must be avoided because of rapid and unpredictable decline in condition. To minimize upset in a small child, IV cannulation should be delayed until after induction, which is usually best done with the child sitting, being comforted by a parent. A moderate degree of CPAP is very effective at keeping the airway patent as anaesthesia deepens. Once deep, and if stable, local anaesthetic spray to the larynx can be helpful in extending the available time for laryngoscopy before airway reflexes return. In epiglottitis, distortion of the epiglottis can make recognition of the glottis very difficult; a useful aid is to press on the child's chest and watch for a bubble of gas emerging from the larynx.
- Whichever technique is used, a full range of equipment should be prepared, including different laryngoscopes, cricothyroidotomy kit, and tubes in various sizes. An endotracheal tube kept on ice will be stiffer and may be useful to get past an obstructing lesion.
- If complete airway obstruction occurs and all conventional attempts to secure the airway fail, emergency surgical access to the airway is the only option. Cricothyroidotomy is preferable to tracheostomy for emergency airway access, as it is quicker to perform, more superficial, and less likely to bleed (above the thyroid gland). (See p. 852).
- In adults awake fibreoptic intubation may be difficult with stenotic lesions as the airway may be completely blocked by the scope during the procedure.

1   Mason RA, Fielder CP (1999). The obstructed airway in head and neck surgery. *Anaesthesia*, **54**, 625–8.

Obstructive sleep apnoea and ENT surgery (see also p. 67)

• Obstructive sleep apnoea (OSA)[2] is the most common form of sleep apnoea syndrome. The airway obstructs intermittently during sleep because of inadequate muscle tone and coordination in the pharynx, the problem usually occurring in association with other factors such as obesity.

• OSA may be encountered as an incidental feature in any setting, but in ENT patients may specifically present for operations to improve known OSA.

• In adults surgery for OSA may include nasal operations or uvulopalato-pharyngoplasty (UPPP), although the role of UPPP in OSA is controversial as it may render the best treatment for OSA, nasal CPAP, less effective in the long term.

• In children OSA usually results from extreme adenotonsillar hypertrophy, and adenotonsillectomy is performed to relieve this.[3]

• Rather than the partial obstruction of simple snoring, OSA produces total obstruction and repeated episodes of hypoxia, leading to arousal (though not awakening) and subsequent re-establishment of airway patency. Multiple episodes can occur each night, with oxygen saturation values falling repeatedly to below 50% in severe cases.

• The repeated interruptions in normal sleep pattern produce daytime lethargy and somnolence whilst the extensive nocturnal hypoxia can lead to pulmonary or systemic hypertension with associated ventricular hyper-trophy and cardiac failure.

• A careful history (from the partner or parent) is the most valuable informa-tion initially. In OSA snoring is interrupted by periods of silent apnoea broken by a 'heroic' deep breath.

• Sleep studies reveal the extent of apnoeas and associated hypoxaemia and will normally already have been done in patients with known or suspected OSA. If the history unexpectedly gives a clear picture of OSA the patient should be referred for sleep studies preoperatively unless surgical urgency dictates otherwise.

• In children with suspected OSA, features of chronic hypoxaemia should be sought. These include polycythaemia and right ventricular strain (large P wave in leads II and V1, large R wave in V1, deep S wave in V6). If features exist, echocardiography and referral for sleep studies should be considered. In severe cases, corrective otolaryngological surgery should be undertaken before unrelated elective surgery.

• Perioperatively the biggest danger is impairment of the respiratory drive and hypoxic arousal mechanisms by the sedative action of drugs adminis-tered, leading to worsening hypoxia.

2 Loadsman JA, Hillman DR (2001). Anaesthesia and sleep apnoea. *British Journal of Anaesthesia*, **86**, 254–66.

3 Warwick JP, Mason DG (1998). Obstructive sleep apnoea syndrome in children. *Anaesthesia*, **53**, 571–9.

- Anaesthetic management is aimed at minimizing periods of sedation and ensuring that ventilation and oxygenation are maintained until the patient is adequately recovered. Specific points include:
  - Preoperative sedative drugs should be avoided.
  - Intubation is usually not a problem (particularly in children) unless other factors are also present.
  - Long-acting opioids should be avoided if possible. Use NSAIDs, paracetamol, or local infiltration where feasible. Codeine phosphate may be preferable to morphine.
  - When needed, long-acting opioids should be given IV and titrated carefully against response.
  - Close overnight monitoring (including pulse oximetry). Admission to HDU or even ITU may be necessary.
  - For nasal surgery a nasopharyngeal airway can be incorporated into the nasal pack and left in place overnight.

Throat packs

- A throat pack (wet gauze or tampons) is often used around the ETT/LMA to absorb blood that might otherwise pool in the upper airway.
- A throat pack is particularly useful during nasal operations where bleeding can be substantial and is not cleared during surgery.
- The pack must be removed before extubation, as it can lead to catastrophic airway obstruction if left. Various systems can be used to ensure removal:
  - Tie or tape the pack to the ETT.
  - Place an identification sticker on the ETT or patient's forehead.
  - Include the pack in the scrub nurse's count.
  - Always perform laryngoscopy prior to extubation.

Nasal vasoconstrictors

- Vasoconstriction is used to reduce bleeding in most nasal surgery. Cocaine (4–10%) and adrenaline (1:100 000–1:200 000) are the most commonly used agents, administered by:
  - spray
  - paste/gel
  - soaked swabs
  - infiltration (not cocaine).
- The recommended maximum dose of cocaine is 1.5 mg/kg, though when applied using swabs higher doses can be used as absorption is only partial. Sympathomimetic activity can result transiently after cocaine absorption.
- In 1947 Moffett described a technique for bathing the nasal mucosa with a solution consisting of:
  - 2 ml cocaine 8%
  - 1 ml adrenaline 1:1000
  - 2 ml sodium bicarbonate 1%.
- Originally the procedure was done with the patient awake and adopting various positions. Moffett's solution is still used (with assorted modifications, e.g. cocaine 10% and bicarbonate 8.4%), though normally after induction and applied either on swabs or prepared as a gel with K-Y Jelly.

Laser surgery of the upper airway

(See also p. 653—anaesthesia for laser surgery.)

- The use of a CO_2 laser may provide advantages for some types of ENT surgery by reducing bleeding or destroying tumour cells or viruses (such as papilloma virus). The intense heat generated, however, may ignite any combustible material such as PVC or rubber endotracheal tubes.
- Techniques available are:
    - Laser-proof tubes: specific tubes (fleximetallic or non-combustible coating) or reflective foil wrap on a regular tube (carefully applied to the part of tube at risk of exposure to laser).
    - No tube (ideal for laryngeal lesions), using jet ventilation or high-frequency jet ventilation through a surgical laryngoscope.
- For laryngeal lesions in children use deep inhalational anaesthesia with halothane by facemask plus LA spray to larynx.

Grommet insertion

Procedure	Myringotomy and grommet insertion, usually bilateral
Time	5–15 min
Pain	+
Position	Supine, head tilted to side, head ring
Blood loss	Nil
Practical technique	FM or LMA, SV

Preoperative

* Usually children (1–8 years) and day case if it is the sole procedure.
* Repeated ear infections therefore check for recent upper respiratory tract infection.

Perioperative

* A face mask is suitable if the surgeon is happy to work round the anaesthetist, but an assistant is needed to adjust the vaporizer, etc. Insert a Guedel airway before draping and ensure that the reservoir bag is visible at all times (a T-piece is ideal if a face mask used).
* The LMA is increasingly used.
* Tape the eyes.

Postoperative

* PRN paracetemol or diclofenac oral/PR—many need no analgesia.

Special considerations

* If the airway is not easy with FM, change early to LMA.
* Reflex bradycardia is occasionally seen related to partial innervation of the tympanic membrane by the vagus.

Tonsillectomy/adenoidectomy – child

Procedure	Excision of lymphoid tissue from oropharynx (tonsils) or nasopharynx (adenoids)
Time	20–30 min
Pain	++
Position	Supine, pad under shoulders, head ring, Boyle–Davis gag with split blade
Blood loss	Usually small, but can bleed postoperatively
Practical techniques	South-facing preformed ETT, SV, or IPPV
	Reinforced LMA, SV, or IPPV (but see below)
	The tube is positioned in the central groove of the blade of a Boyle–Davis gag

Preoperative

- Take a careful history to exclude OSA (see p. 511) or active infection.
- Check for loose teeth.
- Topical local anaesthesia on hands (mark sites of veins).
- Obtain consent for PR analgesia.

Perioperative

- IV induction and intubation using a relaxant of choice or inhalational induction with sevoflurane, with intubation either under deep inhalational anaesthesia or using a relaxant.
- Inhalational induction may be awkward due to the nasopharynx being blocked by the adenoids—a Guedel airway is useful.
- Reliable IV access is essential, though IV fluids are not necessary routinely.
- Use an uncuffed oral tube secured in midline, no pack (obscures surgical field).
- Tape the eyes.
- Meticulous care is needed to ensure that the airway is not obstructed or displaced by the surgeon intra-operatively, particularly after insertion or opening of the Boyle–Davis gag.
- A T-piece is ideal, but ensure that the reservoir bag is not covered so movement can be clearly seen at all times.
- Analgesia with diclofenac PR, morphine or pethidine IV/IM.
- Ensure careful suction (under direct vision) to clear the oropharynx and nasopharynx of blood at the end of the case.
- Insert a Guedel airway and extubate left lateral/head down (tonsil position).

Postoperative

- Keep the patient in the tonsil position until airway reflexes return.
- Deep extubation minimizes coughing/laryngospasm and lessens the risk of bleeding. Careful positioning is vital to prevent aspiration of blood whilst

still deep. Airway problems can occur during emergence, however, and high-quality recovery care is therefore essential if this technique is used.
- Analgesia with PRN paracetamol or diclofenac oral/PR, morphine or pethidine IV/IM.
- Leave the IV cannula in place (flushed with saline) in case of bleeding.

Special considerations
- Blind pharyngeal suction with a rigid sucker may start bleeding from the tonsil bed and should be avoided.
- Use of NSAIDs probably increases bleeding slightly (antiplatelet effect), but the clinical importance is doubtful.
- Local anaesthetic infiltration of the tonsil bed has been used by some.
- Beware continual swallowing in recovery, a sign of bleeding from the tonsil/adenoid bed.
- In suitable circumstances, adenoidectomy alone can be done on a day case basis, with the parents carefully educated to recognize signs of bleeding and able to return quickly in this event. Tonsillectomy has also been done as a day case, but the potentially catastrophic consequences of unrecognized bleeding are likely to limit enthusiasm for this.

Variant Creutzfeldt-Jakob disease
- Prions, which accumulate in lymphoid tissue such as the tonsils and adenoids, are not reliably destroyed during standard methods of surgical sterilisation.
- Inter-patient transmission of prion-borne conditions, including variant Creutzfeldt-Jakob disease (vCJD), via theatre equipment contaminated during tonsillectomy/adenoidectomy is therefore a possible risk, although generally perceived to be small.
- To address this, in January 2001 the UK Department of Health issued guidelines that all relevant surgical and anaesthetic equipment used for tonsillectomy/adenoidectomy should be disposable, including laryngoscope blades and laryngeal mask airways (revoked Dec. 2001).
- It seems sensible, however, to avoid use of the LMA, and utilize a standard disposable oral RAE endotracheal tube.

Bleeding after adenotonsillectomy
- May be detected in recovery or many hours later.
- Blood loss may be much greater than readily apparent (swallowed blood).
- A senior anaesthetist must be involved.
- Problems include:
  - hypovolaemia
  - risk of aspiration (fresh bleeding and blood in stomach)
  - difficult laryngoscopy because of airway oedema and blood
  - residual anaesthetic effect.
- Resuscitate before induction, check Hb (Haemocue® ideal), cross-match, and give blood as needed. Be aware that an early Haemocue® will fall as IV fluids are given.

- Options are:
  - Rapid sequence induction: enables quick intubation to protect the airway, assuming that the glottis is readily recognized at laryngoscopy.
  - Inhalational induction left lateral/head down: allows time for laryngoscopy, but is an unfamiliar technique to many.
- Use a wide-bore gastric tube to empty the stomach after the bleeding point has been stopped.
- Extubate when fully awake.
- Extended stay in recovery for close monitoring.
- A nasopharyngeal pack is occasionally needed (secured via tapes through the nose) if bleeding from the adenoids cannot otherwise be controlled. This is usually very uncomfortable—the patient may need midazolam/morphine to tolerate it.
- Check postoperative Hb.

Tonsillectomy in adults

As for a child, except:

- A nasal tube is preferred by some surgeons.
- The procedure is usually more painful in an adult postoperatively—give morphine in theatre.
- The IPPV-relaxant technique is used more commonly. Mivacurium is useful with a quick surgeon.
- A preoperative oral NSAID avoids suppository use.
- Occasionally patients present with a peritonsillar abscess (quinsy). This is now normally treated with antibiotics and tonsillectomy performed later. If drainage is essential because of airway swelling, it is usually aspirated with syringe and large needle under LA infiltration or refrigeration anaesthesia.

Myringoplasty

Procedure	Reconstruction of perforated tympanic membrane with autograft (usually temporalis fascia)
Time	60–90 min
Pain	+/++
Position	Supine, head tilted to side, head ring, head-up tilt
Blood loss	Minimal
Practical techniques	South-facing preformed ETT, SV, or IPPV.
	LMA (usually reinforced), SV, or IPPV

Preoperative

• Usually young, fit patients.

Perioperative

• Tape the eyes.
• Ensure coughing is avoided during surgery: LA spray to the larynx, monitor the neuromuscular block if an IPPV-relaxant technique is used.
• A dry field improves the surgical view, though this is not as important as for stapedectomy—avoiding hypertension and tachycardia, and a head up tilt are normally sufficient.
• A routine anti-emetic is useful.

Postoperative

• PRN paracetamol or diclofenac oral/PR; may need morphine.
• PRN anti-emetic.

Special considerations

• Use of N_2O may lead to diffusion into the middle ear and a risk of the graft lifting off. Advances in surgical technique have made this less important. Discuss with the surgeon.

Stapedectomy/tympanoplasty

Procedure	Excision/reconstruction of damaged middle ear structures
Time	2–4 h
Pain	+/++
Position	Supine, head tilted to side, head ring, head up tilt
Blood loss	Minimal
Practical techniques	South-facing preformed ETT, SV, or IPPV
	LMA (usually reinforced), SV, or IPPV
	Arterial line sometimes used

Preoperative

- Patients are usually young and fit.
- Avoid the patient arriving anxious and tachycardic by using adequate sedative premedication. Adding oral beta-blocker to the premedication may be helpful (atenolol 25–50 mg)—clonidine has also been used.
- Check for hypertension or other cardiovascular disease, as these will limit the degree to which arterial BP can be lowered.

Perioperative

- A bloodless surgical field enables surgery to proceed with greater accuracy. Use simple measures first: smooth induction, potent opioid preinduction and ensure that coughing at intubation is avoided (LA spray to the larynx is helpful).
- If an IPPV-relaxant technique used, monitor the neuromuscular block to ensure that coughing is avoided during surgery.
- Venous oozing is reduced by the head up tilt. Use of SV lowers the intrathoracic and therefore the venous pressures, but may be at the expense of raised $PaCO_2$.
- If the surgical field is compromised by bleeding, despite simple measures, bleeding can be reduced by lowering arterial BP or heart rate, though if arterial BP alone is reduced, compensatory tachycardia may negate the benefit on the surgical field.
- Give a beta-blocker initially (IV increments of propranolol 1 mg, metoprolol 1 mg, or esmolol infusion) to reduce the heart rate to <60 beats/min, then use a vasodilator (isoflurane, hydralazine, phentolamine, SNP) to keep the mean arterial BP to 50–60 mmHg (in otherwise healthy patients). Alternatively labetalol (combined alpha/beta-blocker, 5 mg increments) can be used, though this gives less individual control of heart rate and BP.
- An arterial line is strongly advised if cardiovascular disease is present or very potent vasodilators (SNP) are used. Adjust the position of the trans-

ducer to level of heart, though head up tilt will further reduce perfusion pressure to the head.

* Tape the eyes.
* Give an anti-emetic routinely—prochlorperazine/cyclizine/ ondansetron.

Postoperative

* Give a regular anti-emetic for 24–48 h.
* PRN paracetemol or diclofenac oral/PR; may need morphine.

Special considerations

* N_2O diffusion into the middle ear may disrupt surgery, though this is less important than in myringoplasty. If avoidance requested, can still be used until 20 min before the end of the case, then discontinued.

Nasal cavity surgery

Procedure	Submucous resection (SMR) of septum, septoplasty, turbinectomy, polypectomy, antral washout
Time	20–40 min
Pain	+/++
Position	Supine, head ring, head up tilt
Blood loss	Usually minor
Practical techniques	South-facing preformed ETT, SV, or IPPV
	LMA (usually reinforced), SV, or IPPV
	Throat pack

Preoperative

- Obstructive airways disease is often associated with nasal polyps.
- Frequently a combination of above procedures is performed.

Perioperative

- Face mask ventilation often needs a Guedel airway due to a blocked nose.
- A nasal vasoconstrictor is usually applied (LA + adrenaline infiltration, cocaine spray/paste, or Moffett's solution).
- Leave eyes untaped for polypectomy (the optic nerve can be close and the surgeon needs to check for eye movement).
- Suck out the pharynx (particularly "Coroner's clot" behind the soft palate) before extubation.

Postoperative

- Position should be left lateral/head down with the Guedel airway in place until airway reflexes return.
- Analgesia with PRN paracetamol or diclofenac oral/PR; may need morphine.
- The nose is usually packed producing obstruction of the nasal airway—if this is disturbing to the patient, or in cases of OSA, a nasopharyngeal airway can be left in overnight with a small pack placed around it.
- Sit up as soon as awake to reduce bleeding.

Special considerations

- Leave the IV cannula in overnight, as can bleed postoperatively.
- Septal correction can be done in combination with rhinoplasty (septo-rhinoplasty).

Microlaryngoscopy

Procedure	Examination of larynx using operating microscope (+ excision/biopsy)
Time	10–30 min
Pain	+
Position	Supine, pad under shoulders, head extended
Blood loss	Nil
Practical techniques	Microlaryngeal tube and conventional IPPV
	TIVA and jet ventilation using Sanders injector (O₂ + entrained air) via a special injector needle attached to the operating laryngoscope, a semi-rigid tracheal catheter, or a cricothyroidotomy needle/cannula

Ventilation during microlaryngoscopy

Microlaryngeal tube and conventional IPPV

* A microlaryngeal tube is a long 5.0 mm ETT with a high-volume/low-pressure cuff.
* Enables maintenance of anaesthesia with inhalational agents.
* Offers protection against aspiration of blood/surgical debris into the lungs but does restrict the surgeon's view of larynx somewhat.
* IPPV is necessary because of the high resistance of the microlaryngeal tube. Use long, slow inspiratory settings on the ventilator to provide adequate tidal volumes.
* The inflation pressure in circuit will be high due to ETT resistance, but the patient's airway pressures distal to the tube should be lower.

Jet ventilation

* Ventilation achieved using a Sanders injector (O₂ + entrained air) via:
  * Injector needle attached (by a small screw clamp) to the proximal end of the operating laryngoscope and ventilation started when correctly aligned with the larynx. Various needle sizes are available with different flow rates. This technique is not suitable if a good view of larynx is unobtainable and has the disadvantage of blowing debris/smoke into trachea with ventilation.
  * Semirigid tracheal catheter (ordinary suction catheter not suitable) with a tip placed mid-way down the trachea. Special catheters are available with a gas sampling port or made from laser-proof material.
  * Cricothyroidotomy needle/cannula placed through the cricothyroid membrane under LA before induction and aimed towards the carina. Several different versions are available commercially; alternatively a Tuohy needle has been used. There is the risk of gas being injected into tissues if the needle is displaced.

- Induce in theatre or use a microlaryngeal tube initially then remove it and change to jet ventilation when all is ready in theatre (the latter technique not possible if using a cricothyroidotomy needle).
- Ensure that the anaesthetic machine in theatre is situated to enable easy FM ventilation at induction/recovery.
- TIVA is needed for maintenance (propofol infusion).
- Ventilate using a normal respiratory rate and adjust inspiratory flow (alter injector settings or change needle size) to that which produces a similar degree of chest expansion to conventional ventilation. Accurate assessment of flows/pressures is not easy during jet ventilation. Barotrauma is a potential risk.
- Ventilation should be stopped intermittently whilst surgical work is being done.
- The main advantage of jet ventilation is the minimal obstruction to the surgical view.
- At the end of the case, either continue jet ventilation until spontaneous ventilation is re-established or discontinue and ventilate by face mask or LMA until spontaneous ventilation recommences.

Preoperative

- Patients are usually smokers and often elderly; CVS/RS problems are common.
- Carefully assess the airway for evidence of obstruction. History, examination, ENT clinic assessment, plain films, and CT scan may all help, but if any degree of stridor is present the obstruction must be substantial (see p. 509).
- Ensure that all equipment is ready before induction, including a cricothyroidotomy kit, and that surgeon is available for emergency tracheostomy if required.

Perioperative

- If airway obstruction is suspected, secure the airway initially using the principles described on p. 509.
- Tape the eyes.
- Short-acting opioids (alfentanil, remifentanil) attenuate the hypertensive response during surgery, which can be profound.
- Muscle relaxation is usually essential: mivacurium or intermittent suxamethonium (glycopyrrolate/atropine to prevent bradycardia with the second dose of suxamethonium).
- LA spray to the larynx reduces the risk of laryngospasm, though airway protection will be impaired, so recover in the left lateral, head down position.

Postoperative

- Analgesia with PRN paracetemol or diclofenac oral/PR.
- May develop stridor postoperatively from oedema of an already-compromised airway—dexamethasone 8–12 mg IV is sometimes used to prevent oedema.

Special considerations

- Jet ventilation is preferable if laser work is planned.

- Microlaryngoscopy can be used to inject inert material (Teflon) into paralysed vocal cords to improve phonation, though this can lead to airway obstruction if it is overdone.
- High-frequency jet ventilation has been used, though it is complex and the ventilation is not easy to assess.

Tracheostomy

Procedure	Insertion of a tracheal tube via neck incision
Time	20–30 min
Pain	+/++
Position	Supine, pad under shoulders, head ring, head up tilt
Blood loss	Normally small, though can bleed from thyroid vessels
Practical techniques	IPPV, ETT with tubing going 'north', changed to tracheostomy tube during case
	LMA if airway is not a problem, IPPV or SV
	Can be done under LA

Preoperative

- Most tracheostomies are done for long-term ITU ventilation or airway obstruction.
- Patients from the ITU will almost certainly already be intubated. If ventilation is difficult and oxygenation critical, set up the ITU ventilator in theatre, using TIVA rather than inhalational agents.
- If tracheostomy is for airway obstruction, the principles described on p. 509 should be used to secure airway access.
- Ensure all equipment is ready before induction, including a cricothyroidotomy kit, and that the surgeon is scrubbed and ready for emergency tracheostomy if required.

Perioperative

- When the trachea is incised, the ETT is withdrawn and a tracheostomy tube inserted by the surgeon under direct vision.
- Secure the ETT with tape in such a way as to allow easy removal during the case, and fix the pilot cuff so it is readily accessible.
- Aspirate the nasogastric tube (if present) and clear the oropharynx of secretions before draping.
- Tape and pad the eyes.
- Drape the patient to allow the anaesthetist access to the ETT for tube change.
- Long tubing is needed for the breathing circuit and gas sampling.
- Before changing to the tracheostomy tube, preoxygenate for 3–4 min (increasing volatile agent as necessary) and check that the neuromuscular blockade is adequate.
- Ensure that the scrub nurse has the correct tracheostomy tube and sterile catheter mount.

- Deflate the ETT cuff before the surgeons incise the trachea, so that it can be reinflated and ventilation continued if problems occur.
- Withdraw the ETT slowly into the upper trachea (do not remove it from the trachea until the tracheostomy is secure and certain) and connect the breathing circuit to the new tracheostomy tube via a sterile catheter mount.
- Beware a false passage created during tracheostomy tube insertion, especially in obese patients. Check the position with capnography or fibreoptic endoscopy if in any doubt.
- If problems occur, remove the tracheostomy tube and advance the ETT back down the trachea.

Postoperative

- Give regular suction to the new tracheostomy (blood, secretions).
- Humidify the inspired gases.
- Analgesia in recovery with diclofenac PR or morphine IV. Usually little analgesia is required thereafter.
- A new tracheostomy often produces protracted coughing—morphine, benzodiazepines, or low-dose propofol are useful for control.
- Give an anti-emetic as required.
- If the tube comes out, reinsertion can very difficult in the first few days—oral endotracheal intubation is often more practical. Two retraction sutures left in the tracheal incision are useful for identifying and opening the stoma.

Special considerations

- Can be done under LA, though this is difficult in a dyspnoeic, struggling patient.
- In ITU the procedure is now commonly done percutaneously using a dilatational technique.
- Tracheostomy is not the ideal route of approach for emergency airway access. Cricothyroidotomy is more accessible and less likely to bleed.
- An LMA can be used if tracheostomy is being done at start of a larger procedure and the upper airway is normal.

Laryngectomy

Procedure	Excision of larynx (epiglottis and glottis)
Time	3–4 h
Pain	++
Position	Supine, pad under shoulders, head ring, head up tilt
Blood loss	Moderate to substantial; cross-match two to four units
Practical techniques	IPPV, ETT with tubing going 'north', changed to tracheostomy tube during case
	Arterial line, urinary catheter, CVP line if surgery likely to be long/complicated or if indicated by cardiac disease

Preoperative

- Some degree of airway obstructionis likely, though the patient will probably have had recent GA (for diagnosis) to guide airway management. Beware a worsening airway if some time has elapsed.
- If no recent GA, assess the airway as for microlaryngoscopy.
- Patients are usually smokers; CVS/respiratory system problems and malnutrition are common.
- The implications of waking up with tracheostomy (communication difficulty, clearance of secretions, coughing produced by tracheostomy tube) must be made clear to the patient preoperatively. The speech therapist will do much of this.

Perioperative

- Tape and pad the eyes and protect pressure points with padding.
- Insert a fine-bore feeding tube at induction and fix securely (can be sutured to the nasal septum).
- Use a warming blanket, humidifier, and fluid warmer.
- Long tubing is needed for the breathing circuit and gas sampling.
- Substantial blood loss can accumulate under drapes at the back of the neck and may not be apparent until the end of the case.
- For CVP access, all neck lines hinder surgery (though the subclavian can be used); the antecubital fossa or femoral are normal routes.
- Antibiotic prophylaxis is needed for at least 24 h.
- When changing to a tracheostomy tube, see the precautions as for tracheostomy, though an 'end-stoma' is created making tracheal access easy and reliable.
- A long tube (armoured or special preformed) is useful via tracheostomy to enable the surgeon to work around the new stoma—beware endobronchial intubation.

Postoperative

- HDU care is ideal. Humidify inspired gases.
- Give regular suction to the new tracheostomy (blood, secretions).
- A new tracheostomy often produces protracted coughing—morphine, benzodiazepines, or low-dose propofol are useful to control this.
- Analgesia with PRN diclofenac PR, morphine IV/IM. Suitable for PCA, although analgesic requirements are surprisingly low normally. Paracetamol suspension (via a nasogastric tube) is often useful after the initial postoperative period.
- Give an anti-emetic as required.

Special considerations

- Beware of air emboli during dissection—early detection is by sudden fall in the $ETCO_2$ level.
- Previous laryngectomy patients presenting for surgery need special management to ventilate via the stoma. Use a paediatric facemask turned through 180°, an LMA applied to the neck, or intubate awake after spraying the tracheal stoma with LA. Insertion of a tracheostomy tube after laryngectomy is usually easy, though check the stoma for stenosis or tumour recurrence and always preoxygenate.
- Partial laryngectomy, with laryngeal reconstruction and temporary tracheostomy, is favoured by some as an alternative to radiotherapy in early laryngeal tumours.

Radical neck dissection

Procedure	Excision of sternomastoid, internal, and external jugular veins and associated lymph nodes
Time	2–4 h
Pain	++
Position	Supine, pad under shoulders, head on ring tilted to side, head up tilt
Blood loss	Moderate to substantial, cross-match two to four units
Practical techniques	IPPV, ETT with tubing going 'north'
	Arterial line, urinary catheter, CVP line if surgery is likely to be long/complicated or if indicated by cardiac disease

Preoperative

- Assess the airway carefully as there may be an associated head and neck tumour or previous major surgery.
- Often done in conjunction with another procedure such as laryngectomy.

Perioperative

- Tape and pad the eyes and protect pressure points with padding.
- Use a warming blanket, humidifier, and fluid warmer.
- Insert a urinary catheter if the procedure is likely to be of long duration.
- Long tubing is needed for the breathing circuit and gas sampling.
- Large bore IV cannula—can bleed briskly from large neck vessels.
- Substantial blood loss can accumulate under the drapes at the back of the neck and not be apparent until the end of the case.
- For CVP access, use the femoral or subclavian vein or the antecubital fossa on the opposite side from surgery (an antecubital line on the same side can enter the neck vein and become transfixed by the surgeon). Head and neck venous drainage postoperatively is via the jugular veins on the opposite side. To avoid possible compromise of flow, they should be avoided for cannulation.

Postoperative

- Venous drainage from the head and neck is markedly impaired by removal of the jugular vein. Head and neck oedema may result for several days. Keep the head up as much as possible and avoid excessive IV fluid administration.
- Analgesia with PRN paracetemol or diclofenac oral/PR, morphine IV/IM. Surprisingly low analgesic requirements normally.
- Give an anti-emetic as required.

Special considerations

- Beware of air emboli during dissection—early detection is by sudden fall in the $ETCO_2$ level
- Surgical manipulation of the carotid sinus can produce unexpected bradycardia.
- If neck dissection has previously been done on the other side, oedema is usually worse and can include the brain. Dexamethasone 8–12 mg IV pre-operatively (then 4 mg IV 6–hourly) is used by many to reduce this.

Parotidectomy

Procedure	Excision of parotid gland, usually preserving the facial nerve
Time	2–5 h
Pain	++
Position	Supine, head ring, head tilted to side and moderately extended, head up tilt
Blood loss	Usually small to moderate, G&S. Greater for malignant tumours
Practical techniques	South-facing preformed ETT and IPPV normally used, though SV can be used for suitable patients
	Reinforced LMA and IPPV or SV suitable for some patients

Preoperative

* Assess whether suitable for SV—not for elderly, obese, or those with respiratory disease.
* Check the mouth opening if there is a malignant parotid tumour.

Perioperative

* The surgeon will often wish to stimulate the facial nerve during the procedure and thus muscle relaxation may need to be avoided at that time.
* To ventilate without relaxant, suppress the respiratory drive with a combination of moderate hyperventilation, substantial doses of short-acting opioid (alfentanil or remifentanil infusion), volatile agent, or propofol infusion.
* If SV is used, ensure that the patient is settled initially using a volatile agent at high levels. Relaxants can by used for first 30–40 min until the facial nerve is reached.
* An LA spray to the larynx is useful to prevent coughing.
* Use a peripheral nerve stimulator to check that the action of the relaxant has ended.
* Tape and pad the eyes and protect pressure points with padding (the surgeon may wish to leave the eye exposed on the side of surgery).
* Use a warming blanket and humidifier, plus a fluid warmer if bleeding.
* Insert a urinary catheter if the procedure is likely to be prolonged.

Postoperative

* To minimize the chance of immediate postoperative wound haematoma, keep the head up in recovery and treat hypertension early.
* Analgesia with PRN morphine IV/IM, paracetemol or diclofenac oral/PR.
* Give an anti-emetic as required.

Special considerations

- During dissection the surgeon uses a nerve stimulator to identify the facial nerve, hence the patient must have no substantial neuromuscular block (two or more twitches present).
- Large-bore IV access at start, as can bleed substantially (especially malignant tumours).

Other ENT procedures

Operation	Description	Time (min)	Pain (+ to +++++)	Position	Blood loss	Notes
Mastoidectomy	Clearance of cholesteatoma from mastoid cavity	90–120	+/++	Head up tilt, head tilted to side on ring	Minimal	Preformed ETT or LMA, SV, or IPPV. Bloodless field needed (see stapedectomy). If disease close to facial nerve, surgeon may request no relaxant used (see parotidectomy)
Drilling of ear exostoses	Excision of external auditory (swimmers') exostoses	60–90	+/++	Head up tilt, head tilted to side on ring	Minimal	Preformed ETT or LMA, SV, or IPPV
FESS	Functional endoscopic sinus surgery	45–60	+/++	Head up tilt, head ring	Small	RAE tube or reinforced LMA, SV, or IPPV, throat pack. Moffett's solution normally used. Moderate hypotension useful to decrease bleeding
MUA of nose	Correction of nasal fracture	1–15	+	Supine	Small	If quick, pre-O₂ + propofol only. If longer, RAE tube or reinforced LMA + throat pack. Occasionally bleeds dramatically

Operation	Description	Time (min)	Pain (+ to +++++)	Position	Blood loss	Notes
Removal of foreign body from nose	Removal of foreign body from nose, usually in child	5–10	ns	Supine, head ring	ns	Gas induction. RAE tube or LMA, throat pack, SV. Avoid FM ventilation if possible (risk of pushing foreign body down into lower airway)
Rhinoplasty	Cosmetic alteration or reconstruction of nose using bone/cartilage graft	60–90	++	Head up tilt, head ring	Small	RAE tube or reinforced LMA, SV, or IPPV, throat pack. Moderate hypotension useful to decrease bleeding
Lateral rhinotomy	Resection of nasal tumour via lateral rhinotomy	90	++	Head up tilt, head ring	Moderate	RAE tube or reinforced LMA, SV, or IPPV, throat pack. Moderate hypotension useful to decrease bleeding
Uvulopalatopharyngoplasty (UPPP)	Excision of uvula and lax tissue from soft palate, sometimes using laser	20–30	+++	Supine, pad under shoulders	Small	RAE tube or reinforced LMA, SV, or IPPV. Laser-proof tube if needed. Regular postop. diclofenac. Precautions for OSA as indicated
Submandibular gland excision	Excision of blocked/infected submandibular gland	45–60	++	Supine, pad under shoulders, head ring	Small	RAE tube or reinforced LMA on opposite side, SV, or IPPV

Operation	Description	Time (min)	Pain (+ to +++++)	Position	Blood loss	Notes
Tracheobronchial foreign body removal	Removal of inhaled foreign body using rigid bronchoscope, usually in child	10–30	+	Supine, pad under shoulders	ns	Deep inhalational anaesthesia using oxygen and halothane, allowing surgeon intermittent access. LA spray, atropine useful to prevent bradycardias. SV possible through ventilating bronchoscope. Avoid ventilation if possible to avoid pushing foreign body further down
Laryngoscopy in child	Examination of larynx in child, usually for recurrent stridor or aspiration	10–15	+	Supine, pad under shoulders	ns	Inhalational induction, LA spray to larynx. Either SV via surgical laryngoscope (circuit connected to scope) or use LMA with bars removed and perform fibreoptic laryngoscopy (ideal for small child and enables larynx to be viewed during emergence)

Operation	Description	Time (min)	Pain (+ to +++++)	Position	Blood loss	Notes
Direct pharyngoscopy	Examination of pharynx using rigid pharyngoscope	10–15	+	Supine, pad under shoulders	ns	Check for reflux. Small (6.5–7) oral RAE tube secured on left, IPPV, mivacurium or intermittent suxamethonium. Risk of bleeding if biopsies done
Endoscopic stapling of pharyngeal pouch	Division of opening to pharyngeal pouch using staple gun endoscopically	15–20	+	Supine, pad under shoulders	ns	RSI, small (6.5–7) oral RAE tube secured on opposite side, IPPV. Surgeon may want oesophageal bougie inserted to help recognise anatomy. NG tube at end and IV fluids as nil by mouth postop
Excision of pharyngeal pouch	Excision of pharyngeal pouch via external approach	45–60	++	Supine, pad under shoulders, head ring	Small	RSI, small (6.5–7) oral RAE tube secured on opposite side, IPPV. Surgeon may want oesophageal bougie inserted to help recognise anatomy. NG tube at end and IV fluids as nil by mouth postop

Operation	Description	Time (min)	Pain (+ to ++++)	Position	Blood loss	Notes
Insertion of (Provox) speaking valve	Insertion of speaking valve via tracheo-oesophageal puncture, following laryngectomy	15	+	Supine, pad under shoulders, head ring	ns	Microlaryngoscopy tube inserted via tracheostomy, IPPV, mivacurium or intermittent suxamethonium, alfentanil, or fentanyl to reduce CVS response
Pharyngolaryngo-oesophagectomy	Resection of larynx, pharynx and oesophagus for tumour of hypopharynx, usually with stomach pull-up. Involves laparotomy ± thoracotomy	6 h	+++	Supine, pad under shoulders, head ring	Major, X-match 4–6 units	No access to patient whatsoever! Prepare as for laryngectomy with all lines, plus double-lumen tube if doing thoracotomy. Consider epidural analgesia for laparotomy/thoracotomy (using plain LA) with PCA IV morphine to cover remaining surgical sites. ITU mandatory postop.

ns = not significant.

Chapter 23
Oral/maxillofacial surgery
Richard Telford

General principles

In common with anaesthesia for ENT surgery, the main concerns with anaesthesia for intraoral/maxillofacial procedures are that of the shared airway plus the potential for difficulties with intubation/airway maintenance. Patients presenting for intraoral procedures vary from the perfectly fit to the medically compromised.

+ Nasal intubation is frequently used in oral surgery, to improve access to the mouth. At the preoperative visit check nostril patency and ask about epistaxis and the use of anticoagulants.
+ If the nasal route is chosen for intubation use a local anaesthetic and/or vasoconstrictor such as cocaine 5–10%, lidocaine (lignocaine) 5% and phenylephrine 0.5% mixture (Co-phenylcaine®), or xylometazoline (Otrivine®).
+ There are many varieties of nasal tube to choose from. One of the best is the 'Polar Preformed North Nasal' from Portex®. These are 'north-facing' tubes made of soft material and cause little nasal trauma. Sizes of 6.0, 6.5, and 7.0 mm should be available. Place in warm water before use to soften the material even further.
+ It may be possible to perform simple intraoral procedures using a reinforced laryngeal mask airway. However, access to the mouth is inevitably compromised and the surgeon tends to dislodge/occlude the airway. Similarly, for unilateral intraoral procedures an oral endotracheal tube placed on the opposite side of the mouth may be acceptable. If in doubt discuss with the surgeon.
+ Access to the airway is limited.
+ Protect the eyes with tape and eyepads.
+ Position the patient with the head at the opposite end to the anaesthetic machine.
+ Stabilize the head with a horseshoe or head ring. For operations on the roof of the mouth use a bolster under the shoulders to extend the neck further.
+ A long breathing circuit is normally required.
+ Throat packs are frequently used to minimize contamination of the airway with blood and debris. Ribbon gauze or tampons may be used. It is important to have a robust system in place to ensure that throat packs are not inadvertently left *in situ*. They should preferably be included in the swab count and careful laryngoscopy should always be performed at the end of the procedure.

Extubation

+ In common with ENT patients, there is a risk of aspiration of blood, pus, and debris. Patients are therefore best extubated in the left lateral position with head down tilt.
+ Some anaesthetists extubate the patient 'deep', having used a spontaneous breathing technique, whereas others use an opioid/relaxant based technique and prefer to extubate awake.
+ The use of a nasotracheal tube, which does not stimulate the gag reflex as much as an oral tube, facilitates the latter approach.

• If a nasal tube has been used do not remove it completely on extubation, but withdraw, cut at the 15 cm mark and insert a safety pin (to prevent migration). This will then serve as a nasopharyngeal airway and also tamponade any potential nasal haemorrhage due to tube insertion.

Cardiac arrhythmias (see also p. 930)

Cardiac arrhythmias are common during tooth extraction under deep inhalational anaesthesia. Contributory factors include hypercarbia, hypoxia, halothane, underlying cardiac disease, light anaesthesia, and injected sympathomimetic agents. Correction of the underlying problem and increasing analgesia is usually effective. If treatment is required beta-blockers are very effective. Arrythmias are much less common with isoflurane or sevoflurane, and the infiltration of local anaesthetic by the surgeon virtually abolishes them.

Free-flap surgery

• Many major maxillofacial reconstructions are performed using tissue/bone free flaps (particularly from the radial forearm).

• These operations are lengthy, 6–18 h.

• Anaesthesia is as for plastic surgery free flaps (see p. 591), with the added complication of a potentially difficult airway, both pre- and postsurgery.

• Surgical tracheostomy may help with the latter, and reduce sedative requirements on ICU.

• HDU or ICU care is usually indicated postoperatively.

Surgical extraction of impacted/buried teeth

Procedure	Removal of teeth
Time	3–45 min
Pain	+
Position	Supine, head ring, bolster under shoulders if teeth to be extracted in the roof of mouth
Blood loss	Minimal
Practical techniques	Nasal tube and IPPV. Extubate awake
	Nasal tube and spontaneous ventilation. Extubate deep
	?LMA and SV

Preoperative

* Make a careful assessment of the airway (see p. 866). Check the nostrils for patency.
* If the patient has a dental abcess there may be marked swelling of the face and severe trismus. Awake fibreoptic intubation may be necessary.
* Obtain consent for an NSAID suppository if planned.

Perioperative

* Consider LMA/oral tube for simple/unilateral extractions.
* Intubate with a preformed nasal tube after applying vasoconstrictor to the nasal mucosa (see above).
* Protect the eyes with tape and pads.
* The surgeon should anaesthetize the appropriate terminal branches of the maxillary division (infraorbital, greater palatine, and nasopalatine) and mandibular division (inferior alveolar, lingual, buccal, and mental) of the trigeminal nerve with a long-acting local anaesthetic (e.g. bupivacaine 0.5 % with adrenaline 1:200 000).
* Give an intraoperative opioid and NSAID.
* IV antibiotics are administered to minimize the risk of infection (benzyl-penicillin 600 mg).
* Steroids (e.g. dexamethasone 8 mg IV) are given to minimize swelling.
* Extubate in the left lateral position with head down tilt.

Postoperative

Balanced analgesia with regular paracetamol and NSAID. Prescribe rescue analgesia with PRN codeine phosphate or tramadol. Write up an antiemetic. Injectable narcotics are rarely required on the ward.

Special considerations

Talk to the surgeon to ascertain the likely length of surgery. Remember that some patients require general anaesthesia only because they are 'dental phobic'. The surgical extractions may be simple and the operative time consequently very short. A short-acting muscle relaxant may be required.

Maxillary/mandibular osteotomy

Procedure	Surgical realignment of the facial skeleton
Time	Lengthy, 4–6 h
Pain	++
Position	Supine, with head up tilt, head ring
Blood loss	Variable. Occasionally can be severe. Cross-match two units
Practical techniques	Nasal tube and IPPV. Extubate awake. Arterial line

Patients presenting for orthognathic surgery may have malformations isolated to one jaw or may be associated with multiple craniofacial deformities as part of a syndrome. They have often had prior dental extractions and preoperative orthodontic work. There are many surgical procedures performed to correct facial deformities. Patients are usually in their late teens or early twenties and are generally fit and well.

Preoperative

* Make a careful assessment of the airway (see p. 866). Check the nostrils for patency.
* Consent for NSAID if planned.
* Check Hb and cross-match blood as per surgical blood ordering schedule (two units).
* Thromboembolic prophylaxis (TEDS, unfractionated or low-molecular-weight heparin). Consider the use of intermittent pneumatic compression boots in theatre.

Perioperative

* Intubate nasally using a preformed nasal tube (see above).
* Have an adequate venous access. Consider the use of invasive pressure monitoring because of the length of surgery.
* Put Lacrilube® onto the eyes then protect them with tape and pads.
* Position the patient very carefully on the operating table. Place the head on a ring and tilt the table head up.
* Use a balanced anaesthetic technique. Aim for an awake, cooperative patient who can maintain their own airway at completion of surgery. Some teams advocate the use of moderate induced hypotension to help minimize blood loss.
* Give IV antibiotics.
* Use steroids (e.g. dexamethasone 8 mg IV) to minimize swelling.
* Keep the patient warm. Measure the central temperature, warm intravenous fluids, and use a heating mattress and/or hot air blower.

- Monitor blood loss carefully. The Hemocue® is an accurate way of tracking haemoglobin concentration in theatre.
- The patient's jaws will frequently be wired together on completion of surgery. Ensure that throat packs are removed and that the oropharynx is cleared of blood and debris before this is done.
- Use an anti-emetic to minimize the risk of nausea and vomiting.
- Extubate the patient once fully awake. Withdraw the nasal tube and cut (15 cm mark at the nostril) to leave as a nasopharyngeal airway.
- Prescribe small doses of intravenous narcotic to be administered in recovery.
- Ensure that you and the nursing staff are familiar with the position of the wires that hold the jaws together. Make sure wire cutters are with the patient at all times.

Postoperative

- Some units send these patients to HDU. Others send them to the ward after a lengthy period in recovery.
- Administer humidified oxygen.
- Ensure all oral analgesics are prescribed in a soluble form. Injectable narcotics are rarely required postoperatively.
- Continue prophylactic antibiotics and steroids postoperatively as per your unit's protocol.
- Prescribe intravenous fluids. Encourage the patient to take fluid by the oral route as soon as possible.

Fractures of the zygomatic complex

These fractures may occur in isolation or may be associated with damage to the eyeball and lacrimal apparatus. There may be limitation of mouth opening due to interference with the movement of the coronoid process of the mandible by the depressed zygomatic complex. Following elevation, the fracture may be stable or unstable and require internal fixation. Most surgery is carried out via a temporal approach or a percutaneous route through the cheek. Intraoral and transantral routes have also been described but are rarely used. Unstable fractures require plating or wiring via skin or intraoral incisions.

Preoperative

• Assess the patient carefully for associated injuries. Treatment of these fractures does not have high clinical priority. The operation is often easier if a period of time elapses (5–7 days) to allow the associated facial swelling to disperse.
• Make a careful airway assessment.
• Obtain consent for an NSAID suppository if planned.

Perioperative

• Intubate the patient with an oral RAE tube. For simple fracture elevations an armoured LMA may be used, but discuss with the surgeon as to likelihood of fixation requirement.
• Lubricate and protect the eyes.
• Position the patient on the operating table with the head at the opposite end to the anaesthetic machine, with the head on a ring.
• Keep the patient warm.
• Give antibiotics and steroids as requested.
• Extubate in the lateral position with the fractured side uppermost.

Postoperative

• IV opioids may be required in recovery.
• Balanced oral analgesia for the ward.

Procedure	Time	Pain	Position	Blood loss	Practical techniques
Elevation of fractured zygomatic complex	10–45 min	+	Supine, head ring	Minimal	Oral RAE tube and IPPV LMA/SV
Internal fixation of fractured zygomatic complex	1–3 h	++	Supine, with head up tilt, head ring	Variable. G&S	Oral RAE tube and IPPV

Mandibular fractures

Procedure	Reduction and fixation of a fractured mandible
Time	2–3 h
Pain	+
Position	Supine, with head up tilt, head ring
Blood loss	Variable. ?G&S
Practical techniques	Nasal tube and IPPV
	Fibreoptic intubation may be required

Mandibular fractures can be treated by either closed reduction and indirect skeletal fixation (using interdental wires, arch bars, or splints) or by open reduction and direct skeletal fixation using bone plates. When indirect skeletal fixation is used the patient's jaws are wired together at the completion of surgery. When direct skeletal fixation is used this is not usually the case.

Preoperative

• Make a careful assessment for associated injuries.
• Make a meticulous assessment of the airway. There may be severe trismus and marked soft tissue swelling (see p. 866).
• Assess nostril patency. Remember to look for evidence of basal skull fracture and CSF leak as these are contraindications to nasal intubation.

Perioperative

• Although planned intubation may appear to be difficult preoperatively (limited mouth opening due to trismus, facial swelling), patients with recent bilateral mandibular fractures are often easy to intubate due to increased anterior jaw movement once anaesthetized.
• However, airway maintenance once anaesthetized may not always be easy, due to increased jaw movement and swelling.
• Gas induction is often difficult due to pain when applying the facemask.
• If in doubt about the airway use preoxygenation with suxamethonium, or awake fibreoptic intubation.

Postoperative

As for patients having maxillary/mandibular osteotomies.

Anaesthesia for dentistry

Despite the Poswillo report (1990), which set safety standards required for monitoring and training in outpatient dental (or dental chair) anaesthesia,[1] the annual mortality in the United Kingdom remained at two deaths per year. In 1998 five dental chair deaths prompted further guidance from the General Dental Council and the Royal College of Anaesthetists. From April 2001, all dental anaesthesia has to be performed in a hospital setting by anaesthetists with appropriate postgraduate training. These reports also stressed the importance of limiting general anaesthesia only for those patients in whom use of local anaesthesia or sedation is not an option.

General anaesthesia for dentistry

General anaesthesia for dental procedures should be reserved for patients who are unable to tolerate local anaesthesia, i.e. young children or adults with mental disability, requiring simple extractions or dental restoration.[2]

Facilities

Facilities should be the same as for any other day surgery procedure. Standard day case selection criteria should be used and patients with significant inter-current disease should be referred for inpatient treatment. Trained staff are required to assist the dentist and the anaesthetist during the procedure and to care for the patient during recovery. Monitoring should continue until the patient is fully awake.

Short procedures

Simple extractions are very quick procedures lasting only a few minutes, allowing rapid recovery and early discharge. Restoration work can take over an hour.

Shared airway

For simple extractions, a nasal mask is commonly used, but laryngeal mask airways (plain or flexible) are an alternative. Once adequate anaesthesia has been achieved, a prop or gag and a mouth pack are inserted by the dentist. The anaesthetist must ensure that the pack does not obstruct the airway and the dentist that the pack is adequately positioned to prevent soiling of the lower airway with blood or dental matter. When the extractions on the first side are complete, the mouth pack is repositioned over the dental sockets to absorb any oozing of blood and a fresh pack inserted to act as a barrier for the second side. During extractions, patency of the airway must be maintained and may require support of the jaw by the dentist. For restoration work, intubation and ventilation are required.

1 Standing Dental Advisory Committee (1990). *Report of an expert working party (Chairman: Professor D Poswillo). General anaesthesia, sedation and resuscitation in dentistry.*

2 Royal College of Anaesthetists (1999). *Standards and guidelines for general anaesthesia for dentistry.*

Positioning

There is no longer a place for 'chair dental anaesthesia'. Postural hypotension can be easily overlooked and it is now standard practice to keep patients supine during anaesthesia.

Arrhythmias

Dental anaesthesia is associated with a high incidence of arrhythmias, usually related to hypoxia, hypercarbia, inadequate anaesthesia, and volatile anaesthetic agents.[3] Arrhythmias are mainly ventricular and may occasionally progress to ventricular fibrillation. Halothane is associated with a frequency of arrhythmia of up to 75% in dental anaesthesia and should be avoided, but isoflurane and sevoflurane can be used safely. The incidence of hypoxia can be reduced by using 100% oxygen for maintenance. $ETCO_2$ is difficult to measure when using a nasal mask but can be monitored properly when using an LMA.

Local anaesthetic infiltration

This should be used where possible to provide analgesia and reduce the incidence of arrhythmias. However, LA may not be suitable in very young children where it may lead to accidental biting and laceration.

Dental labelling

Deciduous teeth are assigned letters A to E in each quadrant and adult teeth are numbered 1 to 8.

Mentally disabled patients

These patients may have difficulty understanding the procedure and are often anxious. A short-acting anxiolytic agent, such as oral midazolam, and topical anaesthetic cream may be helpful. Mental disability may be part of a more complex medical disorder, such as Down's syndrome or other congenital abnormality. It is important to exclude any significant cardiac pathology and to give endocarditis prophylaxis when appropriate (p. 896). Patients requiring extensive extractions or restoration work should be admitted to a day case unit for treatment, but may require an overnight stay if medically compromised.

---

3 Blayney MR, Malins AF, Cooper GM (1999). Cardiac arrhythmias in children during outpatient general anaesthesia for dentistry. *The Lancet* 354, 1864–66.

Anaesthesia for simple dental extractions

Procedure	Dental extractions
Time	2–10 min
Pain	+/++
Position	Supine
Blood loss	Not significant
Practical technique	Nasal mask/LMA

Preoperative

- Patients are usually children aged 3–12 years.
- Patients are screened by the dentist but are not usually assessed by a medical practitioner prior to admission. Beware of undiagnosed pathology, e.g. heart murmurs, which may need prophylactic antibiotic therapy.
- Obtain consent for suppositories.

Perioperative

- Give pre-emptive analgesia if possible, e.g. paracetamol 15–20 mg/ kg PO ± diclofenac 1 mg/kg PO.
- Apply a topical anaesthetic for cannulation if IV induction is planned.
- Propofol for IV induction, sevoflurane for gas induction.
- Tape the eyes.
- Maintenance with a volatile agent (sevoflurane or isoflurane) or propofol.
- Use local anaesthetic infiltration (by the dentist) for difficult extractions, avoid opioids except in longer cases or inpatients.
- Stabilize the head and neck during the procedure.
- Place in the lateral position, slightly head down at the end.

Postoperative

- Advise regular paracetamol for 12–48 h.
- Diclofenac or ibuprofen as indicated.

Special considerations

- During extractions, the dentist may apply considerable pressure and the anaesthetist should apply counter-pressure to support and stabilize the head and jaw.
- Nitrous oxide can be avoided by administration of other analgesic agents, thus enabling the use of 100% oxygen for maintenance, minimizing the risk of hypoxia.
- When using a nasal mask, mouth breathing can occur around the dental pack resulting in decreased uptake of the anaesthetic agent and the patient becoming light. This can be a problem when using short-acting agents such as sevoflurane and can be overcome by using isoflurane or by giving increments of propofol.

- Children with blocked noses can be maintained using an LMA, provided there is no associated upper respiratory tract infection.

Sedation for dentistry

Patients who are unwilling or unable to tolerate dental treatment under local anaesthesia alone can often be managed by a combination technique using sedation. These procedures are usually performed by the dentist in the dental clinic. Oral or intravenous sedation can be provided by short-acting benzodiazepines such as midazolam, but the effects can be unpredictable especially in children. Inhalation sedation can be provided by subanaesthetic concentrations of nitrous oxide (up to 50%) in oxygen.[4] This technique is also known as relative analgesia. Whichever route of administration is used, it is important to ensure that the patient remains conscious throughout.

General considerations

- Ideally patients should be ASA 1 or 2.
- Patients will require an escort for the procedure and to care for them afterwards.
- Written instructions should be provided regarding limitations on driving and operating machinery postoperatively. The patients should also be told to avoid a heavy meal prior to treatment.
- Inhalation sedation cannot be used in patients with nasal obstruction or those unable to cooperate with breathing through a nasal mask.
- Local anaesthetic is used in all patients after the sedation has been established.
- The patient should be able to communicate throughout the procedure.

Suitable regimes

Suitable regimes include:

- Midazolam 2 mg IV, wait 90 s, then give 1 mg every 30 s until sedated.
- 100% oxygen via a nasal mask, add 10% nitrous oxide for 1 min, then 20% for 1 min. Continue increments of 5% (maximum 50%) until sedated.

Special considerations

- Do not use mouth props as the ability to keep the mouth open is an important indicator of consciousness.
- Have flumazenil available to reverse the midazolam if necessary.
- Following IV sedation the patient must be allowed to recover for 1 h before discharge.
- Following nitrous oxide sedation, 100% oxygen must be administered to prevent diffusion hypoxia.
- The patient can be discharged once they are able to stand and walk unaided.

---

4 Holroyd I, Roberts GJ (2000). Inhalation sedation with nitrous oxide: A review. *Dent Update*, 27, 141–6.

Chapter 24
Ophthalmic surgery
Andrew Farmery

Intraocular pressure

Intraocular pressure (IOP) normally ranges between 10 and 20 mmHg, but transient changes occur frequently with posture, during coughing, vomiting, or Valsava manoeuvres. Such transient changes are normal and have no bearing on the intact eye. However, when the globe is open during surgery, such transient changes may cause vitreous extrusion, haemorrhage, or lens prolapse.

Factors affecting IOP

These are in many ways analogous to factors affecting ICP:

- Volume of aqueous humour (determined by the balance of production and drainage).
- Choroidal blood volume (determined by the balance of arterial flow and venous drainage).
- Head up position (via its affect on the above).
- The tone in the extraocular muscles.
- Mannitol and acetazolamide: mannitol (0.5 g/kg IV) reduces IOP by withdrawing fluid from the vitreous. Acetazolamide (500 mg IV) reduces IOP by reducing aqueous production by the ciliary body. Both can be used in the medical management of glaucoma, but the anaesthetist may be required to use them intraoperatively to reduce IOP acutely if surgical conditions require it. As both of these are diuretics, urinary catheterization may be indicated.
- Anaesthetic factors (see Table).

Anaesthetic factors increasing IOP	Anaesthetic factors decreasing IOP
External compression of the globe by a tightly applied facemask	Induction agents, propofol and thiopental, principally by reduction in arterial and venous pressure
Laryngoscopy, through either a pressor response, or from straining in an inadequately relaxed patient	Non-depolarizing muscle relaxants, by reduction in tone of extraocular muscles
Suxamethonium increases IOP transiently through its effect on extraocular muscles	Head up tilt at 15°, assists venous drainage
Large volumes of local anaesthetic solution placed in the orbit. This effect is transient (2–3 min)	Moderate hypocapnia: 3.5–4.0 kPa reduces choroidal blood volume by vasoconstriction of choroidal vessels

Oculomedullary reflexes

These comprise: oculocardiac, oculorespiratory, and oculoemetic reflexes.

* Incidence: 50–80%. Commonly seen in paediatric squint surgery.
* Triggers: traction on the extraocular muscles, pressure on the globe.
* Afferent arc: fibres running with long and short ciliary nerves, via ciliary ganglion, to the trigeminal ganglion near floor of fourth ventricle.
* Efferent arc: vagus, fibres to respiratory and vomiting centre.
* Effects: bradycardia, sinus arrest, respiratory arrest, nausea.
* Prevention: all of these (bradycardia, respiratory arrest, nausea) can be moderated to some extent by use of local anaesthesia (to abolish the afferent arc), avoiding hypercapnia (which appears to sensitize the reflex), and prophylactic glycopyrrolate or atropine.

Preoperative assessment

Many patients presenting routinely for eye surgery are at the extremes of age. The majority of ophthalmic operations (predominantly cataract surgery) are performed as day cases under local anaesthesia, and this proportion is increasing. Most patients are elderly and may have one or more serious systemic diseases. Patients scheduled for general anaesthesia should have routine investigations performed. Patients having cataract extraction under local anaesthesia, however, do not warrant routine investigation. Many centres do not routinely starve such patients and a light meal 2 to 3 h preoperatively may be less disruptive for this elderly population and may facilitate better diabetic control.

Preoperative assessment for local anaesthetic cataract surgery should include:

* Axial length (see p. 565).
* INR/APPT if on warfarin or heparin.
* Blood glucose if diabetic.
* Ability to lie flat for 1 h (heart failure, arthritis, etc.).
* Hearing/comprehension—will the patient be able to hear and understand instructions?
* Anxiety level—will sedation be required?
* Ability to tolerate supplemental oxygen in high concentration—is there a risk of CO_2 retention, requiring delivery of a precise concentration of supplemental oxygen?
* Prophylactic antibiotics are generally not considered to be necessary for patients with cardiac lesions undergoing routine anterior chamber (cataract) surgery.

General anaesthesia versus local anaesthesia

Given the nature of the typical population of ophthalmic patients, there are a number of advantages to avoiding general anaesthesia. These include:

- Minimization of physiological disturbance (including postoperative sleep disturbance).
- Reduced PONV.
- Economic advantages—increased patient throughput (ward admissions and theatre throughput), less demanding on nursing resources, portering, etc.

There are occasions when general anaesthesia is preferable:

- Where patients may refuse the operation under local anaesthesia. Unless there are overwhelming risks, such patients should be offered general anaesthesia providing they are fully informed about the risks and that they accept them.
- In children and patients with learning disabilities or movement disorders.
- Some major and lengthy operations (oculoplastics and vitreoretinal) are also commonly performed under GA since it is unrealistic to expect patients to tolerate them otherwise.
- In patients unable to lie flat and remain motionless for up to 1 h (although most surgeons can operate in a 'deck chair' position rather than true supine).

Local anaesthesia for intraocular surgery

Basic anatomy

The orbit is 40–50 mm deep and pyramidal in shape with its base at the orbital opening and its apex pointing to the optic foramen. Its volume is about 30 ml, 7 ml of which is occupied by the globe and its muscle cone, and the remainder being loose connective tissue through which local anaesthetic solutions can easily spread. The lateral walls of both orbits form an angle of 90° to each other and the angle between the medial and lateral wall of each orbit is 45°. The medial wall is parallel to the saggital plane.

The globe lies in the anterior part of the orbit and sits high and lateral (i.e. nearer the roof than the floor and nearer the lateral than the medial wall). This relationship is important when considering needle access to the orbit, which is usually achieved either medially or inferolaterally where the gap between the globe and orbital wall is greatest. The sclera forms the fibrous bulk of the globe. Its thickness is 1 mm and although tough, is easily penetrated by a sharp needle. Deep to the sclera is the uveal tract, which comprises the ciliary body, the iris, and the choroid layer. Superficial to, and enclosing the sclera, is the membranous Tenon's capsule, lying directly underneath the conjunctiva. It is easily recognized, as it is white and avascular, unlike the vascular sclera below. The four recti and two oblique muscles control eye movement and influence IOP. The lateral rectus is innervated by the abducens nerve (sixth cranial), the superior oblique by the trochlear nerve (fourth cranial), and all the rest by the occulomotor nerve (third cranial) [$(LR_6SO_4)_3$]. The recti muscles form the muscle 'cone' which encloses the sensory and motor nerves, ciliary ganglion, optic nerve, retinal artery, and vein. It is through this cone that peribulbar local anaesthetic drugs must flow or diffuse to effect their action.

The fourth, sixth, and third cranial nerves enter the cone and pierce the muscles on their intraconal surface. These are motor nerves only. The sensory supply is via branches of the trigeminal (fifth) cranial nerve. The first division of the trigeminal (ophthalmic nerve, V^1) enters the orbit via the superior orbital fissure and supplies branches intraconally to the sclera and cornea, and extraconally to the upper lid and conjunctiva after leaving the orbit via the superior orbital notch. The second division (maxillary nerve, V^2) enters the orbit via the inferior orbital fissure. Branches of this nerve are entirely extraconal and supply the lower lid and inferior conjunctiva after leaving the orbit via the inferior orbital foramen.

The ciliary ganglion, lying within the cone, relays sensory fibres from the globe to V^1, receives a parasympathetic branch from the (motor) third cranial nerve, and sympathetic fibres from the carotid plexus.

Ocular block techniques

Retrobulbar block

Local anaesthetic is deposited within the muscle cone (retrobulbar intraconal), blocking the ciliary ganglion, sensory nerves to the sclera and cornea, and motor nerves to the extraocular muscles. This provides anaesthesia and akinesia with a rapid, predictable onset, using a small volume of solution. It is not now recommended because of the following potential complications:

- globe perforation (incidence 0.1% to 0.7%)
- intravascular injection
- haemorrhage (incidence 1%)
- penetration and injection of the optic nerve sheath (incidence 0.27%) with resultant optic nerve damage, subarachnoid spread, brainstem paresis, and cardiopulmonary arrest.

Retrobulbar anaesthesia is not considered further here.

Peribulbar block

First described in 1986. Local anaesthetic solution is deposited within the orbit but outside the muscle cone (peribulbar periconal). The complication rate is therefore reduced.

The most commonly used technique involves an initial inferolateral injection supplemented with a medial injection. A single inferolateral injection is often adequate for anaesthesia, but may not be predictable for complete akinesia.

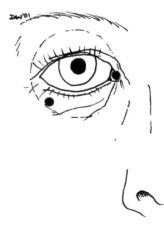

Fig 24.1 Peribulbar block I: inferolateral and medial canthus injection sites.

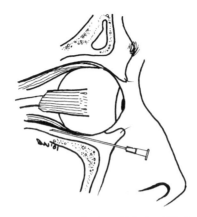

Fig 24.2 Peribulbar block II: inferolateral injection (side view).

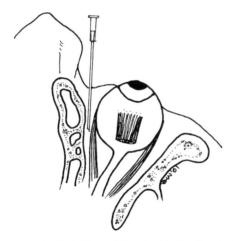

Fig 24.3 Peribulbar block III: medial canthus injection (top view).

Procedure

+ Establish IV access and monitoring.
+ When indicated use minimal sedation, e.g. midazolam 0.5–1.5 mg ± alfentanil 250 μg or fentanyl 50 μg.
+ Instil topical local anaesthetic drops to anaesthetize the conjunctiva. Amethocaine 1% is effective but may cloud the cornea. Oxybuprocaine

0.4% (Benoxinate®) is a better alternative, or proxymetacaine 0.5%, which causes less initial stinging.

* The patient lies supine and is asked to look straight ahead (primary gaze).

* Palpate the junction of the medial two-thirds and lateral third of the inferior orbital rim with the non-dominant hand, where a groove is felt at the junction of the maxilla and zygoma.

* Just lateral to this point, and 1 mm above the rim, insert a 25G 25 mm standard hypodermic needle ('long orange') mounted on a 10 ml syringe, and pass slowly backwards perpendicular to all planes. Needle entry can be either transcutaneous or, by retraction of the lower lid, transconjunctival.

* If the needle tip contacts bone, it is redirected slightly superomedially, to follow the orbit floor once more.

* Advance the needle until its tip is about level with the posterior pole of the globe (i.e. until the hub reaches the plane of the iris). The globe should be observed carefully for any sign of rotation during insertion, indicating scleral contact. Avoid the temptation to wiggle the needle to confirm that the sclera is unengaged. This is likely to increase the risk of haemorrhage.

* After aspiration, slowly inject 6–8 ml of local anaesthetic. The globe can be palpated with the other hand to assess tension. Stop injecting if globe becomes tense/proptosed, or if the upper eyelid falls, as this is likely to indicate retrobulbar injection, requiring a much smaller volume of agent.

* As the needle is withdrawn, a small volume of solution is deposited in the orbicularis of the lower lid.

* Following injection, digital massage or a compression device (Honan balloon) should be applied to dissipate the local anaesthetic and quickly normalize intraocular pressure.

* Assess the block after 5–10 min and if a greater degree of akinesia is required a second injection should be performed. In modern ophthalmic practice a completely akinetic eye is now less often required and a second injection doubles the risk of sharp needle complications. Discuss this requirement with the surgeon.

* Using a similar needle, entry is made at a point just medial to the caruncle. The needle is passed backward with the bevel facing the globe, at an angle of 10° to the saggital plane, directed towards the medial wall of the orbit. If the medial wall is contacted, the needle is withdrawn slightly and redirected laterally.

* If both medial and lateral injections are planned, the volume of solution is 4–5 ml for each.

The larger volumes of solution required for peribulbar block tend to cause proptosis and a temporary increase in IOP. In the intact globe this has no consequence, but will be problematic when the globe is opened for surgery. The raised IOP usually disappears when the solution has dissipated around the globe, alternatively a Honan balloon can be used. This is a tamponade applied to the eye at a set pressure (25 mmHg), which compresses the eye transiently increasing IOP further. However, during compression, the volume of blood and aqueous in the eye is reduced. Upon release of the tamponade, the 'empty' eye becomes hypotonic and remains so for about 15 min, until blood and aqueous volumes are re-established.

Single medial canthus injection

The medial orbital wall runs directly backwards and is separated anteriorly from the optic nerve and major blood vessels by the medial rectus muscle. A single injection technique has recently been advocated using the medial approach to reduce the risk of perforation injury.

- A 25G 22 mm short bevel needle is inserted through the caruncle and advanced directly posteriorly.
- At a depth of 15–20 mm a click is felt (passage through medial check ligament) and the eyeball returns to primary gaze.
- Following aspiration, 8–10 ml of solution is injected.
- Risks of globe perforation and haemorrhage may be reduced using this technique, but a second inferolateral injection may be required (in 10–40% of cases).
- Because needle insertion is parallel to the medial orbital wall, globe perforation is less likely than with the inferolateral approach, and this may therefore be a safer technique when the axial length is greater than 26 mm.
- Chemosis and anterior spread of solution into the soft tissues of the lids is common, but reduces following globe compression, and is rarely a problem.

Contraindications

- INR >2.5. Whenever possible warfarin therapy should be adjusted to reduce the INR to less than 2.5. If this is considered inappropriate (e.g. in patients with artificial heart valves) then the relative risks of a general anaesthetic must be considered. An alternative option is to use a sub-Tenon approach or topical anaesthesia only (see p. 566).
- Axial length >26 mm. In severely myopic patients the globe often has a long anteroposterior diameter ('sausage shaped eyeball'). This increases the likelihood of globe perforation (diagnosed by sudden pain on injection, loss of vision, poor red reflex, or vitreous haemorrhage). Where the axial length is greater than 26 mm, consider single medial canthus injection, the sub-Tenon approach, topical anaesthesia only, or general anaesthesia.
- Perforated or infected eye.
- Patient unable to lie flat or still.

Complications

- As for retrobulbar (above), but lesser incidence.
- The risk of complications from peribulbar anaesthesia, although outweighed by the benefits, are still appreciable: between 1 in 750 and 1 in 360 local anaesthetics have 'life-threatening' and 'serious' complications respectively. The incidence of globe perforation is less than 0.1%.
- Retrobulbar haemorrhage can be recognized by rapid orbital swelling and proptosis. The surgeon should be informed immediately and the pulsation of the central retinal artery should be assessed. If this is compromised, a lateral canthotomy may be required to relieve IOP.
- Globe perforation is not always obvious. It may be noted at the time of surgery if the eye becomes hypotonic, in which case there is a serious risk of retinal haemorrhage and detachment which may require laser retinopexy or vitrectomy.

Sub-Tenon block

This technique is gaining popularity as an easy, safe and effective alternative to retro- and peribulbar anaesthesia. It has the advantage of avoiding 'blind needling' to the orbit, and so has no appreciable risk of the complications discussed above. The technique involves dissecting beneath Tenon's capsule and passing a blunt curved cannula (Southampton cannula) in this space beyond the equator to deposit LA solution. It effectively blocks the ciliary ganglion and the long and short ciliary nerves. Larger volumes deposited more posteriorly are required to block the motor nerves and extraconal branches of the ophthalmic and maxillary nerves.

- Apply topical anaesthesia to the conjuntiva and retract the lower lid using either an assistant or a speculum.

- In the inferonasal quadrant, the conjuctiva is lifted with Moorfield's forceps at a point 5–7 mm from the limbus (awake patients are asked to look up and out).

- A small incision is made in the conjuctiva with (blunt) Westcotts spring scissors which are then used to dissect inferonasally in a plane between the sclera and Tenon's capsule (Tenon's capsule is white and avascular which distinguishes it from the vascular sclera).

- Once in this plane, a blunt curved Southampton cannula is passed backwards beyond the equator and 3–5 ml of local anaesthetic is deposited. Care must be taken to dissect in the right plane. If the cannula is placed subconjunctivally, this will become very apparent on attempting to inject the solution.

- Sub-Tenon block can be used safely in patients with axial lengths >26 mm. It is the block of choice in anticoagulated patients, since any bleeding point can be cauterized directly. It may be most easily performed by the surgeon, although it is increasingly being performed by anaesthetists.

Complications

Conjunctival haematoma. Occurs rarely (less that 0.5%) and is usually easily treated by cautery.

Topical/infiltration anaesthesia

Anterior segment (principally cataract) surgery can be carried out under:

- Subconjunctival injection, where a small volume of local anasthetic is injected near the superior limbus by the surgeon.

- Topical corneoconjunctival anaesthesia, where topical agents can be used to provide anaesthesia. Bupivacaine 0.75% is effective but can sting initially and cloud the cornea. Oxybuprocaine 0.4% (Benoxinate®) or proxymetacaine 0.5% are superior.

For both these techniques, anaesthesia is not as complete as with the formal ocular blocks. The iris and ciliary body retain their sensitivity and akinesia is not a feature. The surgeon and staff will need to ensure that good communication is maintained with the patient at all times. A mild anxiolytic premedication may be useful.

Some surgeons augment these techniques with 0.1–0.5 ml of preservative free lidocaine (lignocaine) 1% into the anterior chamber (intracameral).

Local anaesthetic solutions

- The commonest local anaesthetic solution is a 1:1 mixture of lidocaine (lignocaine) 2% and bupivicaine 0.5–0.75%. Adrenaline adds little to block quality and in best avoided.
- Hyaluronidase should be added to promote spread and reduce IOP. Concentrations of between 10 and 30 units/ml are used.
- Alkalinization and warming of the local agent (to 37 °C) may reduce latency and decrease pain on injection.
- Prilocaine 3% with felypressin has recently been advocated as unsuitable for ocular anaesthesia by the manufacturers, following several cases of optic atrophy.

The Joint Working Party on Anaesthesia in Ophthalmic Surgery[1]

In 1993 the Royal College of Anaesthetists and the College of Ophthalmologists jointly published guidelines on the roles and responsibilities of the anaesthetist in (intraocular) ophthalmic surgery under local anaesthesia. It was agreed that an anaesthetist should be present in such cases to give resuscitation should it be required and to monitor the patient's general condition throughout. In addition, it was recommended that the anaesthetist should be responsible for providing sedation where necessary, administering the local anaesthetic block, and providing intravenous access. These recommendations do not apply to simple infiltration anaesthesia for extraocular surgery.

In 2001 these guidelines were updated with the following recommendations[2]:

- Local anaesthesia should only be administered by appropriately trained staff.
- Surgeons may administer topical, sub-conjunctival and sub-Tenon anaesthesia without an anaesthetist present.
- An anaesthetist must be available when surgery is performed under retro- or peribulbar block.
- An anaesthetist must be present and have sole responsibility for a list in which sedation is used.

1 Royal College of Anaesthetists and College of Ophthalmologists (1993).*Report of the Joint Working Party on Anaesthesia in Ophthalmic Surgery.*

2 Local anaesthesia for intraocular surgery (2001). Royal College of Ophthalmologists and Royal College of Anaesthetists.

General anaesthesia for ophthalmic surgery

The aim is to minimize increases in IOP whilst maintaining cardiovascular stability and avoiding overly deep anaesthesia in a population which is likely to be elderly and with several co-morbidities.

Indications

- Patient preference.
- Other patient factors (e.g. movement disorders, dementia, claustrophobia).
- Long operations (e.g. vitreoretinal).
- Multiple operation sites (e.g. oculoplastics with distant graft donor site).

Preoperative

In addition to routine consultation and investigations, the preoperative visit should identify patients with co-morbidities such as diabetes and cardiovascular disease. Insulin-dependent diabetics will often have reduced their morning dose of insulin and will be fasted. Such patients will require close monitoring of blood glucose, and the institution of a euglycaemic control regimen.

ETT or LMA?

Unless contraindicated, the LMA is ideal. It obviates laryngoscopy with the consequent adverse effects on IOP. It produces minimal stimulation once *in situ* and permits lighter anaesthesia. The quality of emergence is also superior (see below).

IPPV or SV?

For minor and extraoccular surgery spontaneous ventilation is acceptable. Controlled ventilation has a number of advantages in intraocular and more major surgery. It allows more precise control of CO_2 (reducing IOP and desensitizing the oculomedullary reflex) and permits benefits of a balanced technique:

- Ventilating via an LMA is usually uneventful. Avoid high airway pressures (>15 cmH_2O, with the risk of gastric insuflation) if possible by adjusting the tidal volume and using a more symmetrical I:E ratio (i.e. 1:1.5 as opposed to 1:3).
- Always monitor the CO_2 waveform. Any change in the waveform usually heralds a change in ventilation before it is clinically apparent (mal-positioned LMA, inadequate muscle relaxation).
- Use a nerve stimulator routinely. Coughing and gagging are less well tolerated by ophthalmic surgeons than by their orthopaedic colleagues!

Nitrous oxide?

Nitrous oxide should be avoided in vitreoretinal surgery if intraocular gas bubbles of sulphurhexafluoride (SF_6) or similar are planned. Discuss this with the surgeon in advance.

Supplementary local block?

If used as a supplement to GA, the block can be administered after induction. However, since the principal benefit of a local block is that it avoids the necessity of general anaesthesia, if used in addition to GA the risk/benefit ratio for the block is now altered, and it may no longer be justified. Probably the only indication for local block in addition to GA is for vitreoretinal surgery, in which case a sub-Tenon block (with negligible risk) is used.

Emergence without coughing

With an LMA, emergence and LMA removal are usually very smooth. If a tracheal tube is used, spray the cords with lidocaine (lignocaine) at intubation. Unfortunately the effect is short lived and may no longer be effective at extubation. Other techniques are to extubate in a deep plane or administer a bolus of IV lidocaine (lignocaine) (1 mg/kg) or propofol (30–40 mg) 1 min prior to extubation. It is best not to lighten anaesthesia until surgery is complete and the 'sticky drapes' removed (if a block has been used, drape removal may well be the most stimulating part of the operation). Emergence hypertension (and the concomitant raised IOP), if it occurs, can be moderated by the use of IV lidocaine (lignocaine) and/or β blockade.

A standard technique

- IV induction: propofol bolus or TCI.
- Airway: reinforced LMA if appropriate.
- Use IPPV.
- Maintenance: propofol infusion (at around 5 mg/kg/hr in the steady state, or at 2.5 μg/ml if using TCI). Volatile agents are also suitable.
- Ventilate the lungs with oxygen/air or oxygen/nitrous oxide.
- Analgesia provided with either alfentanil/fentanyl or a local anaesthetic block if indicated.

  The following general points should be noted:
- Tape the non-operative eye.
- Access to the airway may be limited by drapes, trays of instruments, and equipment overlying the area. Have a low threshold for moving everyone out of the way to inspect the airway if you suspect difficulties.
- The prophylactic use of glycopyrrolate (200 μg) will reduce the volume of saliva pooling behind the LMA (which can otherwise spill from the corner of the mouth and soak through the surgical drapes). It may also reduce the incidence and severity of 'oculocardic' bradycardias.

Postoperative

Analgesia requirements are usually modest, especially if supplemental local anaesthesia is used. Nausea and vomiting is common in squint surgery, but less so in the majority of other cases. Droperidol (75 μg/kg) has been shown to be effective prophylaxis in squint surgery.

Cataract extraction and Intraocular Lens (IOL) Implant

Procedure	Phacoemulsification of opacified lens, removal and replacement with artificial intraocular implant
Time	20–40 min
Pain	+
Position	Supine
Blood loss	Nil
Practical technique	Local technique
	LMA (armoured), SV/IPPV
	COETT (RAE, armoured), IPPV

Preoperative

- Check the axial length (less than 26 mm for peribulbar block) and INR if necessary. For operations under local anaesthesia, the patient must be able to lie flat and still.
- Often 'day case' surgery.

Perioperative

- Use supplemental oxygen (via nasal cannulas).
- Monitor BP, SpO_2, and nasal expired CO_2 if possible. The latter serves as an indicator of apnoea and is useful if sedation is used. Be aware that the use of sedation may serve to disinhibit rather than sedate some patients.
- If sedation is required, 0.5–1.5 mg midazolam, with 25–50 μg fentanyl or 250 μg alfentanil can be used. This is best employed just before block insertion. The patient should then be allowed to awaken again when in theatre to gain their cooperation and avoid sleeping, snoring, and airway problems.

Postoperative

Simple oral analgesics only are required.

Strabismus surgery

Procedures	Extraocular surgery for correction of squint— may be unilateral or bilateral
Time	60–90 min
Pain	+
Position	Supine
Blood loss	Nil
Practical technique	LMA (armoured), IPPV/SV
	COETT (RAE, armoured), IPPV

Preoperative

- The patient population is mainly children (the commonest ophthalmic operation in children).
- May be 'day case' procedures.
- Preoperative analgesia (20 mg/kg soluble paracetamol).
- Consent for suppositories.

Perioperative

- Higher incidence of oculocardiac reflex; have atropine prepared.
- Suxamethonium should be avoided because tone in the ocular muscles remains abnormal for up to 20 min, making surgical assessment and correction difficult.
- Controlled or spontaneous ventilation, via LMA or tracheal tube, is used. Control of CO_2 may reduce the incidence and severity of the oculocardic reflex.
- All anaesthetics affect eye movement and the position of neutral gaze (Guedel's signs). Propofol may affect this the least, and the rapid recovery it affords allows early assessment of the correction in recovery. Anaesthesia with volatile agents should be of sufficient depth to ensure neutral gaze.
- Rectal diclofenac (1 mg/kg).
- Opioids may be avoided, thereby reducing the incidence of PONV.

Postoperative

- Postoperative pain is mild and can be treated with oral analgesics and topical anaesthetic eye drops.
- There is a high incidence of PONV. Droperidol (75 μg/kg) is effective prophylaxis.

Vitreoretinal surgery

Procedures	Intraocular surgery
	Vitrectomy, cryotherapy, laser, plombage, insertion of oil and/or gas, scleral banding ('explant')
Time	90–180 min
Pain	+/++
Position	Supine
Blood loss	Nil
Practical technique	LMA (armoured), IPPV
	COETT (RAE, armoured), IPPV

Preoperative

* The patient population is generally aged 60–70 years. May have co-morbidities, e.g. hypertension, ischaemic heart disease, and diabetes.
* Patients often present for repeat surgery. They may have undergone failed attempts to improve their vision and their preoperative anxiety may be high.
* May be retinal detachments and therefore semiurgent.

Perioperative

* Surgery is characterized by alternating periods of intense and minimal stimulation. Achieving a depth of anaesthesia and analgesia to accommodate these extremes is not easy without concurrent local block.
* Operations are often prolonged and performed largely in the dark.
* Axial length is usually high (profound myopia causes retinal detachment) so retro/peribulbar blocks are contraindicated. A sub-Tenon block in addition to GA is ideal.
* If necessary, can be performed under local anaesthesia, but the duration of surgery makes this difficult in the majority of patients.
* Controlled ventilation is usual. LMA/propofol/alfentanil technique is ideal.
* Intraocular tamponade with gas (SF_6 or C_3F_8) may be used, usually towards the end of the case. Surgeons vary in their consideration of nitrous oxide. It is often recommended that nitrous oxide be discontinued 20 min beforehand. It may be better to omit it altogether because surgeons seldom give notice and it is probably not wise to interfere with the equilibrium of the anaesthetic at a time when muscle relaxation is being allowed to wear-off.
* Cryotherapy and scleral indentation are very stimulating and should be pre-empted with boluses of alfentanil if a block is not used.
* Beware 'lightening' the patient too soon at the end of surgery. The other eye is often examined, and possibly cryocauterized, at the end of the case.

Postoperative

- With a block the postoperative analgesic requirement is minimal and PONV is rare.
- Otherwise use simple oral analgesics.

Dacrocystorhinostomy

Procedures	Probing of tear duct, insertion of drainage tube, formation of stoma between lacrimal sac and nasal mucosa
Time	30–90 min
Pain	+
Position	Supine, slight head up
Blood loss	Can be relatively bloody, with soiling of nasopharynx
Practical technique	COETT (RAE, armoured), IPPV
	LMA (armoured), IPPV

Perioperative

- Lacrimal surgery can range from simple probing of the tear ducts, to insertion of tubes or formal dacrocystorhinostomy (DCR). The latter is usually done under GA.

- DCR may be bloody. Blood will pass into the nasopharnx and oropharynx. Topical vasoconstrictor solutions (pledgelets soaked in Moffat's solution) placed after induction may minimize this.

- A slight head up tilt and deliberate moderate hypotension (or avoidance of hypertension) further improves the operative field.

- Intubation (oral RAE or reinforced tube) protects the lower airway definitively, but a reinforced LMA is commonly used where topical vasoconstriction, moderate hypotension, and surgical cooperation are available. A throat pack should be used in any case.

- Controlled ventilation, by facilitating moderate hypocapnia, may also contribute to mucosal vasoconstriction and improved operative field. If using an LMA, positive pressure ventilation may reduce the likelihood of blood soiling the lower airway.

Postoperative

- Postoperative analgesia is provided by oral NSAIDs and paracetamol/codeine.

Penetrating eye injury

Procedures	EUA, debridement, closure of punctum.
Time	30–45 min
Pain	+/+++
Position	Supine
Blood loss	+
Practical technique	COETT (RAE, armoured), IPPV
	LMA (armoured), IPPV

Preoperative

* Although relatively straightforward in adults, this can be difficult to manage in children. The essential danger is that elevation of IOP either pre- or perioperatively, risks extrusion of the vitreous, haemorrhage, and lens prolapse.
* Pain, eye rubbing, crying, breath holding, and screaming will elevate IOP. IV sedation may be required to control such a child.
* Give analgesia (oral or rectal paracetamol or NSAIDs). Opioids should be avoided if possible (or at least used cautiously and with an anti-emetic) since vomiting will also affect IOP adversely.
* Patients may have a full stomach. Traumatized children may still have a full stomach several hours postinjury.

Perioperative

* Suxamethonium causes a transient increase in IOP and there is good reason to avoid its use when the eye is open. However, induction agents reduce IOP and so moderate its effects. The risks imposed by suxamethonium should be balanced against the risks imposed by a full stomach. Each case is different and the assessment should include the nature of the eye injury—size of penetration, degree of existing damage.
* If in doubt, use suxamethonium following a large dose of induction agent. There are, however, two practical alternatives to suxamethonium:
  * Wait. If immediate operative repair is not imperative (and it seldom is) the case can be deferred until the stomach is considered safe. Prokinetic agents may be of use.
  * If no airway problems are anticipated, use a rapid sequence technique with rocuronium (1 mg/kg), or 'high-dose' vecuronium (0.15 mg/kg).
  * The pressor response to intubation can be moderated by IV lidocaine (lignocaine) (1 mg/kg), IV esmolol, or prepriming with induction agent immediately prior to intubation.
* Opioids may be used as part of a balanced technique.

Postoperative

Analgesia can be provided by paracetamol/codeine preparations and oral/rectal diclofenac.

Other opthalmic procedures

Operation	Description	Time (min)	Pain (+ to ++++)	Position	Blood loss	Notes
Moh's reconstruction	Plastics procedure on eyelids after excision of basal cell carcinoma	45–60	+	Supine	Nil	May be under local, but may require use of fat or fascia taken from the thigh so GA may be preferred
Enucleation	Removal of globe for tumour or chronic infection	60–90	++	Supine	+	Anaesthetic technique as for vitreoretinal surgery. Local techniques not appropriate
Evisceration	Removal of globe contents for later replacement with prosthesis	60–90	+	Supine	Nil	Anaesthetic technique as for vitreoretinal surgery. Local techniques not appropriate
Syringing of tear ducts in babies		30	+	Supine		Straightforward technique. SV via LMA. Throat pack to absorb any 'wash'
EUA of eyes in babies		10–20	+	Supine		Beware oculocardic reflex. Have atropine 10 µg/kg prepared

Further reading

Hamilton RC (1995). Techniques of orbital regional anaesthesia. *British Journal of Anaesthesia*, 75, 88–92.

Ripart J *et al.* (1996). Medial canthus (caruncle) single injection periocular anesthesia. *Regional Anesthesia and Pain Management*, **83**, 1234–8.

Wong DHW (1993). Regional anaesthesia for intraocular surgery. *Canadian Journal of Anaesthesia*, **40**, 635–57.

Chapter 25
Plastic surgery
Jonathan Warwick

General principles

Anaesthesia for plastic surgery provides many challenges for the anaesthetist owing to the wide spectrum of activity and range of techniques required. Success or failure of surgery may depend on careful manipulation of the patient's physiology to achieve optimal conditions. Close cooperation between anaesthetic and surgical teams is vital.

Procedures encountered on plastic surgery lists may range from simple excision of skin lesions to extensive and lengthy reconstruction following trauma or malignant disease. Operations are often extremely specialized and some procedures may only be performed in designated centres in the United Kingdom.

Anaesthetic technique

Variety of surgery

The complexity of anaesthesia ranges from the routine to the extremely challenging. Some extensive procedures (e.g. free flap repairs or craniofacial reconstruction) may involve invasive monitoring with extensive blood loss, and may require postoperative intensive care support.

Day case anaesthesia

Minor procedures are suitable for surgery as a day case, e.g. correction of prominent ears, Dupuytren's fasciectomy, or the excision of skin lesions.

Regional techniques

Minor body surface procedures may be performed under local anaesthetic infiltration alone. Upper or lower limb surgery is especially suitable for regional or peripheral nerve block. Sedation to supplement a regional technique may be required in anxious patients or for longer procedures. Propofol (1–2 mg/kg/h with addition of alfentanil 20 μg/ml) supplemented with a small dose of midazolam (1–2 mg) is effective. Significant body surface procedures (e.g. excision and grafting of skin tumours) can be accomplished in those unfit for general anaesthesia using extensive infiltration of local anaesthesia and intravenous sedation. Incremental sedation with ketamine (10 mg) and midazolam (1 mg) is a safe and potent analgesic/sedative combination in the elderly.

The difficult airway

Patients with head and neck pathology causing airway difficulty are often encountered. Airway difficulty may arise from anatomical deformity due to tumour, trauma, infection, previous operation, or scarring. Competence in difficult airway techniques (e.g. fibreoptic intubation) is required. The 'shared airway' is regularly a feature of head and neck surgery. Discuss with the surgeon what tube you propose to use, and by what route, to achieve the best surgical access (oral, nasal, conversion to tracheostomy?). How is the tube to be secured (tied, taped, stitched)?

Poor access to patient

The operating site may be extensive (e.g. burns debridement) or multiple (e.g. free flap procedures). This may produce added difficulty with:

- Heat conservation. It may be difficult to achieve enough access to the patient's body surface area to maintain temperature. Heated underblankets are useful.
- Monitoring. ECG leads, the pulse oximeter probe, and blood pressure cuff may all be difficult to position adequately.
- Vascular access. Position cannulas remote from the operative field. Use femoral vessels or the foot if necessary. Long extension sets are needed.

Smooth emergence

Avoid the patient coughing and straining at the end of the procedure. This will put tension on delicate suture lines and increase bleeding and haematoma formation, especially for facial procedures. The combination of propofol maintenance and the laryngeal mask airway produces a particularly smooth emergence.

Attention to detail

Successful anaesthesia for plastic surgery requires thoroughness and careful attention to detail. Patients for aesthetic surgery will have high expectations and will be well informed.

Analgesia

Pain relief is always a challenge to anaesthetists and is a major quality issue. In practice, effective pain control may be more readily achievable in patients recovering from plastic surgery for several reasons:

- Most procedures are performed on the body surface. These tend to be less painful than procedures involving the body cavities and are usually amenable to local anaesthetic infiltration. Continuous catheter techniques may be useful in limb procedures.
- Patients recovering from head and neck procedures are often surprisingly comfortable despite extensive surgery.
- Major body cavities and abdominal musculature are usually not involved. The pain experienced after abdominoplasty is significantly less than pain following laparotomy.
- Plastic surgery procedures seldom involve new fracture of long bones.
- The gastrointestinal tract is usually unaffected. The oral route for drugs is frequently available which may make dosing and administration of analgesics simpler.

Long operations

Patients undergoing complicated reconstructive procedures may be in theatre for many hours. Give careful consideration to:

• Vascular access. Check that line placement will not interfere with the site of surgery. Invasive arterial monitoring is highly desirable to facilitate blood pressure monitoring, to allow regular blood gas estimations, and to avoid frequent blood pressure cuff cycling. A central venous line will assist with estimations of intravascular volume and provide dependable venous access in the postoperative period. Site at least one large-bore peripheral (14–16G) cannula for fluid administration in theatre. A small cannula (20–22G) is helpful for patient-controlled analgesia.

• Blood loss. Ensure blood has been cross-matched. The initial dissection is usually the period of most blood loss and a moderate hypotensive technique may help to limit this. Thereafter losses may be insidious and on-going. Aim to keep track by swab weighing, visual estimation, regular haemoglobin, or haematocrit estimations.

• Fluid balance. Urinary catheterization is essential. Ensure careful monitoring of fluid balance, especially in children and in patients with poor cardio-respiratory function.

• Body temperature. Monitor core temperature (e.g. rectal, nasopharyngeal, or oesophageal). Maintain temperature by using low fresh gas flows, a heat-moisture exchange (HME) filter, warmed IV fluids, a warm ambient theatre temperature (e.g. 24 °C), a heated mattress, or external warming blankets (e.g. 'Bair Hugger'). Take care not to overheat. Consider reducing the temperature of external warming blankets before the desired temperature is reached since overshoot often occurs.

• Positioning. Ensure that structures such as the cervical spine or brachial plexus are not in positions of stress. Take care with pressure areas. Make liberal use of cotton wool padding ('Gamgee') over bony prominences. Raise the heels off the table using foam pads or boots.

• DVT prophylaxis. Venous thromboembolism is often initiated during surgery. All patients should receive perioperative subcutaneous heparin 5000 units twice daily (or daily low-molecular-weight heparin), thromboembolism ('TED') stockings, and intermittent calf compression whilst in theatre.

• Nasogastric tube. Consider emptying the stomach. Children are especially prone to gastric distension during prolonged procedures.

• Eye care. Lightly tape and pad the eyes for protection. Avoid excessive padding, since this may negate the natural protection afforded by the bony orbit. Prophylactic antibiotic ointment is unnecessary. Do not allow corneal abrasion to develop from surface drying.

• ET tube cuff pressure. Cuff pressure will gradually increase if N_2O is used. Where possible, recheck the cuff pressure at intervals during the case. Alternatively, fill the cuff with N_2O-containing gas or saline from the start.

• Postoperative care. Discuss the preferred site of postoperative care with the nursing staff and surgical team. Surgeons often prefer patients to return to the plastic surgery ward where wound care and nursing observation may be more attuned to the specifics of the operation. Closer patient observation, invasive monitoring, and regular blood gas estimation may be more achievable in an intensive/high-dependency unit. In practice, there is seldom conflict. The site for immediate postoperative care is principally dictated by the general condition of the patient.

Breast reduction

Procedure	Reduction of breast size by glandular resection. Usually bilateral
Time	3 h
Pain	++
Position	Supine, 30° head up. Arms may be positioned on boards, or with elbows flexed and hands placed behind the upper part of the buttocks
Blood loss	500 ml, G&S
Practical techniques	IPPV via ETT or LMA

Preoperative

- Bilateral breast reduction is not primarily an aesthetic procedure. These patients may suffer from severe neck and back pain. Participating in exercise and sport is not possible. There may be symptoms of emotional disturbance.

- Patients are usually fit and well, aged 20–40 years. Many surgeons exclude patients with a body mass index >30 due to a higher incidence of wound breakdown, infection, and haematoma formation.

- A mastopexy is a surgical procedure for correcting breast ptosis when breast volume is adequate. Anaesthetic implications are similar. Blood loss is less.

- FBC and group and save. Cross-matching is generally unnecessary except for larger reductions.

- Timing in relation to the menstrual cycle is unimportant.

- All patients should receive DVT prophylaxis (TED stockings and heparin 5000 units SC 12-hourly).

Perioperative

- Patients should receive a balanced GA. IPPV may be preferable since the surgeon often puts pressure on the chest wall during surgery. IPPV will maintain satisfactory chest expansion with good aeration, control of $PaCO_2$ and help minimize blood loss. An LMA is usually satisfactory for IPPV.

- Loosen and remove the theatre gown prior to induction. Place ECG electrodes on the patient's back. Lie the patient on 'incontinence pads' to absorb blood loss.

- Take care to position the patient carefully on the operating table. The anaesthetic machine is usually at the head end. Ensure that the chest and arms are symmetrical. Confirm that the cannulas are firmly positioned and their plastic caps covered with 'gamgee' if the hands are to be positioned behind the buttocks. Local pressure damage to skin may otherwise ensue. Drip extension sets are needed and ensure that the drip runs freely.

- Blood loss depends on surgical technique. Use of cutting diathermy causes less bleeding than a scalpel. Infiltration with dilute adrenaline-containing local anaesthetic helps reduce blood loss. All surgeons have their own recipe. Check the dosage being used, in practice this is seldom a concern (see liposuction).
- Fewer than 5% of patients usually require transfusion. Mild falls in haemoglobin are well tolerated in this predominantly young patient group.
- Moderate reductions may involve removal of 500 g of tissue per breast.

Postoperative

- Bilateral breast reduction does not cause significant postoperative pain. Following a dose of longer-acting opioid towards the end of surgery, regular simple analgesics and NSAIDs are adequate. Intravenous PCA is generally unnecessary. An occasional dose of IM opioid may be required.
- Haematoma formation is an early complication. Occasionally nipple perfusion may be compromised and require decompression of the pedicle. Return to theatre may be indicated. Later complications include wound infection, dehiscence, and fat necrosis.

Special considerations

Occasionally patients for massive breast reduction are encountered (>1 kg tissue removal per breast). Two to four units of blood should be cross-matched. The complication rate is higher. Older patients may have coexisting cardiopulmonary disease and require further investigation. Intubation and IPPV is the preferred technique.

Breast augmentation

Procedure	Bilateral or unilateral augmentation of breast size
Time	90 min
Pain	++/+++
Position	Supine, 30° head up. Arms may be out on boards, or with elbows flexed and hands placed behind the upper part of the buttocks
Blood loss	Minimal
Practical techniques	Spontaneous ventilation or IPPV via LMA

Preoperative

- The availability of this procedure on the NHS depends on clinical need. Breast augmentation may be performed for:
  - Reconstruction following mastectomy.
  - Correction of breast asymmetry. Minor asymmetry is common. In its most severe form there may be unilateral absence of breast tissue and pectoralis major muscle (Poland syndrome).
  - Aesthetic bilateral augmentation. Availability is usually via private funding.
- Patients are usually fit and well. Check FBC.

Perioperative

- Position on the operating table as for breast reduction.
- Conventional augmentation involves creation of a subcutaneous pocket for a silicone implant via an inframammary incision.
- Modern techniques involve initial pocket formation by the insertion of an inflatable capsule mounted on an introducer via a small incision in the anterior axillary line. This is then removed and the implant inserted. Early recovery is good and there is less postoperative discomfort.

Postoperative

- Postoperative discomfort may be related to the size of the implants. Large implants cause more tissue stretching and postoperative pain. In general, breast augmentation appears to cause more discomfort than breast reduction. Give regular NSAIDs and simple analgesics. Opioid analgesia may be needed but PCA techniques are seldom required.
- Haematoma formation may require early return to theatre. Later complications include infection, capsule formation, prosthesis rupture, or skin erosion.

Special considerations

- There has been association made between silicone breast implants and development of systemic symptoms suggestive of connective tissue diseases. This association has not been proven following data from large studies.
- Soybean oil-filled implants have been withdrawn from use in the United Kingdom. There are insufficient data concerning the long-term consequences of soybean oil breakdown. Saline implants are not perceived as sufficiently realistic and are unpopular with many women.
- Breast reconstruction following mastectomy is common. Options include insertion of a breast implant, reconstruction with a pedicled myocutaneous flap (e.g. latissimus dorsi or transverse rectus abdominis muscle 'TRAM'), or a free flap repair (usually TRAM).

Correction of prominent ears

Procedure	Surgical correction of prominent ears, usually caused by the absence of an antehelical fold. May be unilateral
Time	1 h
Pain	+
Position	Supine, 30° head up
Blood loss	Minimal
Practical techniques	Day case anaesthesia, flexible LMA and spontaneous ventilation

Preoperative

* Patients are usually children aged 4–10 years and fit. May not present for surgery until teenage or early adulthood.
* Surgery is offered as child grows older and is aware of prominent ears. Often precipitated by teasing at school. Child may be self-conscious and anxious.
* Obtain consent for suppositories.

Perioperative

* Day case anaesthetic technique.
* Anaesthetic machine usually at the foot end.
* PONV is common. A propofol maintenance is well tolerated.
* Avoid morphine. Use shorter-acting opioids (fentanyl or alfentanil) and NSAIDs.
* The surgeons use extensive LA/adrenaline infiltration to aid surgery. This provides good analgesia.
* 20 ml/kg crystalloid IV may improve the quality of early recovery.

Postoperative

* NSAIDs (e.g. ibuprofen syrup 20 mg/kg/day, or 100 mg three times a day 3–7 years, 200 mg three times a day 8–12 years) and paracetamol 20 mg/kg four times a day prn.
* Dressings should be firm without being excessively tight. Scalp discomfort and itching can be a source of discomfort.
* Excessive pain may be due to haematoma formation and requires a return to theatre for drainage.

Special considerations

Allow time for extensive bandaging at the end of the operation. If a COETT is used early reduction in anaesthetic depth will lead to coughing when the head is manipulated for bandage application. An LMA is ideal.

Facelift (rhytidectomy)

Procedure	Surgical reduction of facial folds and wrinkles to create a more youthful appearance
Time	3–4 h. More extensive procedures 6–8 h
Pain	+
Position	Supine, 30° head up
Blood loss	Minimal
Practical techniques	IPPV via LMA or ETT, hypotensive technique, facial nerve blocks

Preoperative

- NHS funding is not available for these procedures.
- Most patients are aged 45–65 years. Patients are usually fit and well. They may have high expectations of anaesthesia and surgery and may have undergone previous facelift procedures.
- NSAIDs should be discontinued for at least 2 weeks prior to surgery.

Perioperative

- Many surgeons in the United States perform routine facelift procedures under LA infiltration alone. Cost constraints in patients who are self-funding have contributed to this practice. Standard practice in the United Kingdom is for GA. Facelifts should always be regarded as major procedures.
- Incisions are placed in concealed areas (e.g. preauricular, extending up to the temporal region within the hair). The skin is mobilized by subcutaneous undermining and wrinkles/skin folds are improved by traction. Redundant skin is excised. Surgery is adapted to suit the needs of the patient and may include forehead lift, upper and lower blepharoplasty, and removal of submental/submandibular fat. It is occasionally combined with septorhinoplasty.
- Discuss the choice of airway device with the surgeon (e.g. oral tube or nasal north-facing). Consider using a throat pack if there is nasal surgery.
- The anaesthetic machine is usually at the patient's foot end. Long breathing system tubing and drip extension sets are required.
- A moderate hypotensive technique (70–80 systolic) and 30° head up tilt will help minimize blood loss and improve surgical conditions.
- LA infiltration and discrete nerve blocks provide good postoperative pain relief.
- Use a warming blanket.

Postoperative

- A smooth emergence is important to avoid bleeding beneath delicate suture lines. A propofol maintenance and flexible LMA are ideal. Avoid postoperative shivering (treat with pethidine 25 mg IV). Bleeding and haematoma formation may require an early return to theatre.

- Pain is not a prominent feature. Discomfort is attributed to platysma tightening. Postoperative NSAIDs and simple analgesics are required. Marked pain should raise the suspicion of haematoma formation.

Special considerations

- The observed benefits from facelift procedures may only last 3–5 years. Repeat operations are common. Some patients may undergo several facelifts during their lifetime.
- Recent advances have involved more extensive procedures with deeper tissue undermining. These are all performed under GA. The composite facelift mobilizes platysma, cheek fat, and orbicularis occuli muscle. This flap is then repositioned en bloc with the overlying skin. Complications are more frequent.

Free flap surgery

Procedure	The transfer of tissue from a donor site and microvascular anastomosis to a distant recipient site
Time	Variable depending on procedure. Minimum 4 h, often 6–8 h or longer
Pain	+++
Position	Variable. Usually supine. May require position change during surgery
Blood loss	Often 4–6 units
Practical techniques	ET + IPPV, arterial + CVP lines, urinary catheter, epidural catheter for lower limb flaps

Preoperative

* Free flaps are most commonly used to provide tissue cover following trauma or resection for malignancy. It is a widely used reconstructive technique. Understand what operation is proposed and what the aims of surgery are.
* Typical procedures are:
  * Free transverse rectus abdominis muscle (TRAM) myocutaneous flap to reconstruct a breast following mastectomy.
  * Free gracilis muscle flap to cover an area of lower limb trauma with tissue loss.
  * Free radial forearm fasciocutaneous flap to the oropharynx following tumour excision.
* The aim of anaesthesia is to produce a hyperdynamic circulation with high cardiac output, adequate vasodilation, and wide pulse pressure. Patients with lower limb trauma are often young and fit. Patients with head and neck cancer are often smokers with ischaemic heart disease. The elderly or patients with limited cardiorespiratory reserve may not be suitable for surgery.

Perioperative

* Be prepared for a long surgical procedure. All patients should receive a balanced GA. Regional anaesthesia alone is seldom appropriate for these long procedures. Isoflurane is the inhalational agent of choice due to its beneficial effects on systemic vascular resistance (SVR). Propofol maintenance is also ideal since it lowers SVR, is rapidly metabolized, anti-emetic, and may avoid the postoperative shivering particularly associated with volatile agents (there is some in vitro evidence that propofol may be more favourable for microvascular flow by avoiding the effect of volatiles on red cell membrane stiffness).

- A regional block is helpful to supplement anaesthesia. The sympathetic block and dense analgesia produce excellent conditions for graft survival. Lower limb flaps are especially suitable. Surgery on multiple sites may not all be covered by the block. Skin grafts are often taken from the leg to cover a muscle flap.

- Anaesthetic management requires a good practical knowledge of circulatory physiology. Blood flow through the microvasculature must be optimal to help ensure flap survival. Blood flow is primarily influenced by changes in perfusion pressure, calibre of vessel, and blood viscosity (Hagan–Poiseuille formula). We only have a superficial understanding of the physiology of the microcirculation. Much of our anaesthetic management is based on perceived wisdom, rather than on the results of randomized controlled trials.

- Monitor core (e.g. rectal, oesophageal) and peripheral temperature. Insulate the skin probe from any overlying warming blanket. Aim for a normal or even supranormal core temperature and a core-peripheral difference of <2 °C. This must be achieved by the time that microvascular anastomosis is commenced. A widening of the core–peripheral temperature difference may herald vasoconstriction. Local vascular spasm may jeopardize the surgery.

- Correct any preoperative fluid deficit and commence volume loading. Continue maintenance crystalloid, and add 10 ml/kg colloid bolus (e.g. Gelofusine or Hetastarch) as required to expand the intravascular volume. Aim for CVP 12 mmHg (or 2–4 mmHg above baseline), urine output 2 ml/kg/h, widened pulse pressure, and low SVR. Colloid will expand the intravascular volume more effectively than crystalloid. Transplanted tissue lacks intact lymphatics and excess crystalloid may contribute to flap oedema. Take care to avoid excessive volume loading in the elderly who are more prone to develop pulmonary oedema.

- Moderate hypotension and haemodilution during the early phase of dissection may help limit blood loss. Thereafter, maintain systolic arterial pressure (SAP) at >100 mmHg or higher depending on preoperative blood pressure recordings.

- Viscosity is closely related to haematocrit (Hct). Viscosity rises dramatically when Hct >40%. Aim for an Hct of 30%, which in theory gives the best balance between blood viscosity, arterial oxygen content, and tissue oxygen delivery.

- Dextran reduces platelet adhesiveness and factor VIII concentration. It may help maintain graft patency. Depending on surgical preference, give 500 ml Dextran 40 during the procedure, and include 500 ml in the daily IV fluid for 2–3 days.

- Potent vasodilators (e.g. sodium nitroprusside, hydralazine, and phenoxybenzamine) are unnecessary. Sufficient vasodilation can be produced by the anaesthetic agent provided that the patient is warm, volume loaded, pain free, and normocarbic. Nifedepine 10 mg given with the premed and continued three times a day for 5 days in high-risk patients such as smokers, diabetics, and arteriopaths may improve flap survival. Chlorpromazine 1–2 mg IV (dilute a 50 mg ampoule to give a 1 mg/ml solution for injection) is useful to narrow a widened core–peripheral temperature difference when all other factors have been corrected. The surgeon may use pap-averine directly on the vessels to prevent local spasm.

* Prophylactic antibiotics are given at induction and may be repeated during the procedure.

Postoperative

* Aim for a smooth emergence.
* Continue meticulous care well into the postoperative period. Flap observation is a specialized nursing skill and care is often best provided on the plastic surgical ward. The need for HDU/ITU may be dictated by patient factors.
* Vasoconstriction from cold, pain, low circulating volume, hypotension, or hypocapnia will put the flap at risk and needs prompt correction.
* Treat shivering with pethidine 25 mg IV. Continue with warming blanket in recovery.
* The health of the flap is monitored clinically. Hourly observations include a 'flap chart' where temperature, colour, and arterial pulses (using a Doppler probe if possible) are monitored. A pale, pulseless flap with sluggish capillary filling may indicate problems with the arterial supply. A swollen, dusky flap, which blanches easily with a brisk capillary return, indicates a venous outflow problem. An early surgical decision needs to be made concerning re-exploration.
* Analgesia by continuous epidural is ideal for lower limb flaps. An axillary brachial plexus catheter (e.g. continuous infusion of 0.25% bupivacaine 5 ml/h for 2–3 days) is useful for procedures on the forearm and hand.
* Careful consideration should be given as to whether more invasive analgesic techniques are justified for procedures on the upper torso (e.g. thoracic epidural or intrapleural analgesia). Potential risks may outweigh the benefits. These patients often do very well with IV patient controlled analgesia (PCA). For head and neck proedures IV PCA is best.
* Attitudes vary concerning perioperative NSAIDs. They are valuable analgesics and reduce platelet adhesiveness. They may produce increased oozing following lengthy and extensive surgery. Administration postoperatively when clot is more established may be preferable.

Special considerations

* The reimplantation of severed digits or limbs should be managed as for a free flap.
* A 'pedicle flap' is constructed when arteriovenous connections remain intact but the raised flap is rotated to fill a neighbouring defect. Examples include rotation of rectus abdominus muscle to fill a sternal wound, rotation of pectoral muscle to reconstruct a defect in the side of the neck following tumour excision, or pedicled latissimus dorsi breast reconstruction. Whilst the procedure may be technically more simple than free tissue transfer, the anaesthesia requires similar attention to detail.
* Overall free flap survival is >95%. Flap failure will result in further reconstructive procedures. Patients in poor general condition with coexisting disease have the highest risk of flap failure.

Liposuction

Procedure	Vacuum aspiration of subcutaneous fat via a small skin incision and a specialized blunt-ended cannula
Time	Variable 30–90 min
Pain	+
Position	Variable, depending on site. Usually supine
Blood loss	1–40% of the volume of fat aspirated, depending on infiltration technique
Practical techniques	Local infiltration with IV sedation
	LMA and spontaneous ventilation

Preoperative

- Procedure may be used for:
  - lipoma removal
  - gynaecomastia
  - reducing the bulk of transplanted flaps to make them more closely contour the surrounding skin
  - cosmetic removal of subcutaneous fat ('liposculpture') in the abdominal wall, thighs, buttocks, and arms.
- Patients presenting for aesthetic surgery are often fit and well.

Perioperative

- The total amount of fat aspirated depends on patient requirement and surgical judgement.
- Fat is infiltrated with dilute local anaesthetic with adrenaline. Back and forth movement of the cannula disrupts fatty tissue which is then aspirated either by suction apparatus or syringe. Injection of fluid helps fat breakdown and aids aspiration.
- There are several recipes for subcutaneous infiltration solutions: 1000 ml warmed Hartmann's containing 50 ml 1% lidocaine (lignocaine) and 1 ml 1:1000 adrenaline is popular. 1 ml infiltrate per 1 ml aspirate is commonly used (superwet technique).
- The tumescent technique refers to a large volume of LA/adrenaline infiltrate to produce tissue turgor. Developed as an outpatient technique and performed without additional anaesthesia or sedation. 3 ml infiltrate per 1 ml aspirate are often used. There is little evidence that this technique is superior to the superwet technique, and may produce more complications. It may provide unsatisfactory anaesthesia when used alone. Additional sedation or general anaesthesia may be necessary.

- Blood loss depends on the volume of LA/adrenaline infiltrate used. Loss is approximately 1% of the volume of the aspirate for the tumescent technique. This may increase to 40% without subcutaneous infiltration.
- Extensive liposuction physiologically resembles a burn injury and large fluid shifts result. Commence IV infusion for aspirates >1500 ml. Replace aspirate 1:1 with IV crystalloid.

Postoperative

- Pressure dressings are usually applied.
- Monitor urine output.
- Encourage oral fluids.
- Check Hct following extensive liposuction (>2500 ml aspirate).
- Bruising can be considerable.
- Use NSAIDs and simple analgesics for pain relief.

Special considerations

- Dose safety limits for large-volume LA infiltration are controversial. Doses significantly higher than the conventional lidocaine (lignocaine) toxic dose (5 mg/kg) are often used, e.g. 30–70 mg/kg. This may be possible due to the adrenaline producing slower drug absorption, the poor vascularity of fat, and the aspiration of much of the infused solution before the drug has been absorbed.
- Complications are associated with excessive liposuction. In the United Kingdom aspiration is restricted to approximately 2 litres of fat. Considerably higher volume procedures have been reported especially in the United States (in excess of 10 litres). Deaths have occurred from pulmonary oedema and lidocaine (lignocaine) toxicity. Morbidity is related to high aspiration volume and high lidocaine (lignocaine) dosage.

Skin grafting

Procedure	Free skin grafts applied to surgically created raw surfaces following debridement, or to granulating wounds
Time	Variable 30 min–2 h
Pain	++/+++ (especially the donor site)
Position	Variable. Depends on the area to be grafted. Usually supine
Blood loss	Nil for simple grafts. Extensive debridement and grafting of burns may require 6–8 units
Practical techniques	GA/LMA spontaneous respiration (with lateral cutaneous nerve of thigh or femoral 3:1 block if thigh donor site). Spinal for lower limb surgery

Preoperative

- Patient assessment is influenced by the indication for grafting:
  - Patients for simple excision and grafting of isolated lesions may be otherwise well.
  - Elderly patients for excision/grafting of skin lesions or pretibial lacerations may be in poor general health. A local or regional technique may be preferable to a GA.
  - Patients with extensive burns for debridement and grafting require careful assessment. In extreme cases full intensive care may be under way.
  - Skin grafting may be a component of more major surgery, e.g. provision of skin cover to a free muscle flap.
- Assess the status of fluid resuscitation following burns. Note the urine output and fluids currently prescribed. Check Hct and FBC, clotting, U+E, ABGs, chest radiograph.

Perioperative

- Full thickness skin graft (FTSG). Consists of epidermis and dermis. Used in small areas where the thickness, appearance, and texture of skin are important. Usually harvested with a scalpel. The donor site needs to be closed directly:
  - postauricular skin for grafts to the face
  - groin or antecubital fossa to the hand for management of flexion contractures.
- Split skin graft (SSG). Consists of epidermis and variable portion of dermis. Much wider usage than FTSG. Usually harvested with a skin graft knife or power-driven dermatome. Donor sites will heal spontaneously within 2 weeks. Donor sites are chosen according to the amount of skin required, colour and texture match, and local convenience. Meshing is used to

expand the extent of the area that the graft is required to cover. Common donor sites are:

* thigh
* flexor aspect of forearm, upper arm
* abdomen.

* FTSG can be harvested by subcutaneous LA infiltration using 27G needle. Addition of hyaluronidase aids spread (e.g. 1500 IU to 100 ml of LA solution).
* SSG can be harvested using EMLA cream. It should be applied at least 2 h in advance and covered with an occlusive dressing. Anaesthesia does not extend into the deeper dermis so the technique is unsuitable for FTSG. Lateral cutaneous nerve of thigh (LCNT) or femoral 3:1 block provides useful anaesthesia of a thigh donor site.
* Excess harvested skin can be stored at 4 °C for 2–3 weeks.

Postoperative

* The SSG donor site is a potentially painful wound. Supplement with local anaesthesia (LCNT or femoral block) where possible.
* The type of dressing is important for donor site comfort. 'Kaltostat' alginate dressing impregnated with LA (e.g. 40 ml 0.25% bupivacaine) is commonly used. Dressings are difficult to secure on the thigh and frequently slip when the patient mobilizes. A thin adhesive fabric dressing (e.g. sterile 'Mefix') is used by some surgeons and may afford better protection and donor site comfort. The dressing is soaked off after 2 weeks.
* NSAIDs and simple analgesics are usually required for 3–4 days. Itching follows when the acute pain settles and healing is under way.

Special considerations: burns patients

* Extensive debridement and grafting of burns is a major procedure. These patients should receive a balanced GA. Current management is to aim to debride burnt tissue and cover with SSG at the earliest opportunity (often within 48 h). This converts the burn to healthy surgical wound. Potential sources of sepsis are eradicated, fluid shifts are less, and intensive care management tends to be more stable.
* Two anaesthetists may be required. Two surgical teams will considerably speed up the procedure and help minimize complications.
* Blood loss. Ensure 6–8 units are cross-matched. Debrided tissue bleeds freely. Losses can be difficult to estimate particularly in small children. Regularly check Hct and maintain at approximately 30%.
* Temperature control. A large exposed body surface area will lose heat rapidly by radiation and evaporation. Measure core temperature. Use all methods available for heat conservation. Little body surface area may be available for warming blankets. Maintain the operating theatre at 25 °C.
* Monitoring. Placement of non-invasive monitoring devices may be difficult. An arterial line facilitates measurement of blood pressure and blood sampling. A central venous line is valuable to provide reliable venous access for this and future procedures, and help in the management of intravascular volume. Maintain strict asepsis during line insertion.

Cannulas may need to be stitched. Try to place through intact skin. A urinary catheter is essential.

- Suxamethonium is contraindicated except in the first 24 h following burn. Massive K^+ release may cause cardiac arrest.

- Postoperative care. Return to the burns unit. Large body surface area burns (e.g. >40%) or those with additional injury (e.g. smoke inhalation) may need continued ventilation on ITU until warm and stable.

- Analgesia is best provided by IV opioids either as PCA or continuous infusion. Suggest early intervention of the acute pain team. Dressing changes may be helped by Entonox or ketamine/midazolam sedation.

- Antibiotics and early nutrition are important to increase survival.

Burns—early management

General considerations

* The emergency management of severe burns (EMSB) as practised by the Australian and New Zealand Burn Association has been adopted in the United Kingdom by the British Burn Association.
* The initial primary and secondary survey, familiar to all providers of ATLS (Advanced Trauma Life Support), is standard practice no matter what the cause of trauma. EMSB seeks to address the particular needs of the burnt patient.
* Do not allow the burn to detract from the detection and management of injuries that are an immediate threat to life
* Coexisting injury is particularly likely in patients injured by explosions, falls from height, or fire associated with road traffic accidents.
* Fire is the most common cause of burn in adults. Scalding is the most common cause in children.
* Injury may be associated with alcohol intoxication, epilepsy, or a psychiatric illness. Most injuries occur at home. Always consider assault. Burns in children are common non-accidental injuries.
* Mortality is related to patient age, total body surface area (TBSA) burnt, and burn depth.

Airway (with cervical spine control)

* Burns to the head and neck may rapidly cause airway obstruction from massive oedema. Inhalation of hot gases usually causes airway injury above the larynx. Signs of potential airway compromise include singed nasal hairs, hoarse voice, productive 'brassy' cough, and soot in the sputum.
* Clinical judgement is needed to decide if elective intubation, as opposed to continuous observation, is the best course of action in patients with face and neck burns. Maximum wound oedema occurs 12–36 h postinjury, although the airway may be compromised much earlier. If there is any doubt, then there is no doubt—intubate and ventilate without delay. Use an uncut endotracheal tube since oedema can be considerable. Early intubation is a vital intervention before patient transport if the future of the airway is in any question. Delay may result in severe airway difficulty and subsequent intubation may be impossible.

Breathing

* Administer oxygen 15 litre/min via a facemask with a reservoir bag.
* Ventilation may be required in patients:
  * unconscious from coexisting trauma or from the inhalation of toxic substances such as carbon monoxide (CO)
  * developing acute respiratory failure due to smoke inhalation or blast injury
  * in need of extensive resuscitation, sedation, and analgesia following a major burn.

Circulation (with haemorrhage control)

- Hartmann's solution is the internationally accepted resuscitation fluid for burns. It is cost-effective and readily available. Colloid solutions offer no benefit in early fluid management. As wound oedema settles, fluid requirements reduce and tend towards maintenance requirements.
- Burns >25% TBSA produce a systemic inflammatory response. Widespread increase in capillary permeability may result in generalized oedema.
- Remove all jewellery. Insert cannulas through intact skin wherever possible. Institute IV fluids for burns:
  - >15% TBSA in adults
  - >10% TBSA in children.
  - Weigh the patient if feasible. Fluid requirement in first 24 h is 3–4 ml/kg/% TBSA burnt:
  - Give half calculated fluid in first 8 h. Give remainder in next 16 h.
  - Time of injury marks the start of fluid resuscitation.
- Replace bleeding from coexisting trauma with blood. Replace losses from vomiting with normal saline (or dextrose saline in children).
- Fluid requirements are greater in children. Add their daily maintenance needs (as dextrose saline) to the calculated Hartmann's requirement according to:
  - 4 ml/kg/h for the first 10 kg
  - 2 ml/kg/h for the next 10 kg
  - 1 ml/kg/h for each additional kg thereafter.
- All calculated values are a guide only. Monitor urine output and ensure a minimum of:
  - 0.5 ml/kg/h adult
  - 1 ml/kg/h child <30 kg.
- If output is inadequate then give 5–10 ml/kg Hartmann's bolus and increase the next hour's fluids to 150% of the planned volume.
- Test urine for haemochromogens (myoglobin/haemoglobin) arising from muscle damage and red cell breakdown. If positive:
  - Increase urine output to 1–2 ml/kg/h.
  - Alkalinize urine. Add 25 mmol bicarbonate to each litre of Hartmann's.
  - Promote diuresis. Add 12.5 g mannitol to each litre of Hartmann's.

Neurological deficit

- Head injury is common in burns associated with road traffic accidents, falls, blasts, or explosions.
- Carbon monoxide (CO) poisoning is a common cause of altered consciousness (see special circumstances—inhalational injury).
- Other causes of altered level of consciousness include alcohol, epilepsy, and psychiatric conditions.

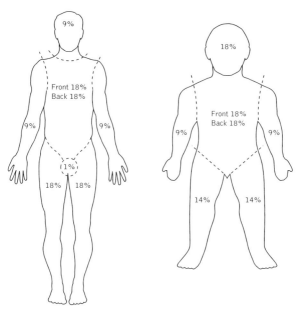

Fig 25.1 Adult and paediatric burn charts.

Exposure (with temperature control)

* Remove all clothing to assess the extent of burn injury. If clothing is stuck to the skin, cut around the area leaving the adherent fabric in place. Keep the patient warm.

* Assess %TBSA burnt by reference to an adult or paediatric burn chart (see Fig. 25.1). The 'rule of 9s' conveniently divides the adult body surface into multiples of 9%. This is inaccurate for small children. The palmar surface of a patient's hand approximates to 1%TBSA.

* Assess burn depth. Burn wounds may be superficial or deep. In practice, most injuries are a mixture of both:
  * Superficial. Consist of burns to the epidermis only (sunburn, flashburns) or involving the superficial part of the dermis (producing a blister). Healing will occur spontaneously without grafting. These burns are painful and pinprick sensation is preserved.
  * Deep. Consist of deep dermal burns (no capillary refill beneath the blister since blood vessels are destroyed) or full thickness (involving entire epidermis and dermis, possibly including underlying structures). Burns may have a white, waxy appearance. Pinprick sensation is lost.

Immediate wound care

- First aid to the burn wound involves cooling the wound with cold running water. This helps reduce production of inflammatory mediators and reduces tissue damage. Continue cooling for at least 20 min. Take care to prevent hypothermia, especially in the young child. Cooling the burn surface is an effective analgesic.
- Burn wounds are initially sterile. Cover with a clean sheet whilst continuing early management.
- Consult with the receiving burn unit concerning the choice of dressings for transfer. Silver sulphadiazine cream may be applied liberally and covered with simple dressings. Clingfilm is useful to limit evaporation and heat loss. Avoid tight dressings. Elevate burned limbs.

Monitoring

- SpO_2, ECG, NIBP. Carbon monoxide poisoning will make the pulse oximeter read towards 100%. Check ABG on a machine with a co-oximeter.
- Use an arterial line for the unconscious, major burns, or inhalational injury.
- Insert a urinary catheter.
- Monitor core temperature.
- Use a nasogastric tube for large burns (>20% adult, >10% child). Gastroparesis is common.
- Take blood for FBC (including haematocrit), urea/creatinine, electrolytes, cross-match, COHb. Check blood sugar (especially in children).

Analgesia

- All burns are painful. Whilst skin sensation is lost over deep burns, the surrounding area is very painful. Most wounds are mixed superficial and deep.
- Severe stress and emotional trauma requires effective sedation/ analgesia.
- Give IV morphine, titrating dose to effect. Use a morphine infusion or PCA to continue.

Escharotomy

- Eschar is the coagulated dead skin of a full-thickness burn. It cannot expand as tissue oedema progresses.
- Circumferential burns to limbs may result in limb ischaemia.
- Circumferential burns to the trunk may reduce chest wall compliance and impede ventilation.
- Escharotomy is performed in theatre. It is the release of the burn wound by incision down to subcutaneous fat. Lines of incision are longitudinally along the medial and lateral sides of limbs. On the trunk, lateral incisions run longitudinally along the anterior axillary line, and extend to the costal margin or upper abdomen. These lines are connected by two anterior incisions. Both are convex upwards, one across the upper chest, and the other across the upper part of the abdomen.
- Ensure blood is available, bleeding can be extreme.
- Patients are often already sedated and ventilated. Conscious patients will need additional sedation and analgesia. Full thickness burns are painless, but incisions will extend onto normal skin for a short distance.

Special circumstances

Inhalation of toxic substances

- CO poisoning is common. Check blood for COHb. It is important for diagnosis. The severity of symptoms may not correlate well with COHb level. Poisoning may mimic alcohol intoxication.

- CO results in reduced O_2 carrying capacity of arterial blood and tissue hypoxia. PaO_2 is normal. CO also binds avidly to other haem-containing compounds, especially the cytochrome system. The half-life of COHb is 250 min when breathing room air, reduced to 40 min when breathing 100% O_2. Oxygen therapy should be continued since a secondary peak of COHb after 24 h occurs and is attributed to washout from cytochromes.

- Symptoms of COHB poisoning are shown in the table:

COHb (%)	Symptoms
0–15	None (smokers)
15–20	Headache, mild confusion
20–40	Nausea and vomiting, disorientation, fatigue
40–60	Hallucinations, ataxia, fits, coma
>60	Death

- Other toxic products of combustion may include: cyanide, ammonia, phosgene, hydrogen chloride, fluoride or bromide, and complex organic compounds. These toxic substances may produce:
  - A chemical burn to the respiratory tract.
  - Interstitial lung oedema, impaired gas exchange, and ARDS.
  - Systemic acid/base disturbances.
  - Hydrofluoric acid binds serum Ca^{2+} and causes hypocalcaemia.

Chemical burn

- Hands and upper limbs are the most frequently affected areas.
- Staff should protect themselves with gloves, apron, and facemask.
- Remove contaminated clothing as early as possible. Store in a secure container for disposal.
- Industrial or household alkalis and acids are commonly used chemicals. Examples include bleach, washing powder, disinfectants, drain cleaner, paint stripper. Immersion in complex hydrocarbons (petrol, diesel) without ignition may cause systemic toxicity. Phosphorus burn may result from fireworks or military applications.
- Tissue damage continues until the chemical is neutralized or diluted by washing with water. Continuous and prolonged (1 h) irrigation with cold water from the outset is vital for all burns (except elemental Na, K, or Li).
- Specific treatments include:
  - Hydrofluoric acid. Highly toxic. Used in the glass industry. 2% TBSA can be fatal. Inactivate toxic F^- ions by application of topical calcium gluconate burn gel, 10% Ca gluconate local injections into the burn wound, and consider intra-arterial or IV (Bier's block) Ca gluconate infusions.

- Phosphorus. White phosphorus ignites spontaneously when exposed to air. It can be extinguished by water. Apply copper sulphate solution which converts phosphorus to black cupric phosphide.
- Bitumen. Common injury in the United Kingdom from road maintenance. It is liquid at 150 °C and causes burns due to the effects of hot liquid. Cool with water. Remove with vegetable or paraffin oil.

Electrical burn

- Low voltage (<1000 V) produces a local contact burn. The 50 Hz A.C. domestic supply is particularly likely to cause cardiac arrest. Muscle spasm may prevent release of the electrical source. There is no associated deep tissue damage.
- High voltage (>1000 V) causes flash burn or deep tissue damage due to current transmission. High-tension cables usually 11 000 or 33 000 V. Produces an entrance and exit wound. May require fasciotomy under GA. Severe renal impairment may result from haemochromogens released from muscle and red cell damage.
- Lightening strike (ultra high tension, high current) has a very high mortality following direct strike. Side flash is more common where a nearby lightening strike produces current that flows over the surface of the victim. Superficial burns may result. Current may flow up one leg and down the other producing an entry and exit wound. Respiratory arrest is common. 'Lichtenberg flowers' is a pathognomonic splashed-on pattern of skin damage resulting from lightening side flash.

Transfer to burn centre

The British Burn Association criteria for transfer to a burn centre are:

- Burn >10%TBSA adult or >5%TBSA child, and any patient with full thickness burn >5%TBSA.
- Burn to special areas: face, hands, feet, genitalia, perineum, major joints.
- Electrical or chemical burns.
- Inhalational injury.
- Circumferential burn to the limbs or chest.
- Patients at the extremes of age.
- Patients with poor medical condition which may complicate management.
- Burns with associated major trauma. Whether the patient is initially managed in a burn centre or a trauma centre will depend on the nature of the coexisting injury.

Other plastic surgical procedures

Operation	Description	Time (min)	Pain (+ to ++++)	Position	Blood loss/ X-match	Notes
Abdominoplasty	Excision of redundant lower abdominal skin	120	++ to +++	Supine	G&S	LMA or ETT, IPPV
Carpal tunnel release	Release of flexor sheath at the wrist to relieve median nerve entrapment	30	+	Supine, arm board	ns (tourniquet)	LA infiltration, or brachial plexus block, or day case GA
Dupuytren's contracture	Excision of contracted palmar fascia	60–90	+	Supine, arm board	ns (tourniquet)	Brachial plexus block, or day case GA
External angular dermoid	Excision of congenital dermoid cyst usually from lateral supraorbital ridge	30	ns	Supine, head ring	ns	LMA and spontaneous ventilation
Flexor/extensor tendon repair	Repair of hand tendons following trauma. Often multiple. May be extensive. May involve nerve/vessel repairs	30–120+	+ to ++	Supine, arm board	ns (tourniquet)	Brachial plexus block ± GA, LMA and spontaneous ventilation, IPPV for extensive repairs
Gynaecomastia	Excision or liposuction of excess male breast tissue	45	+ to ++	Supine	ns	LMA and spontaneous ventilation
Hypospadius repair	Correction of congenital abnormality of male urethra. Usually infant	90	++	Supine	ns	LMA and spontaneous ventilation. Caudal block

Operation	Description	Time (min)	Pain (+ to ++++)	Position	Blood loss/ X-match	Notes
Insertion of tissue expander	Subcutaneous insertion of saline-filled silastic bags, often scalp	45	+ to ++	Supine, head ring	ns	LMA and spontaneous ventilation
Minor body surface procedures	Suture of lacerations, dog bites, excision of small skin tumours, cysts, sinus tracts, lipomas, abcesses, etc.	30	+	Usually supine	ns	LA infiltration or local block. LMA and spontaneous ventilation
Neck, axilla, or groin dissection	Block dissection of regional lymph nodes to excise secondary malignant disease	90–120	++	Supine, head ring	2 units	LMA or ETT, IPPV
Preauricular sinus	Excision of congenital sinus tract, often bilateral	45	+	Supine, head ring	ns	LMA and spontaneous ventilation
Pretibial laceration	Excision of pretibial wound and SSG	45	+ to ++	Supine	ns	Spinal or GA
Repair sacral pressure sore	Debridement and local flap repair	60–90	ns	Lateral or prone	G+S	Beware autonomic hyperreflexia in paraplegics. Variable requirement for anaesthesia. Maybe nil/IV sedation or GA. ETT + IPPV for prone position

Operation	Description	Time (min)	Pain (+ to +++++)	Position	Blood loss/ X-match	Notes
Syndactyly	Release of congenital fusion of two or more digits. Maybe bilateral. May require FTSG	60–180	++	Supine	ns (tourniquet)	LMA and spontaneous ventilation. ETT + IPPV for extensive repairs
Umbilicoplasty	Correction of protruding umbilicus	30	+	Supine	ns	LMA and spontaneous ventilation

ns = not significant.

SSG = split skin graft.

FTSG = full thickness skin graft.

Chapter 26
Gynaecological surgery
John Saddler

General principles

A wide range of patients present for gynaecological surgery. Many are young and fit, will be undergoing relatively minor procedures, and are likely to be going home on the same day. Others will be inpatients undergoing more major surgery, some with gynaecological tumours. Many will be elderly, requiring operations that relieve pelvic floor prolapse.

- Many gynaecological patients are extremely apprehensive, even for relatively minor surgery.
- The general principles of day surgery apply to many gynaecology lists.
- Postoperative nausea and vomiting (PONV) is a particular problem. In some patients this is a major concern. With high-risk patients consider using techniques that may reduce the incidence of PONV, e.g. TIVA and regional anaesthesia. Give prophylactic anti-emetics, particularly to patients with a previous history of PONV.
- Pelvic surgery is associated with deep vein thrombosis (DVT). Ensure that adequate prophylactic measures have been taken to reduce the risk.
- Younger females may be taking the contraceptive pill, which may need to be stopped before some operations. Guidelines are suggested on p. 13.
- Vagal stimulation may occur during gynaecological surgery either during cervical dilatation, traction on the pelvic organs or the mesentery, or during laparoscopic procedures.
- Take care during patient positioning. Patients are often moved up or down the table, when airway devices can be dislodged and disconnections can occur. Many patients will have pre-existing back or joint pain, which may be worsened in the lithotomy position. There is a potential for common peroneal nerve injury if the legs are supported in stirrups.
- An open abdominal wound will rapidly lose heat. Ensure that patients are kept warm during laparotomies. A warmed air mattress is particularly useful.

Minor gynaecological procedures

Procedure	D&C, hysteroscopy, oocyte retrieval
Time	20–30 min
Pain	+
Position	Supine, lithotomy
Blood loss	Nil
Practical technique	LMA, SV, day case

Minor operations that enable access to the endometrial cavity through the cervix include:

- D&C (dilatation and curettage). Largely superseded now by hysteroscopic examination.
- Hysteroscopy: the surgeon is able to visualize the endometrial cavity using a rigid scope. The hysteroscope is flushed with crystalloid to enable better visualization. Fluid volume is measured to ensure there is no uterine perforation (volume recovered less than the volume infused).
- A brief general anaesthetic may be requested for an oocyte retrieval procedure. Patients will have received prior hormonal stimulation to induce the production of oocytes in the ovaries. These are removed with the aid of ultrasound through a transvaginal approach. This may also be performed using heavy sedation.

Preoperative

Many of these patients will be day cases. Premedicate with ranitidine and diclofenac, or obtain permission for rectal administration perioperatively.

Perioperative

Spontaneous ventilation using a facemask or LMA, propofol (infusion or intermittent bolus) or volatile.

Postoperative

Simple oral analgesics, plus anti-emetic of choice.

Special considerations

- Vagal stimulation may occur with cervical dilatation, so have anticholinergic drugs immediately available.
- Stimulation may also induce laryngospasm—ensure adequate depth of anaesthesia.
- There is a risk of uterine perforation through the fundus whenever surgical instruments are introduced through the cervix and into the endometrial cavity. Antibiotics are usually prescribed if this is thought to have occurred. A small perforation can be treated expectantly, larger perforations may require a laparoscopy to evaluate the extent of the perforation.

ERPC, STOP (VTOP)

Procedure	ERPC (evacuation of retained products of conception). STOP/VTOP (suction or vaginal termination of pregnancy)
Time	10–20 min
Pain	+
Position	Supine, lithotomy
Blood loss	Usually minimal
Practical technique	LMA, SV, day case

Preoperative

• ERPC: remaining products of conception may have to be surgically removed after an incomplete miscarriage. This usually occurs between 6 and 12 weeks' gestation. Substantial blood loss may have occurred preoperatively, and may continue perioperatively. IV access and crystalloid/colloid infusion are required if haemorrhage appears anything more than trivial.

• STOP/VTOP is a procedure undertaken up to 12 weeks' gestation.

Perioperative

• LMA or FM, fentanyl. The surgeon usually requests an IV bolus of oxytocin (Syntocinon 5–10 units) to help contract the uterus and reduce bleeding. This drug can cause an increase in heart rate. The use of ergometrine, a vasoconstrictor, for the same purpose is declining because it significantly raises arterial pressure.

• Avoid high concentrations of volatile agents due to the relaxant effect on the uterus. TIVA with propofol infusion, or more usually intermittent bolus, is ideal.

Postoperative

Simple oral analgesics and anti-emetic of choice.

Special considerations

• Pregnancies beyond 12 weeks can be terminated surgically by dilatation and evacuation (D + E). The procedure is similar to a STOP/VTOP, but there is greater potential for blood loss. Larger doses of oxytocin may be required, and intubation should be considered if there are symptoms of reflux oesophagitis.

• If a pregnancy has gone beyond 16 weeks, it may be terminated medically with prostaglandin. These patients may still require an ERPC, and should be managed similarly to a retained placenta (see p. 725).

Laparoscopy/laparoscopic sterilization

Procedure	Intra-abdominal examination of gynaecological organs through a rigid scope ± clips to fallopian tubes
Time	15–30 min
Pain	+/++
Position	Supine, lithotomy, head down tilt
Blood loss	Nil
Practical technique	COETT, IPPV
	LMA, SV, day case

Preoperative

+ Usually young and fit adults.
+ Obtain consent for suppositories

Perioperative

+ Use a short-acting non-depolarizing muscle relaxant. 'Top-ups' may be required. Monitor with a nerve stimulator and use reversal agents if necessary at the end.
+ Intubate with an oral tracheal tube.
+ Give a short-acting opioid (e.g. fentanyl) and PR NSAID (e.g. diclofenac 100 mg).
+ Encourage the surgeon to infiltrate the skin incisions with local analgesia.
+ An alternative technique for uncomplicated short procedures is to use spontaneous ventilation and an LMA. This is only suitable for non-obese patients and the potential for gastric regurgitation and aspiration must be assessed carefully. If gas insuflation is hampered by abdominal muscle tone, deepen anaesthesia or use a small dose of mivacurium, and assist ventilation until the return of SV.

Postoperative

Further opioids (morphine) may be required.

Special considerations

+ As many of these procedures are short and may only take 10–15 min, mivacurium is a logical muscle relaxant to use. Intermittent use of suxamethonium has unwanted side-effects.
+ Bradycardias are common, due to vagal stimulation. Atropine should be readily available. Many anaesthetists administer glycopyrrolate prophylactically at induction.
+ Shoulder pain is common postoperatively due to diaphragmatic irritation. It can be difficult to treat, and is reduced by expelling as much carbon dioxide from the abdomen as possible at the end of the procedure.

- Occasionally, surgical instruments damage abdominal contents, and a laparotomy is required. Severe blood loss may result.
- Very rarely carbon dioxide gas may be inadvertently injected intravascularly, resulting in gas embolus. This results in ventilation/perfusion mismatch, with a fall in $ETCO_2$, impaired cardiac output, hypotension, arrhythmias, and tachycardia. If this is thought to have occurred, the surgeon should be alerted, nitrous oxide should be discontinued, and the patient should be resuscitated (p. 844).
- If contemplating using an LMA premedicate with oral ranitidine (150–300 mg).

Transcervical resection of endothelium (TCRE)

Procedure	Endoscopic resection of endometrium
Time	40 min
Pain	+
Position	Lithotomy
Blood loss	Variable
Practical technique	LMA, SV

Preoperative

* Patients are usually pre-menopausal.
* May have anaemia.

Perioperative

* Spontaneous breathing technique with LMA is usually satisfactory.
* Give a short-acting opioid (e.g. fentanyl) and PR NSAID (e.g. diclofenac).
* Routine IV fluids are unnecessary.
* Take care with positioning (lithotomy position).

Postoperative

* Patients usually stay overnight.
* Stronger opioids (e.g. morphine) are occasionally required.

Special considerations

* A condition similar to 'TURP syndrome' may complicate this procedure. During surgery, the endometrial cavity is irrigated with a pressurized glycine solution and systemic absorption of water may occur. This is more likely with prolonged surgery, or if the endometrium is particularly vascular. The syndrome is characterized by fluid overload, which may compromise cardiac output, cause pulmonary oedema, and result in electrolyte abnormalities, particularly hyponatraemia. Treatment is as for TURP syndrome (p. 628).
* Blood loss is difficult to assess during and after the procedure because of the dilutional effect of the irrigation fluids. Only very rarely is a blood transfusion required.
* Newer techniques are being evolved to reduce the degree of fluid distension of the uterine cavity, making it a safer and shorter procedure.

Abdominal hysterectomy

Procedure	Removal of uterus through abdominal incision (may also include ovaries as bilateral salpingo-oophorectomy)
Time	1 h, often longer
Pain	+++
Position	Supine, head down
Blood loss	250–500 ml, G&S
Practical technique	ETT, IPPV, PCA

Preoperative

- Patients may be anaemic if they have had menorrhagia or postmenopausal bleeding.
- Renal function may be abnormal if an abdominal mass has been compressing the ureters.
- Many patients are anxious and require premedication.
- Postoperative nausea and vomiting (PONV) is common.
- Ensure prophylaxis for deep vein thrombosis (DVT) has been initiated.

Perioperative

- Oral intubation and ventilation.
- If a Pfannensteil ('bikini line') incision is anticipated bilateral ilioinguinal blocks with bupivicaine markedly reduces postoperative pain (the patient must be warned of the possibility of femoral nerve involvement).
- Profound muscle relaxation is required to enable the surgeon to gain optimal access.
- Antibiotic prophylaxis is usually required.
- Head down positioning is often requested which may cause ventilation pressures to rise and diaphragmatic compression. Central venous pressure will increase and gastric regurgitation is also more likely.
- Blood loss is variable; some hysterectomies bleed more than expected. Cross-match blood early if bleeding appears to be a problem.
- Heat loss through the abdominal incision can be significant. Use a warm air blanket over the upper body during the operation.

Postoperative

- Patients usually do well with a PCA supplemented with local anaesthetic blocks or wound infiltration and regular NSAIDs. It is a good idea to add an anti-emetic drug to the opioid to reduce the incidence of PONV. Cyclizine (up to150 mg) or droperidol (5 mg) can be added to a 50 ml syringe with 50 mg morphine.

- Oxygen therapy may be required for 24 h postoperatively or longer. Patients usually tolerate nasal cannulas better than face masks.

Special considerations

- Epidural analgesia is also effective for posthysterectomy pain, particularly in patients who have had midline ('up and down') incisions, and may also reduce the incidence of PONV. However, morbidity from their use prevents many people from using them for routine hysterectomy.

- Wertheim's hysterectomy is undertaken in patients who have cervical and uterine malignancies. The uterus, fallopian tubes, and often the ovaries are removed but, in addition, the pelvic lymph nodes are dissected out. These operations take much longer and there is a potential for substantial blood loss. Invasive monitoring, in the form of central venous access and direct arterial pressure monitoring, should be considered. Epidural analgesia is useful for the postoperative phase.

Vaginal hysterectomy

Procedure	Removal of the uterus through the vagina
Time	50 min
Pain	+/++
Position	Lithotomy
Blood loss	Variable, usually less than 500 ml
Practical technique	LMA, SV, caudal
	Spinal

Preoperative

A degree of uterine prolapse enables the operation to be performed more easily. Patients are therefore usually older and may be frail with underlying cardiac or respiratory problems.

Perioperative

- A spontaneous breathing technique with LMA is usual. Give a longer-acting IV opioid (e.g. morphine 5–10 mg or pethidine 50–100 mg) and supplement with NSAIDs.
- A caudal with 20 ml bupivicaine 0.25% improves postoperative analgesia, but beware toxic levels (see below).
- Spinal anaesthesia (3 ml bupivacaine 0.5%) with or without supplemental sedation is a satisfactory alternative.
- The surgeon usually infiltrates the operative field with a vasoconstrictor to reduce bleeding. Local analgesia infiltration at the same time will aid postoperative analgesia. Monitor the cardiovascular system carefully during this period, and ensure that safe doses of these drugs are not exceeded.
- Take care with positioning. Many patients will have hip and/or knee arthritis, and may have had surgery to these joints. Lloyd-Davis leg slings may be preferable to leg stirrups if leg joints articulate poorly. The common peroneal nerve may be compressed in leg stirrups.
- Keep the patient warm, preferably with a warmed air blanket.

Postoperative

- This operation is much less painful than an abdominal hysterectomy. If opioids, NSAIDs and local analgesia infiltration/caudal have been given intraoperatively, further analgesia needs are often very modest (IM opioids).
- Elderly patients will require supplemental oxygen for at least 24 h postoperatively.

Special considerations

- The procedure is often supplemented by either an anterior or posterior repair which reduces bladder or bowel prolapse through the vagina.

- It is usually not possible to remove the fallopian tubes and ovaries during a vaginal hysterectomy because of the restricted surgical field.
- Laparoscopically-assisted vaginal hysterectomy (LAVH) is designed to enable the uterus, fallopian tubes, and ovaries to be removed through the vagina. The operation begins with a laparoscopy, at which the broad ligament is identified and detached. There is a risk of haemorrhage and ureteric damage at this stage. The anaesthetic principles for laparoscopy apply except that a longer-acting muscle relaxant and an endotracheal tube should be used. Once satisfactory mobility of the gynaecological organs has been achieved at laparoscopy, they are then removed through a vaginal incision. PCA analgesia should be considered postoperatively.

Ectopic pregnancy

Procedure	Laparotomy to stop bleeding from ruptured tubal pregnancy
Time	40 min
Pain	++/+++
Position	Supine
Blood loss	Can be massive, cross-match 2 units
Practical technique	ETT, IPPV, PCA

Preoperative

* The presentation is very variable. At one end of the spectrum a stable patient may have ill-defined abdominal pain and amenorrhoea, and at the other a patient may present with life-threatening abdominal haemorrhage. At least one large-bore IV cannula should be inserted prior to theatre, and crystalloids, colloids, or blood products infused according to the clinical picture.
* FBC, cross-match, and possibly a clotting screen should be requested on admission.
* Seek help from a second anaesthetist if the patient is unstable.

Perioperative

* Rapid sequence induction.
* Careful IV induction if blood loss is suspected. Use etomidate or ketamine if shocked.
* Continue intravenous fluid resuscitation.

Postoperative

* Clotting abnormalities are not uncommon if large volumes of blood have been lost. Send a clotting screen for analysis if necessary, and organize fresh frozen plasma and platelet infusions if indicated.
* Actively warm the patient in the recovery room with heated blankets if possible.
* Set up an intravenous infusion or a PCA device for postoperative analgesia.

Special considerations

* Stable patients may undergo a diagnostic laparoscopy. Be aware that the pneumoperitoneum may impede venous return resulting in hypotension.
* Many centres now perform the whole operation through the laparoscope as a routine, and only convert to a laparotomy if there are any complications.

Other gynaecological procedures

Operation	Description	Time (min)	Pain (+ to +++++)	Position	Blood loss/ X-match	Notes
Simple vulvectomy	Excision of vulva	90	+++	Lithotomy	G&S	
Radical vulvectomy	Excision of vulva and lymph nodes	150	++++	Lithotomy	2 units	Epidural analgesia recommended
Investigative laparotomy	Abdominal assessment of pelvic mass	150	++++	Supine	2 units	Ovarian tumours may be adherent to adjacent structures, e.g. bowel and mesentery. Potentially large blood loss
Sacrocolpopexy	Abdominal repair of vault prolapse	60	+++	Supine	G&S	
Oophorectomy	Removal of ovaries	40	+++	Supine	G&S	
Anterior repair	Repair of anterior vaginal wall	20	++	Lithotomy	Nil	Often combined with vaginal hysterectomy. LMA ± caudal
Posterior repair	Repair of posterior vaginal wall	20	++	Lithotomy	Nil	Often combined with vaginal hysterectomy. LMA ± caudal
Colposuspension	Abdominal procedure for stress incontinence	40	+++	Supine	G&S	COETT, IPPV
Cone biopsy	Removal of the terminal part of the cervix through the vagina	30	++	Supine	G&S	May bleed postoperatively. LMA, SV

Operation	Description	Time (min)	Pain (+ to +++++)	Position	Blood loss/ X-match	Notes
Myomectomy	Abdominal excision of fibroids from uterus	60	+++	Supine	G&S	Blood loss may be greater than expected. COETT, IPPV
Sacrospinous fixation	Vaginal operation for vault prolapse	40	++	Lithotomy	Nil	
Shirodkar suture	Insertion of suture around cervix to prevent recurrent miscarriage	20	++	Lithotomy	Nil	May need to take antireflux precautions (see p. 744)

Chapter 27
Urology and renal surgery

Julia Munn

Anaesthetic considerations for cystoscopic procedures

- Includes cystoscopy, transurethral resection of the prostate (TURP), bladder neck incision, transurethral resection of bladder tumour, ureteroscopy and/or stone removal or stent insertion.

- The majority of patients are undergoing procedures for benign prostatic hypertrophy or carcinoma of the bladder. The incidence of both these conditions increases markedly over the age of 60 years and bladder cancer is smoking-related, so patients frequently have coronary artery disease and chronic obstructive airways disease.

- FBC, creatinine, and electrolytes should be checked preoperatively because bladder cancers can bleed insidiously. Both bladder cancer and benign prostatic hypertrophy can cause an obstructive uropathy/renal impairment and drugs and technique should be chosen accordingly.

- Flexible cystoscopy is largely used for diagnostic purposes, does not require full bladder distension, and can normally be performed under local anaesthetic. Biopsies can be taken this way with only a small amount of discomfort and skilled surgeons can perform retrograde ureteric catheterizations. Occasional patients insist on sedation or GA for flexible cystoscopy. Midazolam or propofol is ideal.

- Rigid cystoscopy requires general anaesthesia, due to scope diameter and the use of irrigating solution to distend the bladder and allow visualization of the surgical field. If large volumes of irrigant are absorbed systemic complications due to fluid overload can result (see TURP syndrome p. 628).

- Spinal anaesthesia works well for rigid cystoscopic procedures, and is commonly used for TURP. Sensory supply to the urethra, prostate, and bladder neck is from S2–S4. Sensory supply to the bladder, however, is from T10–T12 so a higher block is required. Many patients will request sedation. In the elderly population 1–2 mg midazolam ($\pm$ fentanyl 50 μg) is usually adequate. Higher doses may result in loss of airway control, confusion, and restlessness. A low-dose propofol infusion is an alternative.

- Hyperbaric bupivacaine usually produces a higher block than the isobaric solution, especially when the injection is performed with the patient in the lateral position and then turned supine. 3 ml 'heavy bupivacaine' 0.5% usually gives a block to T10. Do not tilt the patient head down unless the block is not sufficiently high. Alternatively 3 ml plain bupivacaine will give an adequate block for TURP, but may not be adequate for transurethral bladder surgery.

- Patients with chronic chest disease tend to cough on lying flat. During surgery under regional block coughing can seriously impair surgical access. Sedation can help to reduce the cough impulse.

- Patients with spinal cord injuries (see p. 180) often require repeated urological procedures. Bladder distension during cystoscopy is very stimulating and prone to cause autonomic hyperreflexia so a GA or spinal is advisable—check previous anaesthetic charts.

- Take particular care positioning elderly patients in lithotomy, especially those with joint replacements.

- Penile erection can make cystoscopy difficult and surgery hazardous. It usually occurs due to surgical stimulation when the depth of anaesthesia is inadequate and can usually be managed by deepening anaesthesia. If the erection still persists small doses of ketamine can be useful.
- Antibiotic prophylaxis is required when there is a proven urinary tract infection or a potential for infection due to an indwelling catheter or urinary obstruction. Patients at risk of acquiring deep-seated infection, i.e. those with abnormal or prosthetic heart valves, prosthetic joints, or aortic grafts will need prophylaxis routinely, with the addition of Gram-positive cover (see p. 896).
- DVT prophylaxis: graduated compression stockings are generally considered adequate in low-risk patients undergoing cystoscopic procedures, as most will mobilize rapidly following surgery. However, low-dose heparin should also be used in patients with additional risk factors or those who have recently undergone other surgery and a period of immobility.

Postoperative complications of rigid cystoscopic procedures

- Perforation of the bladder can occur and can be difficult to recognize, especially in the presence of a spinal block, which may mask abdominal pain. Perforations are classified as extraperitoneal, when pain is said to be maximal in the suprapubic region, and intraperitoneal when there is generalized abdominal pain, shoulder tip pain due to fluid tracking up to the diaphragm, and signs of peritonism. Intraperitoneal perforations need fluid resuscitation and urgent surgery to prevent progressive shock.
- Bacteraemia can have a very dramatic onset with signs of profound septic shock. Usually there is a rapid response to IV fluids and appropriate antibiotics if the diagnosis is made in time. Always suspect this diagnosis with unexplained hypotension after a seemingly straightforward urinary tract instrumentation.
- Bladder spasm is a painful involuntary contraction of the bladder occurring after any cystoscopic technique, most commonly in patients who did not have an indwelling catheter preoperatively. The diagnosis is supported by the failure of irrigation fluid to flow freely in and out of the bladder. It responds poorly to conventional analgesics but is often eased by small doses of IV benzodiazepine, e.g. diazepam 2.5–5 mg or Buscopan (hyoscine butylbromide) 20 mg IV or IM.
- Bleeding and fluid overload are dealt with below under anaesthesia for TURP.

Transurethral resection of the prostate (TURP)

Procedure	Cystoscopic resection of the prostate using diathermy wire
Time	30–90 min, depending on the size of the prostate
Pain	+
Position	Lithotomy ± head down
Blood loss	Very variable (200–2000 ml), can be profuse and continue postop. G&S
Practical techniques	Spinal ± sedation
	GA, LMA, and SV
	GA, ET, and IPPV

Preoperative

* Patients are frequently elderly with coexistent disease.
* Check for renal impairment.
* Uncontrolled heart failure presents a particularly high risk due to fluid absorption.
* Assess mental state and communication—spinal anaesthesia is difficult if the patient is confused or deaf.

Perioperative

* Insert a large cannula (16G) and use warmed IV fluids as rapid transfusion is occasionally necessary.
* Spinal anaesthesia:
  * in theory easier to detect signs of fluid overload (see below)
  * shown in some, but not all, studies to reduce blood loss
  * 2.5–3 ml bupivacaine (plain or hyperbaric) is usually adequate
  * frequent BP check—hypotension unusual with the above doses but can be sudden
  * check BP at end when the legs are down (unmasks hypotension).
* GA:
  * consider intubation if the patient is very obese or has a history of reflux
  * intraoperative fentanyl or morphine plus diclofenac 100 mg PR provides adequate analgesia; unusual to need opioids postoperatively.
* Blood loss can be difficult to assess. In theory can be calculated from measuring Hb of discarded irrigation fluid. In practice it is commoner to visually assess the volume and colour, but this can be very misleading. Checking the patient's Hb with a bedside device (e.g. Haemacue®) is useful. Blood loss is generally related to the size and weight of prostate tissue

excised (normally 15–60 g), the duration of resection, and the expertise of the operator.

- Antibiotic prophylaxis (as above under general considerations).
- Obturator spasm (see below under transurethral resection of bladder tumour).
- Fluid therapy: crystalloid can be used initially. Bear in mind that a significant volume of hypotonic irrigating fluid may be absorbed so do not give excessive volumes and never use dextrose. Consider switching to a colloid if hypotension results from the spinal. Give blood, rather than further clear fluid, if blood loss appears large and the patient is hypotensive.

Postoperative

- There is generally little pain, but discomfort from the catheter or bladder spasm may be a problem (see above under general considerations).
- Bladder irrigation with saline via a three-way catheter continues for approximately 24 h, until bleeding is reduced. Clot retention can give a very distended painful bladder and require washout, sometimes under anaesthetic.
- Bleeding can continue and require further surgery—resuscitation may be necessary preoperatively.
- Measure FBC, creatinine and electrolytes the following day.

Special considerations

- Hypothermia may result when large volumes of irrigation fluid are used (the fluid should be warmed to 37 °C)
- If the prostate is very large (>100 g), a retropubic prostatectomy may carry fewer complications.
- The risk of complications increases with resection times of more than 1 h. If a trainee surgeon embarks on a resection which is likely to take longer than this consider seeking senior surgical assistance or limiting the resection to one lobe only, leaving the other to be done at a later date.

TURP syndrome

- This is a combination of fluid overload and hyponatraemia, which occurs when large volumes of irrigation fluid are absorbed via open venous sinuses. Irrigation fluid must be non-conductive (so that the diathermy current is concentrated at the cutting point), non-haemolytic (so that haemolysis does not occur if it enters the circulation), and it must have neutral visual density, so that the surgeon's view is not distorted. For these reasons it cannot contain electrolytes but cannot be pure water. The most commonly used irrigant is glycine 1.5% in water, which is slightly hypotonic (osmolality 220 mmol/litre).

- Some irrigation fluid is normally absorbed, at about 20 ml/min, and on average patients absorb a total of 1–1.5 litres, but absorption of up to 4–5 litres has been recorded. In clinical practice it is almost impossible to accurately assess the volume absorbed.

- The amount absorbed depends upon the following factors:
  - Pressure of infusion—the bag must be kept as low as possible to achieve adequate flow of irrigant, usually 60–70 cm, never more than 100 cm.
  - Venous pressure—more fluid is absorbed if the patient is hypovolaemic or hypotensive.
  - Duration of surgery/large prostate—problems are more common with surgery lasting more than an hour or with a prostate weighing more than 50 g.
  - Blood loss—large blood loss implies a large number of veins open.

- The syndrome is more likely to occur in patients with poorly controlled heart failure or hyponatraemia. Do not increase the risks of fluid overload by giving an unnecessarily large volume of intravenous fluid.

- The syndrome consists of pulmonary oedema, cerebral oedema, and hyponatraemia. Glycine is a non-essential amino acid which functions as an inhibitory neurotransmitter and it is unclear whether glycine toxicity plays a part in the syndrome. The syndrome carries a significant mortality unless it is recognized and treated promptly. Signs will be detected earlier in the awake patient than in an anaesthetized patient in whom it might not be suspected until the postoperative period.

- Early signs and symptoms will include restlessness, headache, tachypnoea, and may progress to respiratory distress, hypoxia, frank pulmonary oedema, nausea, vomiting, confusion, convulsions, and coma. In the anaesthetized patient the only clue may be tachycardia and hypertension. The diagnosis can be confirmed by finding a low serum sodium. An acute fall to <120 mmol/litre is always symptomatic.

- If detected intra-operatively bleeding points should be coagulated, surgery terminated as soon as possible, and IV fluids stopped. Give furosemide (frusemide) 40 mg and check serum Na and Hb. Support respiration with oxygen or intubation and ventilation if required. Administer intravenous anticonvulsants for fitting.

- If Na <120 mmol/litre consider giving hypertonic saline (NaCl 3%) using the following formula. You are aiming to correct the serum Na to 125–130 mmol/ litre and to reverse neurological changes. The rate of correction should not be more than 12 mmol/litre in the first 24 h. The volume of 3% saline (in ml) which will raise the serum Na by 1 mmol/litre is twice the total body water (TBW) in litres. TBW in men is about 60% of body weight, i.e. for a 70 kg man:

- calculate TBW = $70 \times 0.6 = 42$ litre
- therefore 84 ml 3% saline will raise serum Na by 1 mmol/litre
- 1008 ml 3% saline over 24 h will raise serum Na by 12 mmol/litre.

Transurethral resection of bladder tumour

Procedure	Cystoscopic diathermy resection of bladder tumour
Time	10–40 min
Pain	+/++ and bladder spasm
Position	Lithotomy
Blood loss	0– >500 ml
Practical technique	GA with LMA
	Spinal ± sedation

Preoperative

+ Most common in smokers—check for IHD, COAD.
+ Check Hb, chronic blood loss is common.
+ Check renal function.
+ Refer to previous anaesthetic charts as many patients have repeated surgery.

Perioperative

+ Obturator spasm occurs when the obturator nerve, which runs adjacent to the lateral walls of the bladder, is directly stimulated by the diathermy current. It causes adduction of the leg and can seriously impair surgical access and increase the risk of bladder perforation. It can usually be controlled by reducing the diathermy current.
+ Antibiotic prophylaxis as above.
+ If resection is limited and postoperative irrigation is not planned the surgeon may request a diuretic to 'flush' the bladder—check that the patient is not hypovolaemic.

Postoperative

+ Pain can be a problem with extensive resections—NSAIDs are useful (check renal function).
+ Bladder spasm is common (see p. 625).

Open (retropubic) prostatectomy

Procedure	Open excision of grossly hypertrophied prostate
Time	60–120 min
Pain	+++
Position	Supine
Blood loss	500–2000 ml, cross-match four units
Practical technique	ETT, IPPV, ± epidural

Preoperative

- Elderly men, as for TURP.
- Check renal function.

Perioperative

- Prepare for major blood loss with a large IV cannula, a blood warmer, heated blankets, etc.
- A Pfannenstiel type incision is used.
- Use an epidural cautiously intra-operatively to avoid exacerbating hypotension due to blood loss.
- Cell salvage techniques can be useful where blood loss is expected to be substantial.

Postoperative

- An epidural is useful.
- Ensure adequate chest physiotherapy.

Radical prostatectomy

Procedure	Open complete excision of malignant prostate
Time	120–180 min
Pain	++++
Position	Supine
Blood loss	1000– >3000 ml, cross-match four units
Practical techniques	ETT, IPPV, ± epidural

Preoperative

- Patients are only selected if they are <70 years and reasonably fit.
- Consider booking an HDU bed depending on local practice.

Perioperative

- Prepare for the possibility of very large blood loss with a large IV cannula, blood warmer, etc.
- Consider using arterial and CVP lines, particularly in patients with cardio-vascular disease.
- Ensure bank blood is available and reorder intra-operatively as necessary.
- Take measures to prevent heat loss, e.g. warm air blanket.
- Air embolism is a possible complication.

Postoperative

- Urine output is difficult to measure due to irrigation.

Nephrectomy

Procedure	Excision of kidney for tumour, other pathologies, or live donor
Time	1–2.5 h
Pain	+++/++++
Position	Supine or lateral (kidney position)
Blood loss	Depends on pathology, 300– >3000 ml. G&S/cross-match as required
Practical technique	ETT + IPPV ± thoracic epidural

Preoperative

- Ascertain the pathology before deciding on the technique and monitoring.
- Check Hb—renal tumours can cause anaemia without blood loss.
- Check BP and renal function—'non-functioning' kidney/renovascular disease associated with renal impairment and hypertension.
- Check serum electrolytes—renal tumour can cause inappropriate ADH secretion.
- Check the chest radiograph if there is a tumour—there may be metastases, pleural effusions, etc.

Perioperative

- Common surgical practice in the United Kingdom is for laparotomy via a paramedian or transverse incision for a tumour and a loin incision with retroperitoneal approach for other pathologies or donor nephrectomy.
- Loin incision requires the 'kidney position', i.e. lateral with patient extended over a break in the table—a marked fall in BP is common on assuming this position due to reduced venous return from the legs and possible IVC compression. Further compression during surgery may result in a severe reduction in venous return and cardiac output.
- Ask the surgeon about the predicted extent of surgery—a large tumour may necessitate extensive dissection, possibly via a thoracotomy, or opening of the IVC to resect tumour margins, in which case sudden, torrential blood loss possible. Occasionally the IVC is temporarily clamped to allow dissection and to control haemorrhage; this gives a sudden fall in cardiac output. Inform the surgeon if BP falls suddenly, have colloid and blood checked and available to infuse immediately under pressure, and have a vasoconstrictor or inotrope such as ephedrine prepared.
- Large IV cannulas, blood warmer, CVP and arterial line if the procedure is anything other than an uncomplicated, non-malignant nephrectomy.
- Heminephrectomy is occasionally performed for a well-localized tumour or in a patient with only one kidney (beware precarious renal function). Blood loss can be large as vessels are more difficult to control.

- If an epidural is used a high block will be required postoperatively but use it cautiously intra-operatively until bleeding is under control.

Postoperative

- All approaches are painful—epidurals are useful but need to cover up to T7/8 for a loin incision. PCA or opioid infusion is an alternative.
- Intercostal blocks will give analgesia for several hours.
- NSAIDs are useful if renal function is good postoperatively and the patient is not hypovolaemic.
- Monitor hourly urine output.

Cystectomy

Procedure	Excision of bladder plus urinary diversion procedure (e.g. ileal conduit) or bladder reconstruction (orthotopic bladder formation)
Time	2–3 h (longer with bladder reconstruction)
Pain	++++
Position	Lithotomy + head down
Blood loss	700– >3000 ml, cross-match four units
Practical technique	ETT, IPPV, ± epidural, arterial line/CVP

Preoperative

- Check for IHD, COAD, renal function, and FBC.
- Book an HDU bed depending on local practice and coexisting medical problems.
- Consider autotransfusion intra-operatively.
- Ensure thromboprophylaxis is prescribed.
- Consider preoperative IV hydration to compensate for hypovolaemia due to 'bowel prep'.

Perioperative

- Prepare for major blood loss—large IV cannulas, blood warmer, CVP, and direct arterial monitoring are routine.
- Ensure bank blood is available and reorder intra-operatively as necessary.
- A nasogastric tube is necessary because prolonged postoperative ileus is common.
- May need aggressive fluid replacement (guided by CVP) from the start to compensate for bowel prep and action of the epidural if used.
- Use an epidural cautiously intra-operatively—there will be plenty of time after the main blood-losing episode to establish an adequate block for postoperative analgesia.
- Take measures to prevent heat loss, e.g. warm air blanket.
- Give antibiotic prophylaxis because the bowel is opened.
- Blood loss can be insidious due to loss from pelvic venous plexuses —weigh swabs, but the accuracy of this is poor due to inclusion of saline washes and urine.
- If blood salvage is used discontinue it when the bowel is opened.
- Air embolism is a possible complication as in any major pelvic surgery.

Postoperative

- Epidural or PCA is advisable for at least 2 days.
- NSAIDs are useful, but ensure good renal function before prescribing.

- Use CVP to guide fluid replacement—requirements are usually very large due to intraperitoneal loss and ileus.
- Urine output via a new ileal conduit is difficult to monitor as drainage tends to be positional.
- Leakage from a ureteric anastomosis may present as urine in the abdominal drain—confirm by comparing the biochemistry of the drainage fluid and urine from the conduit.
- HDU or ICU are ideal for the immediate postoperative period.

Percutaneous stone removal

Procedure	Endoscopic excision/lithotripsy of renal stone via nephrostomy
Time	60–90 min
Pain	++/+++
Position	Prone oblique
Blood loss	Variable, 0–1000 ml
Practical techniques	ETT and IPPV

Preoperative

* Usually healthy young and middle-aged adults, but stones may be due to underlying metabolic problem or due to bladder dysfunction from neurological disability.
* Check renal function.

Perioperative

* Patient initially in the lithotomy position to insert ureteric stents, then turned to semiprone to place nephrostomy posterolaterally below the twelfth rib, under radiographic control.
* There is the potential to dislodge lines and for pressure area damage.
* Consider an armoured ETT to prevent kinking, and secure well.
* Tape and pad the eyes.
* Support the chest and pelvis to allow abdominal excursion with ventilation.
* Support and pad the head, arms, and lower legs.
* Check ventilation during and after position changes.
* May need to temporarily interrupt ventilation for radiographs.
* Give antibiotic prophylaxis if there is infected, obstructed urine.

Postoperative

* Pain from nephrostomy is variable.
* NSAIDs (check renal function), IM morphine, or oral codeine/paracetamol.

Special considerations

* Hypothermia can occur if large volumes of irrigation fluid are used.
* Insertion of nephrostomy is often close to the diaphragm with possibility of breaching the pleura, causing pneumothorax or hydrothorax—if in doubt perform a chest radiograph postoperatively.
* Rupture of the renal pelvis is a recognized complication when large volumes of irrigant may enter the retroperitoneal space.
* Gram-negative septicaemia is possible if the urine is infected.

Extracorporeal shock wave lithotripsy

Procedure	Non-invasive fragmentation of renal stones using pulsed ultrasound
Time	20–40 min
Pain	+/++
Blood loss	Nil
Practical techniques	Sedation for adults
	GA, LMA for children

In the early days of extracorporeal shock wave lithotripsy patients were suspended in a water bath in a semi-sitting position, which produced a number of problems for the anaesthetist. Developments in the 1980s meant that a water bath was no longer required and more recent refinements of the ultrasound beam have made it less uncomfortable for the patient so that with some current lithotriptors only a few patients need anaesthesia or sedation.

Preoperative

- Patients often undergo repeated attempts at lithotripsy, so refer to previous treatment records where possible.
- Premedication with oral diclofenac + IM pethidine is usually effective for treatment.

Perioperative

- Put the patient in the lateral position with arms above the head.
- Renal stones are located using ultrasound or an image intensifier and the shock wave focused on the stones.

Postoperative

- Mild discomfort only—oral analgesics or NSAIDs (beware renal function) are adequate.

Special considerations

- The shock wave can cause occasional dysrhythmias, which are usually self-limiting. If persistent the shock waves can be delivered in time with the ECG (refractory period). Judicious use of anticholinergics (glycopyrrolate 200 μg) will increase the heart rate and increase the frequency of delivered shock.
- Pacemakers can be deprogrammed by the shock wave—seek advice from a pacemaker technician.
- Energy from shock waves is released when they meet an air/water interface—it is advised to use saline, rather than air, for 'loss of resistance' if siting an epidural.

Renal transplant

Procedure	Transplantation of cadaveric or live donor organ
Time	90–180 min
Pain	++/+++
Position	Supine
Blood loss	Not significant–500 ml
Practical techniques	ETT and IPPV, CVP

Preoperative

- Usual problems related to chronic renal failure and uraemia (see p. 110).
- Chronic anaemia is common (Hb usually around 8 g/dl).
- There has usually been recent haemodialysis, therefore there is some degree of hypovolaemia and possibly residual anticoagulation.
- Check postdialysis potassium.
- Note sites of any A-V fistulae and avoid potential sites when placing the IV cannula.

Perioperative

- Fluid load prior to induction—wide swings in arterial pressure are common.
- Commonly used agents include isoflurane, atracurium, fentanyl (or morphine) due to renal disease.
- Insert a triple lumen central line with strict aseptic technique and monitor central venous pressure.
- Prior to graft insertion, gradually increase CVP to 10–12 mmHg (using colloids or crystalloids) to maintain optimal graft perfusion and promote urine production.
- Maintain normothermia.
- Most centres use a cocktail of drugs once the graft is perfused to enhance survival (e.g. hydrocortisone 100 mg, mannitol 20% 60 ml, furosemide (frusemide) 80 mg or more). Have these prepared.

Postoperative

- PCA morphine is a suitable analgesic. Epidural is also possible, but there is a danger of bleeding on insertion (residual anticoagulation from haemodialysis, poor platelet function, etc.) and problems with fluid loading and maintaining blood pressure postoperatively.
- Avoid NSAIDs.
- Monitor CVP and urine output hourly. Maintain mild hypervolaemia to promote diuresis.

Other urological procedures

Operation	Description	Time (min)	Pain (+ to +++++)	Position	Blood loss/ X-match	Notes
Ureteroscopy	Investigate obstruction, remove stones	20–60	+	Lithotomy	ns	LMA + SV Check renal function. Antibiotic prophylaxis if urinary obstruction
Insert ureteric stent	To relieve ureteric obsruction, using image intensifier	20	+	Lithotomy	ns	LMA + SV Antibiotic prophylaxis
Remove ureteric stent	Cystoscopy to retrieve stent	10–20	+	Lithotomy	ns	Awake, or LMA + SV Usually possible with flexi scope and LA
Insert suprapubic catheter	Transcutaneous insertion of catheter into full bladder	15	+	Lithotomy or supine	ns	Sedation + LA, or LMA + SV Often patients with neurological disease
Laser prostatectomy	Transurethral laser to prostate	40–90	+	Lithotomy	ns	Spinal. LMA + SV. ET + IPPV Minimal blood loss and absorption of irrigant, suitable for less fit patients
Bladder neck incision	Transurethral diathermy incision of prostate at narrowed bladder neck	15	++	Lithotomy	ns	LMA + SV Younger patients than TURP

Operation	Description	Time (min)	Pain (+ to +++++)	Position	Blood loss/ X-match	Notes
Urethroplasty	Reconstruction of urethra narrowed by trauma or infection—very variable procedure	90–240	++++	Lithotomy	300– 2000 ml	ET + IPPV ± epidural Beware prolonged lithotomy. Consider epidural for postoperative pain
Nesbitt's procedure	Straightening of penile deformation from Peyronie's disease	60–120	+++	Supine	ns	LMA + SV Consider caudal or penile block
Circumcision	Excision of foreskin	20	++	Supine	ns	LMA + SV + LA Caudal or penile block useful. Topical lidocaine (lignocaine) gel to take home. LA alone possible in frail elderly
Urethral dilatation	Stretching of narrowed urethra with serial dilators	10	+	Lithotomy or supine	ns	LMA or spinal
Urethral meatotomy	Incision to widen urethral meatus	10	+	Supine	ns	LMA + SV
Orchidectomy	Remove testis/es—through groin or scrotum depending on pathology	20–45	++	Supine	ns	LMA + SV + ilioinguinal block Need to block to T9/10 if using regional block due to embryological origins

Operation	Description	Time (min)	Pain (+ to ++++)	Position	Blood loss/ X-match	Notes
Vasectomy	Division of vas deferens via scrotal incision	20–40	++	Supine	ns	LA. LMA + SV Often under LA
Pyeloplasty	Refashioning of obstructed renal pelvis via loin incision. Children and young adults	90–120	++++	Lateral 'kidney position'	300– 500 ml	ET + IPPV + epidural/PCA Similar considerations as nephrectomy. May be significant blood loss in children

Further reading

Alexander JP, Polland A, Gillespie IA (1986). Glycine and transurethral resection. *Anaesthesia*, **41**, 1189–95.

Grove TM, Katz RL (1996). Anaesthesia for urological surgery. In: *International practice of anaesthesia*, vol 2/116/1 (eds. C Prys-Roberts, BR Brown), Butterworth Heinemann, London.

Nicholls AJ (2000). Electrolyte imbalance. In: *Perioperative medicine* (eds. A Nicholls, I Wilson), pp. 302–5, Oxford University Press, Oxford.

Peterson GN, Kreiger JN, Glauber DT (1985). Anaesthetic experience with percutaneous lithotripsy. *Anaesthesia*, **40**, 460–4.

Rabey PG (2001). Anaesthesia for renal transplantation. *British Journal of Anaesthesia CEPD Reviews*, **1**, 24–7.

Roberts FL, Brown EC, Davis R, Cousins MJ (1989). Comparison of hyperbaric and plain bupivacaine with hyperbaric cinchocaine as spinal anaesthetic agents. *Anaesthesia*, **44**, 471–4.

Chapter 28
Liver transplantation and liver resection

Mark Bellamy

General principles

Patients presenting for liver transplantation have either acute hepatic failure or end-stage liver disease. The majority of transplants are performed semi-electively in those with end-stage disease. Worldwide, the commonest indication for hepatic transplantation is now hepatitis C cirrhosis.

Preoperative assessment includes investigation/treatment of:

- jaundice, hyponatraemia, ascites, pleural effusions, diabetes
- renal failure
- systemic vasodilatation with hypotension, cardiac failure
- poor nutritional state and decreased muscle mass
- portopulmonary syndromes (associated severe portal and pulmonary hypertension leading to right ventricular failure and potential cardiac arrest intra-operatively)
- hepatopulmonary syndromes (hypoxia and intrapulmonary shunting occurs in 0.5–4% of patients with cirrhotic liver disease)
- varices (oesophageal, gastric, rectal, abdominal wall)
- coagulopathy (prolonged prothrombin time, low platelet count, fibrinolysis).

Haemodynamic instability can result from cardiac involvement in the underlying process (e.g. alcoholic cardiomyopathy), from pericardial effusions, or from circulatory failure due to dilatation and low systemic vascular resistance. Anaemia resulting in a low plasma viscosity further reduces systemic vascular resistance.

Surgical techniques vary, but there are a number of common features.

- Stage one of the operation is dissection (which involves laparotomy) and haemostasis (including tying off varices). The liver is exposed, the anatomy defined, and slings placed around the major vessels.
- Stage two of the operation is the anhepatic phase during which the hepatic artery, portal vein, hepatic veins, and bile duct are divided. The liver, together with its included portion of vena cava, is then removed and the donor liver implanted. Anastomoses are made between donor and recipient vena cava, and recipient and donor portal vein. Venous return during this phase is severely compromised leading to haemodynamic instability. Venovenous bypass is employed in some centres to facilitate venous return from the lower part of the body (femoral vein to right internal jugular or brachiocephalic vein). During this stage, patients with acute liver failure may become profoundly hypoglycaemic, although this is less common in patients being transplanted for chronic liver disease.
- Stage three of the procedure is the postreperfusion phase, beginning with the re-establishment of blood flow through the liver (portal vein to vena cava). This may be accompanied by a massive reperfusion syndrome, comprising release of cytokines, complement activation, transient reduction in core temperature, arrhythmias, and hypotension. Immediately after reperfusion, there is a rapid elevation in plasma K^+ as it is washed out of the liver graft (up to 8–9 mmol/litre).

As the cell membranes of the graft begin to function normally, electrolyte gradients are restored and a fall in plasma K^+ ensues (sometimes producing ventricular ectopics). Hypotension at this stage results from myocardial depression and subsequently from vasodilatation. Myocardial depression usually resolves within 2 or 3 min, but the vasodilatation may persist for 1 to 2 h. Following reperfusion, the hepatic artery is reanastomosed and finally the bile duct reconstructed, either by direct duct-to-duct anastomosis, or by construction of a Roux loop.

Liver transplantation

Procedure	Transplantation of entire liver
Time	4–10 h
Pain	Variable, but less than other comparable procedures (e.g. gastrectomy, thoracotomy). Back pain/shoulder pain may be a feature. PCA (occasionally epidural) effective
Position	Supine, arms out
Blood loss	0–4000 ml, cross-match 10 units (initially, then use uncrossmatched if necessary). Cell saver mandatory (typically reinfuse 2000 ml). FFP— typically 12 units
Practical techniques	ET, IPPV—details below

Preoperative

- Includes investigation and correction of the factors mentioned above.
- Usual tests include: FBC, U&E, clotting, ECG, echo, stress ECG/dobuta-mine stress echo, chest radiograph, liver/chest CT, spirometry, immun-ology, virology, and hepatic angiographic MRI scan.
- Preoperative fluids are not routinely administered except in patients with renal failure/hyperacute liver failure (dextrose-based solutions).

Perioperative

- Establish peripheral venous and arterial access before induction.
- Induce anaesthesia (propofol, thiopental, or etomidate) and relaxant (atracurium). Vasopressors may be required.
- Ventilate to normocapnoea using oxygen-enriched air and volatile agent (isoflurane or sevoflurane). Establish infusion of an opioid agent (alfen-tanil, remifentanil, or fentanyl). Patients undergoing transplantation for fulminant liver failure are at risk of raised intracranial pressure. In this patient group volatile agents must be avoided and TCI propofol used. ICP monitoring may be used depending upon the jaundice–encephalopathy interval (0–7 days always—raised ICP in 70% of cases, 7–28 days occa-sionally—raised ICP in 20%, 28–90 days seldom—raised ICP in 4%).
- Establish central venous and pulmonary arterial monitoring. Transoesopha-geal echocardiography (TOE) may be used in some centres. Insert a large-bore nasogastric tube.
- Lines for venovenous bypass can either be placed by the surgical team using femoral cut downs, or inserted percutaneously, using extracorporeal mem-brane oxygenation lines (21Fr in the right internal jugular and right femoral veins). These are used both for venovenous bypass and large vascu-lar access. Venovenous bypass uses heparin–carmeda bonded circuitry, so systemic anticoagulation is not necessary.

- The patient's temperature must be vigorously maintained as hypothermia easily develops especially during the anhepatic phase, or with massive transfusion. Forced warm air blankets should be placed over the patient's head, upper chest, arms, and another over the legs.

- Fluids are administered by a rapid infusion system and are warmed through a counter-current heating mechanism (e.g. Level-1 system with high-flow disposables and high-flow taps, allowing transfusion of 600 ml/min at body temperature). Perioperatively and postoperatively, the haematocrit is maintained between 0.26 and 0.32 by infusion of blood, and the right end-diastolic volume index maintained at 140 ml/m^2 by infusion of other colloidal fluids as appropriate.

- FFP is transfused approximately two units per unit of blood transfused. Clotting is monitored and fine-tuned by thromboelastography.

- Antifibrinolytic agents are commonly administered—tranexamic acid (15 mg/kg bolus then 5 mg/kg/h by infusion) is given during the anhepatic phase.

- A dextrose-containing solution is infused continuously to maintain blood sugar. K^+ and Ca^{2+} should be monitored regularly during surgery and supplemented when required to maintain normal values. Hypocalcaemia is common during the anhepatic phase as a result of chelation with unmetabolized citrate. This can lead to cardiac depression and poor clotting. Recheck electrolytes immediately prior to graft reperfusion.

- Severe metabolic acidosis is common but rarely needs correction. At the start of reperfusion, a bolus dose of 10 mmol of calcium is administered to protect the patient against the cardiac effects of potassium released from the liver graft. Progressive hypotension follows reperfusion. This may be severe and require small intravenous doses of adrenaline (50 μg) to maintain mean arterial pressure at a clinically acceptable value (above 70 mmHg). In severely ill patients, an infusion may be required.

- Coagulopathy with defibrination and thrombocytopaenia may also occur at graft reperfusion. Treatment includes bolus doses of antifibrinolytic drugs and platelets, as guided by the thromboelastograph. The haemodynamic and biochemical mayhem of graft reperfusion should resolve rapidly in the event of a functioning liver graft. Persisting acidosis or hypocalcaemia are suggestive of graft primary non-function, which represents a transplantation emergency. This may necessitate urgent retransplantation.

- There is no proven strategy for avoiding renal failure, other than optimizing fluid balance and avoiding any nephrotoxins.

Postoperative

- Patients should be managed on the ICU. Early extubation is often feasible. As a result of improved techniques, the mean intensive care stay post-transplant can be reduced to 6 h.

- Analgesia: PCA/epidural/paravertebral blocks have all been used to good effect. Epidural analgesia is possible in only a minority of cases because of coagulopathy. Avoid NSAIDs (interaction with calcineurin inhibitors to induce renal failure).

- Postoperative fluids: maintenance fluid/nasogastric feed at 1.5 ml/kg/h. Give blood/HAS/FFP to maintain CVP at 10–12, haematocrit at 0.26–0.32, and PT <23 s.
- Bleeding postoperatively is relatively uncommon (5–10%).
- Graft primary non-function occurs in up to 5% of cases, requiring retransplantation.
- Hepatic artery thrombosis occurs in 0.5–5% of cases. Thrombectomy may be attempted, but super-urgent regrafting may be necessary.
- Other postoperative problems include sepsis (10–20%) and acute rejection (up to 40%). These are managed medically with good results.
- Immunosuppression is usually started with standard triple therapy (steroid/azathioprine/tacrolimus) and then tailored to the individual. Other drugs in current use include cyclosporin (ciclosporin), mycophenolate mofetil, rapamycin, antilymphocyte globulin, and OKT3.
- Long-term results of liver transplantation are encouraging. One-year survival figures in major centres now run between 85–95%, with a good long-term quality of life.

Hepatic resection

Procedure	Resection of liver tissue
Time	3–12 h
Pain	As for transplantation
Position	Supine, arms out
Blood loss	1000 ml, cross-match 10 units
Practical technique	ET, IPPV. Details below

The major indication for hepatic resection is metastatic colorectal adeno-carcinoma. Most patients presenting for hepatic resection are otherwise relatively fit. Stigmata of liver disease and significant jaundice are unusual except in those presenting for radical hepatic resection for cholangiocarcinoma, where some patients require biliary stenting or drainage preoperatively to reduce jaundice prior to major surgery. The principles underlying anaesthesia for this group of patients are similar to those for any patient undergoing a major laparotomy.

Major liver resection usually results in 75% of the functional hepatic tissue being removed. As the remaining hepatocytes function poorly for some days following surgery, short-acting drugs should be used. Drugs which might compound postoperative hepatic encephalopathy, or which rely on hepatic metabolism, should be avoided (e.g. benzodiazepines). Most resections are accomplished with minimal blood loss but unexpected catastrophic haemorrhage may occur.

Liver resection operations commence with perihepatic dissection and identification of the vascular anatomy. Once this has been defined (in particular the relationship of lesions to the hepatic veins), resection of the liver can take place. Intra-operative diagnostic ultrasound is often used to pinpoint lesions requiring resection. Bleeding occurs either from vascular inflow to the liver (portal vein, hepatic artery), or by venous back bleeding from the hepatic venous system. Usually, branches of the hepatic artery and portal vein to the segment of liver to be resected have been ligated, so inflow bleeding should not be a major problem. In practice, the line of resection often passes through a watershed area, between vital and devitalized tissue, and remaining inflow bleeding may require additional control by intermittent cross-clamping of vascular inflow to the rest of the liver. This results in a degree of ischaemia-reperfusion injury to the remaining liver tissue, and potentially poor postoperative liver function.

Very radical liver resections are now possible where the liver is totally excised, along with its included portion of vena cava, and dissected *ex vivo* on the bench following perfusion with ice-cold preservation solution. Healthy parts of the liver are then attached to a Goretex vena cava graft and reimplanted. The anaesthetic technique for this prolonged and difficult procedure is very similar to that for liver transplantation.

Preoperative

* As for any major abdominal surgery, but including screening of liver function and coagulation.

Perioperative

- All patients undergoing major liver resection should be invasively monitored and have large venous access. Either a 12Fr high-flow central line or a pair of 7.5Fr Swan–Ganz introducer catheters may be substituted.
- Thoracic epidural analgesia is utilized to good effect postoperatively.
- The anaesthetic technique employed should be aimed at preserving hepatic blood flow and minimizing liver injury. Artificial ventilation of the lungs with oxygen-enriched air and a volatile agent is the best way of achieving this. Isoflurane and desflurane are associated with the best preservation of hepatic blood flow.

Fluid management

- Maintenance of a high central venous pressure used to be common to reduce the risk of air embolism but it is associated with an increased risk of venous back bleeding.
- A reduced central venous pressure substantially reduces venous back bleeding, but there is a theoretically increased risk of air embolus. This approach has dramatically reduced transfusion requirements, with no reported adverse consequences. Techniques for reducing the central venous pressure include epidural boluses and head up (reverse Trendelenburg) tilt. Aim for CVP of 0–2 mmHg and systolic BP of 70–80 mmHg.
- Intra-operative blood sampling allows accurate transfusion replacement. Fresh frozen plasma is occasionally also required in cases of massive haemorrhage, in cases where there is a prolonged hepatic inflow cross-clamp time, or where very little hepatic tissue remains. As with patients undergoing liver transplantation, active warming measures should be taken to maintain the patient's temperature and minimize any coagulopathy.

The overall results of radical hepatic resection are very encouraging with many cases treated that were previously considered inoperable. Many remain disease free 5 years following resection. In those cases where recurrences arise, further hepatic resection is often possible.

Chapter 29
Laser surgery

John Saddler

General principles

* Laser is an acronym for Light Amplification by Stimulated Emission of Radiation. Laser light represents an intense beam of energy that is capable of vaporizing tissues. Lasers have numerous medical and surgical applications, but also create unique hazards to patients and staff.
* Light is a form of radiant energy that spans the mid-range of the electromagnetic spectrum. It is released as photons and travels as a wave.
* In a laser tube, the application of an energy source on a lasing medium creates stimulated emissions of photons. These bounce back and forth between carefully aligned mirrors, and are focused into a high-intensity beam. The light produced is monochromatic (all the same wavelength) and coherent (all the wave peaks moving synchronously at the same amplitude).
* Lasers are defined by their wavelengths, which also determines their colour. Some lasers are outside the visible spectrum. The wavelengths and colours of currently available medical lasers are outlined in the table.

Laser wavelength and colour

Laser type	Wavelength (nm)	Colour
Dye laser	360–670	Blue to red
Argon	488–515	Blue/green
Helium–neon	633	Red
Ruby	694	Red
Nd–YAG	1064	Near-infrared
Carbon dioxide	10 600	Far-infrared

* Laser light striking a tissue surface may be:
  * Reflected. Reflection off shiny surfaces may damage the eyes of staff in the vicinity.
  * Transmitted to deeper layers. Lasers pass through tissues to a variable depth, which is partially determined by the wavelength.
  * Scattered. Shorter wavelengths induce greater scattering.
  * Absorbed. This produces the clinical effect, when the absorbed light is converted to heat. Organic tissue contains various substances capable of absorbing light. These are termed chromophores, and include haemoglobin, collagen, and melanin. Each substance has a particular absorption spectrum, which is determined by its chemical structure. For example, oxyhaemoglobin, which is targeted in vascular lesions, has absorption peaks at 418 nm, 542 nm, and 577 nm. Laser light at or close to these frequencies will be the most effective.

Safety aspects

- A designated trained laser safety officer (usually a trained member of the nursing or medical staff) should be present at all times when a laser machine is in use. An illuminated light should display outside the theatre when the laser is in operation.

- Laser light can be reflected off mirror-like surfaces. Medical instruments used with lasers should have matt, rather than shiny, surfaces.

- The eye is the most susceptible tissue to injury by laser light. Retinal and corneal damage can occur, depending on the frequency of the beam. All operating room personnel must wear safety glasses appropriate for the laser in use. These should have side shields to protect the lateral aspect of the eye. If an anaesthetized patient is receiving laser radiation near the eyes, protective matt metallic eye covers can be applied.

- Damage to skin can occur, depending on the type of laser in use. Theatre workers do not normally need to protect against skin damage, as they will be able to move away from the path of an aberrant beam. Apart from the area being treated, anaesthetized patients must have all exposed skin covered with drapes. These should be made of absorbable material and not plastic, which is potentially combustible. Tissue adjacent to the lesion can be protected with moistened pads or swabs. In all cases, the eyes should be taped closed and covered with moist swabs. Plastic tape is much more combustible than canvas-type tape and should be avoided.

- Some skin preparation fluids are flammable, and should not be used during laser surgery.

- Laser light can ignite plastic and rubber materials. During laser therapy to lesions within the airway careful consideration has to be given to the method of airway maintenance during the procedure. The simplest approach is to avoid using a tracheal tube altogether, and to employ Venturi ventilation. This involves the use of a high-pressure oxygen source and entrainment of atmospheric air. The injector is placed in the lumen of a rigid laryngoscope or bronchoscope which is open at both ends, and permits entrainment of oxygen-enriched air during inspiration and escape of carbon dioxide and exhaust gases during expiration. This system of a 'tube within a tube' is safe, and reduces the chance of barotrauma-induced pneumothorax or pneumomediastinum. Intravenous anaesthesia is usually employed to ensure an adequate depth of anaesthesia during Venturi ventilation. It is also important to prevent the patient from moving or coughing during this procedure, so a suitable muscle relaxant should be administered, and neuromuscular transmission monitored with a nerve stimulator.

- If the use of an endotracheal tube cannot be avoided, unmodified conventional tubes cannot be used because they support combustion and can potentially cause airway fires. Specifically-prepared non-flammable laser tubes are available, e.g Laser-Trach™ tracheal tubes (Sheridan). Alternatively, tracheal tube protectors, e.g. Laser-Guard™ (Xomed) can be wrapped around conventional tubes. These have an adhesive inner silver foil and an outer sponge covering, which is saturated in saline prior to use. The cuffs of both these tubes are vulnerable, and should be protected by damp pledgets. The cuff should be filled with saline, which can be mixed with methylene blue so that it becomes obvious if the cuff is punctured.

- Both nitrous oxide and oxygen support combustion. If using a circuit rather than an oxygen injector, 30% oxygen and air is a sensible choice. If air is not available, oxygen and nitrous oxide can be used, but take special care to protect the tube cuff.

- A laser plume, composed of smoke and gas, accompanies the use of medical lasers. Efficient smoke evacuation must be maintained close to the operative site.

- If a fire occurs in an airway during laser surgery, the flow of anaesthetic gases (including oxygen) should be stopped, and the tube removed. The area should be flushed with water, followed by ventilation with 100% oxygen. Spontaneous breathing in a sitting position should be the main objective, but reintubation may be necessary if airway oedema is severe. A tracheostomy may also be necessary.

Examples of medical lasers

Pulsed dye laser

This was developed with the aim of selective absorption by blood vessels. The light is emitted at a wavelength that targets red blood corpuscles within blood vessels. The energy is dissipated within the dermis, and causes only minimal epidermal scarring. This type of laser is used mainly for treating port wine skin lesions. Children requiring laser therapy to these lesions will often be subjected to multiple treatments, usually under general anaesthesia. Post-operative pain may be a problem, particularly if large areas are treated. Combinations of paracetamol and NSAIDs may be effective, but occasionally opioid analgesics are required.

Carbon dioxide laser

These lasers have a long wavelength (10 600 nm) which is outside the visible spectrum, and are preferentially absorbed by water. Target cells are heated to the point of vaporization by the beam. They penetrate to only a very shallow depth, so tissue damage can be directly observed. They are used in aesthetic facial surgery, to reduce the wrinkling associated with ageing, and in ENT practice to vaporize vocal cord and airway lesions. Care must be taken to avoid eye and airway injury (see above).

Nd–YAG laser

This laser is also outside the visible range, and, unlike the CO_2 laser, is transmitted through clear fluids and absorbed by dark matter. It can penetrate to a depth of 1 cm. It has multiple applications, including airway neoplasms, vascular malformations and ophthalmic surgery.

Chapter 30
CT and MRI imaging

David Sanders

General principles

The anaesthetist working in the medical imaging department may be expected to use old or unfamiliar equipment in a strange and potentially 'hostile' environment isolated from the support normally available in a theatre suite:

- The same standard of care (e.g. preoperative assessment, trained assistant, minimum monitoring standards, resuscitation facilities, and recovery care) must be provided irrespective of where the anaesthetic is given.
- Patients need accommodation for assessment and postprocedure recovery —a day case ward is ideal if not too far from the medical imaging department.
- All anaesthetists should undertake an accompanied familiarization session before working 'solo' in the imaging department.
- Discuss your needs with the radiographers and ask about their requirements.

Indications for anaesthesia

- Infants or uncooperative children.
- Older children or adults with psychological, behavioural, or movement disorders.
- Intubated patients such as acute trauma victims and patients receiving intensive care.
- Analgesia, sedation, or anaesthesia may also be required for interventional procedures performed under CT or possibly MRI guidance.
- Small babies (under 2 months) will often sleep through a scan if given a feed and wrapped up well.

Patient considerations

- Most are children so appropriate skills in paediatric anaesthesia are essential.
- Some patients (e.g. children with CNS tumours) required repeated scans and benefit from consistency in staff and techniques.
- Patients for elective scans are rarely 'normal'. Check the indications for scan and the nature of the underlying pathology—developmental delay, epilepsy, malignancy, psychiatric, and movement disorders. Significant cardiovascular and respiratory problems are uncommon but beware of 'syndromes' with CVS manifestations.

Anaesthesia—general points

- A preanaesthetic visit, assessment, and any investigations should be completed before the patient arrives in the imaging department.
- Take a look around the department and locate the nearest resuscitation facilities (self-inflating bag and mask, portable oxygen, 'crash' trolley, and defibrillator)—confirm that your assistant and the radiographers also know where these are!
- Have a plan for managing an 'arrest' situation. Access for resuscitation in scanners is usually poor. Ask the radiographers how to get the patient out rapidly—they should practice this regularly.

- Check whether the anaesthetic machines are using piped gases or cylinders. If using cylinders confirm that a full spare oxygen cylinder is immediately available.
- Make sure you understand fully how any unfamiliar equipment works—especially the ventilator and disconnect alarms. Do not proceed until you are happy.
- Plan the location of the anaesthetic machine, suction, and monitoring and the configuration and routing of the breathing system in advance.
- Decide where to induce the patient—a dedicated induction area may not be available or may be very small.
- Certain equipment configurations (e.g. anaesthetic machine in scan room and monitors in control room) may require two anaesthetists to manage the patient safely.
- Ensure satisfactory recovery facilities are available, i.e. an appropriately equipped recovery bay and an experienced recovery nurse near the scanner or arrangements for safe transfer of the patient to an operating department recovery room.

Anaesthesia for computed tomography (CT)

A CT scanner uses a rotating X-ray beam and detector coupled to a controlling and signal-processing computer to generate images of transverse 'slices' of body tissues. Older machines scan the slices in a series of discrete steps, but modern 'spiral' CTs acquire image data in a single continuous pass. In modern machines individual scans take a few seconds and a complete study may only require 5–10 min.

Equipment
- The CT scanning environment does not restrict the type of equipment used, but space is often limited so compact anaesthetic machines and monitors are more practical.
- Patient, anaesthetic machine, and monitors must all be visible from the control room.

Techniques
- The patient's head is usually accessible during CT scanning so an LMA may be used if the patient does not require IPPV or airway protection.
- A variety of anaesthetic (and sedation) techniques can be used—inhalation or intravenous induction and maintenance with spontaneous or controlled ventilation. The final choice should be determined by the equipment available and the patient's needs, e.g. airway protection, control of raised intracranial pressure, or respiratory support.
- Only 'light' anaesthesia to produce immobility and lack of awareness is required.

Hazards
- CT scanning generates potentially harmful ionizing radiation so it is preferable for the anaesthetist to monitor the patient from outside the scan room. If it is necessary to remain near the patient wear appropriate radiation protection.
- Cannulas, catheters, drains, and endotracheal tubes can be pulled out during transfers and by movement of the patient through the scanner—ask the radiographer how far the table will move and check that lines and breathing system do not snag other equipment.

Contrast media
- Modern intravascular contrast media for X-ray imaging utilize highly iodinated, non-ionic, water-soluble compounds.
- Common agents are iohexol (Omnipaque™) and iopamidol (Niopam™), which are monomeric, and the dimeric compound iodixanol (Visipaque™). Concentrations equivalent to 300–320 mg of iodine per ml are typically used.
- You may be asked to administer intravenous contrast to anaesthetized patients. The volume required varies with the preparation, investigation, age, and body weight but may be up to 150 ml (see Table).

	Volume (ml)	
Investigation	**Adult**	**Child**
CT head	50–100	10 + 2 ml/kg (up to adult dose)
CT body	100–150	10 + 2 ml/kg (up to adult dose)
Aortography	100	–
Urography	2–3 ml/kg	2–3 ml/kg

- Contrast is viscous and can be difficult to inject through small cannulas or injection ports (take the bung off and inject via the hub of the cannula).
- Check the timing of injection with the radiographer because some 'dynamic' investigations (e.g. aortography) require contrast to be administered as the scan is occurring.
- Intravenous iodine-containing contrast media occasionally trigger allergic reactions (ask about iodine sensitivity).
- These agents may cause renal failure in patients who are dehydrated or have impaired renal function so ensure adequate hydration in patients who have been starved for GA. Lactic acidosis can be precipitated in patients taking biguanides (metformin) and these oral hypoglycaemics should be stopped 48 h before the scan.

Practical considerations

- Metal-containing objects such as ECG leads, pressure transducer cables, or clips lying in the X-ray beam will cause artefacts so route them away from the area to be scanned.
- Scans of the thorax or abdomen may require brief periods of apnoea, i.e. 'breath-holds', to reduce artefacts caused by respiratory movement. Both paralysed and spontaneously breathing patients can be ventilated manually at this point and their lungs held in inspiration for the few seconds needed to perform each individual scan.
- The patient's arms usually need to be positioned above the head during thoracic or abdominal scans. Wide adhesive tape is useful for securing the limbs (keep a roll on the anaesthetic machine).
- Intensive care patients requiring CT scans should be managed like any inter-ICU transfer with full transport monitoring and ventilatory support. Ideally the ICU resident or consultant should supervise the patient and review the scan with the reporting radiologist. Getting such patients into and out of the scanner can be a slow process.

Anaesthesia for magnetic resonance imaging (MRI)

MRI is a versatile imaging tool free from the dangers of ionizing radiation. A computer creates cross-sectional or three-dimensional images from minute radio-frequency signals generated as hydrogen nuclei are flipped in and out of alignment with a powerful magnetic field by high-frequency magnetic pulses.

- Non-invasive but has unpleasant aspects—the subject has to lie motionless in a long narrow noisy tunnel with the part of body to be imaged closely surrounded by an 'aerial coil' creating a very claustrophobic environment.
- A typical sequence of scans lasts 15–25 min but complex scans may take much longer.
- Up to 3% of adults cannot tolerate scanning without sedation or anaesthesia.
- Provision of safe anaesthesia for MRI requires specialized equipment and careful organization—unlike CT you cannot simply take a standard machine and monitor to the MRI scanner.

Hazards

Combining MRI with anaesthesia creates several problems—some arise from the effects of the magnetic fields on anaesthetic equipment and some from the effects of anaesthetic equipment on the scanner.

- Most scanners use a superconducting magnet to generate a high-density static magnetic field, which is always present. Field strength is measured in tesla (T)—most scanners use 0.5–1.5 T magnets (about 10 000 times the Earth's magnetic field).
- Near the scanner (>5 mT) the static field exerts a powerful attraction on ferromagnetic materials (e.g. scissors, gas cylinders, laryngoscopes) which can become projectiles. Electric motors (e.g. in syringe drivers) may run erratically and any information stored on magnetic media (credit cards, cassette tapes, or floppy disks) will be erased. The magnetic field decreases as distance from the scanner increases—beyond the 0.5 mT boundary or outside the scan room can be considered safe.
- Devices (e.g. hypodermic needles) made from stainless steel, which is not ferromagnetic, can be taken into the scan room. If you are unsure about an object don't risk it!
- Oscillating magnetic fields induce eddy currents in electrical conductors (e.g. ECG leads, metallic implants). These currents may disrupt or damage electronic equipment (including pacemakers) and cause heating effects that can result in burns.
- Large masses of metal (e.g. anaesthetic machines, gas cylinders) near the scanner or small amounts of non-ferrous metals within the three-dimensional volume being scanned can distort the magnetic fields causing poor quality images.
- The scan room is usually shielded to prevent external electrical interference from swamping the MR signals. All electrical equipment within the scan room must also be fully shielded and electrical conductors entering the room (e.g. monitoring cables) require special radio-frequency filters.

- Rapidly changing magnetic fields cause mechanical vibrations and extremely loud 'knocking' noises, which can potentially damage hearing.

Equipment

Two alternative approaches are feasible:

- specialized 'MRI compatible' equipment within the scan room, or
- conventional equipment outside the scanner's magnetic field in the control room.

Standardizing on one option keeps anaesthetist, anaesthetic machine, and monitors together. Choice depends upon space, funds, expected frequency of GAs, and individual preference. Using conventional equipment at a distance avoids crowding the scanner, is less expensive, and allows faulty monitors to be substituted. The anaesthetist can regulate the anaesthetic and monitor the patient without being in the scan room and hazards can be reduced by applying the simple rule that 'nothing enters the scan room except the patient and the trolley'.

A typical set-up is as follows:

- Induction area adjacent to but outside the scan room (beyond the 0.5 mT boundary) equipped with a compact conventional anaesthetic machine and monitoring.
- Piped gases, scavenging, and suction in both the induction area and the control room.
- Non-magnetic tipping trolley for patient transfer into the scanner.
- Compact (e.g. wall mounted) anaesthetic machine and ventilator in the control room with a 10 m coaxial (Bain) breathing system.
- Respiratory gas/agent analyser with capnograph display fitted with an extended sampling tube (increases the response time by 5–10 s).
- MRI-compatible pulse oximeter (fibreoptic patient probe and shielded cable).
- ECG with MRI-compatible (carbon fibre) patient leads and electrodes.
- NIBP machine with an extended hose, non-metallic connectors, and a range of cuffs.

Practical considerations and techniques

- Physically and 'magnetically' restricted access makes patient observation and treatment difficult so a secure airway is a priority.
- Neonates and young babies (< 2 months) will often sleep through a short scan if fed, wrapped up, and placed on their side in the scanner.
- Babies and small children (< 15 kg), any patient with an intracranial space-occupying lesion, suspicion of raised ICP, or needing a protected airway—use intubation and IPPV.
- Larger children and adults (if no risk of raised ICP)—use LMA and spontaneous ventilation.
- If intubating a patient for a head scan use a RAE tube. It keeps the connectors and breathing system clear of the head coil.
- Tape the valve on the pilot tube of a cuffed ETT or LMA so that it lies outside the volume to be scanned or the metal of the spring will distort the images.

- Sedation with oral or IV benzodiazepines may be used by radiologists for healthy but claustrophobic adults. Patients with severe back or root compression pain may also require strong analgesia to tolerate positioning for a scan.
- The role of sedation for MRI scanning in children is unclear. Some children's centres have reported successes with structured sedation programmes run by dedicated sedationists. However, the safety of having heavily sedated children in the medical imaging department without direct anaesthetic supervision has been questioned.

Tips for IPPV through a 10 m long breathing system

- Use a system which functions as a 'T-piece' (Mapleson D or E) so dead space is unaffected by length. Ayres T-piece and coaxial Bain systems work well and are both suitable for ventilating babies and small children.
- Airway pressures measured near the ventilator may not accurately represent distal pressures at the endotracheal tube.
- Tidal volume delivered to the lungs will be reduced by 'compression losses' of the gas within the system and by expansion of the tubing during inspiration.
- As a result of these effects IPPV using a simple pressure generator (e.g. Penlon Nuffield 200 with a Newton valve) may not be effective in children weighing more than 15 kg.
- Tidal volume loss in the system can make it difficult to compensate for significant leaks round uncuffed tracheal tubes—change to a slightly larger tube so the leak is minimal.
- Increased expiratory resistance of some systems (e.g. Ayres T-piece) generates a positive expiratory pressure which increases with the fresh gas flow.

Scanning intensive care patients

- The same considerations apply as for CT scanning (see above) but potential hazards are greater so the risk/benefit balance should be assessed carefully.
- Do not scan patients who are haemodynamically or otherwise unstable.
- Electronic pressure transducers, metal-containing ICP 'bolts', temporary pacing wires, and conventional ECG leads must be removed before the patient enters the scan room.
- Full checks (and if necessary plain radiographs) must be performed to confirm there are no hazardous metallic implants or foreign bodies present.
- Patients who are stable on inotrope infusions can be scanned but the infusion pumps must remain at a safe distance from the magnet—ideally outside the scan room. Prepare duplicate pumps in the control room with extended infusion lines threaded with the breathing system into the scan room. Connect the patient to the running infusions while outside the room, check they are stable, and then move them into the scanner.

Patient and staff safety

- To avoid accidental injury all patients having an MRI scan must complete a screening/consent form. In the case of children or sedated ICU patients these must be completed on their behalf by relatives or staff.

- To prevent injury and property damage all staff must similarly complete a screening questionnaire and leave metallic objects, pagers, credit cards, etc. outside the room.

- The greatest dangers arise from ferromagnetic implants or foreign bodies—certain types of artificial heart valves, old cerebral aneurysm clips, or steel splinters in the eye, where movement could disrupt valve function or precipitate intracranial or vitreous haemorrhage respectively.

- Patients and staff with cardiac pacemakers must remain outside the 0.5 mT boundary.

- Anaesthetized and sedated patients should have their ears protected to prevent noise-induced auditory damage.

- Intravenous MRI contrast media are paramagnetic but do not contain iodine and have a high therapeutic ratio. Side-effects include headache, nausea and vomiting, local burning and weals (incidence 2.4%). Severe hypotension/anaphylactoid reactions are rare (approximately 1:100 000).

- Commonly used agents are Magnevist™ (gadopentetate) at a dose of 0.2–0.4 ml/kg and Omniscan™ (gadodiamide) at 0.2 ml/kg.

Cardiac arrest

- Do not attempt advanced life support in the scan room.

- Do NOT allow the cardiac arrest team into the scan room.

- Start basic life support with a non-metallic self-inflating bag and chest compressions.

- Remove the patient from the scan room on a non-magnetic trolley and continue resuscitation outside the 0.5 mT boundary.

Further reading

Edwards M-B (1998). *Prosthetic heart valves implanted in the United Kingdom 1986–1997*, 2nd edn. UK Heart Valve Registry.

Hatch DJ, Sury MRJ (2000). Sedation of children by non-anaesthetists. *British Journal of Anaesthesia*, **84**, 713–14.

Menon DK, Peden CJ, Hall AS, Sargentoni J, Whitwam JG (1992). Magnetic resonance for the anaesthetist Part I: physical principles, applications, safety aspects. *Anaesthesia*, **47**, 240–55.

Peden CJ, Menon DK, Hall AS, Sargentoni J, Whitwam JG (1992). Magnetic resonance for the anaesthetist Part II: anaesthesia and monitoring in MR units. *Anaesthesia*, 47, 508–17.

Shellock FG (1996). *Pocket guide to MR procedures and metallic objects: update 1996*. Lippincott-Raven, Philadelphia.

Chapter 31
Electroconvulsive therapy

Suzie Tanser

Physiological effects of ECT

- Cardiovascular
  - Immediate: parasympathetic stimulation (bradycardia, hypotension)
  - Later (after 1 min): sympathetic stimulation (tachycardia, hypertension, increased myocardial oxygen consumption, dysrhythmias)
- Cerebral effects
  - increased cerebral oxygen consumption
  - increased cerebral blood flow
  - increased intracranial pressure.
- Other
  - increased intraocular pressure
  - increased intragastric pressure.

Preoperative assessment

- ECT is commonly carried out in elderly patients who may have a variety of coexisting disease processes. A careful preoperative assessment should always be undertaken.
- The majority of patients will be taking psychiatric drugs, many of which have the potential to interact with anaesthetic agents (p. 205).
- Patients are commonly poor historians and care should be taken to assess compliance with preoperative fasting.
- ECT is a repeated procedure so always study the previous anaesthetic notes to see the effect of the anaesthetic on seizure modification.
- ECT is commonly carried out at isolated sites and appropriate personnel and resuscitative facilities must be available.
- Sedative premedication is not indicated and may prolong recovery.

Contraindications to ECT

- Absolute: recent myocardial infarction, recent CVE, intracranial mass lesion.
- Relative: uncontrolled angina, congestive cardiac failure, severe osteoporosis, major bone fractures, glaucoma, retinal detachment.

Anaesthesia for ECT

- Aims. Rapid induction, attenuation of undesirable physiological effects, appropriate seizure modification, rapid recovery.

- Induction. Preoxygenation should be performed prior to induction. Methohexitone (0.75 mg/kg) was, for years, the most commonly used induction agent, but has now been withdrawn. Propofol (1–2 mg/kg) is now the agent of choice, giving rapid onset and offset and obtunding of the cardiovascular response. Thiopental, ketamine, and etomidate have all been successfully used.

- Muscle relaxants. Suxamethonium (0.5 mg/kg) is most commonly used. Low-dose mivacurium (0.08 mg/kg) has been tried, but although recovery was found to be good, seizure modification was inadequate. If mivacurium is used, the dose should be at least 0.15 mg/kg and reversal will probably be necessary. Longer-acting agents are not generally suitable.

- Airway maintenance. Providing there are no risk factors for aspiration the airway can normally be maintained with an oral airway and mask unless longer-acting muscle relaxants are used. Assisted ventilation with 100% oxygen is recommended until spontaneous respiration has returned. A bite block is commonly used during the seizure period to prevent damage to the lips, tongue, or teeth.

- Atropine premedication was commonly used to prevent the bradycardic response seen in the immediate phase response. Bradyarrythmias are particularly common during stimulus titration, where subconvulsive stimuli are used to determine seizure threshold, but routine atropine premedication is no longer recommended due to the detrimental effects of atropine on myocardial work and oxygen demand.

- Sympathetic attenuation. Sympathetic stimulation in patients with cardiovascular disease may be undesirable. Various agents such as GTN, sodium nitroprusside, hydralazine, and propanolol have been tried but there is no consensus on their use. Pretreatment with beta-blockers may be useful (e.g. oral atenolol 50 mg preoperatively) or esmolol infusion (50–200 µg/kg/min) may be used intra-operatively.

- Recovery. The post-ictal stage is occasionally associated with a period of agitation, confusion or aggressive behaviour. Avoidance of excessive stimulation during the recovery phase may help attenuate this. Sedation with benzodiazepines or haloperidol may be required.

- Side-effects. Exacerbation of ischaemic heart disease, cardiac rupture, long bone fractures, inhalation of teeth, etc. have all been reported. Mortality following ECT is reported as 0.03%.

Further reading

Cheam EW, Critchley LA, Chui PT, Yap JC, Ha VW (1999). Low dose mivacurium is less effective than succinylcholine in electroconvulsive therapy. *Canadian Journal of Anaesthesia*, **46**, 49–51.

Mayur P, Shree R *et al.* (1998). Atropine premedication and the cardiovascular response to electroconvulsive therapy. *British Journal of Anaesthesia*, **81**, 466–7.

Royal College of Psychiatrists (1995). *The ECT handbook (Council Report CR 39)*. Gaskell, London

Chapter 32
Military anaesthesia

Matthew Roberts

General principles

Anaesthesia for the unprepared battlefield patient encompasses the skills of resuscitation, anaesthesia, postoperative intensive care, and patient transfer. Surgery for less severely injured and semielective cases, such as the delayed primary suture of wounds, demand anaesthetic techniques that allow rapid recovery and early onward evacuation. Anaesthesia is conducted in the austere, isolated, and potentially very mobile environment of the field surgical team or field hospital associated with the ever-present threat of personal injury.

The austere environment
To allow military surgery and anaesthesia of an acceptable standard requires:
- shelter
- electricity for light, heating, and equipment
- water supply (clean).

The battle casualty
Although the majority of military personnel are fit, the stress of military operations may reveal previously undiagnosed disorders such as ischaemic heart disease. The battle casualty is likely to be:
- cold, exhausted, dehydrated, and filthy
- in haemorrhagic shock
- frightened or suffering from post-traumatic stress
- temporarily deaf from high explosive.

Injuries suffered may be blunt trauma from vehicle accidents and falls or high-velocity penetrating missile injuries. These wounds are often extensive, multiple, and always contaminated. Repeated operations for debridement, delayed primary suture, and skin graft are required. Most casualties reaching the surgical team alive will have limb injuries. Burns are particularly common, and explosions may result in pulmonary and intestinal blast injury.

Anaesthetic equipment
Ideally all equipment used in the field should be:
- robust
- compact and lightweight
- simple to use
- accord with United Kingdom and international standards.

Power source
The electricity supply in a field medical unit is from generators that must be of sufficient power to cope with maximal demands. Ideally all electrical items should have an independent battery supply as back up.

Oxygen
The logistical problem of the supply of medical gases in the field is complex. Cylinders or oxygen concentrators may be utilized. Where oxygen supplies are limited, ventilators should be electrically driven and oxygen added to the circuit as needed. This allows scarce oxygen to be reserved for preoxygenation, the immediate postoperative period, and the critically ill.

Refrigeration

Refrigeration is required for the storage of blood and temperature-sensitive drugs.

Anaesthetic technique—inhalational anaesthesia

Draw-over anaesthesia is the most suitable inhalational technique for use in the field; it can be employed using spontaneous or controlled ventilation, is not dependent on a compressed gas supply, and requires only light portable equipment. The requirements are:

* one-way patient valve and self-inflating bag
* low-resistance vaporizer, e.g. OMV or Ohmeda PAC
* oxygen T-piece and reservoir (a length of tubing).

As most casualties are unprepared for surgery, rapid sequence induction, intubation, and controlled ventilation is employed. A standard balanced inhalational technique for battle casualties involves:

* Assessment and resuscitation—with oxygen if available.
* Preoxygenation—5 litre/min of 90% oxygen from a concentrator administered with a drawover circuit will give an FiO_2 of 40–50%.
* Rapid sequence induction with cricoid pressure. Ketamine is the favoured induction agent in potentially shocked patients, although it may not be appropriate in patients with head or eye injuries.
* Controlled ventilation. Maintain neuromuscular blockade with vecuronium.
* Draw-over anaesthesia with isofluorane or halothane in air.
* Oxygen supplementation as required.
* Supplementary opioid analgesia, usually morphine.
* Reverse and then extubate awake, head down lateral.
* Alternatively transfer sedated and ventilated to intensive care if available.

In non-emergency cases such as planned delayed primary suture or change of dressings a spontaneous breathing draw-over technique can be used with a facemask or laryngeal mask airway. Oxygen supplementation will be required as respiratory depression will occur.

Circle anaesthesia could have advantages in the field in terms of savings in oxygen and volatile agent. However, monitoring of inspired oxygen, $ETCO_2$, and anaesthetic agent is mandatory, which adds complexity.

Anaesthetic technique—total intravenous anaesthesia

Ketamine as a sole anaesthetic agent

- Ideal for 'roadside anaesthesia'.
- Can be administered IV 1–2 mg/kg or IM 10 mg/kg or a combination of IV/IM.
- Sympathetic tone is maintained.
- Airway control is not usually lost (although this should not be assumed).
- Emergence phenomena can be unpleasant and may be reduced by concurrent use of midazolam. This diminishes some of the safety features of ketamine.
- Causes increases in intracranial and intraocular pressures.

Ketamine and midazolam by infusion

- A technique for use with controlled ventilation.
- IV induction: midazolam 0.07 mg/kg + ketamine 1 mg/kg.
- Maintenance by infusion. Mix ketamine 200 mg, midazolam 5 mg, and 0.9% saline to a volume of 50 ml.
- Infusion rate in ml/h = (patient's body weight in kg)/2.
- The mixture has a shelf life of 72 h.
- Unpleasant dreams or hallucinations are rare.
- Blood pressure and pulse rate tend to be maintained.

Propofol and alfentanil

- A technique for use with controlled ventilation in casualties with an uncompromised circulation.
- IV induction with standard doses of alfentanil and propofol.
- Mix propofol 500 mg and alfentanil 2.5 mg.
- Initial infusion of approximately 10 mg/kg/hr of propofol.
- Reduce gradually to 5 mg/kg/h according to clinical signs.
- Rapid clear-headed recovery with low incidence of nausea.

Regional techniques

Nerve blocks can be of value in providing an adjunct to postoperative pain but are of limited value as a sole method of anaesthesia as war wounds do not respect anatomical boundaries. Local anaesthetic infiltration by the surgeon is encouraged. Spinal anaesthesia is contraindicated in shock. Epidural anaesthesia may have a place in the rear hospital where asepsis can be confidently observed.

Analgesia in the field—a simple approach

The following approach is applicable to postoperative patients as well as the casualty arriving in the resuscitation department of the field hospital:

• Resuscitate as required.
• Morphine IV 2 mg every 3 min until comfortable.
• Assess, dress, and splint wounds. Apply traction to fractures.
• Morphine 10 mg IM 2–hourly PRN so long as the respiratory rate is >8/min, the systolic blood pressure is >90 mmHg, and the casualty is responsive and in pain.
• Consider nerve blocks if practical.
• Consider Entonox or ketamine for manipulations.
• Reassess frequently, and remember that worsening pain may indicate a developing complication, e.g. compartment syndrome or sepsis.

Chapter 33
The critically ill patient

Julia Munn

The ICU patient going to theatre

The planning, transfer, and monitoring of a critically ill patient on intensive care, who needs surgery, can be a challenge for the anaesthetist. Physiological instability should be anticipated, detected, and acted upon promptly and effectively.

In some instances the surgery may be planned a day or two in advance, such as in the multiple trauma patient who needs further orthopaedic work. In such cases the patient should be in a reasonably stable state at the time of planned surgery. Other types of surgery may be of a much more urgent nature, e.g. peritonitis or haemorrhage. These cases are more likely to be septic or hypovolaemic and may decompensate intra-operatively. Both senior anaesthetists and surgeons should be involved.

Consent

The decision to operate must be taken by the surgeon and intensivist after considering all the risks and benefits of surgery in a critically ill patient. Informed consent is often impossible as the patient may be sedated or comatose. Whilst the family is not able to give consent in law, their support is invaluable, and whenever possible the reasons for surgery and risks should be discussed with them.

Preoperative assessment

- Do not forget routine aspects of the preoperative assessment just because the patient is already critically ill, i.e. history of previous anaesthetics, chronic medical conditions, allergies, etc.

- Assess the patient's current condition from discussion with ICU medical and nursing staff and from information on the observation charts. If the patient is ventilated check the depth of sedation and doses of drugs used.

- Assess haemodynamic stability and note the current fluid requirements and rate/concentration of inotrope infusions. Ensure that there is an adequate supply of inotrope prepared for theatre. Consider which vasopressors may be required.

- Note the patient's oxygen requirement and, if ventilated, the compliance, minute volume, and PEEP etc. to predict the ventilator settings that will be necessary in theatre. If the patient has severe ARDS with critical oxygenation and poor compliance the theatre ventilator may be inadequate and it may be necessary arrange to use an ICU ventilator. Current policy in many ICUs is to use high PEEP, if necessary, to achieve oxygenation in ARDS but to keep peak pressure <30 cmH$_2$O. This commonly results in hypercapnia, but as long as the arterial pH is >7.25, is considered preferable to worsening lung injury.

- Check intravenous access and consider if any additional cannulas may be required. Many ICU patients have had all peripheral access removed.

- Assess the patient's fluid balance and decide whether additional monitoring will be helpful.

- Check which antibiotics the patient is receiving and whether any doses will be due in theatre.

- Check the most recent FBC, U&E, and blood gases, and ensure that blood has been cross-matched and is available.

- If you are taking the patient to a more remote facility such as the X-ray department, ensure that you have adequate anaesthetic assistance and bear in mind the difficulties in patient access and monitoring.

Transfer to theatre

- You are responsible for the safe transfer of the patient to and from theatre.
- Familiarize yourself with the transport equipment and ensure it is functioning before you leave the ICU.
- If the patient is already ventilated establish on the transfer ventilator before leaving the ICU to ensure adequate ventilation can be maintained. Most current transfer ventilators have a PEEP facility.
- If the transfer may be painful or distressing to the patient, consider deepening the level of sedation.
- If the patient is not already sedated and ventilated decide whether to induce in ICU, the anaesthetic room, or theatre. Factors to influence your decision should be safety aspects, available assistance, haemodynamic instability, and patient comfort.
- Monitor the patient as fully as possible en route.
- Take time to disentangle all lines, re-establish full monitoring, and check IV access before the start of surgery. Access to the patient can very difficult under the drapes.

Perioperatively

- The patient is likely to require additional anaesthetic. This can be TIVA or a volatile agent, plus a muscle relaxant. If an epidural is already in situ and the patient is stable, this can be 'topped up' to provide analgesia, but it is rarely practical or particularly advantageous to site an epidural at this stage if prolonged postoperative ventilation is anticipated.
- Anticipate and prepare for a worsening of the patient's haemodynamic state due to additional anaesthetic, blood loss, or sepsis.
- Anticipate the need for rapid transfusion and ensure a stock of colloid solutions and blood in theatre with pressure bags or a rapid infusion device.
- Continue all invasive monitoring and act swiftly to reverse any deleterious changes. Judge fluid requirements using CVP or PCWP, measured losses, and urine output rather than blood pressure.
- If surgery is prolonged check Hb, clotting, and acid–base status regularly.
- Give antibiotics as indicated.
- Complete an anaesthetic chart and record all fluids given, blood loss, inotrope changes, etc.

Transfer back to ICU

- Inform ICU when surgery is about to finish to plan staffing or assist in the transfer.
- Ensure the patient is stable before leaving theatre.
- Take the same care establishing ventilation and monitoring as on the trip to theatre.
- Ensure you give a full verbal and written handover to the ICU medical and nursing staff and communicate the surgeon's postoperative requirements.
- Ensure the patient is safely established on the ICU ventilator and haemodynamically stable before passing on responsibility to the ICU team.

Anaesthesia for the septic patient

In the management of a patient who is haemodynamically unstable due to sepsis, or blood loss the anaesthetist has a key role in improving and maintaining tissue oxygenation perioperatively. A prolonged period of poor organ perfusion may lead to multiple organ failure, which carries a very high mortality.

Most cases of sepsis will be intra-abdominal requiring a laparotomy for a perforated viscus. Other cases will include surgery for soft tissue infections, urological or gynaecological sepsis, and intrathoracic sepsis. Patients requiring a laparotomy for gastrointestinal obstruction or bleeding may also be unstable due to hypovolaemia and the same principles of resuscitation apply, although they are less likely to develop a systemic inflammatory response syndrome (SIRS) than the septic patient.

Definition

* Sepsis, and the body's response to it, has been defined by consensus conference of the American College of Chest Physicians and Society of Critical Care Medicine as a combination of two or more of the following conditions occurring as the response to infection:
  * temperature >38 °C or <36 °C
  * heart rate >90 beats/min
  * respiratory rate >20/min or $PaCO_2$ <4.3 kPa
  * WBC >12 000/mm^3 or >10% immature forms.
* Severe sepsis is defined as sepsis plus hypoperfusion, organ dysfunction or hypotension.
* Septic shock is defined as sepsis plus hypotension, despite adequate fluid resuscitation, plus organ perfusion abnormalities.
* Systemic inflammatory response syndrome (SIRS) has the same definitions as sepsis but can occur as a response to a number of insults other than infection, e.g. pancreatitis, multiple trauma.

Pathology

The response to sepsis involves a large number of chemical mediators, acting via complex and interactive pathways, some of which are pro- and others anti-inflammatory. In a septic patient, the severity of illness is determined more by the nature of the inflammatory response than by the infection itself.

Most abdominal sepsis is caused by Gram-negative bacteria which contain endotoxin in their outer membrane. Endotoxin is a lipopolysaccharide implicated in macrophage and monocyte activation and the release of numerous mediators including tumour necrosis factor-α (TNF-α), interleukin 1 (IL-1) and other cytokines, plus prostaglandins, leukotrienes, the complement and fibrinolytic systems, platelet-activating factor, and nitric oxide (NO).

Pathological effects caused by these mediators include vasodilatation, increased capillary permeability, impaired tissue oxygen utilization, and myocardial depression.

Preoperative assessment

* Classical signs of sepsis are pyrexia, tachycardia, warm bounding peripheries, and hypotension.

- These signs are not always seen, particularly in:
  - young children
  - the very elderly
  - patients with pre-existing pathology, e.g. severe cardiac failure
  - patients on steroids or beta-blockers
  - patients moribund from advanced sepsis.
- Other signs may include confusion, drowsiness, cool peripheries, tachypnoea, hypoxia, and oliguria.

Interpretation of investigations in the septic patient

- FBC: expect high WBC with neutrophilia (a low WBC is evidence of overwhelming sepsis). A low platelet count is common in severe sepsis.
- U&E: urea and sodium raised proportionately more than creatinine indicates dehydration, disproportionately high creatinine indicates renal impairment.
- Coagulation screen: increased INR indicates septic coagulopathy (unless on warfarin).
- Blood sugar: usually raised, low sugar indicates advanced sepsis or hepatic dysfunction.
- Arterial blood gases: metabolic acidosis is common; there may be compensatory hyperventilation unless the patient is very obtunded. Hypoxia is common in severe sepsis.
- Blood lactate: high, confirming tissue hypoxia as the cause of acidosis. If acidotic with normal lactate check creatinine and urine output (renal failure is the most likely cause of non-lactic acidosis in the septic patient, another cause is diabetic ketoacidosis).
- The chest radiograph may show 'wet lungs' or non-cardiogenic pulmonary oedema, which may progress to changes of ARDS.
- The combination of clinical signs plus investigations should give an indication of the severity of illness, resuscitation required, and necessary postoperative support.

Resuscitation, monitoring, and planning

- Anticipate and prepare for a deterioration in the patient's condition intraoperatively. Anaesthesia will reverse any haemodynamic compensation by its vasodilatory and negative inotropic effects. Surgery may initially worsen the septic state by further releasing bacteria, endotoxins, and cytokines, in addition to blood and fluid loss.
- For these reasons patients in septic shock will benefit from time spent improving their filling status and establishing monitoring preoperatively. If you consider that the patient requires further resuscitation plan where and how to undertake it. It may be possible on the ward but is usually more efficient and effective if undertaken by the anaesthetist in the anaesthetic or recovery room.
- Plan the patient's postoperative care as far as possible in advance. If there are no ICU beds available consider requesting a prolonged stay in theatre recovery. The more notice the nurses are given to arrange staffing the more likely any of these options are to be possible. A recurrent recommendation in reports of the Confidential Enquiry into Perioperative Deaths (CEPOD)

is for increased provision of HDU beds and for better use to be made of them. The 1999 CEPOD report specifically states that the surgical and anaesthetic management for sick elderly patients must include the planning of appropriate postoperative care, in an HDU if necessary.

- The following vascular access and monitoring should be established during the resuscitation phase, before induction of anaesthesia:
  - two functioning, large-bore intravenous cannulas
  - CVP line
  - arterial line
  - urinary catheter
  - consider a pulmonary artery catheter or other means of monitoring cardiac output (e.g. oesophageal Doppler) in advanced sepsis, or if there is pre-existing cardiac failure or severe respiratory disease which would make interpretation of the CVP potentially misleading.

- While establishing monitoring administer oxygen and continue giving fluid. Fluids can be crystalloid or colloid, preferences vary between institutions and between countries. Colloids are likely to remain in the circulation longer, particularly in the septic patient with 'leaky' capillaries, and to result in a smaller total volume of fluid infused.

- Ensure blood is cross-matched and available—transfuse the patient with blood if anaemic or actively bleeding. Hb will also fall due to haemodilution and there may be excessive blood loss due to a septic coagulopathy.

- If antibiotics have not been started, check that blood cultures are taken first.

- Give antibiotics at the correct time and in the correct dose; check the ward chart as doses are not infrequently missed when patients are being prepared for theatre. Unless the infecting organism has already been identified use 'best guess' antibiotics (see p. 902). If the patient has recently received an appropriate course of antibiotics switch to your hospital's 'second line' choice. Several antibiotics can accumulate and produce toxic side-effects in renal failure but a normal dose should be used initially to ensure that a therapeutic level is reached. It is much better to start with a broad range of antibiotics at high doses, which can be rapidly reduced when the patient shows signs of improving, than to provide inadequate cover to a very sick patient.

Induction and maintenance of anaesthesia

- Rapid sequence induction should be used in any patient who is acutely ill due to sepsis from any source as gastric stasis is common.
- Any induction agent is likely to cause an exaggerated fall in BP so use cautiously.
- Insert a nasogastric tube if one is not already in place.
- The use of epidural blockade is controversial in sepsis:
  - a potential bacteraemia may be considered to be a contraindication
  - coagulopathy may preclude siting of the epidural
  - hypotensive effects are likely to be exaggerated and difficult to reverse

- if siting of an epidural not contraindicated by other factors, consider inserting a catheter but waiting until the patient is stable before establishing the block.
- Either a volatile or TIVA can be used but a shocked patient will probably have a reduced requirement to maintain anaesthesia and any agent will have a more pronounced effect on BP than usual.
- The effects and duration of action of opioids may be increased due to impaired hepatic and renal perfusion; use cautiously if the patient is to be extubated postoperatively. Additional opioid can be given on emergence from anaesthesia when opioid effects can be assessed.
- Avoid NSAIDs in patients who are persistently hypotensive or septic.

Importance of tissue oxygenation maintenance intra-operatively

- Do not wait until the patient arrives in ICU postoperatively before instituting the principles of organ support—any delay in reversing shock will only increase the chances of multiple organ failure and death.
- Intra-operative hypotension should be treated promptly and appropriately as it is poorly tolerated in the elderly and patients with pre-existing medical conditions.
- Inadequate fluid replacement and intra-operative hypotension is cited in several CEPOD reports as a major factor in postoperative mortality.
- Remember that a normal ECG does not exclude significant coronary artery disease and a normal serum creatinine does not exclude renal impairment. Renal function can fall by 80% before serum creatinine increases above normal.
- Patients with pre-existing renal impairment are far more likely to develop renal failure after a period of hypoperfusion.
- Renal blood flow falls dramatically below a mean arterial BP of 60–80 mmHg. This threshold is higher in patients who are normally hypertensive.
- Normal BP does not indicate adequate organ perfusion, as BP may be maintained by vasoconstriction at the expense of adequate perfusion.
- Maintenance of hepatosplanchnic perfusion is probably most important in the prevention of multiple organ failure, but also the most difficult to monitor.

Means of monitoring tissue oxygenation in theatre

- Urine output (aim for 0.5 ml/kg/h in adults).
- Arterial blood gases (aim to reduce metabolic acidosis).
- Mixed venous oxygenation if PA catheter in situ. Normal $S\bar{v}O_2$ >75%; this is reduced in shock with inadequate tissue oxygen delivery or increased utilization. However, in septic shock, reduced tissue oxygen extraction can occur and give normal or high $S\bar{v}O_2$. The trend in values is more useful than a one-off measurement.
- Peripheral–core temperature difference (normal <2 °C), more useful in low cardiac output states/hypovolaemia than hyperdynamic sepsis.

Means of restoring and maintaining tissue oxygenation in theatre

Fluids

* Continue to give fluids aiming for CVP 8–10 mmHg, PCWP >12 mmHg.
* Pulmonary oedema is possible in septic patients due to increased capillary permeability. However, as long as ICU facilities are available, there is generally a better outcome and faster recovery from pulmonary oedema than from multiple organ dysfunction resulting from inadequate fluid resuscitation.
* Theoretically, colloid should stay in the circulation longer than crystalloid and reduce the risk of pulmonary oedema.
* Estimate blood loss, monitor Hb regularly, and give blood to keep Hb at 9–10 g/dl.

Inotropes/vasoconstrictors

* If BP and urine output remain low, despite an adequate CVP, an inotrope or vasoconstrictor should be started.
* Increments of ephedrine or metaraminol are a reasonable choice initially but only have a short-lived effect. Consider an infusion of adrenaline/noradrenaline (epinephrine/norepinephrine).
* In sepsis a high-output, vasodilated state is likely, making noradrenaline (norepinephrine) the first choice. If a mixed picture (with cardiac depression) is more likely, or you are treating 'blind' without a pulmonary arterial catheter, adrenaline (epinephrine) may be more appropriate. Where the major feature is one of an inadequate output with a raised SVR, dobutamine may be considered. However, dobutamine may result in hypotension during anaesthesia and is often less easy to use than adrenaline (epinephrine) until the full haemodynamic picture can be measured.

Oxygen and PEEP

* Oxygenation may be impaired by non-cardiogenic pulmonary oedema due to increased capillary permeability in sepsis.
* Increase FiO_2 until SaO_2 is at least 95%.
* Consider adding positive end expiratory pressure (PEEP), 5 cmH$_2$O initially, if the patient is still hypoxic when FiO_2 0.5. Most modern anaesthetic machines have a PEEP facility, either integral with the ventilator or as an optional valve. Increase PEEP to 10 cmH$_2$O if required following an alveolar recruitment manoeuvre (hold lungs on inspiration at 40 cmH$_2$O for 5–10 s).
* On the latest anaesthetic machines pressure control inverse ratio ventilation is sometimes available and should be considered if the patient remains hypoxic on high FiO_2 and PEEP.

Ventilation

* Increased capillary permeability in sepsis may reduce lung compliance and produce high airway pressures or low tidal volumes if pressures are limited.
* If the patient was acidotic preoperatively he was likely to be hyperventilating in compensation. If a high minute volume is not supplied by mechanical ventilation intra-operatively the acidosis may worsen and cause a further deterioration.

- There is increasing evidence in ARDS that the shear forces caused by ventilation with normal or high pressures/tidal volumes can exacerbate lung injury. In patients with early ARDS, peak airway pressure should be limited to 30 cmH_2O and tidal volume to <10 ml/kg, unless there is risk of resultant hypoventilation causing a profound acidosis (pH <7.2).

Further reading

Extremes of age. Report of the National Confidential Enquiry into Perioperative Deaths (1999).

Takala J (1999). Multiple organ failure: clinical features and pathogenesis. In *Intensive care medicine* (ed. J Bion), pp. 22–34. BMJ Books, London.

Transferring the critically ill

Safe transfer demands experienced staff and careful preparation. Several studies have demonstrated that patients are often inadequately resuscitated and monitored during transfer. Specialized transport teams have been shown to improve outcome but are not always available or appropriate.

Reasons for transfer

- Intrahospital transfer, e.g. from the emergency department to the operating theatre, radiology, or ICU.
- Interhospital transfer, e.g. from the district general hospital to neurosurgery or paediatric ICU for specialist therapy or investigation.

Dangers of transfer

- Deranged physiology worsened by movement (acceleration/ deceleration leads to cardiovascular instability).
- Cramped conditions.
- Isolation.
- Temperature and pressure changes.
- Vehicular accidents.
- 15% of patients develop avoidable hypoxia and hypotension.

Principles of safe transfer

- Staff experienced in intensive care and transfer (usually consultant or registrar plus experienced nurse)
- Specialist transport teams may improve outcome, but may cause delay.
- Use of appropriate equipment and vehicle.
- Extensive monitoring.
- Careful stabilization.
- Continuing reassessment.
- Direct handover.
- Documentation and audit.

The transfer vehicle

- Should be customized with adequate space, light, gases, electricity, and communications.
- Mode—consider urgency, mobilization time, geography, weather, traffic, and costs.
- Consider air if over 150 miles (remember decreasing PaO_2 at altitude, expanding air spaces requiring naso/orogastric tube, temperature, noise, and vibration).

Problems during transfer

- Vibration leads to failure and innacuracy of non-invasive BP, and invasive monitoring should be used if at all possible.
- Access to the patient may be limited.
- Acceleration/deceleration may lead to cardiovascular instability.

- Hypothermia, particularly during transfer between vehicles, may be a problem.
- Pulse oximeters may be unreliable in cold, moving patients.

Aeromedical transfer

- Hazards depend on whether the craft is rotary (helicopter) or fixed wing (aircraft).
- Helicopters fly at relatively low altitude and therefore avoid some of the problems of aircraft.
- High altitude decreases the partial pressure of oxygen—at 1500 m arterial PaO_2 is about 5.6 kPa (75 mmHg). Most aircraft are pressurized to 1500–2000 m.
- Decreased barometric pressure leads to an expansion of gas-filled cavities (patients should have nasogastric tubes and may need chest drains).
- Pressurizing the cabin pressure to sea level can decrease these problems but this increases fuel costs!
- Air in the endotracheal tube should be replaced by saline.

Advantages/disadvantages of different modes of transport

	Road	Helicopter	Airplane
Best distance	<50 miles	50–150 miles	>150 miles
Speed	Slow	Fast, particularly if direct	Fast—may be slowed by numbers of transfers
Cost	Low	Expensive	Very expensive
Patient access	Good	Usually poor	Good
Noise and vibration	Moderate	Poor	Moderate—poor on takeoff/landing
Altitude	None	Low	High

Specific paediatric considerations

- Hypothermia is a greater risk, particularly in the infant. Central temperature should be monitored and warming mats, 'bubble wrap', hats, etc. employed to maintain temperature.
- Secure IV access is paramount prior to departure.

Equipment

- Must be robust, lightweight, and battery operated.
- A portable ventilator with adequate disconnection and high-pressure alarms, plus the ability to alter minute volume, FiO_2, I:E ratio, and positive end expiratory pressure.
- An oxygen supply sufficient for the trip and a reserve of 1–2 h.
- A portable monitor for ECG, invasive pressures, non-invasive blood pressure, oxygen saturation, $ETCO_2$, and temperature.

- Adequate battery supply for monitor and infusion pumps—a transformer may allow ambulance power supply to be used.
- Defibrillator and suction source (usually fitted in the ambulance).
- Transfer drug and intubation boxes (already prepared)—separate ones for adult and paediatric use.
- A mobile phone.
- A warming blanket.
- A check list, observations sheet, and pens.

Calculating oxygen reserves

Size of oxygen cylinder (volume (litres))	Operation time (min) for different minute volumes at FiO_2 1.0		
	Minute volume 5 litre/min	Minute volume 7 litre/min	Minute volume 10 litre/min
D (340)	56 min	42 min	30 min
E (680)	113 min	85 min	61 min
F (1360)	226 min	170 min	123 min

Battery life

- This can vary greatly, depending on manufacturer, but must be known.
- Remember the charge time is usually considerable.
- Battery life will vary depending on the rate of infusion.

Battery life for pump running at 5–10 ml/h

Type	Battery life (estimated) (h)	Charge time (estimated) (h)
Graseby 3100	3	14
Alaris IVAC	6	24
Graseby Omnifuse	8	18

Preparation

- Ensure meticulous stabilization prior to transfer.
- Take a full history and make a thorough examination.
- Full monitoring including invasive BP and CVP where indicated.
- Blood tests, radiographs, and CT prior to transfer.
- Explain procedure to patient and family.

Check list for preparation

A: airway

- Is the airway safe? If in doubt intubate.

* Cervical spine control—this must be adequate if there is a history of trauma.

B: breathing

* Portable ventilator—mode, inspired oxygen concentration, minute ventilation. Check blood gas on the portable ventilator prior to departure.
* Self-inflating (AMBU®) bag in the event of a ventilator/oxygen failure.
* Suction.
* Adequate sedation, analgesia, and relaxation
* Adequate O_2 reserves.
* Insert a chest drain if there is any chance of a pneumothorax (e.g. fractured ribs).

C: circulation

* Two large-bore IV cannulas and restored blood volume.
* Control external bleeding.
* Invasive BP, CVP, and PAWP when indicated.
* Inotropes—if in doubt have them mixed and ready to run.
* Insert a urinary catheter and monitor output.

D: disability

* GCS (mannitol, IPPV).
* Note pupillary signs.
* Naso/orogastric tube.

E: exposure

* Temperature loss.
* Splint long bones.
* Pumps and batteries.

F: forgotten?

* All notes, referral letter, results, radiographs (including CT scans), and blood products.
* Inform the receiving unit that you are leaving the base hospital.
* Inform relatives.
* Take contact numbers.
* Take warm clothing, mobile phone, food, and credit card/money for the team!
* Plan for the return journey.
* Medical indemnity and insurance for death or disability of transfer staff.

Equipment and drug box guidelines

Airway and breathing

Suction equipment	Stethoscope
Face masks, airways, self-inflating bag with reservoir	Gum elastic bougie
Endotracheal tubes, connectors, and ties	Tracheostomy tubes and tracheal dilators (if appropriate)
Laryngoscopes, spare batteries	

Circulation

Cannulas + IV dressings and tape	Syringes and needles
IV fluids and giving set	Mini sharps receptacle

Resuscitation drugs

Adenosine	Hydrocortisone
Adrenaline	Lidocaine (lignocaine)
Amiodarone	Metoprolol
Atropine	Naloxone
Calcium chloride	Noradrenaline
Diazemuls®	Salbutamol nebulizers
Dextrose	Sodium bicarbonate
Furosemide (frusemide)	Sodium chloride 0.9% ampoules
GTN spray	Plain drug labels

Sedation/muscle relaxants

Propofol	Atracurium or vecuronium
Midazolam	Suxamethonium

Paediatric equipment—extras

Paediatric oxygen mask with reservoir bag	Small cannulas
Appropriate self-inflating bag with reservoir (for size of patient). Masks and airways	Intraosseus needle
Endotracheal tube selection	10% dextrose 500 ml for infusion
Laryngoscope and stylets	Paediatric drug doses book and resuscitation card
McGill forceps and suction catheters	

Further reading

Intensive Care Society (1997). *Guidelines for transfer of the critically ill adult in the UK*. Intensive Care Society, London.

Guidelines Committee of the American College of Critical Care Medicine (1993). Guidelines for the transfer of critically ill patients. *Critical Care Medicine*, **21**, 931–7.

Wallace PGM, Ridley SA (1999). Transport of critically ill patients. British Medical Journal, **319**, 368–71.

Section III
Obstetric anaesthesia and analgesia

Chapter 34
Obstetric anaesthesia and analgesia
James Eldridge

Physiology and pharmacology

From early in the first trimester of pregnancy, a woman's physiology changes rapidly, predominantly under the influence of increasing production of progesterone by the placenta. The effects are widespread:

• Cardiac output increases by approximately 50%. Diastolic blood pressure falls in early to mid-trimester and returns to prepregnant levels by term. Systolic pressure, although following the same pattern, is less affected. Central venous and pulmonary arterial wedge pressures are not altered by pregnancy.

• Cardiac output increases further in labour, even with effective epidural analgesia. Cardiac output peaks immediately after delivery. It is in this period, when the preload and afterload of the heart are changing rapidly, that women with impaired myocardial function are at greatest risk.

• Uteroplacental blood flow is not autoregulated and so is dependent on the uterine blood pressure.

• Aortocaval occlusion occurs when the gravid uterus rests on the aorta or the inferior vena cava. Even in the absence of maternal hypotension, placental blood supply may be compromised in the supine position. After the 20th week of gestation, a left lateral tilt should always be employed. If either mother or fetus is symptomatic, the degree of tilt should be increased.

• The plasma volume increases 50% by term while the red cell mass only increases by 30%, resulting in the physiological anaemia of pregnancy.

• Pregnant women become hypercoagulable early in the first trimester. Antepartum maternal deaths from pulmonary embolism occur most commonly in the first trimester. Plasma concentrations of factors I, VII, VIII, IX, X, and XII are all increased. Antithrombin III levels are depressed.

• Arterial carbon dioxide partial pressure falls to approximately 4.0 kPa. The functional residual capacity is reduced by 20% resulting in airway closure in 50% of supine women at term. This, in combination with a 60% increase in oxygen consumption, renders pregnant women at term vulnerable to hypoxia when supine.

• In labour painful contractions and excessive breathing of Entonox can result in further hyperventilation and marked alkalosis may occur. An arterial pH in excess of 7.5 is common.

• Gastric emptying and acidity are little changed by pregnancy. However, gastric emptying is slowed in established labour and almost halted if systemic opioids are administered for analgesia in labour. Barrier pressure (the difference in pressure of the stomach and lower oesophageal 'sphincter') is reduced, but the incidence of regurgitation into the upper oesophagus during anaesthesia, in otherwise asymptomatic individuals, is not significantly different in the first and second trimesters.

• By 48 h postpartum, intra-abdominal pressure, gastric emptying, volume, and acidity are all similar to non-pregnant controls. Although lower oesophageal sphincter tone may take longer to recover, mask anaesthesia is acceptable 48 h after delivery in the absence of other specific indications for intubation.[1]

1   Bogod DG (1994). The postpartum stomach–when is it safe? *Anaesthesia*, **49**, 1–2.

- Renal blood flow increases by 75% by term and glomerular filtration rate by 50%. Both urea and creatinine plasma concentrations fall.
- Neurological tissue has a greater susceptibility to the action of local anaesthetics during pregnancy. MAC is reduced in pregnancy.
- The volume of distribution increases by 5 litres, affecting predominantly the polar water-soluble agents. Lipid-soluble drugs are more affected by changes in protein binding. The fall in albumin concentration increases the free active portion of acidic agents, while basic drugs are more dominantly bound to α_1 glycoprotein. Some specific binding proteins such as thyroxine binding protein increase in pregnancy.
- Although plasma cholinesterase concentration falls by about 25% in pregnancy, this is counteracted by an increase in volume of distribution, so the actual duration of action of agents such as suxamethonium is little changed in pregnancy.

Analgesia for labour

Maternal satisfaction in labour is multifactorial. While analgesia in labour is important to many women, it is not a requirement for a positive experience of childbirth. Various coping strategies and support methods are available, including prepared childbirth, support from a partner, known midwife or 'doula' (a senior female companion who is experienced in childbirth), water baths, aromatherapy, and massage. These can greatly increase maternal satisfaction.

The most commonly employed 'analgesics' are transcutaneous electrical nerve stimulation (TENS), inhaled nitrous oxide, opioids, and regional techniques. Although some women find TENS helpful in labour, randomized studies show only weak evidence of analgesia. Opioids in labour, although simple to administer and cheap, act predominantly as sedatives and amnesics–pain scores are minimally changed. Entonox is more efficacious than pethidine, but complete analgesia is never attained.

Regional analgesia provides the most effective pain relief. Provided hypotension is avoided, fetal condition in the first stage of labour may be improved as maternal sympathetic stimulation and hyperventilation are reduced. However, a degree of maternal motor block is almost universal, and most randomized studies comparing regional and parenteral analgesia demonstrate an association between epidural analgesia and prolonged labour together with a higher incidence of instrumental deliveries. Careful obstetric management of labour and appropriate anaesthetic management of analgesia may negate this effect.[2]

Uterine pain is transmitted in sensory fibres which accompany sympathetic nerves and end in the dorsal horns of T10–L1. Vaginal pain is transmitted via the S2–S4 nerve roots (the pudendal nerve). Spinal, combined spinal/epidural (CSE), and epidural analgesia have largely replaced other regional techniques (paracervical, pudendal, caudal block). In 1997/8 24% of all parturients in the United Kingdom used regional analgesia. Neuraxial techniques can be expected to provide effective analgesia in over 85% of women.

Acceptable analgesia must be provided, but minimizing the incidence of hypotension and motor blockade is important. Reducing the degree of motor block increases maternal satisfaction and may decrease the incidence of assisted delivery. Motor block can be reduced by:

- Using synergistic agents such as opioids and the α_2 agonist, clonidine, to reduce the dose of local anaesthetic administered.

- Establishing regional analgesia with low-dose epidural local anaesthetic and opioid or low-dose intrathecal local anaesthetic and opioid.

- Using patient-controlled epidural analgesia (PCEA) or intermittent top-ups to maintain analgesia. In general, infusions deliver a greater total dose of local anaesthetic than intermittent top-ups, while PCEA delivers the smallest total dose.

---

2   Russell R (2000). Editorial–the effect of regional analgesia on the progress of labour and delivery. *British Journal Anaesthesia*, **84**, 709–12.

The choice of local anaesthetic may also affect motor block. At equimolar doses, ropivacaine produces less motor block than bupivacaine but it is not as potent as bupivacaine, and the relative motor block at equipotent doses remains controversial.

Indications for regional labour analgesia

+ Maternal request.
+ Expectation of operative delivery (e.g. multiple pregnancy, malpresentation).
+ Maternal disease– in particular conditions in which sympathetic stimulation may cause a deterioration in maternal or fetal condition.
+ Specific cardiovascular disease (e.g. regurgitant valvular lesions, myocardial ischaemia).
+ Severe respiratory disease (e.g. cystic fibrosis).
+ Specific neurological disease (intracranial AV malformations, space occupying lesions, etc.).
+ Obstetric disease (e.g. pre-eclampsia).
+ Conditions in which general anaesthesia may be life-threatening, particularly if rapid regional anaesthesia may be difficult to institute (e.g. morbid obesity).

Contraindications for regional labour analgesia

+ Maternal refusal.
+ Allergy (true allergy to amide local anaesthetics is rare so always take a careful history).
+ Local infection.
+ Uncorrected hypovolaemia.
+ Coagulopathy. (Although guidelines suggest that with a platelet count >80×10^9/litre and INR <1.4 neuraxial procedures are safe, clinical judgement for each individual patient remains of paramount importance. The cause of the clotting abnormality and the indication for the procedure have to be considered.)

Relative contraindications for regional labour analgesia

+ Expectation of significant haemorrhage.
+ Untreated systemic infection (provided that systemic infection has been treated with antibiotics, the risk of 'seeding' infection into the epidural space with neuraxial procedures is minimal).
+ Specific cardiac disease (e.g. severe valvular stenosis, Eisenmenger's syndrome, peripartum cardiomyopathy). Although regional analgesia has been used for many of these conditions, extreme care must be taken to avoid any rapid changes in blood pressure, preload, and afterload of the heart. Intrathecal opioid without local anaesthetic may be advantageous for these patients.
+ Bad backs and previous back surgery do not contraindicate regional analgesia/anaesthesia, but scarring of the epidural space may limit the effectiveness of epidural analgesia and increase the risk of inadvertent dural puncture. Intrathecal techniques can be expected to work normally.

Consent

Most anaesthetists do not take written consent before inserting an epidural for labour analgesia, but 'appropriate' explanation must be given. The information offered varies according to local guidelines and with the degree of distress of each individual woman. The explanation and, in particular, the possible hazards discussed must be documented, as many women do not accurately recall information given in labour. Information about labour analgesia should always be available antenatally.

Epidural analgesia for labour

- Scrupulous attention to sterile technique is required. Mask and gown should be worn.[3]

- Establish IV access. In the absence of previous haemorrhage or dehydration, when low-dose local anaesthetic techniques are used, large fluid preloads are unnecessary.

- Position either in a full lateral or sitting position. Finding the midline in the obese may be easier in the sitting position. Accidental dural puncture may be slightly lower in the lateral position.

- Fetal heart rate should be recorded before and during the establishment of analgesia. Whether regional analgesic technique requires routine continuous fetal heart rate monitoring after analgesia has been established is controversial.

- Skin sterilization with chlorhexidene is more effective than with iodine.

- Locate the epidural space (loss of resistance to saline may have slight advantages in both reduced incidence of accidental dural puncture and reduced incidence of 'missed segments' compared with loss of resistance to air).

- Introduce 4–5 cm of catheter into the epidural space. (Longer has an increased incidence of unilateral block and shorter increases the chance that the catheter pulls out of the space.) Multihole catheters have a lower incidence of unsatisfactory blocks.

- Check for blood/CSF.

- Give an appropriate test dose. An 'appropriate' test remains controversial. Using 0.5% bupivacaine significantly increases motor block. Using 1:200 000 epinephrine to detect intravenous placement of a catheter has both high false-positive and false-negative rates. Many anaesthetists will use 10–15 ml of 0.1% bupivacaine with a dilute opioid (2 μg/ml fentanyl) as both the test and main dose. This will exclude intrathecal placement, but may give false negatives if the catheter is intravenous. The failure of analgesia after such a test dose should therefore warn of possible intravenous cannulation.

- If required give further local anaesthetic to establish analgesia. There should be no need to use concentrations >0.25% bupivacaine.

- Measure maternal blood pressure every 5 min for at least 20 min after every bolus dose of local anaesthetic.

Once the epidural is functioning the epidural can be maintained by one of three methods:

- Intermittent top-ups of local anaesthetic administered by midwives (5–10 ml 0.25% bupivacaine or 10–15 ml 0.1% bupivacaine with 2 μg/ml fentanyl).

- A continuous infusion of local anaesthetic (5–12 ml/h of 0.0625–0.1% bupivacaine with 2 μg/ml fentanyl).

---

3 McLure HA., Talboys CA *et al.* (1998). Surgical face masks and downward dispersal of bacteria. *Anaesthesia*, **53**, 624–6.

- Intermittent top-ups of local anaesthetic administered by a patient controlled device (PCEA) (5 ml boluses of 0.0625–0.1% bupivacaine with 2 μg/ml fentanyl and a 10–15 min lockout period).

Whichever technique is used, review frequently to ensure that the epidural is effective. Poorly functioning epidurals should be corrected early, particularly if a surgical procedure may be required.

Combined spinal/epidural analgesia for labour

A combination of a low dose of subarachnoid local anaesthetic and/or opioid together with subsequent top-ups of weak epidural local anaesthetic produces a rapid onset with minimal motor block and effective analgesia. An epidural technique alone can produce a similar degree of analgesia and motor block, but may take 10–15 min longer to establish. CSE can be performed as a needle-through-needle technique or as separate injections:

- Locate the epidural space at the L3/4 interspace with a Tuohy needle. Pass a 25–27G pencil-point needle through the Tuohy needle to locate the subarachnoid space.
- Inject subarachnoid solution (e.g. 0.5–1.0 ml of 0.25% bupivacaine with 5–25 µg fentanyl). Do not rotate epidural needle. Insert the epidural catheter.

or

- Perform spinal at L3/4 with a 25–27G pencil-point needle.
- Inject subarachnoid solution.
- Perform the epidural once analgesia has been established.

Caution: The epidural catheter cannot be effectively tested until the subarachnoid analgesia has receded.

- When the first top-up is required (usually 60–90 min after the spinal injection), give the epidural test dose (e.g. 10–15 ml of 0.1% bupivacaine with 2 µg/ml fentanyl).

Further management of the epidural is the same as for epidural analgesia alone.

Dealing with a poorly functioning epidural

Look for the pattern of failure. Remember that a full bladder may cause break through pain. Ask the midwife if a full bladder is likely. Carefully assess the spread of the block. It is important to be confident that the epidural could be topped up for a caesarean section if required. Therefore, if in doubt, re-site the epidural.

Pattern of failure	Remedy
Global failure	
No detectable block despite at least 10 ml 0.25% bupivacaine (or equivalent)	Resite epidural
Partial failure	
Unilateral block: Feel both feet to assess whether they are symmetrically warm and dry. See if the pattern matches the distribution of pain	Top-up epidural with painful side in a dependent position. (Use local anaesthetic and 50–100 µg fentanyl.)
	Withdraw catheter 2–3 cm and give a further top-up
	Resite epidural
Missed segment: True missed segments are rare. Commonly a 'missed segment' is felt in the groin and is usually a unilateral block or inadequate block on one side	Top up with opioid (i.e. 50–100 µg fentanyl). The intrathecal mode of action will minimize segmental effects
	Continue as per 'unilateral block'
Back pain: Severe back pain is associated with an occipitoposterior position of the fetus, and may require a dense block to establish analgesia	Top up with more local anaesthetic and opioid
Perineal pain	Check sacral block and that the bladder is empty
	Top up with more local anaesthetic in sitting position
	Continue as per unilateral block

Complications of epidural analgesia

Hypotension

In the absence of fetal distress, a fall in systolic blood pressure of 20% or to 100 mmHg (whichever is higher) is acceptable. However, uterine blood flow is not autoregulated and prolonged/severe hypotension will cause fetal compromise. Preload is not routinely required when using low doses of local anaesthetic, but patients should not be hypovolaemic before instituting regional analgesia. When hypotension is detected it should be treated quickly:

- Avoid aortocaval occlusion–make sure that the patient is in the full lateral position.
- Measure the blood pressure on the dependent arm.
- Give an intravenous fluid bolus of crystalloid solution.
- Give 6 mg IV ephedrine and repeat as necessary.

Remember that brachial artery pressure may not reflect uterine artery blood flow. If fetal distress is detected, and is chronologically related to a regional anaesthetic procedure, treat as above even in the absence of overt hypotension.

Subdural block[4]

Subdural block occurs when the epidural catheter is misplaced between the dura mater and arachnoid mater. In obstetric practice, the incidence of clinically recognized subdural block is less than 1 in 1000 epidurals. However, subdural blocks may be clinically indistinguishable from epidural blocks. Definitive diagnosis is radiological. The characteristics of a subdural block are:

- A slow onset (20–30 min) of a block that is inappropriately extensive for the volume of local anaesthetic injected. The block may extend to the cervical dermatomes and Horner's syndrome may develop.
- The blocks are often patchy and asymmetrical. Sparing of motor fibres to the lower limbs may occur.
- A total spinal may occur following a top-up dose. This is likely to be a consequence of the increased volume rupturing the arachnoid mater.
- If a subdural is suspected, resite the epidural catheter.

Total spinal

The incidence of total spinal is variously reported to be between 1 in 5000 and 1 in 50 000 epidurals. Usually the onset is rapid, although delays of 30 min or more have been reported. Delayed onset may be related to a change in maternal position, or a subdural catheter placement. Symptoms are of a rapidly rising block. Initially difficulty in coughing may be noted (commonly seen in regional anaesthesia for caesarean section), then loss of hand and arm strength, followed by difficulty with breathing and swallowing. Respiratory paralysis, cardiovascular depression, unconsciousness, and finally fixed

---

4 Reynolds F, Speedy H (1990). The subdural space: the third place to go astray. *Anaesthesia*, **45**, 120–3.

dilated pupils ensue. Unsurprisingly total spinals are reported more often after epidural anaesthesia rather than analgesia, as larger doses of local anaesthetic are employed.

Management of total spinal is as follows:

• Maintain airway and ventilation, avoid aortocaval compression, and provide cardiovascular support.

• Even if consciousness is not lost, intubation may be required to protect the airway.

• Careful maternal and fetal monitoring is essential and, if appropriate delivery of the fetus. In the absence of fetal distress, caesarean section is not an immediate requirement. Ventilation is usually necessary for 1–2 h.

Accidental intravenous injection of local anaesthetic

'Every dose is a test dose.' Avoid injecting any single large bolus of local anaesthetic intravenously. Remember that intravenous or partial intravenous positioning of epidural catheters occurs in at least 5% of epidurals. The risk can be minimized by:

• Meticulous attention to technique during placement. Always check for blood in the catheter.

• Always being alert to symptoms of intravenous injection with every dose of local anaesthetic, even when previous doses have been uncomplicated.

• Divide all large doses of local anaesthetic into aliquots.

• Use appropriate local anaesthetics. Lidocaine (lignocaine) and the single enantiomer local anaesthetics are safer than bupivacaine.

Dural puncture[5]

When loss of CSF is greater than production, as might occur through a dural tear, CSF pressure falls and the brain sinks, stretching the meninges. This stretching is thought to cause headache. Compensatory vasodilation of intracranial vessels may further worsen symptoms. The incidence of dural puncture should be less than 1% of epidurals. All midwives, as well as obstetric and anaesthetic staff, should be alert to the signs of post dural puncture headaches, as symptoms may not develop for several days. If untreated, headaches are not only unpleasant, but on rare occasions can be life-threatening, usually as a result of intracranial haemorrhage or coning of the brainstem.

Management of accidental dural puncture can be divided into immediate and late.

Immediate management

The initial aim is to achieve effective analgesia without causing further complication.

Either:

* If a dural puncture occurs, pass the 'epidural' catheter into the subarachnoid space.
* Label the catheter clearly as an intrathecal catheter and only allow an anaesthetist to perform top-ups.
* Give intermittent top-ups through the catheter (1 ml of 0.25% bupivacaine ± 5–25 μg fentanyl. Tachyphylaxis may occur with prolonged labour).

This technique has the following advantages:

* The analgesia produced is likely to be excellent.
* There is no possibility of performing another dural puncture on reinsertion of the epidural.
* The unpredictable spread of epidural solution through the dural tear is eliminated.
* The incidence of post dural puncture headache is reduced (but only if the catheter is left in for more than 24 h).

It has the disadvantages of:

* The catheter cannot be used to perform an early blood patch.
* A theoretical risk of introducing infection.
* The catheter may be mistaken for an epidural catheter.

Or:

* Remove the epidural catheter.
* Reinsert the epidural at a different interspace–usually one interspace higher. If the reason for tap was difficult anatomy, a senior colleague should take over.
* Run the epidural as normal but beware of intrathecal spread of local anaesthetic. The anaesthetist should give all top ups.

5   Reynolds F (1993). Dural puncture and headache. Avoid the first but treat the second. *British Medical Journal*, **306**, 874–5.

With either technique the patient should be informed at the earliest opportunity that a dural puncture has occurred and of the likely sequelae. Labour itself may be allowed to continue normally. Arrangement must be made for daily postnatal follow-up.

Late management

Following a dural puncture with a 16–18G Tuohy needle, the incidence of post dural puncture headache is approximately 70%. Not all dural punctures are recognized in labour so be alert to the possibility, even in women who had uncomplicated epidural analgesia. Headaches in the postnatal period are common. The key differentiating factor between a 'normal' postnatal headache and a post dural puncture headache is the positional nature of the latter.

Common features of post dural puncture headache include:

- Typically onset is 24–48 h post dural puncture. Untreated they usually last 7–10 days.
- Characteristically worse on standing. Headache is often absent after overnight bed rest, but returns after mobilizing.
- Usually in the fronto-occipital regions and radiates to the neck, with associated neck stiffness.
- Photophobia, diplopia, and difficulty in accommodation common. Hearing loss, tinnitus, and VIth nerve palsy are possible.
- Nausea occurs in up to 60% of cases.

Treatment is either to alleviate symptoms while waiting for the dural tear to heal itself, or to seal the puncture. Epidural blood patching is the only commonly used method of sealing dural tears, although neurosurgical closure has been reported.

Prophylactic treatment

- The most effective prophylactic treatment is blood patching. At the end of labour, 20 ml of blood can be injected through the epidural catheter (having removed the epidural filter). All residual block must have worn off before performing a prophylactic patch as radicular pain is an indication to stop injecting. However, early blood patching has a lower success rate and bacteraemia is common immediately after delivery (7% rising to 80% with uterine manipulation).
- Bed rest alleviates symptoms, but the incidence of post dural puncture headache after 48 h is the same for those that mobilized throughout. Because of the risk of thromboembolism, bed rest should not be routinely encouraged in asymptomatic women.
- Epidural infusion of saline (1 litre/24 h) will compress the dural sac and can alleviate symptoms. It may also reduce the flow of CSF through a dural tear. After 24 h of continuous infusion the incidence of post dural puncture headache is marginally reduced. However, radicular pain in the lower limbs may occur and patients are immobilized.

Symptomatic treatment

- Simple analgesics are the mainstays of symptomatic treatment. They should always be offered, even though they are unlikely to completely relieve severe post dural puncture headache.

- Adequate fluid intake is to be encouraged, although there is no evidence that hydration reduces the incidence of post dural puncture headache.
- Caffeine/theophyllines. These act by reducing intracranial vasodilation, which is partially responsible for the headache. Symptoms are improved, but not cured. Both oral and IV caffeine are efficacious. A suitable regimen is 600 mg caffeine/day in divided doses. (One cup of coffee contains roughly 150 mg caffeine.)
- Sumatriptan. Although this cerebral vasoconstrictor is of benefit, it is expensive, is given subcutaneously (6 mg) and may cause coronary artery spasm. Its use is best reserved for those in whom blood patching is contra-indicated.
- ACTH. Case reports suggest ACTH can effectively alleviate symptoms of post dural puncture headache, probably by increasing the concentration of β endorphin and intravascular volume.
- Abdominal binders. These relieve symptoms of post dural puncture headache presumably by increasing epidural vein blood flow, which in turn compresses the dural sac. However, they are uncomfortable and have fallen out of use. Abdominal compression can be used to assess a patient. If abdominal pressure effectively relieves a headache it suggests that the headache is due to a dural tear.

Epidural blood patch[6]

Epidural blood patch performed around 48 h postpartum has a 60–90% cure rate at the first attempt (recent studies that have followed women for more than 48 h have found lower success rates). The mechanism of action is two fold:

- Blood injected into the epidural space compresses the dural sac and raises the intracranial pressure. This produces an almost instantaneous improvement in pain.
- The injected blood forms a clot over the site of the dural tear and this seals the CSF leak.

Blood injected into the epidural space predominantly spreads cephalad, so blood patches should be performed at the same or lower interspace as the dural puncture. Suggestions that labour epidurals after blood patching may be less effective, have not been confirmed.

- Consent must be obtained. The patient should be apyrexial and not have a raised white cell count.
- Two operators are required. One should be an experienced 'epiduralist', the other is required to take blood in a sterile manner.
- The patient should have a period of bed rest before performing the patch to reduce the CSF volume in the epidural space.
- Aseptic technique must be meticulous both at the epidural site and the site of blood letting–usually the antecubital fossa.

6 Carrie LE (1993). Post dural puncture headache and extradural blood patch. *British Journal of Anaesthesia*, **71**, 179–80.

- An epidural should be performed at the same or a lower vertebral inter-space as the dural puncture with the woman in the lateral position to mini-mize CSF pressure in the lumbar dural sac.

- Once the epidural space has been identified, 20–30 ml blood are obtained.

- Inject the blood slowly through the epidural needle until pain occurs (commonly in the back or legs) or to a maximum of 20–25 ml. If pain occurs, pause and if the pain resolves, try continuing slowly. If the pain does not resolve or recurs then stop.

- To allow the clot to form, maintain bed rest for at least 2 h and then allow slow mobilization.

- As far as possible, the patient should avoid straining, lifting, or excessive bending for 48 h, although there are obvious limitations when a woman has a newborn infant to care for.

- Follow-up is still required. Every woman should have clear instructions to contact the anaesthetists again if symptoms recur even after discharge home.

- Serious complications of blood patching are rare. However, backache is common, with 35% of women experiencing some discomfort 48 h post epidural blood patch and 16% of women having prolonged backache (mean duration 27 days). Other reported complications include repeated dural puncture, neurological deficits, epileptiform fits, and cranial nerve damage.

Anaesthesia for caesarean section

With all caesarean sections, it is vital that the obstetrician clearly communicates the degree of urgency to all staff. A suggested classification is:[7]

- Immediate: There is immediate threat to the life of woman or fetus.
- Urgent: Maternal or fetal compromise that is not immediately life-threatening.
- Early: No maternal or fetal compromise, but needs early delivery.
- Elective: Delivery timed to suit woman and staff.

For all emergency caesarean sections, the patient must be transferred to theatre as rapidly as possible. Fetal monitoring should be continued until abdominal skin preparation starts. In most centres, general anaesthesia is used when an 'immediate' caesarean section is required, but 'urgent' caesarean sections are usually performed under regional anaesthesia. There is an expectation that the decision to delivery time should be less than 30 min when the indication for caesarean section is fetal distress. However, delivery before this time limit is no guarantee of a successful outcome and delivery after this limit does not necessarily mean disaster. Each case must be individually assessed and the classification of urgency continuously reviewed.

Regional anaesthesia for caesarean section

Regional anaesthesia for caesarean section was initially driven by maternal preference. However, regional anaesthesia is also more than 16 times safer than general anaesthesia.[8]

Advantages of regional anaesthesia include:

- Both mother and partner can be present at delivery.
- Improved safety for mother with minimal risk of aspiration and lower risk of anaphylaxis.
- The neonate is more alert, promoting early bonding and breastfeeding.
- Fewer drugs are administered, with less 'hangover' than after general anaesthesia.
- Better postoperative analgesia and earlier mobilization.

Three techniques are available–epidural, spinal, and combined spinal epidural. Epidural is most commonly used for women who already have epidural analgesia in labour. Spinal is the most popular technique for elective caesarean section, although in some centres combined spinal/epidurals are preferred. Whatever technique is chosen, a careful history and appropriate examination should be performed. This should include checking:

- Blood group and antibody screen. Routine cross-matching of blood is not required unless haemorrhage is expected or if antibodies that interfere with cross-matching are present.

7   Lucas DN, Yentis SM et al. (2000). Urgency of caesarean section: a new classification. *Journal of the Royal Society of Medicine*, **93**, 346–50.

8   Hawkins JL, Koonin LM et al. (1997). Anesthesia-related deaths during obstetric delivery in the United States, 1979–1990. *Anesthesiology*, **86**, 277–84.

- Ultrasound reports to establish the position of the placenta. A low-lying anterior placenta puts a woman at risk of major haemorrhage, particularly if associated with a scar from a previous caesarean section.

An explanation of the technique must also be offered. Although caesarean section under regional becomes routine for the anaesthetist, it is rarely routine for the mother. Reassurance and support are important. The possibility of complications must also be mentioned–in particular, the possibility of intra-operative discomfort and its management. Pain during regional anaesthesia is now the leading obstetric anaesthetic cause of maternal litigation. Document all complications that are discussed.

Neonates are usually more alert after regional than general anaesthesia. However, the speed of onset of sympathectomy that occurs with spinal anaesthesia (as opposed to epidural anaesthesia) results in a greater fall in maternal cardiac output and blood pressure and may be associated with a more acidotic neonate at delivery. In conditions where sudden changes in afterload may be dangerous (i.e. stenotic valvular heart disease) the speed of onset of a spinal block can be slowed by:

- Careful positioning during the onset of the block (see below).
- Using an intrathecal catheter and incrementally topping up the block
- Using a combined spinal epidural approach and injecting a small dose of intrathecal local anaesthetic. The block can be subsequently extended using the epidural catheter.

While a slow onset of block may be preferable in elective caesarean section, a rapid onset is necessary for emergency caesarean sections. Spinal anaesthesia provides a better quality of analgesia and is quicker in onset than epidural anaesthesia.

Epidural anaesthesia for caesarean section

Advantages	Disadvantages
Easy to top up labour epidural	Slow onset
Stable BP	Large doses of LA
Intra-operative manipulation possible	Poorer quality of block than spinal anaesthesia
Epidural can be used for postop. analgesia	

Indications for caesarean section under epidural anaesthesia:

◆ Women who already have epidural analgesia established for labour.

◆ Severe pre-eclampsia (controversial see p. 737).

◆ Specific maternal disease (e.g. cardiac disease) where rapid changes in systemic vascular resistance might be problematic.

Technique

◆ History/examination/explanation and consent.

◆ Ensure that antacid prophylaxis has been given.

◆ Establish 16G or larger IV access. Give 10–15 ml/kg crystalloid preload.

◆ Insert an epidural catheter at the L2/3 or L3/4 vertebral interspace.

◆ Test dose then incrementally top up the epidural with local anaesthetic and opioid:

  ◆ 5–8 ml boluses of 2% lidocaine (lignocaine) with 1:200 000 adrenaline every 2–3 min up to a maximum of 20 ml (mix 19 ml 2% lidocaine (lignocaine) with 1 ml 1:10 000 adrenaline rather than using a preparatory mixture which contains preservative and has a lower pH and therefore slows onset of the block) or

  ◆ 5 ml 0.5% bupivacaine or levobupivacaine or ropivacaine every 4–5 min up to a maximum of 2 mg/kg in any 4 h period. (the single enantiomer local anaesthetics may offer some safety advantage; however, lidocaine (lignocaine) is still safer than both ropivacaine and levobupivacaine).

◆ Opioid (e.g. 100 μg fentanyl or 2.5 mg diamorphine) improves the quality of the analgesia and a lower level of block may be effective if opioid has been given.

◆ Establish an S4 to T4 block (nipple level) measured by light touch. Always check the sacral dermatomes, as epidural local anaesthetic occasionally does not spread caudally. Anaesthesia to light touch is more reliable at predicting adequacy of block than loss of cold sensation.[9] Document the level of block obtained and the adequacy of perioperative analgesia.

9   Russell IF (1995). Levels of anaesthesia and intraoperative pain at caesarean section under regional block. *International Journal of Obstetric Anaesthesia*, **4**, 71–7.

- Position the patient in the supine position with a left lateral tilt or wedge. Give supplemental oxygen by facemask. (This is very important in obese patients who may become hypoxic when supine, and may benefit a compromised fetus).
- Treat hypotension with:
  - fluid
  - 6 mg ephedrine IV bolus (if tachycardia must be avoided then 50 µg phenylephrine may be used, but expect a reflex bradycardia)
  - increasing the left uterine displacement.
- At delivery give 5–10 IU syntocinon IV bolus. If tachycardia must be avoided then a slow IV infusion of 30–50 IU syntocinon in 500 ml crystalloid is acceptable.
- At the end of the procedure give an NSAID unless contraindicated (100 mg diclofenac PR).

Spinal anaesthesia for caesarean section

Advantages	Disadvantages
Quick onset	Single shot
Good quality analgesia	Limited duration
Easy to perform	Inadequate analgesia difficult to correct
	Rapid changes in BP and cardiac output

Spinal anaesthesia is the most commonly used technique for elective caesarean sections. It is rapid in onset, produces a dense block, and with intrathecal opioids can produce long-acting postoperative analgesia. However, hypotension is much more common than with epidural anaesthesia.

Technique

- History/examination/explanation and consent.
- Ensure that antacid prophylaxis has been given.
- Establish 16G or larger IV access. Give 10–15 ml/kg crystalloid preload.
- Perform spinal anaesthetic at L3/4 interspace using a 25G or smaller pencil-point needle. With the orifice pointing cephalad inject the anaesthetic solution (e.g. 2.5 ml 0.5% hyperbaric bupivacaine with 250 µg diamorphine, 15 µg fentanyl, or 100 µg morphine. Use of morphine has little intra-operative benefit but provides prolonged postoperative analgesia. However, it carries a higher incidence of postoperative nausea and vomiting, plus a theoretically increased risk of respiratory depression.)
- Continue as for epidural anaesthesia for caesarean section (p. 713).

Rapid onset of block may be associated with fetal acidaemia. Slowing the speed of onset may be desirable for non-urgent caesarean section. This can be achieved using the 'Oxford position' (Fig. 34.1) and hyperbaric local anaes-

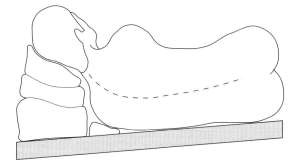

Fig 34.1 The 'Oxford' position.

thetic. With this technique, the spinal injection is performed with the woman in a full left lateral position with a slight head down tilt, but a wedge under the shoulders and head to lift the upper thoracic and cervical spines. This ensures a horizontal spinal column along which hyperbaric local anaesthetic will flow. Spread above T4–T6 is prevented by the upward curvature of the spine at this point. Following subarachnoid injection the woman is turned into the full right lateral position with the same wedging technique until the block is adequate for surgery. The 'Oxford position' minimizes aortocaval occlusion and slows the onset of block compared with both a lateral to lying and a sitting to lying technique.[10]

10 Stoneham M, Eldridge AJ *et al.* (1999). Oxford positioning technique improves haemodynamic stability and predictability of block height of spinal anaesthesia for elective caesarean section. *International Journal of Obstetric Anesthesia*, **8**, 242–8.

Combined spinal/epidural anaesthesia for caesarean section

Advantages	Disadvantages
Quick onset	Rapid change in BP and cardiac output
Good quality analgesia	Technically more difficult with higher failure rate of spinal injection
Intra-operative manipulation possible	Untested epidural catheter
Epidural can be used for postop. analgesia	

In some centres CSE has become the technique of choice. Indications include:

- Prolonged surgery.
- The epidural catheter may be left in situ and used for postoperative analgesia.
- When limiting the speed of onset of block is particularly important. A small intrathecal dose of local anaesthetic can then be supplemented through the epidural catheter as required.

Technique

- History/examination/explanation and consent.
- Ensure that antacid prophylaxis has been given.
- Establish a 16G or larger IV access. Give 10–15 ml/kg crystalloid preload.

The intrathecal injection may be performed by passing the spinal needle through the epidural needle (the 'needle-through-needle' technique) or by performing the intrathecal injection completely separately from the epidural placement either in the same or a different interspace. The needle-through-needle technique is associated with an increased incidence of failure to locate CSF with the spinal needle, but only involves one injection. If a two-injection technique is used, the epidural is usually sited first because of the time delay that may occur in trying to locate the epidural space with a Tuohy needle after the spinal injection. The risk of damaging the epidural catheter with the spinal needle is theoretical.

With either technique, beware of performing the spinal injection above L3/4, as spinal cord damage has been reported.

Needle-through-needle technique

- Position the patient and locate the epidural space with a Tuohy needle. Pass a long (12 cm) 25G or smaller pencil-point needle through the Tuohy needle into the intrathecal space. Inject anaesthetic solution with the needle orifice pointing cephalad. (e.g. 2.5 ml 0.5% hyperbaric bupivacaine with 250 μg diamorphine or 15 μg fentanyl or 100 μg morphine).
- Insert the epidural catheter. Aspirate the catheter carefully for CSF. Testing the catheter with local anaesthetic before the intrathecal dose has receded

may be unreliable. However, using the catheter intra-operatively is reasonable, as the anaesthetist is continuously present to deal with the consequences of an intrathecal injection. This may not be true if opioids are given through the catheter for postoperative analgesia at the end of the procedure before the block has receded–see below.

Two-needle technique

• Position the patient and perform an epidural. After the catheter is in position perform a spinal injection at L3/4 or below with a 25G or smaller pencil-point needle.

• If the block is inadequate, inject local anaesthetic or 10 ml normal saline through the epidural catheter. Normal saline works by compressing the dural sac, causing cephalad spread of intrathecal local anaesthetic.

• Continue as for epidural anaesthesia for caesarean section (p. 713).

Inadequate anaesthesia

Every patient should be warned of the possibility of intraoperative discomfort and this should be documented. Between 1–5% of attempted regional anaesthetics for caesarean section are inadequate for surgery. The majority should be identified before operation commences. Careful documentation of management is required, especially if pain occurred after surgery started. These patients must be followed in the postoperative period and if required further explanations and reassurance given.

Preoperative inadequate block

Epidural

- If no block develops then the catheter is incorrectly positioned. It may be reinserted, or a spinal performed.
- If a partial but inadequate block has developed, the epidural may be resited or withdrawn slightly. Should the toxic limit for the local anaesthetic agent have been reached, elective procedures can be abandoned, but for urgent procedures a general anaesthetic or a spinal anaesthetic will be required. If a spinal is chosen exceptional care with positioning and observation of the block level is required, as high or total spinal can occur. Use a normal spinal dose of hyperbaric local anaesthetic, as this should ensure adequate anaesthesia, but control the spread with careful positioning.

Spinal

- If no block develops, a repeat spinal may be performed.
- If a partial but inadequate block develops, an epidural may be inserted and slowly topped up.
- Use a GA if required.

Intraoperative inadequate block

In this situation good communication with the mother and surgeon is essential. If possible stop surgery. Identify the likely cause of pain (i.e. inadequately blocked sacral nerve roots, peritoneal pain, etc.). Try to give the mother a realistic expectation of continued duration and severity of pain. Treat as below. If the patient requests GA, in all but exceptional circumstances, comply. If the anaesthetist feels that severity of pain is not acceptable, persuade the patient that GA is required.

Spinal

Give reassurance if appropriate. Treat with:

- Inhaled nitrous oxide.
- Intravenous opioid (e.g. 25–50 µg fentanyl repeated as necessary). Inform the paediatrician that opioids have been given, but this dose is usually inconsequential to the fetus.
- Surgical administration of local anaesthetic (take care with total dose).
- GA.

Epidural/CSE

Treat as per spinal anaesthesia but in addition epidural opioid (e.g. 100 µg fentanyl) and/or more epidural local anaesthetic can be used.

Preload

A fluid preload is a traditional part of the anaesthetic technique for regional anaesthesia. It has two functions:

- to maintain intravascular volume in a patient who is likely to loose 500–1000 ml blood
- to reduce the incidence of hypotension associated with regional anaesthesia.

However, it is questionable how effectively it prevents hypotension. Volumes as large as 30 ml/kg or more of crystalloid solution do not reliably prevent hypotension. In some women, particularly those with severe pre-eclampsia, large preloads are harmful as the rise in filling pressures and the reduced colloid osmotic pressure will predispose to pulmonary oedema. The ineffectiveness of preload may in part be due to the rapid redistribution of fluid into the extravascular space. There is evidence that colloids, such as hetastarch, may be more effective, but these are expensive, carry a small risk of anaphylactic reactions, and may interfere with the clotting mechanism. They are not therefore recommended for routine use.

Preload should be:
- Timely (given immediately before or during the onset of the regional technique to minimize redistribution).
- Limited to 10–15 ml/kg crystalloid. Larger volumes should be avoided as they offer little advantage and may be harmful.
- More fluid should only be given if clinically indicated.
- Consider colloid if excessive fluid load is likely to be harmful.

Emergency caesarean section should not be delayed to allow a preload to be administered.

General anaesthesia for caesarean section

Elective general anaesthesia is now rare, limiting opportunities for training. The majority of complications relate to the airway, as failed intubation is much more common in obstetric than non-obstetric anaesthesia (1:250 versus 1:2000 respectively). All obstetric theatres should have equipment to help with the difficult airway and all obstetric anaesthetists should be familiar with a failed intubation drill.

Indications for general anaesthesia

- Maternal request.
- Urgency of surgery. (In experienced hands and with a team that is familiar with rapid regional anaesthesia, a spinal or epidural top-up can be performed as rapidly as a general anaesthetic.)
- Regional anaesthesia contraindicated (e.g. coagulopathy, maternal hypovolaemia, etc.).
- Failed regional anaesthesia.
- Additional surgery planned at the same time as caesarean section.

Technique

- History and examination. In particular assess the maternal airway–Mallampati score, thyromental (see p. 866).
- Antacid prophylaxis.
- Start appropriate monitoring (see below).
- Position supine with left lateral tilt or wedge.
- Preoxygenate for 3–5 min or, in an emergency, with four vital capacity breaths with a high flow through the circuit. A seal must be obtained with the facemask. At term, women have a reduced FRC and a higher respiratory rate and oxygen consumption. This reduces the time required for denitrogenation, but also reduces the time from apnoea to arterial oxygen desaturation.
- Perform rapid sequence induction with an adequate dose of induction agent (e.g. 5–7 mg/kg thiopental). Isolated forearm techniques suggest that awareness without recall may be common when the dose of induction agent is reduced. A 7.0 mm endotracheal tube is adequate for ventilation and may make intubation easier.
- Ventilate with 50% oxygen in nitrous oxide. If severe fetal distress is suspected then 75% oxygen or higher may be appropriate. Maintain $ETCO_2$ at 4.0–4.5 kPa.
- Use 'overpressure' of inhalational agent to rapidly increase the end tidal concentration of anaesthetic agent to at least 0.75 of MAC (e.g. 2% isoflurane for 5 min, then reduce to 1.5% for a further 5 min).
- At delivery:
  - Give 5–10 IU syntocinon IV bolus. If tachycardia must be avoided then a slow IV infusion of 30–50 IU syntocinon in 500 ml crystalloid.
  - Administer opioid (e.g. 15 mg morphine).

- Ventilate with 35% inspired oxygen concentration in nitrous oxide. Inhalational agent can be reduced to 0.75 MAC to reduce uterine relaxation.
- At the end of the procedure give an NSAID (e.g. 100 mg diclofenac PR). Bilateral ilioinguinal nerve blocks are also effective for postoperative analgesia.
- Extubate awake in the head down left lateral position.
- Give additional IV analgesia as required.

Effect of general anaesthesia on the fetus

Most anaesthetic agents, except for the muscle relaxants, rapidly cross the placenta. Thiopental can be detected in the fetus within 30 s of administration with peak umbilical vein concentration occurring around 1 min. The umbilical artery to umbilical vein concentration approaches unity at 8 min. Opioids administered before delivery may cause fetal depression. This can be rapidly reversed with naloxone (e.g. 200 μg IM). If there is a specific indication for opioids before delivery they should be given, and the paediatrician informed. Hypotension, hypoxia, hypocapnia, and excessive maternal catecholamine secretion may all be harmful to the fetus.

Failed intubation

(For failed intubation drill see p. 874.)

When intubation fails but mask ventilation succeeds, a decision on whether to continue with the caesarean section must be made. A suggested grading system is:[11]

- Grade 1: Mother's life dependent on surgery.
- Grade 2: Regional anaesthetic unsuitable (e.g. coagulopathy/haemorrhage).
- Grade 3: Severe fetal distress (e.g. prolapsed cord).
- Grade 4: Varying severity of fetal distress with recovery.
- Grade 5: Elective procedure.

For Grade 1 cases surgery should be continued and for Grade 5 the mother should be woken. The action between these extremes must take account of additional factors including the ease of maintaining the airway, the likely difficulty of performing a regional anaesthetic, and the experience of the anaesthetist.

11 Harmer M (1997). Difficult and failed intubation in obstetrics. *International Journal of Obstetric Anaesthesia*, **6**, 25–31.

Antacid prophylaxis

Animal data suggest that to minimize the risk from aspiration, the gastric volume should be less than 25 ml, non-particulate, and with a pH >2.5. Various strategies are available to achieve this:

Elective surgery

- 150 mg ranitidine orally 2 and 12 h before surgery.
- 10 mg metoclopramide orally 2 h before surgery.
- 30 ml 0.3 M sodium citrate immediately before surgery.

(pH >2.5 is maintained for little more than 30 min after 30 ml 0.3 M sodium citrate. If a GA is required after this, a further dose of citrate is required.)

Emergency surgery

If prophylaxis has not already been given:

- 50 mg ranitidine by slow IV injection immediately before surgery.
- 10 mg metoclopramide IV injection immediately before surgery.
- 30 ml 0.3 M sodium citrate orally immediately before surgery.

Postoperative analgesia

Most postpartum women are very well motivated and mobilize quickly. However, effective analgesia does allow earlier mobilization. The mainstays of postoperative analgesia are opioids and NSAIDs. The route that these are given is dependent on the intra-operative anaesthetic technique.

Opioids

- IV patient controlled analgesia or an IM opioid can be used, although these are not as effective as neuraxial analgesia. A small quantity of opioid may be transferred to the neonate through breast milk, but with a negligible effect.

- Intrathecal/epidural opioid:
  - When given as a bolus at the beginning of surgery, fentanyl lasts little longer than the local anaesthetic and provides almost no postoperative analgesia. Epidural fentanyl maybe given as an infusion or as intermittent postoperative boluses (50–100 μg up to 2–hourly for two to three doses) if the epidural catheter is left *in situ*.
  - Intrathecal diamorphine (250 μg) can be expected to provide 6–18 h of analgesia. More than 40% of women will require no other postoperative opioid. Pruritus is very common (60–80%) although only 1–2% have severe pruritus. This can be treated with 200 μg naloxone IM or 4 mg ondansetron IV/IM.
  - Epidural diamorphine (2.5 mg in 10 ml normal saline) provides 6–10 h of analgesia after a single dose. Intermittent doses may be given if the epidural catheter is left *in situ*.
  - Intrathecal 100 μg preservative-free morphine provides long lasting analgesia (12–18 h). Doses above 150 μg are associated with increased side-effects without improved analgesia. However, pruritus and nausea are common. The low lipophilicity of morphine may increase the risk of late respiratory depression. Epidural morphine (2–3 mg) provides analgesia for 6–24 h, but pruritus is again common and nausea occurs in 20–40%.

NSAIDs

NSAIDs are very effective postoperative analgesics, reducing opioid requirements. They should be administered regularly whenever possible.

Clonidine

- The α_2 adrenergic agonist clonidine given intrathecally (75–150 μg) or epidurally (150–600 μg) acts presynaptically at the dorsal horns and possibly centrally in the brain stem to produce analgesia. Sedation and hypotension are troublesome side-effects.

Retained placenta

- Check IV access with 16G or larger cannula has been obtained.
- Assess total amount and rate of blood loss and cardiovascular stability. Blood loss may be difficult to accurately assess. If rapid blood loss is continuing then urgent cross-match and evacuation of placenta under general anaesthetic is required.
- If blood loss is <1000 ml and cardiovascularly stable then either regional or general anaesthesia can be used. Generally regional anaesthesia is preferred, but do not use a regional technique if hypovolaemia is suspected.
- Remember antacid prophylaxis.
- For general anaesthesia a rapid sequence induction technique with cuffed ET will be needed to protect the airway from possible regurgitation.
- Regional anaesthesia can either be obtained by topping up an existing epidural, or by performing a spinal (e.g. 2 ml 0.5% hyperbaric bupivacaine intrathecally). Traditionally a sacral to T10 block has been considered as adequate but recent data suggest that a T7 level more reliably ensures analgesia.[13]
- Occasionally uterine relaxation is required. Under general anaesthesia increasing the halogenated vapour concentration can provide this, and under regional anaesthesia 0.1 mg intravenous aliquots of glyceryl trinitrate is effective (dilute 1 mg in 10 ml normal saline and give 1 ml bolus repeated as required). With either technique expect transitory hypotension.
- On delivery of the placenta give 10 IU syntocinon ± syntocinon infusion.
- At the end of the procedure give an NSAID unless contraindicated.

---

13 Broadbent CR, Russell R (1999). What height of block is needed for manual removal of placenta under spinal anaesthesia? *International Journal of Obstetric Anesthesia*, **8**, 161–4.

Summary of dosing regimes

Procedure	Technique	Suggested dose
Labour	Epidural loading dose	20 ml 0.1% bupivacaine with 2 μg/ml fentanyl
	Epidural infusion	10 ml/h 0.1% bupivacaine with 2 μg/ml fentanyl
	Top ups	10–20 ml 0.1% bupivacaine with 2 μg/ml fentanyl
	CSE	Intrathecal: 1 ml 0.25% bupivacaine with 5–25 μg/ml fentanyl
		Epidural: top up and infusion as above
	PCEA	5 ml bolus of 0.1% bupivacaine with 2 μg/ml fentanyl with a 10–15 min lockout
LSCS	Spinal	2.5 ml 0.5% bupivacaine in 8% dextrose ('heavy') + 250 μg diamorphine
	Epidural	20 ml 2% lidocaine (lignocaine) with 1:200 000 adrenaline (1 ml of 1:10 000).
	CSE	Normal spinal dose (reduce if slow onset of block is required). If required top up the epidural with 5 ml aliquots of 2% lidocaine (lignocaine)
Post LSCS analgesia	GA	Bilateral ilioinguinal nerve blocks at end of surgery. Intravenous aliquots of morphine until comfortable. Parenteral opioid (IM or PCA as available)
	GA or regional	100 mg diclofenac PR at end of surgery, followed by 75 mg diclofenac PO 12-hourly. Simple analgesics as required (i.e. cocodamol, codydramol, etc.)
	Regional	Epidural diamorphine (2.5 mg) in 10 ml normal saline 4 hrly prn

LSCS = lower segment caesarian section

Neonatal resuscitation

Physiology

A term neonate needs to generate a negative pressure of more than 40 cmH$_2$O with its first breath. It must also clear its lungs of 100 ml fluid. The opening of alveoli and changes in oxygenation reduce pulmonary vascular resistance and promote closure of the ductus arteriosus. A distressed fetus has characteristic breathing movements that correlate with the severity of distress. The fetus may progress through these stages before delivery. As acidosis develops the fetus will initially start breathing movements, which become quicker and deeper and then cease. This interruption of breathing is called primary apnoea. During this phase, heart rate falls and peripheral circulation is shut down (a white baby). The duration of primary apnoea is variable but is followed by a period of slow deep breaths (6–10 breaths/min). When these breaths cease, a period of secondary apnoea is entered. Secondary apnoea is followed by cardiac arrest.

A neonate that is not breathing at delivery may be in primary or secondary apnoea.

At delivery

- If meconium is suspected, then to prevent aspiration (particularly of solid matter), the pharynx should be aspirated as soon as possible. The pharynx should be inspected and if meconium is present then the trachea should be intubated and suctioned before ventilation is commenced.
- Dry the baby. A wet baby will lose heat extremely rapidly.
- Assess the baby's colour, heart rate, and respiratory pattern.

Condition	Action
Pink, heart rate >100 beats/min, regular respiration	Normal — keep warm and dry
Cyanosed or white, heart rate >100 beats/min, irregular respiration	Give oxygen and continue to observe
Cyanosed or white, heart rate <100 beats/min, irregular or absent respiration	Resuscitate as below

Resuscitation

Airway

Clear the airway, intubation is rarely required initially.

Breathing

- The first breaths need to be slow and deep. Give five 2 s ventilations with inflation pressure of 30 cmH$_2$O. Little chest movement may be evident with the first two to three breaths as fluid is cleared form the lungs.
- Continue ventilation at a rate of 30–40 breaths/min.

Circulation

- Circulatory problems in the neonate are almost always a consequence of failed oxygenation, and when oxygenation is corrected, cardiac recovery is usually rapid.
- If the heart rate is less than 60 beats/min then start cardiac compression (compress the sternum with thumbs or two fingers) at a rate of 120/min. Assess heart rate every two minutes. When heart rate >80 beats/min stop compressions.
- If the heart rate is 60–80 beats/min continue to assess. If the heart rate has not improved within 2 min of starting ventilation then commence cardiac compressions as above.
- Continue to assess the heart rate until the heart is beating consistently greater than 100 beats/min.
- If the heart rate does not recover then consider drug therapy:
  - Adrenaline 10 μg/kg.
  - Bicarbonate. Consider using in the proven acidotic fetus. Adrenaline has a reduced effect on receptors in an acidotic milieu. Dose 1–2 mmol/kg (1–2 ml/kg 8.4% HCO_3).
  - Fluid: 10–20 ml/kg normal saline or colloid. The fetus may become acutely hypovolaemic with antepartum haemorrhage, vasa praevia, or trauma.
  - Naloxone. If opioids have been given and the neonate is drowsy, 200 μg naloxone IM can be given. Smaller doses are effective for short periods but the neonate may become sedated again as the opioid may last longer than the naloxone.

If the above measures have all proven ineffective then other causes of poor outcome must be assessed. Congenital heart disease, diaphragmatic hernias, or pneumothorax may all occur.

Placenta praevia and accreta

Placenta praevia

Placenta praevia occurs when the placenta implants between the fetus and the cervical os. The incidence is about 1 in 200 pregnancies, but is higher with previous uterine scars and multiparity. The subclassification of placenta praevia is variously defined. A simple classification is:

* Marginal–when the placenta extends to the os without crossing it.
* Partial–when the placenta partially covers the os.
* Complete–when the placenta fully covers the os.

Of more importance is whether a vaginal delivery is possible (unlikely if the placenta extends to within 2 cm of the os) and if it isn't, whether the placenta covers the anterior lower segment of the uterus. If it does, the obstetrician will have to divide the placenta to deliver the fetus and blood loss can be expected to be large, particularly if there is a previous uterine scar.

Diagnosis is usually made by ultrasound, often after a small painless vaginal bleed. Obstetric management is aimed at preserving the pregnancy until the 37th gestational week. Premature labour, excessive bleeding, or fetal distress may necessitate delivery. In most circumstances, women with placenta praevia are admitted to hospital and cross-matched blood kept continuously available. If at 37 weeks' gestation a vaginal delivery is not possible, a caesarean section is performed.

Placenta accreta

Placenta accreta occurs with abnormal implantation of the placenta. Usually the endometrium produces a cleavage plane between the placenta and the myometrium. In placenta accreta vera the placenta grows through the endometrium to the myometrium. In placenta increta the placenta grows in to the myometrium, and in placenta percreta the placenta grows through the myometrium to the uterine serosa and on into surrounding structures. Because the normal cleavage plane is absent, following delivery the placenta fails to separate from the uterus, which can result in life-threatening haemorrhage.

Incidence is rising, possibly as a result of the increasing numbers of caesarean sections performed. Placenta accreta is much more common when the placenta implants over a previous scar (5% of women with placenta praevia and no previous scar, rising to 50% of women with two previous scars–two thirds of these will require caesarean hysterectomy).[14] Diagnosis of percreta is occasionally made with ultrasound or the presence of haematuria, but usually placenta accreta and increta are diagnosed at surgery.

Anaesthetic management

Anaesthetic management is dictated by the likelihood of major haemorrhage, maternal preference, and obstetric/anaesthetic experience levels. Patients with placenta praevia are at risk of haemorrhage because:

14 Clark SL, Koonings PP, Phelan JP (1985). Placenta previa/accreta and prior cesarean section. *Obstetrics and Gynecology*, 66, 89–92.

- the placenta may have to be divided to facilitate delivery
- the lower uterine segment does not contract as effectively as the body of the uterus so the placental bed may continue to bleed following delivery.

Further increase in risk occurs sequentially with placenta accreta, increta, and percreta. Caesarean hysterectomy is required in 95% of women with placenta percreta, with a 7% overall mortality rate.

Although the sympathectomy that occurs with regional anaesthesia may make control of blood pressure more difficult, practical experience shows regional anaesthesia can be safely used for placenta praevia, provided that the patient is normovolaemic before the neuraxial technique is performed. Even in caesarean hysterectomy, the degree of hypotension and blood loss is the same with regional and general anaesthetic techniques. However, if significant haemorrhage does occur, hypotensive and bleeding patients will require reassurance and this may divert the anaesthetist from providing volume resuscitation. Regional anaesthesia should therefore only be undertaken by experienced anaesthetists who have additional help available.

Technique

- Experienced obstetricians and anaesthetists are essential.
- All patients admitted with placenta praevia should be seen and assessed by an anaesthetist.
- When caesarean section is to be performed two to eight units of blood should be cross-matched, depending on the anticipated risk of haemorrhage.
- Obstetric staff experienced in caesarean hysterectomy should be immediately available.
- Two 14G cannulae should be inserted and equipment for massive haemorrhage must be present.
- If regional anaesthesia is used, a CSE may offer advantages as the surgery may be prolonged.
- For bleeding patients a general anaesthetic is the preferred choice.
- Have a selection of uterotonics to hand (see p. 733). Even if massive haemorrhage is not encountered, an infusion is advantageous (e.g. syntocinon 30–50 IU in 500 ml crystalloid over 1–2 h).
- If massive bleeding does occur, hysterectomy may be the only method of controlling bleeding. Excessive delay in making this decision may jeopardize maternal life.
- Do not forget surgical methods of controlling haemorrhage– bimanual compression of the uterus, ligation of internal iliac arteries, temporary compression of the aorta.
- Even if no significant bleeding occurred intra-operatively, continue to observe closely in the postnatal period as haemorrhage may still occur.

Massive obstetric haemorrhage

The gravid uterus receives 12% of the cardiac output and thus when haemorrhage occurs it can be extremely rapid. In the developing world, haemorrhage is the leading cause of maternal death. Placental abruption, postpartum haemorrhage, and placenta praevia are the principal causes of massive haemorrhage.

The fetus is at greater risk from maternal haemorrhage than the mother. Hypotension reduces uteroplacental blood flow and severe anaemia will further reduce oxygen delivery. In addition, abruption may directly compromise blood supply. Fetal mortality may be as high as 35%. Standard protocols for major haemorrhage should be available in every delivery suite.

Aetiology of obstetric haemorrhage

Antenatal

- Placental abruption. Bleed is often associated with pain. Blood loss may be concealed with retroplacental bleeding. Fetal compromise is common. Small bleeds may be treated conservatively.
- Placenta praevia/accreta. Usually a small painless bleed. May be catastrophic.
- Uterine rupture. Fetal distress is the most reliable indicator. Classically uterine rupture is said to be painful, but painless dehiscence of a previous uterine scar is not uncommon.

Postnatal

Defined as blood loss of greater than 500 ml post delivery. Estimates of 'normal' blood loss after vaginal delivery are of the order of 250– 400 ml, and after caesarean section around 500–1000 ml. Blood loss is usually underestimated.

- Uterine atony. Associated with chorioamnionitis, prolonged labour, and an abnormally distended uterus (e.g. polyhydramnios, macrosomia, multiple gestation, etc.).
- Retained placenta. Haemorrhage may be massive, but is usually less than 1 litre and occasionally minimal.
- Retained products of conception. This is the leading cause of late haemorrhage, but is rarely massive.
- Genital tract trauma. Vaginal and vulval haematomas are usually self limiting, but retroperitoneal haematomas may be extensive and life-threatening.
- Uterine inversion. This is a rare complication in the Western world. It is associated with uterine atony and further relaxation may be required to enable replacement. After replacement uterotonics should be administered.

Diagnosis

Diagnosis of haemorrhage is usually self-evident, although be aware that concealed bleeding may occur, especially with placental abruptions. In addition signs of cardiovascular decompensation may be delayed, as women are usually young, fit, and start with a pregnancy-induced expansion of their intravascular volume. Beware of the woman with cold peripheries–this is abnormal in pregnancy. Hypotension is a late and ominous sign.

Management

In the event of a major haemorrhage requiring surgery, do not delay operation until cross-matched blood is available.

- Call for help.
- Give supplemental oxygen. If laryngeal reflexes are obtunded, intubate and ventilate. In antenatal patients avoid aortocaval occlusion.
- Insert two 14G cannulas and take blood for cross-matching. Request type-specific blood (this can be retrospectively cross-matched.)
- Fluid resuscitate with crystalloid and/or colloid.
- If required give group O rhesus negative blood (i.e. blood loss of 2–3 litres and ongoing without the imminent prospect of cross-matched blood being available and/or the presence of ECG abnormalities).
- Start appropriate monitoring of mother and fetus. Urine output and invasive monitoring of central venous and arterial pressures may be indicated depending on the rate of blood loss and maternal condition. However, early monitoring of CVP is not essential as hypotension is almost always due to hypovolaemia.
- Treat the cause of haemorrhage.
- If surgery is required:
  - do not perform a regional technique if the patient is hypovolaemic
  - beware of coagulopathies in the presence of concealed abruption.
- With continuing haemorrhage further equipment including warming devices and rapid transfusion devices should be available.
- Correct coagulopathy with platelets, fresh frozen plasma, and cryoprecipitate as indicated.
- Once blood loss has been controlled, continue care on a high-dependency unit or intensive care unit.

Specific treatment for haemorrhage

Treatment may be with uterotonics or surgery or both depending on the cause:

- Uterotonics can only be used in the postnatal period.
- Most postnatal haemorrhage is due to uterine atony and can be temporarily controlled with firm bimanual pressure while waiting for definitive treatment.

Commonly used uterotonics and doses

Drug	Dose	Notes
Oxytocin (Syntocinon®)	5–10 IU bolus. 30–50 IU in 500 ml crystalloid and titrated as indicated	Synthetically produced hormone causing uterine contraction, peripheral vasodilation and has very mild antidiuretic hormone actions. (Early preparations made from animal extracts had significant ADH activity)
Ergometrine	0.5 mg IM or 0.125 mg by slow IV injection and repeat	An ergot alkaloid derivative. Produces effective uterine constriction but nausea and vomiting are very common. Systemic vasoconstriction may produce dangerous hypertension in at-risk groups (e.g. pre-eclampsia, specific cardiac disease)
Carboprost (Hemabate®) (15-methyl prostaglandin F2α)	0.25 mg intra-myometrially or IM every 10–15 min to a max. of 2 mg	Effective uterine constrictor. Also causes nausea, vomiting, and diarrhoea. May produce severe bronchospasm, alter pulmonary shunt fraction, and induce hypoxia

Pregnancy induced hypertension, pre-eclampsia, and eclampsia[15]

Pre-eclampsia remains a leading cause of maternal death. It is a systemic disorder. The precise aetiology is complex. Immunological factors, genetic factors, endothelial dysfunction, as well as abnormalities in placental implantation, fatty acid metabolism, and coagulation and platelet factors have all been implicated. The earlier in gestation that pre-eclampsia manifests itself, the more severe the disease.

Definitions

- Hypertension. A sustained systolic BP >140 mmHg or diastolic BP >90 mmHg.
- Chronic hypertension. Hypertension that existed before pregnancy.
- Pregnancy induced hypertension. Hypertension that develops in pregnancy. In the absence of other signs of pre-eclampsia, this has a minimal effect on pregnancy but may be indicative of a tendency to hypertension in later life.
- Pre-eclampsia. Pregnancy induced hypertension in association with renal involvement causing proteinuria (>300 mg /24 h or 2+ on urine dipstick). Incidence is 6–8% of all gestations.
- Severe pre-eclampsia. Pre-eclampsia in association with any of the following: a sustained BP >160/110; proteinuria >5 g/24 h or 3+ on urine dipstick; urine output <400 ml/24 h; pulmonary oedema or evidence of respiratory compromise; epigastric or right upper quadrant pain; hepatic rupture, platelet count <100×10^9/litre; evidence of cerebral complications. Incidence is 0.25–0.5% of all gestations.
- Eclampsia. Convulsions occurring in pregnancy or puerperium in the absence of other causes. Almost always occurs in the presence of pre-eclampsia, although signs of pre-eclampsia may not be manifest until after a fit.

Pathophysiology

Cardiorespiratory

- Hypertension and increased sensitivity to catecholamine and exogenous vasopressors.
- Reduced circulating volume, but increased total body water.
- In severe pre-eclampsia systemic vascular resistance is increased and cardiac output reduced. However, some women with have elevated cardiac output with normal or only marginally increased systemic vascular resistance. Fetal prognosis is improved in this group.
- Poor correlation between central venous and pulmonary capillary wedge pressure.

15 Brodie H, Malinow AM (1999). Anaesthetic management of pre-eclampsia/ eclampsia. *International Journal of Obstetric Anesthesia*, **8**, 110–24.

- Increased capillary permeability which may result in:
  - Pulmonary oedema. In pre-eclampsia the most common mode of maternal death is pulmonary oedema and ARDS. Be very careful with fluid therapy!
  - Laryngeal and pharyngeal oedema. Stridor may result.

Haematological

- Reduced platelet count with increased platelet consumption, hypercoagulability with increased fibrin activation and breakdown. Disseminated intravascular coagulation may result.
- Increased haematocrit resulting from the decreased circulating volume.

Renal function

- A reduced glomerular filtration rate.
- Increased permeability to large molecules resulting in proteinuria.
- Decreased urate clearance with rising serum uric acid level.
- Oliguria in severe disease.

Cerebral function

- Headache, visual disturbance, and generalized hyper-reflexia.
- Cerebrovascular haemorrhage. Deaths due to intracranial haemorrhage are declining with improved control of blood pressure.
- Eclampsia (resulting from cerebral oedema or cerebrovascular vaso-constriction).

Fetoplacental unit

- Reduced fetal growth with associated oligohydramnios.
- Poor placental perfusion and increased sensitivity to changes in maternal blood pressure.
- Reduction of umbilical arterial diastolic blood flow and particularly reverse diastolic flow is indicative of a very poor fetal outcome without early intervention.

Management of pre-eclampsia

- There is no effective prophylactic treatment to prevent pre-eclampsia. Some obstetricians may use low-dose aspirin in selected high-risk pregnancies, but the benefit is unproven.
- In established pre-eclampsia the only definitive treatment is the delivery of the placenta. Symptoms will usually start to resolve within 24–48 h.
- When pre-eclampsia develops at term there is no advantage to delaying delivery. If pre-eclampsia develops before term, a compromise has to be made between maternal and fetal health. Maternal blood pressure is controlled for as long as possible to allow fetal growth to be optimized. If the fetal or maternal condition deteriorates, delivery must be expedited.
- Antihypertensive therapy–blood pressure should be controlled to below 160/110 to prevent maternal morbidity, particularly from intracranial haemorrhage, encephalopathy, and myocardial ischaemia and failure:
  - Established oral antihypertensive drugs include oral methyldopa/ nifedipine preparations and beta-blockers (particularly the combined alpha-

and beta-blocker labetalol). Prolonged use of beta-blockers may reduce fetal growth.

- ACE inhibitors are associated with oligohydramnios, still birth, neonatal renal failure and should be avoided.

- Rapid control of severe hypertension can be achieved with:
  - Hydralazine (5 mg IV aliquots to a maximum of 20 mg).
  - Labetalol (5–10 mg IV every 10 min).
  - Oral nifedipine (sublingual nifedipine should be used with caution because of associated rapid changes in placental circulation which may compromise fetal condition).
  - In cases resistant to treatment, infusions of sodium nitroprusside or glyceryl trinitrate may be needed. If used, arterial pressure monitoring is required.

- Magnesium prophylaxis in pre-eclampsia is controversial because, although it is effective at reducing the incidence of eclampsia, fetal effects have been variously reported as beneficial and deleterious.

- Fluid management in severe pre-eclampsia is critical. Intravascular volume is depleted but total body water is increased. Excessive fluid load may result in pulmonary oedema, but underfilling may compromise fetal circulation and renal function. General principles are:
  - Individual units are encouraged to develop and follow protocols for fluid management.
  - A named individual should have overall responsibility for fluid therapy in severe pre-eclampsia.
  - Measure hourly urine output.
  - Beware of excessive fluid loads being delivered with drug therapy (i.e. oxytocin or magnesium). Increased concentrations may be required.
  - Be cautious with preload before caesarean section and avoid preload before regional analgesia.
  - A common approach is to use a small background infusion of crystalloid, and to treat persistent oliguria with 250–500 ml of a colloid. If oliguria continues, further fluid management is usually guided by central venous pressure.

- Invasive arterial pressure monitoring is indicated in severe pre-eclampsia for:
  - Monitoring the response to laryngoscopy and surgery during general anaesthesia.
  - Taking repeated arterial blood gases.
  - Monitoring rapidly acting hypotensive agents (such as sodium nitroprusside).

- Central venous pressure monitoring is indicated in severe pre-eclampsia:
  - For persistent oliguria (<0.5 ml/kg/h) unresponsive to small fluid challenges.
  - If pulmonary oedema develops.

Although central venous pressure does not always correlate well with pulmonary arterial wedge pressure, a low CVP is almost never associated with a high PCWP.

Analgesia for vaginal delivery

- Effective epidural analgesia controls excessive surges in blood pressure during labour and is recommended.
- Check the platelet count before performing an epidural. If the maternal condition is rapidly deteriorating or if the platelet numbers are falling then a count must be performed immediately before placement. The 'acceptable' level of platelet count is debatable and based on little evidence. However, common general guidelines are:
  - If the platelet count is $<100 \times 10^9$/litre, then a clotting screen is also required.
  - If the platelet count is $>80 \times 10^9$/litre and the clotting screen is normal then regional techniques are acceptable.
  - With a platelet count of $<80 \times 10^9$/litre, a very careful assessment from a senior individual is required and the potential risks and benefits should be discussed with the patient.
  - Thromboelastography may offer a better method of assessing bleeding potential, but as yet its place is unproven.
- Preload before regional analgesia is not required, but monitor the blood pressure and fetus carefully and treat changes in blood pressure promptly with 3 mg increments of ephedrine.

Anaesthesia for caesarean section

General anaesthesia or regional anaesthesia may be used. General anaesthesia is indicated if significant thrombocytopenia (see above) or coagulopathy has developed.

General anaesthesia

- Assess the airway carefully. Obvious oedema may be apparent. Sometimes partners may be better able to assess the onset of facial oedema. A history of stridor is of major concern. A selection of small tube sizes must be available. Consider awake fibreoptic intubation in severe cases.
- Obtund the hypertensive response to laryngoscopy. (e.g. alfentanil 1–2 mg, but inform the paediatrician that opioids have been used, or labetalol 10–20 mg before induction). In very severe pre-eclampsia, intra-arterial pressure monitoring is required before induction.
- If magnesium has been used, expect prolongation of action of non-depolarizing muscle relaxants. Use a reduced dose and assess muscle function with a nerve stimulator.
- Ensure adequate analgesia before extubation. The hypertensive response to extubation may also need to be controlled with antihypertensive agents.
- Effective postoperative analgesia is required, but avoid NSAIDs as these patients are prone to renal impairment and may have impaired platelet count or function. When the proteinuria has resolved, which is often within 48 h, NSAIDs may be introduced.
- Continue care in a high-dependency area or intensive care.

Regional anaesthesia

Depleted intravascular volume may make severe pre-eclamptic patients more vulnerable to the hypotensive effect of the rapid onset of spinal as opposed to epidural anaesthesia. Recent studies suggest that pre-eclamptic women are actually less prone to hypotension than normal individuals and no difference in fetal outcome could be demonstrated between spinal and epidural anaesthesia. Spinal anaesthesia is known to consistently produce better analgesia.

- As with regional analgesia, platelet count and if necessary clotting screen needs to be assessed (see above).
- A reduced volume of preload should be used (possibly with colloid).
- Expect ephedrine to have an increased effect.
- A slow onset of block is desirable. This can be achieved with epidural spinal, or combined spinal epidural (see regional anaesthesia for caesarean section).
- Effective postoperative analgesia is required, but avoid NSAIDs as these patients are prone to renal impairment and may have impaired platelet count or function.
- Care should be continued on a high-dependency or intensive care unit.

Eclampsia

- Incidence is 1 in 2000 of pregnancies in the United Kingdom,[16] but there are wide international variations.
- Most fits occur in the third trimester, and nearly one-third occur post-partum, usually within 24 hours of delivery.
- Eclampsia is a life-threatening event.
- Management is aimed at immediate control of the fit and secondary prevention of further fits.

Immediate management

- Airway (left lateral position with jaw thrust), breathing (bag and mask ventilation and measure saturation), circulation (obtain IV access and measure blood pressure when possible, avoid aortocaval compression).
- Control of fits is with 4 g of magnesium given intravenously over 10–20 min

Prevention of further fits[17]

- Magnesium infusion at 1 g/h for 24 h.
  - Therapeutic level 5–7 mg/dl (2–4 mmol/l). Magnesium levels may be monitored clinically (loss of reflexes (8–10 mg/dl), reduced respiratory rate (10–15 mg/dl), or with laboratory monitoring). Reduce the infusion rate with oliguria.
  - Subsequent fits should be controlled with an additional bolus of 2 g magnesium.
  - Patients on calcium channel antagonists are at particular risk of toxicity. Toxicity can be treated with intravenous calcium (i.e. 10 ml of 10% calcium chloride).

16 Douglas KA, Redman CWG (1994). Eclampsia in the United Kingdom. *British Medical Journal*, **309**, 1395–9.

17 The Eclampsia Trial Collaborative Group (1995). Which anticonvulsant for women with eclampsia? Evidence from the Collaborative Eclampsia Trial. *The Lancet*, **345**, 1455–63.

After the initial fit has been controlled, if eclampsia has developed antenatally a decision has to be made as to when delivery is to be performed. In general the patient should be stabilized on a magnesium infusion and then consideration given to vaginal or operative delivery. Eclampsia is not an indication for emergency caesarean section. If general anaesthesia is required, expect prolongation of the action of non-depolarizing muscle relaxants. After delivery patients should be observed on a high-dependency or intensive care unit.

The HELLP syndrome

Haemolysis, Elevated Liver enzymes, and Low Platelets comprise the HELLP syndrome. It is usually associated with pre-eclampsia or eclampsia, but these are not a prerequisite for diagnosis. Severe HELLP syndrome has a 5% maternal mortality. HELLP rarely presents before the 20th week of gestation, but one-sixth present before the third trimester and a further third present postnatally (usually within 48 h of delivery). Symptoms are sometimes of a vague flu-like illness, which may delay diagnosis. Maintain a high index of suspicion.

Features include

- Evidence of haemolysis (a falling haemoglobin concentration without evidence of overt bleeding, haemoglobinuria, elevated bilirubin in serum and urine, elevated LDH).

- Elevated liver function tests–AST (serum aspartate aminotransferase), ALT (serum alanine aminotransferase), alkaline phosphatase, and g-glutamyl transferase. Epigastric or right upper quadrant abdominal pain are present in 90% of women with HELLP. Liver failure and hepatic rupture may occur. Extreme elevation in AST is associated with poor maternal prognosis. Most women with right upper quadrant pain and a platelet count of $<20 \times 10^9$/litre will have an intrahepatic or subcapsular bleed.

- A falling platelet count. Counts of less than 100×10^9/litre are of concern while a count of less than 50×10^9/l is indicative of severe disease.

- Hypertension and proteinuria is present in 80% of women with HELLP. 50% suffer nausea and vomiting. Convulsions and gastrointestinal haemorrhage are occasional presenting features.

  The only definitive treatment is delivery of the placenta, although high-dose steroids may delay progress of the disease. If the maternal condition is not deteriorating rapidly and the fetus is profoundly premature, delivery may be delayed by 48 h to allow steroids to be administered to promote fetal lung maturity.

- The method of delivery depends on maternal condition and the likelihood of successfully inducing labour. Severe HELLP syndrome will require an urgent caesarean section.

- The risk of epidural haematoma may preclude the use of regional analgesia/anaesthesia. Consideration must be given to both the absolute platelet number as well as rate of fall in platelet count. All patients require a clotting screen.

- Be prepared for major haemorrhage.

- Further management is supportive, with appropriate replacement of blood products as required.

- Invasive monitoring is dictated entirely by the clinical condition of the patient.

- ARDS, renal failure, and disseminated intravascular coagulation may develop.

- After delivery of the placenta, recovery can be expected to start within 24–48 h. These patients should all be on a high-dependency or intensive care unit.

Incidental surgery during pregnancy

One to two per cent of women require incidental surgery during pregnancy.[18] Surgery is associated with increased fetal loss and premature delivery, although this probably reflects the underlying condition that necessitated the surgery rather than the anaesthetic or the surgery itself. The risk of teratogenicity is very small.

General considerations

* When possible delay surgery until the postnatal period or alternatively into the second trimester, when teratogenic risks to the fetus are reduced. The fetus is at greatest risk from teratogenicity in the period of organogenesis, which continues to the 12th week of gestation.

* Make sure that the obstetric team are aware that surgery is planned.

* Remember gastric acid prophylaxis.

* Remember DVT prophylaxis. Pregnant women are hypercoagulable.

* Consider regional anaesthesia. The combination of a mother maintaining her own airway together with a minimal fetal drug exposure, is desirable However, data demonstrating that regional anaesthesia is safer than general anaesthesia are lacking.

* Airway management in the first and early second trimester is controversial. In asymptomatic women with no other indication for intubation, it is acceptable not to perform a rapid sequence induction up to the 18th week of gestation. However, be aware that lower oesophageal sphincter tone is reduced within the first few weeks of pregnancy and intra-abdominal pressure rises in the second trimester. If patients have additional risk factors for regurgitation, use a rapid sequence induction.[19]

* Every effort must be made to maintain normal maternal physiological parameters for the gestational age of the fetus throughout the perioperative period.

* Treat haemorrhage aggressively. Avoid hypovolaemia and anaemia as both impact on fetal oxygenation.

* From the 20th week of gestation use left lateral tilt to reduce aortocaval compression. Remember that although upper limb blood pressure may be normal, uterine blood flow may still be compromised in the supine position.

* If general anaesthesia is employed, use adequate sleep doses of inhalational agents. Light anaesthesia is associated with increased catecholamine release, which reduces placental blood flow. The tocolytic effect of inhalational agents is advantageous.

18 Mazze RI, Kallen B (1989). Reproductive outcome after anesthesia and operation during pregnancy: a registry study of 5405 cases. *American Journal of Obstetrics and Gynecology*, **161**, 1178–85.

19 Vanner RG (1992). Gastro-oesophageal reflux and regurgitation during general anaesthesia for termination of pregnancy. *International Journal of Obstetric Anesthesia*, **1**, 123–8.

- Fetal monitoring may be beneficial although its value remains unproven. I fetal distress is detected, maternal physiology can be manipulated to optimize uterine blood flow.
- The primary risk to the fetus is premature labour in the postoperative period Detection and suppression of premature labour is vital. Women should be told to report sensations of uterine contractions so that appropriate tocolytic therapy can be instituted (100 mg indometacin PO/PR provides effective short-term tocolysis while awaiting further advice from obstetric staff).
- Effective postoperative analgesia is required to reduce maternal catecholamine secretion. Although opioids can be used, they may result in maternal hypercarbia. Regional analgesia with local anaesthetic agents may be preferential. If this would prevent the mother from detecting uterine contractions, consider external uterine pressure transduction ('tocodynamometry'). For minor surgery, local anaesthesia and simple analgesics such as paracetamol and codeine may be used. Chronic dosage with NSAIDs should be avoided, in the first trimester because of increased fetal loss and in the third trimester because of the possibility of premature closure of the fetal ductus arteriosus.

Teratogenicity

The fetus is at greatest risk of teratogenesis in the period of major organogenesis. This is predominantly in the first 12 weeks of gestation, although minor abnormalities may still occur after this. Causes of teratogenicity are diverse and include infection, pyrexia, hypoxia, and acidosis as well as the better-recognized hazards of drugs and radiation. The association of drugs with teratogenicity is often difficult. Epidemiological studies have to be large to establish associations, while animal experiments may not reflect either human dose exposure or human physiology. Although none of the commonly used anaesthetic agents are proven teratogens specific concerns are addressed below.

Premedication

- Benzodiazepines. Case reports have associated benzodiazepines with cleft lip formation, but this has not been substantiated by more recent studies. A single dose has never been associated with teratogenicity. Long-term administration may lead to neonatal withdrawal symptoms following delivery, and exposure just before delivery may cause neonatal drowsiness and hypotonia.
- Ranitidine and cimetidine are not known to be harmful but caution is advised with chronic exposure to cimetidine because of known androgenic effects in adults.

Induction agents

- Thiopental. Clinical experience with thiopental suggests that this is a very safe drug to use, although formal studies have not been conducted.
- Propofol is not teratogenic in animal studies. Its use in early human pregnancy has not been formally investigated. Propofol is safe to use during caesarean section at term.
- Etomidate is also not teratogenic in animal studies. It is a potent inhibitor of cortisol synthesis, and when used for caesarean section, neonates have reduced cortisol concentrations.

- Ketamine should be avoided in early pregnancy as it increases intrauterine pressure, resulting in fetal asphyxia. This increase in intrauterine pressure is not apparent in the third trimester.

Inhalational agents

- Halothane and isoflurane have been used extensively in pregnancy and are safe. At high concentrations, maternal blood pressure and cardiac output fall resulting in a significant reduction in uterine blood flow. The halogenated vapours also cause uterine relaxation, which may be beneficial for surgery during pregnancy.
- Despite early concerns, recent epidemiological studies suggest that nitrous oxide is safe. However, nitrous oxide is consistently teratogenic in Sprague Dawley rats if they are exposed to 50–75% concentrations for 24 h during their peak organogenic period. Given that anaesthesia can be safely delivered without nitrous oxide it is sensible to avoid this agent.
- Muscle relaxants. Because these agents are not lipophilic, only very small quantities cross the placenta and so fetal exposure is limited. These agents are safe to use.
- Anticholinesterase inhibitors: These agents are highly ionized and so, like muscle relaxants, do not readily cross the placenta and are safe to use. Chronic use of pyridostigmine to treat myasthenia gravis may cause premature labour.

Analgesics

- Opioids readily cross the placenta, but brief exposure is safe. Long-term exposure will cause symptoms of withdrawal when the fetus is delivered. Animal studies suggest possible fetal teratogenicity if prolonged hypercapnia or impaired feeding develop as side-effects of opioid exposure.
- Chronic exposure to NSAIDs in early pregnancy may be associated with increased fetal loss and in the third trimester may cause premature closure of the ductus arteriosus and persistent pulmonary hypertension of the newborn. Single doses are unlikely to be harmful. These agents are also used to suppress labour, particularly in the second trimester.
- Bupivacaine and lidocaine (lignocaine) are safe. When used near delivery, bupivacaine has no significant neonatal neurobehavioural effects, while lidocaine (lignocaine) may have a mild effect. Cocaine abuse during pregnancy increases fetal loss and may increase the incidence of abnormalities in the genitourinary tract.

Cervical cerclage (Shirodkar suture)

Procedure	Surgical treatment of incompetent cervical os
Time	20 min
Pain	+
Position	Lithotomy
Blood loss	Nil
Practical techniques	Spinal/epidural
	GA with RSI/cuffed ET if >18 weeks' gestation or reflux

An incompetent cervix may be caused by congenital abnormalities, cervical scarring or hormonal imbalance. Premature dilation of the cervix and fetal loss may result, usually in the second trimester. Cervical cerclage is performed to prevent this premature dilation and is one of the commonest surgical procedures performed in pregnancy. Although occasionally inserted before conception, it is usually performed between the 14th and 26th weeks of gestation. Emergency cerclage may be required in the face of a dilating cervix and bulging membranes. Unsurprisingly, emergency cerclage is less successful in maintaining a pregnancy than prophylactic cerclage.

Preoperative

- The risks of cerclage include membrane rupture (which is much more common if the membranes are already bulging), infection, haemorrhage, and inducing premature labour.
- Careful assessment of airway, gestation, symptoms of reflux, and supine hypotension.
- Remember antacid prophylaxis.
- Explain risks of teratogenicity/spontaneous miscarriage (see p. 742).

Perioperative

- Both regional and general anaesthesia may be used.
- If general anaesthesia is used and uterine relaxation is required to allow bulging membranes to be reduced, the halogenated vapour concentration can be increased.
- For regional anaesthesia, a T8–T10 level is required for intraoperative comfort. If uterine relaxation is required, 100 µg aliquots of intravenous glyceryl trinitrate may be used and repeated as necessary, although transient hypotension is to be expected.

Postoperative

- In the postoperative period women should be observed closely for premature labour.
- Vaginal cervical cerclage sutures are usually removed at the 38th week of gestation.

Special considerations

- Various permutations on cervical cerclage are available. These are broadly divided into transvaginal procedures and transabdominal procedures.
- The transabdominal procedure requires two operations—one for insertion and a caesarean section for delivery and removal of the suture. It also carries a greater risk of ureteric involvement.
- Transvaginal procedures are much more common. Shirodkar and McDonald procedures are the two commonest methods. They both require anaesthesia for insertion but can be removed without anaesthetic.

Breast feeding and maternal drug exposure

If a drug is to be transferred from mother to neonate through breast feeding, it must be secreted in the milk, absorbed in the neonatal gastrointestinal tract, and not undergo extensive first-pass metabolism in the neonatal liver. In general, for breast-fed infants, neonatal serum concentration of a drug is less than 2% of maternal serum concentration resulting in a subtherapeutic dose. Most drugs are therefore safe. However, there are some exceptions to this rule—either because transfer is much higher or because transfer of even minute quantities of a drug is unacceptable. Drugs with high protein binding may displace bilirubin and precipitate kernicturus in a jaundiced neonate.

Factors that make significant transfer more likely include:
- Low maternal protein binding.
- Lipophilicity or, with hydrophilic drugs, a molecular weight of <200 Da.
- Weak bases (which increases the proportion of ionized drug in the weakly acidic breast milk leading to 'trapping').

Transfer to the fetus can be minimized by breastfeeding before administering the drug, and if the neonate has a consistent sleep period, administering the drug to mother at the beginning of this.

Although many drugs are excreted in minimal quantities in breast milk with no reports of ill-effects manufacturers will often recommend avoiding agents during breast feeding.

Remember that breast feeding constitutes a metabolic and fluid load for the mother, so if surgery is contemplated then keep the mother well hydrated and if surgery is elective, have the patient first on the list. Try to minimize nausea and vomiting.

The following table gives information on some agents, but a full list of drug compatibility with breast feeding is beyond the scope of this book.

Drug	Comment
Opioids	Minimal amount delivered to neonatal serum. Minor concern about the long duration of action of pethidine's metabolite nor-pethidine
NSAIDs	Most NSAIDs are considered safe in breast feeding. Some would advise caution with aspirin because of unsubstantiated concerns about causing Reye's syndrome in the neonate
Antibiotics	Penicillins and cephalosporins are safe, although trace amounts may be passed to the neonate
	Tetracycline should be avoided (although absorption is probably minimal because of chelation with calcium in the milk)
	Chloramphenicol may cause bone-marrow suppression in the infant and should be avoided
	Ciprofloxacin is present in high concentrations in breast milk and should be avoided
Antipsychotics	It is generally suggested that these should be avoided although the amount excreted in milk is probably too small to be harmful. Chlorpromazine and clozapine cause infant drowsiness
Cardiac drugs	Amiodarone is present in milk in significant amounts and breast feeding should be discontinued
	Most beta-blockers are secreted in minimal amounts. Sotalol is present in larger amounts. Avoid celiprolol.
Anticonvulsants	While carbamazepine does not accumulate in the infant, phenobarbital and diazepam may. Infants should be observed for evidence of sedation.

Controversies in obstetric anaesthesia

Feeding in labour

In the 1950s the Confidential Enquiries into maternal deaths highlighted aspiration as a major cause of maternal death. As a result a policy of starvation during labour became widespread. Although airway problems continue to be implicated in maternal deaths, aspiration as a cause of death is now rare. Some have argued that this is due to improved training and equipment and the starvation policy is purely incidental, particularly as starved individuals may have a significant volume of gastric secretions in the stomach.

In addition starvation may adversely affect the progress of labour. Ketosis and hypoglycaemia are common when starvation is combined with the physical effort of labour. This may reduce the likelihood of a spontaneous vaginal delivery. A widely quoted study by Ludka supports this. She noted a 38% increase in caesarean section rate, a 500% increase in the use of oxytocics, and a 69% increase in the need for neonatal intensive care in a 6–month period when a nil by mouth policy was introduced in to her delivery suite. When the starvation policy was relaxed the rates returned to their previous level. However, this study did not report on the number of women included nor have these results been repeated at other centres.

Scrutton randomized women to feeding or starvation in labour and found that ketosis and hypoglycaemia were less common when women were fed. However, gastric volume was greater in the fed group, and there was no difference in the duration of first or second stages of labour, oxytocic requirements, or mode of delivery.[20]

Most women do not want to eat when in established labour. However, if feeding is to be instituted, suggested recommendations are:

- Only 'low-risk' women should be permitted to eat. However, identification of 'low-risk' women in early labour is notoriously inaccurate.

- Stop all intake of solids if any opioid, epidural, or oxytocic is used.

- Allow only 'low-residue' foods that rapidly empty from the stomach (cereals, toast, low-fat cheese, and semisweet biscuits). Very cold foods such as ice creams are known to delay gastric emptying.

- As particulate matter is known to be especially problematic in the event of aspiration, isotonic sports drinks may offer the ideal solution. These effectively prevent ketosis without increasing gastric volume.

Backache and neurological damage after neuraxial techniques

In the early 1990s two retrospective studies by MacArthur[21] and Russell[22] suggested an association between epidural analgesia in labour and subsequent

20 Scrutton MJL, Metcalfe GA *et al.* (1999). Eating in labour. A randomised controlled trial assessing the risks and benefits. *Anaesthesia*, **54**, 329–34.

21 Macarthur A, Macarthur C et al. (1997). Is epidural anesthesia in labor asscoiated with chronic low back pain? A prospective cohort study. *Anesthesia and Analgesia*, **85**, 1066–70.

22 Russell R, Dundas R et al. (1996). Long-term backache after childbirth: prospective search for causative factors. *British Medical Journal*, **312**, 1384–8.

new backache and headache. Prolonged abnormal posture permitted by effective analgesia was the proposed mechanism. This received widespread media coverage and spurred several prospective studies. These prospective studies established that previous studies had underestimated the incidence of antenatal backache. None of the prospective studies have found an increased incidence of 'new' backache at the time of delivery in association with regional anaesthesia. (This excludes a period of short-term backache at the site of needle puncture. The incidence of local tenderness at the site of epidural insertion is roughly 50%, but this usually resolves within a few days.)

Neurological damage does occur after childbirth, but establishing cause and effect is difficult. Neurological sequelae following delivery under general anaesthesia are as common as in delivery under regional anaesthesia, suggesting that obstetric causes of neurological sequelae are probably more common than any effects from the regional technique. Prolonged neurological deficit after epidural anaesthesia occurs of the order of 1 in 10 000 to 1 in 15 000 cases.

Epidurals, dystocia, and caesarean section[23]

It has been recognized for many years that epidurals are associated with caesarean section. However, argument continues as to whether this is a causative association. Various possible mechanisms have been proposed. These include:

- Reduced maternal expulsive effort resulting from abdominal muscle weakness.
- Change in the way in which the force of contraction is transferred to the pelvic floor when relaxed by an epidural.
- Change in the uterine force of contraction (this is not substantiated by recent studies).
- Interference with the Ferguson reflex (increased oxytocic production with pressure on the pelvic floor in the second stage of labour). This is controversial, as the Ferguson reflex has not been clearly demonstrated in humans.

'Impact studies' (studies of changes in caesarean section rates when there is a dramatic change in epidural analgesia rates) have not found a causative association, and of the many large randomized controlled comparisons of epidural versus narcotic analgesia, only two[24] have noted an association. Both of these studies were criticised for methodological problems.

Approximately 50% of randomized studies did find an association with assisted vaginal deliveries and regional analgesia. This may be minimized by reducing the total dose of local anaesthetic administered.

'Walking' epidurals in labour[25]

Effective analgesia with minimal motor block of the lower limbs can be readily produced with low doses of epidural or intrathecal local anaesthetic usually in

23 Chestnut DH (1997). Epidural analgsia and the incidence of cesarean section. Time for another close look. *Anesthesiology*, **87**, 472–5.

24 Thorp JA, Hu DH *et al.* (1993). The effect of intrapartum epidural analgesia on nulliparous labor: a randomized, controlled, prospective study. *American Journal of Obstetrics and Gynecology*, **169**, 851–8.

25 Morgan BM (1995). 'Walking' epidurals in labour. *Anaesthesia*, **50**, 839–40.

combination with an opioid (e.g. subarachnoid injection of 1 ml of 0.25% bupivacaine with 10–25 μg fentanyl or an epidural bolus of 15–20 ml of 0.1% bupivacaine with 2 μg/ml fentanyl. Subsequent epidural top-ups of 15 ml of the same solution as required). In some centres women with minimal motor blockade are encouraged to mobilize. The possible advantages of these techniques include:

- The vertical position, without epidural anaesthesia, is associated with shorter labour, possibly less fetal distress, and greater maternal preference. However, the vertical position and mobility do not reduce the need for forceps delivery and the advantages have not been substantiated when walking with epidural analgesia.

- The minimal motor block associated with these techniques increase maternal satisfaction scores. Intrathecal, as opposed to epidural, techniques produce a more rapid onset of analgesia, possibly a more rapid cervical dilation and a marginal reduction in assisted delivery.

Mobilization has been criticized because:

- While women usually have adequate leg strength, it is rarely complete, and is likely to become increasingly compromised with repeat doses of epidural local anaesthetic.

- Impaired proprioception may make walking dangerous even when leg strength has been maintained. Whilst dynamic posturography suggests that following an initial intrathecal dose of 2.5 mg bupivacaine and 10 μg fentanyl, proprioception is adequate for safe walking, this may no longer be true after repeated epidural top-ups.

- Intrathecal narcotics may cause temporary fetal bradycardia, probably by altering uterine blood flow through a change in maternal spinal reflexes.

- Assessing fetal condition is difficult when the mother is mobile.

In practice, when a technique that is likely to permit walking is used, only approximately 50% of women who could walk actually choose to do so. Despite this, most women prefer the added sense of control that is engendered by retaining leg strength. If women are to be allowed to walk, always wait at least 30 min from the initiation of the block before attempting mobilization. Then:

- Check strength of straight leg raising in bed.

- Ask the woman if she feels able to stand.

- When the woman first stands, have two assistants ready to offer support if required.

- Perform a knee bend.

- Ask the women if she feels safe.

- Allow full mobilization.

- After each top up the same sequence must be repeated.

Herpes simplex infection

- Infection with herpes simplex virus is common. The risk to the fetus is minimal provided that active genital infection is not present during delivery. In the presence of active infection delivery should be by caesarean section. Regional anaesthesia is not contraindicated provided no active lesions are present at the site of insertion.

- In 10% of infected women, herpes infection is reactivated by intrathecal or epidural morphine. The mechanism has not been elucidated. Theories relating to pruritus have been proposed, but have not been substantiated. Generally reactivation occurs 2–5 days after the epidural administration. There are isolated case reports of recrudescence after neuraxial pethidine and fentanyl, but it is not likely that this is indicative of a causative effect.

Previous subarachnoid haemorrhage

- Arteriovenous fistulae and intracranial aneurysms may be at greater risk of haemorrhage during pregnancy due to risk of the increased blood flow. Hypertensive disorders of pregnancy do increase the risk of intracranial bleeds.
- When an intracranial bleed has been surgically corrected these patients can be treated as 'normal' unless intracranial shunts are present. When ventriculoperitoneal shunts have been formed, it is sensible to avoid the subarachnoid space because of the risk of introducing infection.
- If no definitive surgical treatment has been performed, the delivery needs to take account of the size, position, and risk of further bleeding. If elective caesarean section is planned, regional anaesthesia is safe, and obviates the risk of a hypertensive response to intubation. Regional techniques should be avoided with arteriovenous malformations of the cord.
- If a vaginal delivery is contemplated, epidural analgesia is recommended and pushing in the second stage should be minimised.

Maternal resuscitation

Maternal cardiac arrest is fortunately rare. The basic algorithms for adult resuscitation are appropriate for maternal resuscitation with several important differences:

- After 20 weeks' gestation, the mother must be tilted to minimize aortocaval occlusion. The tilt is ideally provided by a wooden support, but if this is not available an assistant can kneel beside the arrested individual. The hips can then be wedged on to the knees of the assistant.
- After 20 weeks' gestation the fetus should be delivered as soon as possible. This improves the chance of maternal survival and that of a term fetus as aortocaval compression severely limits the effectiveness of chest compressions. The fetus is likely to be severely acidotic and hypoxic at delivery.
- Remember that pregnant women have reduced oesophageal sphincter tone and that cricoid pressure and intubation should both be performed as rapidly as possible.
- Normal resuscitation drugs should be used. Adrenaline is the drug of choice despite its effect on uterine circulation.
- Adrenaline is also the drug of choice in major anaphylactic or anaphylactoid reactions. Severe hypotension associated with anaphylaxis results in a very poor fetal outcome. Early delivery is vital for the fetus.
- Consideration should be given to the diagnosis and treatment of obstetric causes of maternal arrest.

Common causes of maternal arrest include:
- haemorrhage
- pulmonary embolism
- amniotic fluid embolus
- cerebral haemorrhage
- intracranial haemorrhage
- myocardial infarction
- iatrogenic events:
  - hypermagnesaemia–treat with 10 ml of 10% calcium chloride
  - high or total spinal–supportive treatment
  - local anaesthetic induced arrhythmia.

Amniotic fluid embolism

Amniotic fluid embolism is the third most common cause of maternal death in the United Kingdom. It is clinically diagnosed (although aspiration of fetal tissue from pulmonary catheters may subsequently confirm the diagnosis) and estimates of its incidence vary widely, but are of the order of 1in 25 000 live births. It is unclear whether the devastating effects of amniotic fluid embolism are due to the amniotic fluid itself or due to an anaphylactic response to fetal tissue that has been introduced into the maternal circulation. Within the first 30 min after amniotic fluid embolism, intense pulmonary vasoconstriction occurs and is associated with right heart failure, hypoxia, hypercarbia, and acidosis. This is followed by left heart failure and pulmonary oedema. A coagulopathy is to be expected.

Incidence of amniotic fluid embolism is increased with:

- age >25 years
- multiparous women
- obstructed labour, particularly in association with uterine stimulants
- multiple pregnancy
- short labour.

Clinical features include:

- sudden collapse with acute hypotension and fetal distress
- pulmonary oedema (>90%) and cyanosis (80%)
- coagulopathy (80%) (haemorrhage may be concealed)
- fits (50%)
- cardiac arrest (occurs in nearly 90% of women).[26]

Little advance has been made on treatment of this devastating condition, although care with the use of uterine stimulants and timely diagnosis of obstructed labour may help to reduce the incidence. Once amniotic fluid embolism has occurred, treatment is purely supportive:

- Airway, breathing, and circulation.
- Senior individuals should be present (obstetric, anaesthetic, paediatric and midwifery).
- Haematology services should be alerted, as large quantities of blood products may be required.
- Early delivery of the fetus is vital for both maternal and fetal survival.
- Pulmonary arterial catheterization may be useful to guide ionotropic support and measure right and left side filling pressures.
- Measure coagulation profile regularly. Platelets, fresh frozen plasma, and cryoprecipitate may all be required.
- Intensive care will be required for those that survive the initial insult.

Early mortality is high (50% within the first hour). Even in those that survive, long-term neurological problems are common.

26 Clark SL, Hankins GDV *et al.* (1995). Amniotic fluid embolism: analysis of the national registry. *American Journal of Obstetrics and Gynecology*, 172, 1156–69.

Cardiac disease and pregnancy

Cardiac disease is the leading cause of indirect maternal death in pregnancy. Although rheumatic disease is now rare, the increasingly elderly maternal population and the increased survival into child-bearing years of the previous generation of patients with complex congenital cardiac malformations, may increase the frequency with which cardiac disease is encountered. Pregnancy and labour often present a severe stress test to these women. As a generality, if a woman was symptomatic with minimal activity before pregnancy, particularly if symptomatic at rest (New York Heart Association Classification III and IV), the course of pregnancy is likely to be stormy and mortality of the order of 20–30% is to be expected. The period of greatest stress is in the immediate postpartum period.

It is beyond the scope of this book to give anything but the broadest plans of how to manage women with cardiac disease during pregnancy:

- Early assessment is vital.
- Plan the delivery–with severe disease, elective caesarean section offers advantage as appropriate personnel can be guaranteed to be present. A combination of obstetricians, anaesthetists, cardiologists, and paediatricians will need to be involved in decision-making.
- Investigations should be performed as indicated. The risk to the fetus from procedures such as chest radiographs are vanishingly small.
- Make sure that the woman is in an appropriate place for delivery (this may be the normal delivery suite or it may be the cardiac theatres in a tertiary centre).
- Remember cardioprophylactic antibiotics both for labour and delivery.
- Avoid ergometrine.
- Use oxytocin only with extreme caution because of its vasodilating effect, which may decompensate an already compromised individual. If oxytocin must be given, use a slow infusion.
- Expect the period of highest risk to be in the 1–2 h post delivery (cardiac output peaks, autotransfusion plus blood loss leads to a variable effect on pre- and afterload).
- Continue management on intensive care if appropriate.

General principles

- Conditions associated with pulmonary hypertension have a very high maternal mortality in pregnancy (>70%).
- Extreme caution is required to avoid sudden changes in afterload for patients with fixed cardiac output.
- Cyanotic heart lesions (i.e. right to left shunts) will not tolerate reductions in systemic vascular resistance. Nevertheless epidural analgesia is sometimes used to minimize the stress of labour, but onset of analgesia must be slow, and phenylephrine is used to maintain afterload. General anaesthesia is probably the technique of choice for caesarean section.
- Aortic stenosis may become symptomatic during pregnancy. Serial echocardiography is often used. Tachycardia and reduction in afterload should be avoided. Loss of sinus rhythm should be treated promptly. General or

slow onset regional anaesthesia have both been advocated for caesarean section. The technique is probably less important than the skill with which it is applied.

- Valvular insufficiencies are usually well tolerated during pregnancy.
- Women with symptomatic Marfan's disease, particularly if the aortic root is dilated, have a high risk of aortic dissection. They are usually maintained on beta-blockers. Unexplained severe chest pain is an indication for a chest radiograph and an echocardiogram.
- Myocardial infarction during pregnancy has a 20% mortality. Infarction occurs most commonly in the third trimester. If possible delivery should be delayed at least 3 weeks after infarction. Both elective caesarean section and vaginal delivery have been advocated. In either case, cardiac stress should be minimised with effective analgesia.

Paediatric and neonatal anaesthesia

Chapter 35
Paediatric and neonatal anaesthesia

Simon Berg

Neonatal/infant physiology

The practice of paediatric anaesthesia embraces a range of patients from the premature neonate to the adolescent. Major differences exist in the anatomy, physiology, and pharmacological response of children and adults. In anaesthetic terms special considerations apply to the neonate. Children pose a different set of problems but these differences become clinically less significant with age.

A neonate is defined as a baby within the first 44 weeks of postconceptual age. The previous definition of the first 4 weeks of life may be misleading for the premature baby. An infant is by convention a child in the first year of life.

Respiratory considerations

- The neonate has limited respiratory reserve.
- Each terminal bronchiole opens into a single alveolus instead of fully developed alveolar clustering. The alveoli are thick-walled and constitute only 10% of the adult total.
- The ribs are horizontally aligned so that the 'bucket handle' action of the adult thorax is not possible. Intercostal muscles are poorly developed and the diaphragm has a more horizontal attachment reducing mechanical advantage. Respiratory muscle fatigue is also more likely.
- Ventilation is essentially diaphragmatic. Abdominal distension may cause splinting of the diaphragm leading to respiratory failure.
- Alveolar minute volume is therefore rate dependent. The resting respiratory rate and oxygen consumption in neonates are approximately double that of adults.
- Closing volume occurs within tidal breathing in the neonate. Minor decreases in functional residual capacity (FRC) increase the pulmonary shunt and lead to lung collapse. The application of continuous positive airway pressure (CPAP) improves oxygenation and reduces the work of breathing.
- The narrow airways result in increased resistance up to the age of 8 years. Nasal resistance represents almost 50% of total airway resistance, accentuating the problem of children with nasal congestion who are obligate nasal breathers.
- Apnoea is a common postoperative problem in preterm neonates. Apnoea is significant if the episode exceeds 15 s or if cyanosis or bradycardia occur. Caffeine given intravenously (10 mg/kg) at induction reduces the incidence of apnoeic episodes by 70%. CPAP may be helpful by the action of distending pressure triggering stretch receptors on the chest wall.
- Due to the higher metabolic rate and alveolar minute volume, volatile agents achieve a more rapid induction and emergence than with adults. They are profound respiratory depressants and as a consequence most anaesthetized neonates require intubation and controlled ventilation.
- A neonate has a PaO_2 of approximately 10 kPa but an oxygen saturation of 97% due to the increased oxygen affinity of HbF (the predominant haemoglobin type at term); pH and $PaCO_2$ are normal within 24 h. Tidal volume and dead space have comparable adult values by the end of the first week of life.

Parameter	Neonate	Adult
Tidal volume (spontaneous) (ml/kg)	7	7–10
Tidal volume (IPPV) (ml/kg)	7–10	10
Dead space (ml/kg)	2.2	2.2
V_D:V_T ratio	0.3	0.3
Respiratory rate	30	15
Compliance (ml/cmH$_2$O)	5	100
Resistance (cmH$_2$O/litre/s)	25	5
Time constant (s)	0.5	1.1
Oxygen consumption (ml/kg/min)	7	3

Parameters for children over 2 years approximate to adult values. The respiratory rate can be estimated from the formula: 24–age/2.

Cardiovascular considerations

- The neonatal heart has small ventricles with reduced contractile mass and poor ventricular compliance. The foramen ovale closes by day one and the ductus arteriosus after 4 weeks.

- Cardiac output is high (200 ml/kg/min) and rate dependent; the neonate can tolerate heart rates of up to 200 beats/min without ill-effect.

- Bradycardia will occur in response to hypoxia and should be managed with oxygenation rather than atropine. A resting neonatal heart rate of below 60 beats/min cannot provide an adequate cardiac output and external cardiac compression should be commenced.

- Pulmonary vascular resistance (PVR) falls at birth in response to rises in PaO$_2$ and pH and a fall in PaCO$_2$. Pulmonary arterial pressure reaches adult levels by 2 weeks.

- Hypoxia and acidosis will increase PVR leading to pulmonary hypertension and the possibility of a right to left shunt through the ductus arteriosus and foramen ovale (transitional circulation).

- A systolic blood pressure of 70–90 mmHg is normal in the term neonate because of the low systemic vascular resistance and may be even lower in the premature baby. Autoregulation of the cerebral circulation is present from birth in the term infant.

- At term autonomic and baroreceptor control is fully functional, although vagally mediated parasympathetic tone predominates. The electrical conducting system is also fully formed.

- The QRS axis is deviated to the right, but a normal axis develops by the end of the neonatal period.

- The incidence of congenital heart disease is 7–8 per 1000 live births, the commonest type of major congenital abnormality; 10–15% of these children have an associated non-cardiac abnormality. All neonates with midline defects should be assessed for related cardiac disease.

Age (years)	Pulse	Mean systolic blood pressure (mmHg)	Mean diastolic blood pressure (mmHg)
Neonate	80–200	50–90	25–60
1	80–160	85–105	50–65
2	80–130	95–105	50–65
4	80–120	95–110	55–70
6	75–115	95–110	55–70
8	70–110	95–110	55–70
10	70–110	100–120	60–75
12	60–110	110–130	65–80

- Mean systolic blood pressure over 1 year can be calculated from the formula:

  90 + (age in years × 2).

Lower limit (5th centile) is:

  70 + (age in years × 2).

Gastrointestinal considerations

- The liver is immature at birth and this is accentuated in prematurity. Metabolic enzyme systems have matured by 12 weeks but some drugs are metabolized more slowly and others by different enzyme pathways from adults. The action of barbiturates and opioids in the neonate is prolonged and enhanced.
- Bilirubin metabolism is affected by a poorly developed glucuronyl transferase system. Rises in unconjugated biliribin may lead to neonatal jaundice or kernicterus by crossing the blood–brain barrier. Some drugs, e.g. sulphonamides, diazepam, vitamin K, displace bilirubin from plasma proteins and exacerbate jaundice.
- Carbohydrate reserves are low in neonates. The premature baby and stressed or sick neonate is vulnerable to hypoglycaemia. Treatment should include 4-hourly blood glucose measurements and an initial intravenous infusion of 10% dextrose although higher concentrations are sometimes required.
- Vitamin K-dependent factors are low at term. The routine administration of vitamin K may prevent haemorrhagic disease of the newborn and should be mandatory before surgery in the first week of life.

Renal considerations

- Nephron formation is complete at term, but renal function is immature. The glomerular filtration rate achieves adult values by 2 years and tubular function by 6–8 months. Renal blood flow is reduced due to high renal vascular resistance.
- Neonates cannot excrete a large solvent or sodium load. Additionally they can only concentrate urea to half its adult capacity as a response to dehydration.

Haematological consideratons

* Circulating blood volume is calculated as follows:
  * neonate: 90 ml/kg
  * infant: 85 ml/kg
  * child: 80 ml/kg.
* Postdelivery haemoglobin concentrations range from 13–20 g/dl (average 18 g/dl) depending on the degree of placental transfusion. Subsequently the haemoglobin concentration falls as the increase in circulating volume exceeds the growth in marrow activity, the 'physiological anaemia of infancy' which usually varies from 10–12 g/dl.
* The predominant haemoglobin type at term is HbF (80–90%). By 4 months this has fallen to 10–15% and been replaced by HbA. HbF has a higher oxygen affinity with a reduced 2,3-diphosphoglycerate (2,3-DPG) level and the oxygen dissociation curve is shifted to the left. In a ventilated neonate, an alkalosis by moving the oxygen dissociation curve further to the left will reduce oxygen availability.
* Conventionally, blood is transfused intra-operatively at 15% blood loss. Ideally transfused blood should be fresh, warmed, filtered, and cytomegalovirus (CMV) negative. However, in most centres fresh whole blood is not available. It can be administered either via a burette or using a syringe and three-way tap.
* A preoperative haemoglobin less than 10 g/dl is abnormal and should be investigated. Cancellation is not always necessary, for example in an ex-premature infant who is otherwise well with no haemodynamic compromise.

Central nervous system considerations

* Neurons are complete at term. Dendritic proliferation, myelination, and synaptic connections develop in the third trimester and first 2 years of life.
* The blood–brain barrier is more permeable in neonates; barbiturates, opioids, antibiotics, and bilirubin all cross more readily.
* The brain contains a high proportion of fat, which may allow volatile agents to reach higher concentrations more rapidly. The minimal alveolar concentration (MAC) of volatile agents is lower in neonates and higher in children relative to adult values.

Weight

Approximate weights can be determined from the following formula:

birth: 3–3.5 kg

3–12 months: weight (kg) = [age (months) + 9]/2

1–6 years; weight (kg) = [age (years) + 4] × 2.

All paediatric patients should, however, be accurately weighed preoperatively, and drug dosing based upon this actual value.

Thermoregulation

- Neonates have a poorly developed thermoregulatory mechanism. They have a high surface area to volume ratio with minimal subcutaneous fat and poor insulation. The vasoconstrictor response is limited and the neonate is unable to shiver.

- Non-shivering thermogenesis is achieved by the metabolism of brown fat found in the back, shoulders, legs, and lagging the major thoracic vessels. However, this metabolism considerably increases oxygen consumption and may worsen pre-existing hypoxia. Brown fat is deficient in premature infants.

- Neonates lose heat during surgery by conduction, convection, and evaporation but predominantly by radiation. The neutral thermal environment is one in which oxygen demand, heat loss, and energy expenditure are minimal. This optimal ambient temperature depends on age, maturity, and weight. Average temperatures are 34 °C for the premature baby, 32 °C for the neonate, and 28 °C in the adult.

- General anaesthetics depress the thermoregulatory response in children and adults; heat is lost from the core to the cooler peripheral tissues. Prolonged hypothermia can lead to a profound acidosis and impaired perfusion. Platelet function is decreased, but clotting factor function remains normal above 32 °C. The duration of opioids and muscle relaxants is prolonged. There is also a reduced ability for wound repair, depressed immune function, and an increased risk of infection.

Measures to conserve heat loss

- Theatres should be heated some time before surgery to warm the walls and raise the ambient temperature. A temperature of 21 °C is adequate for larger children but infants and neonates may require an ambient temperature of 26 °C. In practice this is too hot; a theatre temperature of 21 °C is an adequate compromise if active measures are taken to reduce heat loss and maintain the 'microclimate' around the patient. Doors should stay closed to avoid draughts.

- Avoid exposure of the child; this applies particularly in the anaesthetic room. The head is relatively large in infants and should be covered with a bonnet, gamgee, or even polythene. The rest of the body can also be insulated with warm gamgee.

- Use an active warming device. These include a warming mattress or convective warm air blanket; an overhead radiant heater may be suitable for neonates.

- Humidify and warm anaesthetic gases. Heated water vapour humidifiers are available, but disposable heat and moisture exchangers are usually satisfactory. Use of a circle breathing system also provides a means of warming and humidifying anaesthetic gases.

- Perioperative fluids, especially blood, should be prewarmed.

- Cleaning fluids should be kept warm.

- Temperature measurement is essential in neonatal surgery, paediatric surgery of intermediate to long duration, or where major fluid and blood loss is expected.

Neonatal/infant pharmacology

General principles

* Drugs can be administered by any conventional route. Intramuscular injection is unnecessarily painful and should be avoided if possible. Subcutaneous infusion of opioids is a useful well-tolerated technique for pain relief in the absence of hypovolaemia. In an emergency, fluid resuscitation and anaesthetic drugs can be effectively administered via the intraosseous route.
* Body water content is high, falling to adult values of 60% by 2 years. Fat constitutes 10% by weight at term and reaches 25% at 1 year. Thus the volume of distribution of both hydrophilic and lipophilic drugs will be affected by age.
* The liver is the principal site of drug metabolism, but at birth, the enzyme systems are not fully developed. Glucuronidation activity is particularly reduced in the neonate and does not reach adult levels until 1 year.
* Neonatal morphine metabolism results in morphine-3-glucuronide rather than morphine-6-glucuronide, the principal adult metabolite.

Premedication

* Benzodiazepines are widely used to achieve anxiolysis, a smooth induction, and for their amnesic qualities. Oral midazolam (0.5 mg/kg) has a noticeable effect within 20 min but has worn off after 2 h. Intranasally, the effect is more rapid but it is unpleasant to administer. Temazepam and diazepam are both still commonly used. The longer duration of action makes lorazepam unsuitable for day case surgery.
* Phenothiazines are long acting and have antiemetic and anticholinergic properties. Trimeprazine (2 mg/kg) and promethazine (1 mg/kg) are declining in use.
* Droperidol (0.05–0.1 mg/kg) is only weakly anxiolytic and is given in combination with other premedicant drugs for its anti-emetic effect.
* Choral hydrate and triclofos are used more for sedation than premedication.
* Ketamine 2 mg/kg IM may assist in anaesthesia of the uncooperative child who refuses to accept oral premedication (it can be given orally in doses of 5–6 mg/kg). Its action starts within 15 min but it may be associated with excess salivation and emergence delirium.
* Clonidine given orally (4 μg/kg) produces good conditions for induction and may reduce postoperative analgesic requirements but it is associated with hypotension and a delayed recovery.
* Antisialogogues are no longer used routinely but are reserved for patients with excessive secretions, e.g. Down's syndrome, cerebral palsy, the suspected difficult airway, and co-administration with ketamine. Absorption can be variable if given orally.
* Opioids have declined in use because of the need for intramuscular injection. Their main indication is in cardiac surgery where they may be given in combination with other drugs, e.g. pethidine compound (see p. 815). Fentanyl is available in the United States for use by the oral transmucosal route.

Inhalational agents

- Induction and awakening are more rapid than in the adult.
- Compared with an adult, MAC values are lower in the preterm, roughly equivalent at term and reach higher values between 6 months and 1 year, a rise that is sustained until adolescence.
- All inhalational agents are respiratory depressants. Tidal volume is reduced in a dose-dependent manner and the ventilatory response to CO_2 is obtunded. Hypoxia in the neonate tends to depress rather than stimulate ventilation.
- Nitrous oxide should be avoided in congenital lobar emphysema, pneumothorax, and certain abdominal conditions including necrotizing enterocolitis because of its ability to expand enclosed air spaces.
- Halothane remains a popular anaesthetic. It is well tolerated and provides conditions for a smooth induction. Although 20% is metabolized, there is a negligible incidence of halothane hepatitis in children. Cardiac arrhythmias are more common, especially associated with adrenaline. Its greater solubility and longer duration of action makes it a suitable agent for airway endoscopy.
- Enflurane is mildly irritant and produces a less smooth induction. Respiratory depression is greater than with halothane with little compensatory increase in respiratory rate. Enflurane should be used with caution in children with epilepsy.
- Isoflurane has a pungent odour and is relatively more difficult as an agent for inhalational induction. It is an excellent maintenance agent with rapid awakening.
- Sevoflurane is an ideal inhalational induction agent for children. It is nonirritant and initial concentrations can start as high as 8%. It is more stable haemodynamically than halothane, but bradycardia and apnoea have both been reported at high concentrations. There are reports of emergence delirium with sevoflurane, but the clinical significance of this is unclear.
- Desflurane is the least metabolized of the volatile agents. It requires a special vaporizer and is too pungent to be suitable for induction. However, it is an excellent maintenance agent with a more rapid recovery than sevoflurane.

Induction agents

- Thiopental is still in common use in paediatric practice. It is indicated for neonatal induction but at a reduced dose of 2 mg/kg in the first week of life, approaching normal values by the end of the neonatal period. The infant dosage is higher (4–6 mg/kg) but approaches adult values by 2 years.
- Propofol is now licensed for use as an induction agent for children over 1 month, but not for infusion below 3 years. The TCI pump is not configured for paediatric use. Children up to 8 years may require almost double the adult dosage (3–5 mg/kg). There is a reduction in heart rate, particularly below 2 years, probably related to attenuation of the baroreceptor reflex. There are also larger falls in blood pressure compared with equipotent doses of thiopental. Respiratory depression and the incidence of apnoea are greater than with thiopental, although laryngeal mask insertion is easier due to depression of laryngeal reflexes. Propofol is not contraindicated in epilepsy.

- Ketamine (2 mg/kg) is indicated for induction of the compromised cardiac or neonatal patient, usually in conjunction with fentanyl. It is widely used as a sole agent in developing countries. Ketamine has a favourable haemo-dynamic profile. The dose should be reduced in neonates because of reduced clearance and prolonged metabolism. Emergence phenomena are less common in children, especially in combination with midazolam, but the incidence of PONV and salivation is higher. Ketamine can also be used as part of a sedation technique with midazolam for short procedures such as line insertion, lumbar puncture, and bone marrow aspiration—a drying agent may be required.

- Etomidate is rarely used in paediatric practice. Its indications are for the haemodynamically compromised patient. The end point of induction is not always as clear as other agents and it is associated with increased PONV.

Opioids

- Morphine is less effective than fentanyl in obtunding the surgical stress response. It has a slower onset as it is less lipophilic, and a longer duration of action. It should be used cautiously in neonates because of the risk of respiratory depression. Its principal application is for postoperative analgesia. The administration of morphine increases the incidence of PONV by over 30% and it should be avoided in day surgery.

- Fentanyl is commonly used as an intra-operative opioid (1–5 μg/kg). Dosages of up to 25 μg/kg may be required to obtund the stress response in cardiac surgery. At high concentrations bradycardia, hypotension, respiratory depression, and chest-wall rigidity are all well recognized complications. The neonate is particularly prone to bradycardia, probably from depression of the baroreceptor reflex.

- Alfentanil and remifentanil are comparable in use to adults. They should also be used cautiously in neonates. Bradycardia and hypotension are well-recognized side-effects and can be reduced by slow administration, infusion, or when necessary a vagolytic agent.

Muscle relaxants

- Suxamethonium is still the most rapid onset muscle relaxant with optimal conditions for intubation. In infants, the dose required is double that of adults (2 mg/kg) due to increased volume of distribution.

- With the exception of pancuronium, infants are more sensitive while children are more resistant, to non-depolarizing relaxants compared with adults. Pancuronium appears to have a similar dose profile across all ages. In practice variation in individual response is more important than age-dependent sensitivity and relaxant dosages approximate to adult values.

Fluid balance

* In the neonate, 80% of total body weight is water; the value is higher in the preterm infant and reaches an adult level of 60% by 2 years. Extracellular water constitutes 45% of total body water at term, over 50% in the preterm but attains an adult value of 35% by early childhood. Plasma volume tends to stay constant at 5% of total body weight independent of age.
* The turnover of water is over double that of the adult. Forty per cent of extracellular water is lost daily in infants as urine, faeces, sweat, and insensible losses. A small increase in loss or reduction in intake can rapidly lead to dehydration.
* Fluid maintenance is calculated from calorie requirement, 100 kcal/ kg for the infant, with older children requiring 75 kcal/kg and adults 35 kcal/kg. Each kilocalorie requires 1 ml of water for metabolism.

	Neonatal fluid requirement (ml/kg/day)	
	Term	**Preterm**
Day 1	60	60
Day 2	90	90
Day 3	120	120
Day 4	150	150
Day 5	150	180

Neonatal fluid requirements

* Fluid is initially given cautiously as the kidneys cannot easily excrete a water or sodium load. If under a radiant heater or undergoing phototherapy, 30 ml/kg is added to the regime.
* The fluid of choice is 10% dextrose. This is adjusted in increments of 2.5% to achieve normoglycaemia ideally between 3.5–4 mmol/litre. A blood sugar below 2.6 mmol/litre is treated with 2 ml/kg of 10% dextrose.
* Electrolytes are routinely added as sodium 3 mmol/kg/day and potassium 2 mmol/kg/day. Other electrolytes including calcium are added as indicated.

Paediatric fluid requirements

* The fluid of choice is 4% dextrose/0.18% saline. Maintenance is calculated using the '4–2–1' regime:
  * 4 ml/kg/h (100 ml/kg/day) for each of the first 10 kg
  * 2 ml/kg/h (50 ml/kg/day) for each of the second 10 kg
  * 1 ml/kg/h (25 ml/kg/day) for each subsequent kg.

For example a 5 kg infant needs 20 ml/h or 500 ml/day and a 25 kg child needs 65 ml/h (40 + 20 + 5 ml/h) or 1550 ml/day (1000 + 500 + 50 ml/day).

* Maintenance requirement makes no allowance for extra losses from gastroenteritis, intestinal obstruction, and insensible loss from pyrexia. Additional sodium and potassium may also be required.

- Intra-operative fluid replacement will comprise basic maintenance requirement plus additional amounts to replace other observed fluid losses. These losses are replaced by isotonic crystalloid, i.e. normal saline, Hartmann's solution, colloid, or blood according to clinical need. Regular blood glucose measurement is essential in neonatal surgery.

- Colloid solutions including albumin, gelofusine, and haemaccel are all routinely used in paediatric practice. The recent meta-analysis implicating the use of albumin in increased mortality did not include any studies looking at intra-operative albumin use.

- Blood transfusion is required after 15% blood loss. Blood volume should be calculated prior to surgery. Swabs should be carefully weighed and suction recorded. For convenience blood can be rapidly transfused using a syringe and three-way tap.

Fluid resuscitation

- Assessment of dehydration and hypovolaemia is made predominantly on clinical grounds. Increased capillary refill and core–peripheral temperature gap with a thready pulse are early signs of hypovolaemia. An increased heart rate is not always helpful and may reflect pain, anxiety, or fever. Oliguria and a reduced level of consciousness are late signs. Hypotension does not occur until over 35% of the blood volume is lost.

- Resuscitation in the first instance consists of administering fluid boluses of 20 ml/kg of either isotonic crystalloid or colloid and then reassessing the patient. Blood may also be required and should be transfused to give a haemoglobin concentration greater than 10 g/dl.

- The swing of the arterial or pulse oximeter trace is a valuable aid in assessing intravascular loss.

Anaesthetic equipment

Although principles are similar to adult practice, there are a range of sizes and specific differences in the equipment used in paediatric anaesthesia.

Oropharyngeal airway

- These range in size from 000 to 4 (4 to 10 cm in length).
- They are rarely useful in neonates who are obligate nasal breathers but may be advantageous in mask ventilation to prevent gastric distension. The oropharyngeal airway is often of benefit in syndromic children with suspected airway problems.
- Estimating the size of the airway is crucial. An incorrect size will worsen airway obstruction. The correct length is equal to the distance from the corner of the mouth to the angle of the jaw.
- The airway should not be inverted during insertion in infants as this may potentially damage the palate.

Nasopharyngeal airway

- The nasopharyngeal airway has limited application in paediatric practice. It is tolerated at lighter levels of anaesthesia than an oropharyngeal airway and may be of use during induction and recovery of some congenital airway problems and in children with obstructive sleep apnoea.
- It should be well lubricated prior to insertion; bleeding is a recognized complication from mucosal or adenoidal trauma.
- The appropriate length is equal to the distance from the tip of the nostril to the tragus of the ear.
- If an ET tube is used as a modified nasopharyngeal airway then the size is calculated from the formula age/4 + 3.5.

Facemasks

- Clear plastic masks with an inflatable rim provide an excellent seal for spontaneous and assisted ventilation.
- They have a greater dead space than the traditional black rubber Rendell–Baker masks but they are less threatening and easier to position.
- They are manufactured in a round or tear-drop shape; the round shape is suitable only for neonates and infants. They are also available as flavoured masks.
- The transparent design allows for observation of cyanosis and regurgitation, the presence of breathing, and a qualitative estimate of tidal volume.
- The size is estimated to fit an area from the bridge of the nose to the cleft of the chin.

The laryngeal mask airway (LMA)

- There are a range of sizes suitable for paediatric use (see table below).
- Both the indications and insertion techniques are similar to adult use. An alternative method of insertion used in paediatric practice is to advance the LMA upside down and partially inflated behind the tongue before rotating through 180°.

- Bite blocks should be used with a reinforced LMA to prevent occlusion if the child bites down on the tube. The size 1 LMA is only suitable for short procedures.
- The intubating laryngeal mask airway (ILMA) is now available in size 3 which is potentially useful for older children.

Size of LMA	Weight (kg)	Cuff volume (ml)
1	0–5	2–5
1.5	5–10	5–7
2	10–20	7–10
2.5	20–30	12–14
3	Large child >30	15–20

Laryngoscopes

- Laryngoscope blades are available in different lengths from size 0 to 3 according to the size of the child.
- In addition to the curved Macintosh style blade, a straight-bladed Magill laryngoscope also exists to facilitate infant intubation. There are many eponymous straight blades and preference is a matter of personal choice.
- Polio and McCoy blades are also available as paediatric laryngoscopes.

Endotracheal tubes

- Paediatric endotracheal tubes should be uncuffed until at least 8 years of age.
- Uncuffed tubes are available from 2 mm to size 7 mm. Cuffed tubes start from 5.5 mm.
- Paediatric versions of the RAE, armoured, and laser tubes all exist. Additionally the Cole tube is designed for neonatal resuscitation and a north-facing uncuffed preformed tube has been developed for routine paediatric surgery.
- Unlike adults, the paediatric trachea is conical. Its narrowest part is at the level of the cricoid ring, the only part of the airway completely surrounded by cartilage. If the tracheal tube is too large, it will compress the tracheal epithelium at this level, leading to ischaemia with consequent scarring and the possibility of subglottic stenosis.
- The correctly sized tube is one in which ventilation is adequate but a small audible leak of air is present when positive pressure is applied at 20 cmH$_2$O.
- Paediatric 8.5 mm connectors can be used in addition to the standard 15 mm connector. Catheter mounts should be avoided because of the large dead space involved.

* Infant tube sizes can be estimated as follows:

Weight or age	Tube size (mm)
>2 kg	2.5
2–4 kg	3.0
Term neonate	3.5
3 months–1 year	4.0
Over 2 years	Tube size = age/4 + 4

* Tube size may also approximate to the size of the little finger or diameter of the nostril.
* Tube placement needs to be meticulous to avoid endobronchial intubation or inadvertent extubation.
* Tube length in cm can be calculated as follows:

  age/2 + 12 – oral tube

  age/2 + 15 – nasal tube.
* To assess the length of tube required to be passed below the vocal cords, either the thick black guide line at the distal end of the tube can be used or the approximate distance is equal to the tube size in cm. Ultimately the decision must be confirmed clinically.

Anaesthetic breathing systems

Ayre's T-piece with Jackson–Reece modification

* The Jackson–Reece modification of the Ayre's T-piece (Mapleson F) is the most commonly used circuit in paediatric anaesthetic practice. It is suitable for all children up to 20 kg beyond which it becomes inefficient.
* It is a low-resistance, valveless, lightweight circuit. The expiratory limb exceeds tidal volume to prevent entrainment of room air during spontaneous ventilation.
* The open-ended 500 ml reservoir bag or Jackson–Reece modification allows:
  * an assessment of tidal volume
  * an ability to partially occlude the bag for CPAP or PEEP
  * the potential for assisted or controlled ventilation
  * a qualitative appreciation of lung compliance
  * a reduction in dead space during spontaneous ventilation (fresh gas flow washes out expired gas during the pause after expiration).
* Scavenging is limited. However, newer versions of the T-piece incorporate a closed bag with an expiratory valve and scavenging attachment.
* Requirements for fresh gas flow (FGF) are higher in spontaneous than controlled ventilation. Recommendations are two to three times alveolar minute volume for spontaneous breathing or 1000 ml + 200 ml/kg in controlled ventilation.
* In practice FGF is dependent on the respiratory pattern. A rapid respiratory rate with minimal expiratory pause allows no time for the FGF to flush out the expiratory limb before the next breath ensues and a higher FGF is

required. Conversely, an end expiratory pause during controlled ventilation will help reduce FGF.

- Most children require a minimum FGF of 3 litres, which can then be adjusted to achieve normocapnia and an inspired carbon dioxide concentration of less than 0.6 kPa. Partial rebreathing allows conservation of heat and humidification.

- End tidal carbon dioxide concentration may be underestimated in children below 10 kg from dilution of expired gases. Sampling should be as distal in the circuit as possible.

Humphrey ADE system

- This hybrid system incorporates the Mapleson A, D, and E circuits in one breathing system.

- Studies indicate that the E mode behaves similarly to the T-piece and that the A mode is efficient in children over 10 kg. Both the D and E modes are suitable for controlled ventilation.

- The expiratory valves are of low resistance and do not add appreciably to the work of breathing.

Circle absorption systems

- Low-flow anaesthesia is cost-efficient, reduces atmospheric pollution (nitrous oxide is a greenhouse gas), and conserves warmth and moisture. The reaction of carbon dioxide with soda lime is exothermic producing heat and water.

- The ability to monitor inspiratory and expiratory levels of oxygen, nitrous oxide, carbon dioxide, and volatile agent is mandatory.

- Paediatric circle systems using 15 mm lightweight hose are suitable for children over 5 kg. The unidirectional valves may increase resistance to breathing and should not be allowed to become damp.

- During controlled ventilation, the leak around the endotracheal tube may require gas flows to be increased.

- There is no evidence that compound A, formed by the action of sevoflurane on soda lime, is nephrotoxic in children.

Mechanical ventilation

- Standard adult ventilators are suitable down to 20 kg.

- Below 20 kg, a paediatric ventilator should be able to deliver small tidal volumes, rapid respiratory rates, variable inspiratory flow rates, and different I:E ratios.

- Calculation of tidal volume is meaningless because of compression of gases in the ventilator tubing and a variable leak around the endotracheal tube. More sophisticated ventilators may, however, be capable of measuring expired tidal volume which is of more practical value.

- Some ventilators are designed to work with specific breathing systems. The Newton valve converts the Nuffield Penlon 200 ventilator from flow generator to pressure generator and can be attached directly to the expiratory limb of the Ayre's T-piece. Many new anaesthetic workstations incorporate integral ventilators attached to circle systems suitable for paediatric practice.

- Pressure controlled ventilation is commonly used in paediatric practice and reduces the risk of barotrauma and pneumothorax. This mode will compensate for a leak around the endotracheal tube, but not for changes in lung compliance, partial or complete tube obstruction, or bronchospasm.

- Volume control can make an allowance for changes in lung compliance but at a potential cost of high peak airway pressures.

- Ultimately, setting ventilator parameters is based on clinical observation. Inspiratory flow, pressure, or volume is gradually increased until adequate chest movement is observed. Measurement of capnography and pulse oximetry confirms normocapnia and adequate oxygenation. The peak airway pressure is kept to a minimum. A ventilator alarm is mandatory.

- Most children can be ventilated adequately with inspiratory pressures of 18–20 cmH$_2$O and a respiratory rate between 16 and 24/min. The rate can be adjusted accordingly to achieve normocapnia.

- The ability to hand ventilate using the Ayre's T-piece is essential to paediatric practice. A circuit should always be available in the event of ventilator failure or unexpected desaturation. Mechanical ventilation may be inadequate for the small premature neonate. In the baby with gastroschisis or exomphalos, hand ventilation can be used to assess changes in lung compliance and determine how much of the abdominal contents can be reduced back into the abdominal cavity. Hand ventilation during repair of a tracheo-oesophageal fistula can be timed to allow the surgeon maximum exposure and time to effect the repair.

Conduct of anaesthesia

Preoperative assessment

The preoperative visit is essential in establishing a rapport with both parents and children and in helping to dissipate anxiety. Communication should be simple, informative and truthful:

- Avoid wearing a white coat. Involve the parents, but try to question the child directly when appropriate and stay at eyelevel if possible.
- A preadmission visit reduces parental anxiety and is beneficial to children over 6 years. Play therapists can help provide an informal setting and informatively prepare the child by describing the course of events from the ward to induction of anaesthesia. A collection of photographs or a video may be helpful.

History

- Problems with previous anaesthetics, e.g. PONV, poor pain relief, or difficult venous access. Include a family history to exclude malignant hyperpyrexia and suxamethonium apnoea.
- Previous hospital admissions.
- Current medical conditions.
- Cardiovascular assessment—known heart murmurs, whether blue or breathless on exercise, or failure to thrive if neonate.
- Respiratory assessment—asthma, frequent colds, obstructive sleep apnoea. The patient may have a current chest infection (see p. 774).
- Neonatal history—problems at delivery, prematurity, admission to special care baby unit including duration and severity of problem.
- Drug history.
- Allergy—drugs, latex.
- Immunization—children may develop a viral-like malaise and pyrexia following certain vaccinations. Surgery should be avoided for 1 week following DTP (diphtheria/tetanus/pertussis) and Hib (Haemophilus influenzae type B) and 2 weeks after MMR (measles/ mumps/rubella).

Examination

- Airway—check mouth opening, loose teeth, drooling, large tongue, enlarged tonsils, micrognathia, short neck.
- Cardiovascular system—check colour (consider pulse oximeter), heart murmurs.
- Respiratory system—check nasal secretions, wheeze or added breath sounds, shape of thorax, kyphoscoliosis or other spinal deformity.
- Central nervous system—check loss of airway reflexes, hypotonia.

Preoperative investigations

Routine preoperative haemoglobin is indicated for:

- neonates
- ex-premature infants under 1 year
- children at risk of sickle cell disease

- children for whom intra-operative transfusion may be necessary
- children with systemic disease.
- A preoperative Hb of less than 10 g/dl does not necessarily entail cancellation if the child is otherwise well.

Routine biochemistry is required for:

- children with metabolic endocrine or renal diseases
- children receiving intravenous fluids.

The child with a cold

- The preschool child develops an average of six to eight upper respiratory tract infections (URTI) per year. Almost 25% of children have a runny nose for the majority of the year. This group may have seasonal rhinitis or chronically infected adenoids.
- Anaesthesia in the presence of an intercurrent URTI is associated with a higher risk of complications. There is an increased incidence of excess secretions, airway obstruction, laryngospasm, and bronchoconstriction. This risk is increased five-fold using an LMA and by a factor of 10 if the child is intubated. Complications are also higher with infants.
- Children with moderate to severe chest infections should be postponed. This will include those with productive cough, purulent chest or nasal secretions, pyrexia, and signs of viraemia or constitutional illness, including diarrhoea and vomiting with loss of appetite.
- The child with a mild cold is always a difficult problem. The history in these cases is crucial. It is important to decide whether the child is at the beginning or end of the URTI. Other members of the family or children at school may have already experienced the same infection and this can provide useful information.
- A child deemed to be postviral, apyrexial, with no chest signs, and constitutionally well is probably fit for surgery even if they have a runny nose.
- An intercurrent URTI requires postponement for 2 weeks, but this should be 4 weeks if lower respiratory tract involvement is suspected. A diagnosis of bronchiolitis or measles warrants a delay of at least 6 weeks.

The child with a murmur

The majority of pathological murmurs are diagnosed neonatally and these children will already be under the care of a cardiologist. Antibiotic prophylaxis will apply in certain conditions. Previously unreported murmurs are commonly heard at 2–4 years. The majority are functional. If the murmur is pansystolic with normal heart sounds in a child with a normal oxygen saturation and no limitation in exercise tolerance, it can be assumed to be innocent. If there are any doubts, surgery should be deferred until a formal assessment has been made by a paediatric cardiologist.

Consent

- Allow time at the end of preoperative assessment for parents to ask questions.
- Discuss the options of intravenous or inhalational induction and obtain consent for a suppository and regional or peripheral nerve block, if indicated, including attendant risks.

- Discuss the risks associated with general anaesthesia. Anaesthesia for a fit child is as safe as travelling in an aeroplane.
- Signed written consent is the preferred option.

Local anaesthetic creams

- The availability of topical local anaesthetic preparations reduces the pain of venepuncture and greatly facilitates intravenous induction.
- Emla Cream is a eutectic mixture of 5% lidocaine (lignocaine) and 5% prilocaine in a 1:1 ratio. It should be applied for at least 45 min and can produce vasconstriction. Emla should be avoided in children under 1 year because of the risk of methaemoglobinaemia from absorbed prilocaine due to reduced levels of methaemoglobin reductase.
- Ametop is a 4% gel formulation of amethocaine. There is a shorter onset time of 30 min and prolonged duration of action (4 h) compared with Emla. It is licensed from 4 weeks of age and has vasodilating properties. There may be a higher incidence of allergic reactions.
- It is important to identify the veins to be anaesthetized and not blindly apply the cream to the dorsum of each hand. Veins in the wrist and on the dorsum of the foot should not be forgotten.
- Keep the area bandaged to prevent removal or licking of cream!

Preoperative fasting (see also p. 9)

- Fasting instructions are designed to minimize the risk of regurgitation of gastric contents and consequent pulmonary aspiration.
- Fasting minimizes gastric volumes but does not guarantee an empty stomach. Ideally gastric pH should be greater than 2.5 and gastric fluid should be less than 0.4 ml/kg. Prolonged fasting does not further reduce the risk of aspiration and in infants can easily lead to dehydration and hypoglycaemia.
- Infants may be at greater risk of regurgitation. There is reduced lower oesophageal sphincter tone and an increased tendency to distend the stomach during mask ventilation. However, the incidence of pneumonitis following aspiration in children is much less common than in adults.
- Clear fluids can be given safely up to 2 h preoperatively. The intake of fluids given as either water or a fruit squash drink should be encouraged. It reduces the incidence of dehydration. Children are less irritable at induction and there may be a reduction in postoperative nausea and vomiting.
- The data for milk and solid food are less clear. Breast milk is cleared from the stomach more rapidly than formula milk in infants and both have shorter transit times than solid food.
- Current evidence suggests that children may safely be given either breast or formula milk up to 4 h preoperatively while solid food requires a minimal 6 h fast.

Fasting guidelines

	Minimum fasting time (h)
Clear fluid	2
Breast milk	4
Formula/cows' milk	4–6
Solid food	6

- Every unit should have fasting guidelines which should be sent to parents some days before planned admission for surgery. Close liaison with the ward staff ensures that children receive adequate clear fluid preoperatively and that milk feeds for neonates and infants are appropriately timed.
- Surgeons should be encouraged not to change the list order. This is unacceptable with neonates and small infants, but the ability to take clear fluid may afford some flexibility with older children.

Premedication

- Routine sedative premedication for all children is unnecessary.
- Some children will require preoperative sedation. They include the excessively upset child, children with previous unpleasant experiences of anaesthesia and surgery, and certain children with developmental delay. Older children or adolescents may request premedication.
- Infants have not yet developed a fear of strangers and appear relatively undisturbed when separated from their mothers. The preschool child is most at risk. They are vulnerable to separation anxiety in a strange environment but without the ability to reason.
- Even when anaesthesia and surgery are uneventful, there may be a disturbingly high incidence of postoperative psychological problems. Sleeping disturbance, nightmares, bed-wetting, eating disorders, and behavioural changes have all been reported. Some authors suggest that sedative premedication especially in the preschool age group may reduce parental anxiety, improve patient compliance, and reduce the incidence of some of these postoperative behavioural changes.
- Oral midazolam (0.5 mg/kg) is an ideal premedicant. It acts within 15–30 min to reduce anxiety leading to a more cooperative child, but with minimal delay in recovery. The intravenous formulation is used, but is extremely bitter and should be diluted in concentrated fruit juice (paracetamol elixir is also suitable and has the merit of incorporating an analgesic component to the premedicant).
- Alternative premedicants are listed on p. 815. They tend to be less predictable and longer lasting. Some such as trimeprazine have the advantage of including both a drying and antiemetic action.
- Modern anaesthetic agents do not require the routine use of anticholinergic agents.
- Antisialogogue drugs are indicated for the suspected problem airway and the excessively drooling child. Some anaesthetists still routinely give drying agents for neonates and the smaller child.
  - The absorption of orally administered atropine (40 µg/kg) is variable.
  - To ensure efficacy administer atropine 20 µg/kg IM 30 min preoperatively or 10 µg/kg IV at induction. Atropine should also precede administration of suxamethonium to protect against possible bradycardia.
- Children undergoing cardiac surgery are traditionally heavily premedicated. Choices include morphine, which may prevent right ventricular infundibular spasm in uncorrected Fallot's tetralogy, or a combination of drugs, e.g. Peth Co, which comprises a mixture of pethidine, promethazine, and phenergan.

Parents in the anaesthetic room

- In the United Kingdom a parent is routinely allowed into the anaesthetic room while their child is anaesthetized. It is now accepted that enforced separation disempowers the parent and is an emotionally traumatic experience for both parent and child.
- Parents are naturally anxious over loss of control, a strange environment, and the possibility of adverse events. Unfortunately this parental anxiety may communicate itself to the child.
- Parental presence should not be compulsory. It is not always beneficial and may even be counterproductive with a very anxious parent. Evidence of benefit has only been demonstrated for children older than 4 years with a calm parent attending the induction.
- Preschool children are especially at risk of behavioural disturbance, probably because of difficulties in reasoning. In contrast some adolescents may not wish their parents to accompany them.
- Anaesthetic induction appears to be the most distressing event experienced by parents. Separation from the child after induction, watching the child become unconscious, and the degree of stress experienced by the child before induction are all important factors.
- The parent should always be accompanied by a nurse who can comfort them and escort them out of the anaesthetic room once the child is asleep. It is extremely unusual to allow more than one parent into the anaesthetic room. There may rarely be extenuating circumstances but these should be discussed beforehand with the anaesthetist.

Induction of anaesthesia

- Induction should occur in a child-friendly environment.
- A dedicated paediatric theatre is not always an option. An alternative is a customized paediatric anaesthetic trolley incorporating a comprehensive range of airway and vascular equipment.
- Prepare drugs and equipment before the child arrives. Recheck the weight, using the formula: weight (in kg) = (age + 4) × 2. Precalculate the dose of atropine and suxamethonium in prepared syringes should the need arise to administer these drugs urgently.
- The pulse oximeter is the minimum monitoring acceptable in the anaesthetic room, although it will not read accurately on the agitated child. However, many children will tolerate an ECG and BP cuff prior to induction.

Inhalational induction

- It is important to learn more than one method. Not all children are susceptible to the same technique.
- Sevoflurane is the volatile agent of choice. It is rapidly acting, giving a smooth induction with less cardiovascular depression than halothane. It is not odourless, but is relatively non-irritant. Start the induction with 8% sevoflurane in 70% nitrous oxide with 30% oxygen.
- Halothane is an alternative agent, but induction should proceed through incremental increases in halothane concentration.
- Involve the parent as much as possible. This may involve holding the child or even participating in the induction.
- Position the child either supine on the trolley or across the lap of the parent so that the parent or anaesthetic assistant can gently restrain the arms if necessary. Warn the parent that the child's head will become floppy and need support.
- For smaller children, a cupped hand method is useful. Occlude the end of the bag to direct all the fresh gas flow towards the patient's mouth and nose.
- A facemask is often tolerated by older children. This can be held by the parent, child, or anaesthetist and the child can be encouraged to blow up the bag 'like a balloon'. A flavoured facemask may be useful initially but the volatile agent rapidly becomes the dominant smell within the facemask.
- The parent should be warned of abnormal movements when the child is nearly anaesthetized.
- Once anaesthesia is achieved and the eyelash reflex is absent, anaesthesia can be maintained with another volatile agent if desired.

Intravenous induction

- Although IV induction has been made easier with the advent of local anaesthetic cream, it should not be attempted if venous access is obviously difficult.
- The smaller child sits across the parent's lap and the arm is placed under and through the parent's axilla, thereby obstructing the child's view. The anaesthetic assistant gently squeezes the arm to occlude venous but not

arterial supply and the skin is stretched. Alternatively the anaesthetist compresses the wrist with the non-cannulating hand. The older child will usually lie on the trolley with the parent on one side of the trolley holding the child's hand, while the other is cannulated.

- The induction agent of choice is propofol 3–5 mg/kg with 1% lidocaine (lignocaine) (1 ml/10 ml) added to reduce pain on injection.

- Thiopental at a dose of 3–5 mg/kg is a suitable alternative and is licensed for neonates.

- Ketamine 2 mg/kg is reserved for haemodynamically compromised patients or those with severe cardiovascular disease, usually in conjunction with fentanyl 1–2 µg/kg.

Comparison of intravenous and inhalational induction

- IV induction is simple and safer but is associated with more hypoxia. This may be because children are rarely preoxygenated.

- Inhalational induction produces more coughing and laryngospasm.

- Psychological studies suggest that inhalational induction may be more traumatic to the child but the majority of children under 8 years choose this technique if given the choice.

- In practice it seems prudent to opt for IV induction if possible unless the child actively chooses an inhalational method.

Tips for cannulation

- Problems in securing IV access can be difficult even for paediatric anaesthetists! It is important to realize this, relax, and send for help if necessary. Good lighting, competent anaesthetic assistance, and a selection of cannulas with prepared saline-flush syringes are all essential.

- Neonates often have surprisingly good superficial veins on the hand or wrist. Otherwise healthy children between 3 months and 2 years can be notoriously difficult because of the fat pad over both the hand and foot.

- Compression of a limb should act as a venous rather than arterial tourniquet. The skin is often mobile and should be gently stretched.

- Examine the wrists and dorsum of feet for superficial veins. The scalp is a possibility for neonates but it is difficult to secure. The long saphenous and cephalic veins may be palpated.

- In some children, most commonly in the feet, the skin is surprisingly tough and a small nick in the skin with a 21G needle may be necessary especially with small cannulas. Loosening the cap of the cannula will permit flashback of blood in small veins.

- Unlike adults transfixion is possible in smaller children. It is a potentially useful technique for all veins but especially in 'blind' long saphenous and femoral vein cannulation.

- If all else fails, intraosseous access can be an invaluable alternative. Observing aseptic precautions, prepare an area of skin over the anteromedial aspect of the tibia 1 cm below and medial to the tibial tuberosity. The intraosseous needle is inserted perpendicularly to the skin and advanced in a twisting pushing movement against the bone until there is a sudden loss of resistance. The position is confirmed if the needle remains upright without support, marrow can be aspirated, and fluid can be administered without subcutaneous swelling around the entry site. Children can be successfully anaesthetized via this route although thiopental should be avoided because of its irritant properties. The intraosseous route is particularly useful in fluid resuscitation of the shocked child before definitive intravenous access can be gained.

- The surgical cut-down is rarely needed, often technically difficult, and should be reserved as an absolutely last resort.

Airway management

- Airway complications including coughing, laryngospasm, and upper airways obstruction are more common in children.
- The cornerstone to airway management as with adults is the triple manoeuvre of head tilt, chin lift, and jaw thrust.
- Hyperextension of the neck in the neonate often worsens the airway and a neutral position is usually more successful. For older children, the adult 'sniffing the morning air' position should be adopted.
- Smaller children do not require a pillow; this may lead to unwanted head flexion.
- The paediatric facemask should be accurately sized and held gently but firmly on the face with the thumb and forefinger. The other fingers should curl around and grip the mandible. It is important to avoid pressing on the floor of the mouth, which will push the tongue forward and obstruct the airway.
- Early use of an oropharyngeal airway may be useful in older children.
- A nasopharyngeal airway may be attempted. This should be well lubricated. It is indicated in cases of micrognathia and can be inserted at lighter levels of anaesthesia.
- The most important technique in management of the airway is judicious use of CPAP. Ensure a good seal with the facemask then partially occlude the bag on the Ayre's T-piece.

Laryngospasm

- Laryngospasm is more common in children than adults. Additional risk factors include inhalational induction, asthma, chronic lung disease, and an intercurrent upper respiratory tract infection.
- Children become cyanosed more rapidly than adults because of increased metabolic rate/oxygen consumption and reduced FRC.
- Contrary to the old adage, children do not 'always take a final breath'. Bradycardia is a premorbid event indicating inadequate cardiac output and a significant risk of cerebral hypoxia.
- Partial laryngospasm management:
  - 100% oxygen
  - CPAP
  - gentle assisted ventilation
  - propofol 1–2 mg/kg bolus.
- Complete laryngospasm management:
  - 100% oxygen
  - CPAP
  - assisted ventilation may exacerbate the condition by inflating the stomach and forcing the arytenoids and false cords against the true vocal cords.
  - Early administration of suxamethonium 2 mg/kg and atropine 10 µg/kg may be necessary.

Intubation

◆ Neonatal intubation is not difficult, only different. The neonatal head is proportionately larger than the adult's with a shorter neck, large tongue, and small mandible. The larynx is more anterior and superior at a level of C3–C4 compared with C5–C6. The epiglottis is large, floppy, and V-shaped. Awake intubation for neonates is no longer acceptable. In the absence of medical conditions with recognized airway complications, paediatric intubation is usually straightforward.

◆ Below 6 months of age, use a straight-bladed laryngoscope. The head should be in a neutral position and the shoulders supported if necessary. Advance the laryngoscope blade past the larynx then withdraw slowly until the larynx becomes visible, i.e. the blade is posterior to the epiglottis. Gentle cricoid pressure is often helpful. If nasal intubation is required use a laryngoscope blade with minimal guttering to allow more room for instrumentation in the oropharynx.

◆ Over 6 months of age a curved blade is usually easier. Intubation can be performed in the conventional adult position with the blade resting in the vallecula.

◆ Most intubated neonates will also require a nasogastric tube (8–10FG).

◆ The formulae used to calculate tube size and length represent approximations. It is important to have a range of endotracheal tubes available including a half size above and below the original estimation.

◆ Complications are common in children. Oesophageal and endobronchial intubation, extubation, kinking of the tube, and disconnection should all be anticipated. Secretions are far more likely to cause obstruction because of the smaller tube sizes involved, and periodic suction may be necessary.

◆ Intubation increases the work of breathing. The reduction in cross-sectional area of the neonatal trachea with a size 3.5 tube in situ increases airway resistance by a factor of 16. As a result of this and the respiratory depressant effects of volatile agents, most intubated infants should undergo controlled ventilation as part of the anaesthetic technique.

Tube fixation

◆ Tube fixation is crucial. The neonatal trachea is only 4 cm in length. Inadvertent extubation and endobronchial intubation is common.

◆ The tube should be secured in a 'three-point fixation' to prevent movement of the tube in all three planes.

◆ Two pieces of trouser-shaped Elastoplast may be used with one 'leg' across the upper lip while the other 'leg' is wrapped around the tube. An oropharyngeal airway helps splint the tube.

◆ There are numerous other methods of fixation, all equally valid. Wherever possible the tube should be secured to the maxilla rather than the more mobile mandible.

◆ The preformed north-facing uncuffed endotracheal tube is easy to use, facilitates tube fixation, and reduces the incidence of endobronchial intubation.

The difficult intubation

* The key to difficult intubation is to identify the at-risk patient and plan an elective induction accordingly with appropriate help, assistance, and equipment. Some conditions are well known to be associated with airway problems (e.g. Pierre–Robin, Treacher–Collins, and Goldenhar syndromes). Other patients can be identified by assessment of the airway preoperatively.

* The child should be premedicated with atropine 20 µg/kg IM or glycopyrrolate 5 µg/kg IM 30 min preoperatively, to dry secretions, and ephedrine or pseudoephedrine nose drops. Sedative premedication should be avoided.

* Airway management may be difficult (see earlier). The traditional method is deep inhalational anaesthesia with CPAP, and an IV in situ. Laryngoscopy and intubation are attempted with the patient breathing spontaneously. Halothane is more suitable than sevoflurane at this stage allowing more time for intubation. McCoy and polio blades are both available in paediatric sizes.

* A blind nasal approach to intubation is possible, but experience in the technique is declining.

* The LMA will often secure the airway adequately without the need for intubation.

* If intubation is still necessary, it may be possible to pass a bougie through the LMA into the trachea and then railroad an endotracheal tube. A fibreoptic bronchoscope can be employed using the same technique. A size 3 ILMA is available and may be suitable for a larger child.

* Fibreoptic intubation is not usually necessary. Children will still need to be anaesthetized but a propofol infusion is a good alternative method to volatile anaesthesia. The smaller size neonatal and paediatric bronchoscopes do not all have a suction channel and should be checked to confirm that the selected tracheal tube will fit over them.

* Conventional tubes may present problems in railroading because of the angles involved and armoured tubes should be used. Alternatively a guidewire can be inserted into the trachea using the suction channel and the tube passed over it.

* Tracheostomies are rarely required. They are exceedingly difficult as an emergency procedure. Paediatric cricothyroidotomy cannulas are available at 18G and 16G sizes and should be present in the anaesthetic room.

Rapid sequence induction

- The indications for rapid sequence induction (RSI) in children are the same as in adults.
- Ranitidine and metoclopramide are not routinely prescribed.
- Preoxygenation does not usually present problems with infants and older children but may be more difficult in preschool age children. Inhalational induction may on occasion be necessary.
- The administration of suxamethonium should be preceded by atropine to prevent bradycardia. There is little experience as yet with rocuronium.
- The application of cricoid pressure often facilitates intubation. If intubation cannot be achieved initially, mask ventilation should recommence while cricoid pressure is maintained.
- A nasograstric tube should be routinely used. If already in situ in the neonate it should remain in place rather than being removed. There is no consensus for older children.
- Since the endotracheal tube is uncuffed, a throat pack may help prevent intra-operative aspiration but has no application in the higher-risk periods of induction and reversal.
- The child should be extubated awake in the left lateral position.

Maintenance

- Position the infant and smaller child with both arms raised at the level of the head. Exposure of the hand allows assessment of the pulse, peripheral temperature, colour, and capillary refill. A blocked IV infusion may be more easily cleared and a new cannula may be easier to site.

- The pulse oximeter probe should be sited on the same arm as the IV infusion and contralateral arm to the BP cuff. Avoid oximeter probes on the feet as the trace is usually lost once abdominal surgery commences.

- Check that the endotracheal tube is still in situ and securely fixed and the lungs are ventilating adequately and equally. The connections should all be secure and the tube and breathing circuit supported if necessary.

- Confirm that the cannulas are secure, working, and accessible, especially if sited on the feet; extension tubing may be necessary. A three-way tap allows administration of drugs and fluid volume when necessary. Avoid allowing air bubbles into the IV lines by using a bubble trap. Neonatal surgery requires a minimum of two cannulas, for maintenance and volume. Blood sugar should be checked regularly.

- The theatre temperature should be 21 °C and it should have been preheated for at least 30 min. The child's head should be covered and body exposure reduced to a minimum. It is easier to prevent hypothermia than to treat it. Methods of warming the child include an electric warming mattress, overhead radiant heater, and convective warm air blanket. Both intravenous and cleaning fluid should be warmed.

- Routine monitoring will include ECG, blood pressure (with appropriate size cuff), pulse oximeter, capnography, and full gas monitoring with a ventilator alarm when indicated. Temperature measurement is important and the neonate requires routine use of a precordial or oesophageal stethoscope.

- Electronic monitoring is often unreliable with the sick or shocked neonate. It should support but not replace clinical observation. The oesophageal or precordial stethoscope permits a continuous qualitative assessment of heart sounds and ventilation. More importantly, it 'ties' the anaesthetist to the patient.

- Do not let the surgeon start operating until you are ready.

- Anaesthetic complications in paediatric practice are as common during maintenance as at induction or in the postoperative period.

Reversal

- At the end of surgery, the child should be warm, well saturated, normocarbic, and pain free. A cold acidotic neonate will not breathe postoperatively.

- The LMA can be removed either deep or awake. If an armoured LMA is in situ a bite block will be needed. There is often a stage shortly before waking when the mouth opens slightly to resemble a small yawn; this is an ideal opportunity to deftly remove the LMA.

- Most children should be extubated awake. If warm, and with adequate analgesia, this is tolerated well. Exceptions include tonsillectomy and other procedures when coughing is to be avoided. In these cases, deep extubation is preferable.
- Neonates should be extubated awake preceded by an assisted ventilation to prefill the lungs with 100% oxygen.

Postoperative pain relief

- The same principles as in adult patients apply to paediatric practice including the application of multimodal analgesia and specialized pain charts.
- Paracetamol and NSAIDs are widely prescribed for minor cases and day surgery and also for their morphine-sparing effects for major surgery. The loading dose of rectal paracetamol should be at least 30 mg/kg.
- Caudal analgesia and peripheral nerve blocks are useful for day cases. Epidural blockade is of proven benefit in abdominal surgery. Below 6 months it is technically easier and possibly safer to insert the catheter via the caudal route.
- Morphine infusions can be administered cautiously to neonates and as nurse-controlled analgesia (NCA) for smaller children. Patient-controlled analgesia (PCA) can be used effectively in children as young as 6 years, although most regimes include a background infusion.
- Liaison with the ward staff is crucial and a standardized pain management approach is the ideal (see below). More detailed analgesic protocols are included in paediatric drug guidelines (see p. 816).

Example of pain management regime

Pain intensity	Treatment
Mild	Paracetamol or diclofenac
Moderate	Paracetamol + diclofenac
Moderate +	Paracetamol + diclofenac + codeine phosphate
Moderate ++	Paracetamol + diclofenac+ oromorph
Severe	Morphine infusion or NCA or PCA
	Consider epidural infusion

Postoperative nausea and vomiting

- Postoperative nausea and vomiting (PONV) is uncommon under the age of 2 years.
- Children particularly at risk include those having adenotonsillectomy or squint surgery, a positive history of travel sickness and a previous history of PONV. Morphine increases the risk of PONV by 30%.
- There is no proven benefit to employing a total intravenous technique in children.
- Combinations of antiemetics and the use of 5-HT$_3$ antagonists with low-dose dexamethasone may be more efficacious than simple monotherapy.
- Children at risk from PONV should receive ondansetron 0.1 mg/kg IV prophylactically in the first instance.

Regional anaesthesia

- Successful regional blockade provides conditions for light and haemodynamically stable general anaesthesia. The stress response is attenuated and early pain-free emergence is possible leading to a smooth postoperative recovery.
- Unlike adults, few children tolerate these techniques awake and the majority of regional blocks are performed with anaesthetized patients. Because of this, motor blockade is unnecessary and lower concentrations of local anaesthetic can be used. The most widely used solutions are 0.25% bupivacaine and 0.2% ropivacaine.

Caudal block

- Caudal extradural analgesia (CEA) has a wide application in children. The technique is easier than with adults with a higher success rate of approximately 95%.
- CEA can achieve a higher dermatomal block than adults. Epidural fat is less dense and less tightly packed with the result that local anaesthetic can spread more easily.
- CEA is used for a range of surgical and orthopaedic procedures below the umbilicus.

Technique

- Position the patient in the left lateral position with the legs flexed at the hip. Aseptic technique is a prerequisite.
- Identify the sacral hiatus as the apex of an equilateral triangle with the base formed by a line joining the posterior superior iliac spines.
- Alternatively with the hips flexed at 90° a line extended from the mid-line of the femur will intersect with the sacral hiatus. The natal cleft does not always correspond to bony midline structures.
- Define the boundaries of the sacral hiatus. This is again a triangle with the base formed by a line joining the sacral cornua and the apex representing the lower part of the fourth sacral vertebra. The sacral hiatus is covered by the sacrococcygeal membrane.
- Make a small nick in the skin with a needle to reduce the possibility of a dermoid. Direct a blunt, short-bevel (regional block) needle at 60° to the skin from the midpoint of the line joining the sacral cornua. Alternatively use a 22G or 20G cannula depending on the size of the child. A small 'give' indicates penetration of the sacrococcygeal membrane. Flatten the cannula or needle slightly, then advance. If using a cannula, withdraw the stylet to just behind the cannula before advancing the cannula into the caudal space. Do not advance the needle or cannula any more than is necessary.
- Advancement of a cannula rather than needle may reduce the incidence of inadvertent dural or vascular puncture. Easy progression of the cannula is a good prognostic indicator of success.
- Test aspiration should be gentle; vessel walls can collapse producing a false negative result. Aspiration should then be repeated during injection of the local anaesthetic. A 'whoosh' test using air should be avoided because of the risk of air embolus.

- The commonest reason for a failed attempt is from positioning the needle too caudally.

Dosage

- The Armitage regime (using 0.25% bupivacaine or 0.2% ropivacaine)

Required block	Volume (ml/kg)
Lumbasacral	0.5
Thoracolumbar	1
Mid thoracic	1.25

- If the calculated volume is greater than 20 ml, use 0.19% bupivacaine (three parts local anaesthetic to one part saline).
- The duration of the block averages 4–8 h using this regime.
- Caudal blockade can be extended with:
  - clonidine 1 µg/kg
  - diamorphine 30 µg/kg
  - ketamine 0.5 mg/kg (preservative-free)
  - morphine 50 µg/kg (preservative-free).
- Adrenaline has been implicated in cases of spinal ischaemia and should be avoided. Clonidine produces postoperative sedation. Morphine and diamorphine increase the incidence of urinary retention and should be reserved for surgery in which catheterization is required.

Advantages/complications

- Simple, safe, successful, with a wide range of indications.
- Motor block, paresthesiae, hypotension, urinary retention, inadvertent dural puncture or intravascular injection can all occur. All these complications are rare using a single-shot caudal technique.

Continuous caudal epidural analgesia

- A single-shot caudal injection is restricted in its duration of action. A catheter can be introduced into the epidural space via the caudal route; it is a safe and effective method of administering epidural analgesia in infants.
- The single curve of the back allows the catheter to thread predictably into the epidural space; the tip of the catheter should be close to the level of the dermatomes that need to be blocked.
- Over 2 years of age, the development of a lumbosacral curvature tends to lead to a higher failure rate. However, some authors claim comparable success rates at this age.
- Because of the proximity of the perineum, a caudal catheter should not be left in situ for longer than 36 h.

Epidural block

- The technique of epidural blockade is technically more difficult in children and requires experience. The ligamentum flavum is less well developed and the intervertebral spaces are narrower. In infants, the epidural space is rarely located at a depth greater than 15 mm and often as superficially as 10 mm from the skin.

- The technique is similar to that used in adults; either a midline or paramedian approach is acceptable. Severe neurological complications including fatalities have been reported in association with using air to find the epidural space. Reported complications are generally higher in infants. The caudal route may represent a safer alternative with this group.
- Dosage:
  - Loading dose: 0.75 ml/kg of 0.25% bupivacaine for lumbar epidural (0.5 ml/kg thoracic epidural).
  - Infusion: 60 ml of 0.125% bupivacaine + 1 mg preservative-free morphine (or 2 μg/ml fentanyl).
  - Rate: 0.1–0.4 ml/kg/h.
- Epidural needle: 18G for infants/children, 19G for neonates/infants (catheter 'end-hole' only).

Subarachnoid block

- Spinal anaesthesia is rarely performed in children. One of the few indications is for herniotomy in the high-risk neonate, e.g. the oxygen-dependent premature or ex-premature infant with chronic lung disease.
- Expert assistance is crucial. The infant needs to be firmly gripped in the lateral or sitting position. The technique needs to be precise. The needle should be directed at right angles to the skin in the midline below L3 with L5–S1 reported as the safest approach. Prior infiltration of local anaesthetic into the skin will help prevent patient movement.
- The block has a rapid onset but a duration rarely greater than 40 min. If sedation is required during the surgery, the incidence of postoperative apnoea is comparable with a general anaesthetic technique.
- Dosage: 0.1 ml/kg 0.5% 'heavy' bupivacaine + 0.06 ml for the needle dead space or 0.13 ml/kg 0.5% 'heavy' bupivacaine.
- Spinal needle: 5 cm 21G.

Ilioinguinal and iliohypogastric nerve block

- This is a useful alternative to caudal blockade in herniotomy, hydrocele, and orchidopexy. It should be avoided for neonatal herniotomy as the local anaesthetic may obscure the operating field. The block can be performed under direct vision by the surgeon.
- Technique: At a point 1 cm medial to the anterior superior iliac spine, direct a regional block needle or blunted 21G needle at right angles to the skin. There is resistance at the aponeurosis of external oblique. At this point 'bounce' the needle until a loss of resistance is encountered.
- Dosage: 0.75 ml/kg 0.25% bupivacaine. Retain 1–2 ml for a subcutaneous fan injection laterally, medially, and inferiorly.
- Advantages: It is an easy block to perform. It decreases the level of anaesthesia and reduces postoperative analgesic requirement.
- Disadvantages: It does not block visceral pain from traction of the spermatic cord or peritoneum and is unsuitable for a high undescended testis. There is a 10% incidence of femoral nerve block.

Dorsal nerve block of penis

* This block is indicated for distal surgery to the penis, including circumcision, meatoplasty and simple hypospadias repair.
* Technique:
    * Raise two subcutaneous swellings of local anaesthetic either side of the midline, each 5 mm from the pubic symphysis at the dorsal base of the penis. Use a 23G or 21G needle.
    * Alternatively a simple ring block at the base of the penis can be performed using a 25G needle.
* Dosage: 2–6 ml 0.25% of bupivacaine. Avoid adrenaline.
* Advantages: These techniques are safe, simple, and predictable. They avoid the need for injection deep to Buck's fascia close to the corpora cavernosa and penile vessels.
* Disadvantages: Haematoma and ischaemia are very unlikely using the superficial technique.

Axillary block

* This block is indicated for hand and lower arm surgery.
* Technique:
    * Position the patient supine with the arm abducted to 90° and the elbow flexed.
    * Direct a 23G or 25G needle with attached extension tubing just above and parallel to the axillary artery. The needle is advanced until it pulsates. The position can be confirmed with a nerve stimulator or alternatively the nerve stimulator is used from the beginning. A click or loss of resistance are not always elicited in children.
* Dosage: 0.5 ml/kg 0.25% bupivacaine.
* Advantages: Safe and effective.
* Disadvantages: Upper arm and shoulder surgery cannot be performed. The axillary artery may be difficult to palpate.

Local infiltration

* This is administered at the end of the operation by the surgeon but may be more efficacious if administered prior to the initial incision.
* It is suitable for small incisions and can help provide good postoperative pain relief.
* Dosage: 1 ml/kg of 0.25% bupivacaine.

Diaphragmatic hernia

Procedure	Repair of defect in diaphragm either by suturing to abdominal wall or with a synthetic graft
Time	1–2 h
Pain	+++
Position	Supine
Blood loss	Usually minimal to moderate
Practical techniques	GA + IPPV, arterial line

Preoperative

- Incidence varies between 1 in 3000 and 1 in 4000 deliveries, affecting left side in 85% of cases. May be other associated anomalies.
- Characteristically present in respiratory distress with tachypnoea, cyanosis, and a scaphoid abdomen. The chest radiograph is diagnostic. The diagnosis is usually made antenatally on ultrasound.
- Overall mortality of 50% from lung hypoplasia, abnormal pulmonary vasculature, and pulmonary hypertension.
- Gas exchange should be optimal preferably with FiO_2 <0.5 before surgery. This is not always possible.
- Mainly transfer from special care baby unit already intubated and ventilated. May require more advanced ventilatory modes such as high-frequency oscillation.

Perioperative

- Avoid ventilation via a face mask.
- Nasogastric tube, two IV cannulas, arterial line. Oesophageal stethoscope with temperature probe. Consider CVP measurement.
- Avoid nitrous oxide to prevent distension of the gut within the thorax.
- Ventilate using rate rather than pressure to reduce barotrauma.
- High-dose fentanyl (25 µg/kg) may reduce the pulmonary vasoconstriction response to surgical stress.
- An arterial line essential.

Postoperative

- Postoperative ventilation for at least 24 h, then attempt to wean.
- Infant may deteriorate within 12 h due to pulmonary hypertensive crises.
- Rarely, if minimal defect, can extubate immediately.

Special considerations

- Pulmonary hypertension is treated by assisted hyperventilation with 100% oxygen and fluid boluses if necessary. Prostacyclin or inhaled nitric oxide can be used successfully and should not be stopped abruptly for surgery. Extra-corporeal membrane oxygenation (ECMO) is a last resort but has also been successful.
- To assist weaning a thoracic epidural may be of benefit either inserted conventionally or via the caudal route.

Gastroschisis/exomphalos

Procedure	Replacement of abdominal contents into the abdominal cavity
Time	2 h
Pain	++/+++
Position	Supine
Blood loss	Moderate
Practical technique	GA + IPPV

Preoperative

- Obvious neonatal diagnosis from birth. Now usually diagnosed in utero. Overall incidence varies between 1 in 3000 and 1 in 4000.
- Gastroschisis is defect in anterior abdominal wall usually on the right causing herniation of abdominal contents without a covering sac.
- In exomphalos, there is a failure of the gut to return to the abdominal cavity during fetal development resulting in persistent herniation through the extra embryonal part of the umbilical cord, which covers it. This may include other abdominal organs.
- There is an increased incidence of associated anomalies including cardiac disease in exomphalos. A full cardiology assessment should be performed.
- Exposed abdominal contents result in large evaporative heat and water losses and predispose to infection. It should initially be covered with clingfilm or an equivalent.

Perioperative

- May already be intubated and ventilated. Otherwise intubate conventionally.
- Nasogastric tube and oesophageal temperature/stethoscope.
- Two IV cannulas for maintenance and volume.
- Arterial monitoring is useful.
- Heat conservation is important. Warm the theatre and use a warming mattress or hot air mattress, radiant heater. Keep the patient's head covered. Use warmed fluids.
- Fluid losses may be considerable.
- Intraoperative analgesia: fentanyl 5–10 µg/kg or epidural if extubation within 48 h is contemplated.

Postoperative

- Postoperative ventilation, especially if the abdomen is tense, should be in the head up position.
- Pay assiduous attention to fluid balance. There may be large losses into the abdomen of crystalloid and protein.

Special considerations

- Lines should be sited in the arms as abdominal distension may impair venous return from the lower body.
- It is simpler to insert a percutaneous long line at this stage for later parenteral feeding. Postoperatively, progressive oedema makes cannulation more difficult.
- Manual ventilation is useful to assess the effect of replacement of abdominal contents on lung compliance to determine the correct degree of abdominal reduction.
- Complete reduction is not always possible. A silo is then created around the extra-abdominal contents to be gradually reduced on the intensive care unit. Fluid loss and infection are major issues.

Tracheo-oesophageal fistula

Procedure	Ligation of fistula + anastomotic repair of oesophageal atresia
Time	2 h
Pain	+++
Position	Left lateral for right thoracotomy
Blood loss	Moderate
Practical technique	GA + IPPV ± manual ventilation

Preoperative

- Incidence of 1 in 3500. Commonest type (85%) is oesophageal atresia with a distal fistula. The majority of cases are now diagnosed in utero. It should always be excluded in cases of hydramnios.
- High incidence of prematurity (30%) and cardiac disease (25%).
- Presents clinically with choking and cyanotic episodes on feeding with an inability to pass a nasogastric tube.
- Constant risk of pulmonary aspiration. A double-lumen 'Replogle' tube in the oesophagus allows irrigation and suction.

Perioperative

- Inhalational or IV induction.
- Careful ETT placement. Confirm symmetrical ventilation with the tube distal to the fistula.
- Two IV cannulas for maintenance and volume.
- An arterial line is useful.
- Allow intra-operative access to pass the transanastomatic tube nasally to facilitate oesophageal repair.
- Manual ventilation may be necessary to assess lung compliance after ligation of the fistula, to assist in repair of oesophagus, and to periodically reinflate left lung. Surgical restriction may impede ventilation and blood or secretions can block the tube.
- Intraoperative analgesia: fentanyl (5–10 µg/kg) or epidural either by the thoracic or caudal route if early weaning is anticipated.
- Ensure active heat conservation.
- The operation is usually via an extrapleural approach.

Postoperative

The majority of cases are ventilated postoperatively, especially if the oesophageal repair may be under tension. The nasogastric tube or transanastamotic tube must be secured.

Special considerations

- Pay attention to positioning of the ETT to avoid ventilating the stomach via the fistula. Preoperative bronchoscopy may be useful. The fistula may at times be close to the carina. The tube may need to be advanced, withdrawn, or the bevel rotated.
- Classically these cases were intubated awake because of possible difficulties in ventilation. This is no longer common practice but manual ventilation at induction should be gentle to minimize gastric distension.

Patent ductus arteriosus

Procedure	Ligation or clipping of ductus arteriosus
Time	1 h
Pain	+
Position	Left thoracotomy
Blood loss	Usually minimal. Occasionally massive if the vessel is torn
Practical technique	IPPV, fentanyl

Preoperative

- Small premature babies. 25% of premature infants <1.5 kg recovering from hyaline membrane disease have a patent ductus arteriosus. It is associated with other cardiac anomalies.
- Indications are for ventilator dependence and developing broncho-pulmonary dysplasia.

Perioperative

- High-risk group. Operation may be undertaken on the special care baby unit.
- The patient is usually already ventilated with full monitoring.
- Arterial monitoring is not usually necessary.
- IV access is required.
- IPPV with oxygen nitrous oxide and fentanyl up to 10 µg/kg with a low dose of volatile agent. Replace nitrous oxide with air if frail.
- Active heat conservation.
- Avoid saturations >96% because of retinopathy of prematurity. Local infiltration for analgesia.

Postoperative

Give postoperative ventilation until stable, then attempt to wean.

Special considerations

- Sudden ligation of the ductus may precipitate an acute rise in systemic blood pressure and increase the risk of intraventricular haemorrhage. The duct should be clamped gently or alternatively the concentration of the volatile agent can be temporarily increased.
- Older children requiring patent ductus arteriosus occlusion tend to be fit, although some present with cardiac failure. Increasingly these procedures are being performed non-surgically as day cases by interventional cardiologists via a percutaneous femoral approach.

Pyloric stenosis

Procedure	Splitting the pylorus muscle longitudinally down to the mucosa
Time	30 min
Pain	+
Position	Supine
Blood loss	Minimal
Practical technique	GA + IPPV, ?RSI

Preoperative

* Incidence of 1 in 350 births, may be commoner in first born males. 80% are male, 10% are premature.
* Often present with biochemical abnormalities, notably hypochloraemic alkalosis. The operation is never urgent and full resuscitation should occur.
* Electrolytes, particularly chloride and bicarbonate, and pH should be within normal limits. Chloride is the most important ion for assessment and must be greater than 90 mmol/litre.

Perioperative

* No complete agreement, but there is a risk of pulmonary aspiration from gastric outflow obstruction.
* A nasogastric tube is compulsory and will be in situ. Aspirate and do not remove. It does not reduce the effect of cricoid pressure and may act as an escape valve if mask ventilation increases intragastric pressure.
* IV is usually in place. Induction may be rapid sequence or non-depolarizing relaxant for which some anaesthetists use cricoid pressure. Consider rapid sequence if there is excessive nasogastric loss (>2ml/kg/h).
* Fentanyl (1 μg/kg) + paracetamol suppository (20–30 mg/kg) + local infiltration up to 1 ml/kg of 0.25% bupivacaine.
* Extubate awake in the left lateral position.

Postoperative

* Remove the nasogastric tube at the end of the procedure.
* Give paracetamol PO/PR.
* Feed within 6 h but maintain fluids until feeding is established.
* Use an apnoea alarm overnight.

Special considerations

* Resuscitation: 0.45% saline + 20 mmol/litre KCl. Replace nasogastric loss with normal saline + 20 mmol/litre KCl. Use colloid if hypovolaemia is present. Mild cases may respond to 5% dextrose with 0.45% saline (bicarbonate <32 mmol/litre), more severe cases will require normal saline.
* May be performed laparoscopically.

Intussusception

Procedure	Reduction of invaginated (usually ileocolic) bowel
Time	1–2 h
Pain	+++
Position	Supine
Blood loss	Moderate, may be large
Practical technique	RSI + IPPV

Preoperative

- Intussusception is the commonest cause of obstruction in infants over 2 months of age; incidence 2 in 1000 births.
- Invagination of the bowel into an adjacent lower segment, usually at the terminal ileum or ileocolic valve. Rarely caused by polyp or Meckel's diverticulum (5% of cases).
- Present with paroxysmal pain, blood and mucus in stool (redcurrent jelly stool), and sausage-shaped mass in right abdomen.
- 70% of cases are reduced by air or barium enema.
- The child may be profoundly shocked. Urgent fluid resuscitation with gastric decompression and electrolyte correction will be needed. Colloid and blood may be required. Delay may result in perforated or necrotic bowel. Fluid loss may be greater than expected.

Perioperative

- Rapid sequence induction. Retain the nasogastric tube in situ.
- Fentanyl 2–5 µg/kg + volatile agent. Consider an epidural if stable.
- Two secure cannulas of adequate size. A central line is often useful in severe cases.
- Routine monitoring, temperature measurement probe, and urinary catheter.
- Prolonged intussusception with ischaemic gut requiring resection often leads to metabolic acidosis and septic shock. Admission to a paediatric ICU will be required.

Postoperative

Local wound infiltration + morphine NCA.

Special considerations

No concensus as to whether the child should receive surgery at the base hospital or be transferred to a regional centre. If transferred, this should not delay resuscitation or blood cross-match, which can be sent with the patient.

Herniotomy

Procedure	Excision of patent processus vaginalis
Time	20 min
Pain	++
Position	Supine
Blood loss	Minimal
Practical technique	SV + LMA, caudal or regional block
	IPPV, caudal or local infiltration
	Spinal or caudal block

Preoperative

- Otherwise fit ASA 1 children.
- 20% of preterm babies present for surgery at approximately 40 weeks post-conceptual age or when ready to leave the special care baby unit.
- Obtain consent for suppository and block. Discuss risks and complications.

Perioperative

- If >5 kg inhalational or IV induction with laryngeal mask, then caudal or ilioinguinal block and intra-operative opioids if necessary.
- If <5 kg, intubate with controlled ventilation. In neonates, avoid ilioinguinal block as the spread of local anaesthetic may obscure the surgical field. Use either caudal or postoperative infiltration.
- Diclofenac (1 mg/kg) suppository (>1 yr) or paracetamol (20–30 mg/kg) suppository if under 1 year.

Postoperative

- Day case: PRN paracetamol and diclofenac.
- Neonate: PRN paracetamol. Admit overnight.

Special considerations

- The majority of herniotomy repairs are in healthy children and suitable as day cases.
- There is no consensus as to the most appropriate regional block. Caudal blockade is indicated for bilateral herniotomy repair and children up to 20 kg. Ilioinguinal block is effective in children over 5 kg.
- The ex-premature baby may be small for dates and oxygen-dependent with chronic lung disease. Postoperative apnoea and bradycardia are documented risks associated with general anaesthesia for this group. Hypocarbia and hypothermia should be avoided and an oxygen saturation between 90% and 95% is acceptable. Caffeine (10 mg/kg IV) given at induction reduces the risk of apnoea by 70%.

- To avoid general anaesthesia a spinal technique may be used (0.1 ml/kg of 0.5% 'heavy' bupivacaine + 0.06 ml for needle dead space). This may be technically difficult and complicated by a bloody or dry tap. It is too short acting for bilateral repair. A single-shot caudal is an alternative method. Supplementary sedation results in the same risk of postoperative apnoea as with general anaesthesia.

- Term babies in the first 6 weeks of life and ex-premature infants up to 60 weeks' post-conceptual age should be admitted overnight for oxygen saturation and apnoea alarm monitoring.

- A strangulated hernia that does not reduce is an emergency and requires fluid resuscitation and a nasogastric tube. Precautions should be taken against regurgitation and aspiration.

Circumcision

Procedure	Removal of prepuce or foreskin
Time	20 min
Pain	++
Position	Supine
Blood loss	Minimal
Practical technique	SV, LMA, caudal/penile block/ring block

Preoperative

* Common day case procedure, but move towards more conservative management including simple stretch or preputioplasty.
* Obtain consent for suppository and regional block. Discuss complications and risks.

Perioperative

* Inhalational or IV induction. Laryngeal mask.
* Regional block: caudal, penile block, or ring block.
* Diclofenac suppository (1 mg/kg) (>1 yr) or paracetamol (30 mg/kg) if under 1 year.

Postoperative

* PRN paracetamol 20 mg/kg
* Topical lidocaine (lignocaine) gel can be applied frequently without exceeding the toxic dose.

Special considerations

* A regional block must be performed prior to the surgery.
* Circumcision is one of the most painful postoperative day case procedures; parents should be warned and advised to apply topical gel regularly and continue paracetamol for several days.
* There is no consensus as to the optimal strategy for pain relief. All methods are effective. Caudal is technically easier in infants and penile block may be more suitable in children over 5 kg. Ring block is technically easy in boys greater than 5 kg, producing excellent and consistent analgesia.

Orchidopexy

Procedure	Release of undescended testis into scrotum
Time	30 min
Pain	++
Position	Supine
Blood loss	Minimal
Practical technique	SV, LMA + regional block

Preoperative

* Boys, usually over 2 years (2% of population).
* Common day case procedure.
* Obtain consent for suppository and regional block. Discuss risks and complications.

Perioperative

* Inhalational or IV induction. Laryngeal mask.
* Regional technique: caudal, ilioinguinal block or local infiltration.
* Diclofenac suppository (1 mg/kg) (>1 year) or paracetamol suppository (30 mg/kg) if <1 year.
* Give supplementary opioids if indicated.

Postoperative

PRN diclofenac, paracetamol, codeine phosphate, and anti-emetic.

Special considerations

* Adequate analgesia is difficult if the testis is high. Caudal block should be high volume with lower concentration (bupivacaine 0.19% is three parts 0.25% bupivacaine to 1 part saline). A mid thoracic level is obtained from 1.25 ml/kg of this mixture.
* If ilioinguinal block is used, only the anterior third of the scrotum is anaesthetized—use local infiltration for the scrotal incision.
* Testicular traction even with seemingly adequate blockade may lead to intra-operative bradycardia or mild laryngospasm especially with the ilioinguinal block. Surgery should be stopped and anaesthesia deepened; supplementary opioids may be required.
* Suspected torsion of the testis is a surgical emergency and the need for a rapid sequence induction will have to be considered. Analgesic techniques are as before.
* A high testis may need surgery in two stages. The first procedure is to identify the testis and if possible bring it down to the inguinal ring. This is usually performed laparascopically and will require intubation, controlled ventilation with intra-operative opioids, and rectal diclofenac or paracetamol.

Hypospadias

Procedure	Restoration of proximal urethral opening to the tip of the penis
Time	1–3 h
Pain	++
Position	Supine
Blood loss	Minimal
Practical technique	SV/IPPV + regional block

Preoperative

- Usually an isolated problem, but there may be an association with certain rare dysmorphic syndromes.
- Obtain consent for suppository and regional block. Discuss complications and risks.

Perioperative

- Inhalational or IV induction.
- If procedure <1 h use LMA + SV.
- If procedure >1 h use LMA or ETT + IPPV.
- Extended caudal 1 ml/kg 0.25% bupivacaine + ketamine, clonidine, morphine, or diamorphine to prolong the duration of the block (see p. 790).
- Diclofenac suppository (>1 yr) or paracetamol (30 mg/kg) if under 1 year.
- Employ heat conservation measures.

Postoperative

- Regular NSAIDs/paracetamol. Consider morphine NCA (not always necessary).
- Opioids can be used in caudal block since the patient will be catheterized.
- If opioid is used in the caudal space the patient must be admitted overnight.

Special considerations

- May be simple procedure, e.g. meatal advancement and glanduloplasty, or extensive involving buccal mucosa graft. The anaesthetic technique can be adjusted accordingly.
- Avoid erection with regional block plus an adequate depth of anaesthesia.

Cleft lip and palate

Procedure	Repair of defect in upper lip and palate
Time	1–2 h
Pain	++
Position	Supine, head ring, shoulder support
Blood loss	Minimal for cleft lip. Moderate for cleft palate
Practical technique	IPPV. Armoured or RAE tube

Preoperative

- Incidence of between 1 in 300 and 1 in 600 births but can be 1 in 25 where there is a family history.
- Both lip and palate are involved in 50% of cases. Cleft palate alone has a high incidence of associated anomalies.
- It is an isolated defect in 90% of cases.
- Associated syndromes often involve a difficult airway, e.g. Pierre–Robin, Treacher–Collins, and Goldenhar syndromes. Therefore make a careful assessment of the airway.
- Discuss risks and complications. Obtain consent for suppository.
- Administer IM atropine 20 μg/kg 30 min preoperatively if a difficult airway is suspected.

Perioperative

- Inhalational or IV induction. When there is a suspected airway problem, use inhalational induction with sevoflurane and then maintain with halothane. CPAP will be useful. Intubate deep with child breathing spontaneously or following muscle relaxant once a safe airway has been established.
- A preformed RAE may be obstructed or kinked by the gag, especially the smaller sizes. A reinforced tube will resist compression but needs to be carefully secured at correct length.
- Use IPPV.
- Use a throat pack and make sure the eyes are protected.
- The surgeon usually places the gag. Encourage local anaesthetic infiltration.
- Fentanyl 2–4 μg/kg + suppository (paracetamol 30 mg/kg <1 year or diclofenac 1 mg/kg >1 year) + local infiltration with adrenaline.
- Codeine phosphate 1 mg/kg IM prior to reversal.

Postoperative

- Extubate awake. Suction the pharynx early and carefully to prevent damage to the repair.
- Nasal tubes may be inserted to maintain patency of the airway. A tongue stitch is rarely used.

- Routine postoperative analgesia to include regular paracetamol, diclofenac, or ibuprofen and codeine phosphate.

Special considerations

- Intubation is usually uncomplicated.
- The laryngoscope blade rarely lodges in the cleft. If there is a problem, a roll of gauze can fill the gap.
- Prolonged surgery may cause swollen tongue from pressure of mouth gag.
- With airway problems, opioids should be given cautiously. Postoperative monitoring should include pulse oximetry and apnoea alarm.
- Cleft lip is usually repaired at 3 months, cleft palate at 6 to 9 months. The lip may be repaired at the neonatal stage to improve the scar and assist maternal bonding. There is no evidence to support this.

Congenital talipes equinovarus

Procedure	Correction of club foot abnormality
Time	45 min–1 h
Pain	++
Position	Supine, sometimes prone for posterior release
Blood loss	Minimal
Practical technique	SV, LMA, caudal
	If prone then ETT + IPPV, caudal

Preoperative

* Occurs in 1 in 1000 births.
* It is usually an isolated anomaly but may occur in association with some myopathic diseases and therefore there may be an increased risk of malignant hyperthermia.
* Obtain consent for a suppository and regional block. Discuss risks and complications.

Perioperative

* Inhalational or IV induction with LMA. If prone intubate and ventilate. Give additional opioids if indicated.
* Caudal blockade: 1 ml/kg 0.25% bupivacaine.
* Rectal diclofenac 1 mg/kg (>1 year), rectal paracetamol 30 mg/kg if <1 year.

Postoperative

Give regular diclofenac, paracetamol, codeine phosphate + anti-emetic for the first day. Oramorph may be a useful alternative.

Special considerations

For prolonged pain relief either top-up the caudal at the end of the procedure by using an indwelling 22G or 20G cannula or extend the duration of the block by adding preservative-free ketamine (0.5 mg/kg) to the initial dose of bupivacaine. Diamorphine and clonidine will also extend the block. However, the former may lead to urinary retention and the latter inappropriate levels of drowsiness.

Femoral osteotomy

Procedure	Stabilizing the hip in congenital dislocation by making a cut through the proximal femur
Time	2 h
Pain	+++
Position	Supine
Blood loss	Moderate/potentially large
Practical technique	SV + LMA or IPPV + caudal/epidural

Preoperative

• Usually an isolated defect. Commoner in girls or where there is a family history.
• Obtain consent for a suppository and regional block. Discuss risks complications.

Perioperative

• Inhalational or IV induction. SV or IPPV with LMA or intubate + IPPV i <10 kg.
• Caudal block + preservative-free ketamine or clonidine. Avoid cauda opioids because of the risk of urinary retention. Alternatively give a lumbar epidural. Intraoperative opioids may be useful.
• Employ heat conservation measures.
• Attention to blood loss.

Postoperative

• Extended caudal or morphine NCA with regular NSAIDs or paracetamol Consider enteral morphine preparation.
• A hip spica provides support and helps with pain relief.

Special considerations

• Blood loss may be extensive if it is repeat surgery.
• A hip spica complicates urinary retention in girls.

Inhaled foreign body

Procedure	Removal of foreign body from bronchial tree
Time	30 min
Pain	+
Position	Supine
Blood loss	Nil
Practical technique	SV or IPPV

Preoperative

* The commonest reason for bronchoscopy in the 1–3 year age group.
* A foreign body in the upper airways may present as an emergency acute airway obstruction.
* Obstruction of the lower airways may follow a history of coughing after several days. Peanut oil is an irritant and leads to mucosal oedema and chemical pneumonitis. A chest radiograph shows characteristic hyperinflation during expiration, but the foreign body is not usually visible.
* Treat symptoms as indicated, e.g. dehydration, pneumonia, wheeze.
* Obtain consent, and discuss risks and complications.

Perioperative

* Inhalational induction is usual to avoid pushing the object further in— 100% oxygen with sevoflurane or halothane.
* Deep inhalational maintenance with halothane (sevoflurane gives too rapid an awakening).
* Apply topical anaesthesia to the vocal cords (2% lidocaine (lignocaine)) and consider a drying agent.
* Rigid bronchoscopy—the Storz bronchoscope has attachment for a T-piece.
* If the foreign body is in the lower airway, then use IPPV with a muscle relaxant since the object will be pushed distally by the bronchoscope until it can be grasped by forceps. Give assisted ventilation via a T-piece or high-frequency jet ventilation.
* This may be a difficult procedure.

Postoperative

* If bronchoscopy is traumatic, give dexamethsone 0.25 mg/kg IV then two doses 8-hourly of 0.125 mg/kg.
* Consider physiotherapy and antibiotics as indicated.

Special considerations

* If tracheal or ball-valve obstruction is suspected, IPPV is contraindicated.
* Intubation may assist lung ventilation and sizing of the bronchoscope if a tracheal foreign body is excluded.

Medical problems

Acute laryngotracheobronchitis (croup)

* Croup occurs predominantly in epidemics in the autumn and early spring. The peak age of incidence is 6 months to 2 years. It is viral in aetiology; the majority of cases being due to parainfluenza, but influenza and respiratory syncitial virus can also cause this condition.
* The symptoms are coryzal for the first few days but then progress to a characteristic barking cough and hoarseness with profuse secretions and occasional dysphagia. Pyrexia is mild or absent.
* The larynx, trachea, and bronchi are all involved and become more oedematous leading to the onset of stridor. An anxious child will exacerbate the condition, as the trachea will tend to collapse on inspiration.
* The majority of children respond to conservative measures and reassurance. There is no evidence to support the use of humidified steam tents. In severe cases, steroids and nebulized adrenaline are required.
* 10% of children are admitted and 1% will require intubation.
* The majority of children have a single isolated episode.

Acute epiglottitis

* This is an acute life-threatening infection caused by Haemophilis influenzae type B (Hib). It most commonly presents at 2 to 3 years.
* There is a rapid onset of oedema of the epiglottis and aryepiglottic folds. The child has a high temperature, usually greater than 39.5 °C and presents sitting or leaning forwards, drooling saliva, unable to swallow, with the tongue pushed forwards. Inspiratory and expiratory stridor is rapidly progressive and a late sign.
* Acute epiglottitis is a medical emergency. The antibiotic of choice is cefotaxime (50 mg/kg twice daily). Intubation will be indicated in 60% of these children; in some centres all cases are routinely intubated.
* Following the introduction of the Hib vaccine, this condition is now rare.

Anaesthetic management

* The differential diagnosis between croup and epiglottitis is not always obvious. If epiglottitis is even remotely suspected, there must be consultation with an ENT surgeon at consultant level.
* Induction occurs in the anaesthetic room or operating theatre with the full range of appropriate equipment and monitoring available.
* Traditionally, obtaining IV access has been contraindicated prior to induction because of the risk of acute glottic closure. However, the use of topical cream facilitates atraumatic venepuncture. Unless access is obviously difficult, cannulation should proceed before anaesthesia.
* An inhalational induction is performed in the sitting position with sevoflurane or halothane in 100% oxygen, the choice depends solely on the experience of the operator. Once anaesthetized, the child can be moved to a supine position and maintained with halothane up to concentrations of 5% if needed. Halothane permits a more prolonged attempt at laryngoscopy. CPAP should be routinely applied, but the airway is not usually difficult to maintain.

- In croup laryngoscopy is usually straightforward, but the endotracheal tube required may be surprisingly narrow. Start with one size smaller than normal. Croup tubes exist which are of extra length for a given internal diameter making them suitable for older children. If possible, once the airway is secure, the child should be reintubated nasally since this is better tolerated. Profuse secretions are always a problem and frequent suction is necessary.

- With epiglottitis intubation may be exceedingly difficult. Laryngoscopy often reveals abnormal anatomy with no obvious glottic opening. Careful inspection may reveal movement of small amounts of mucous indicating tidal flow. If the child is deep enough careful injection of saline onto the glottis may demonstrate air bubbles. The child should be intubated using a stylet so that the tracheal tube can be immediately railroaded if necessary.

- During anaesthesia, the ENT surgeon should be scrubbed in theatre with the tracheostomy set open.

- Once intubation has been achieved, oedema rapidly settles and by demonstrating a leak around the tube, extubation is normally possible within 36 h. Dexamethasone is often given prior to extubation to reduce laryngeal oedema.

Sedation

- The expansion of imaging techniques together with new diagnostic and therapeutic interventions has led to a rise in demand for sedation services.
- Compared with general anaesthesia, sedation is neither cheaper nor safer. Safety is paramount and the requirements in terms of personnel and resuscitation equipment are the same.
- The adult concept of sedation where verbal contact is maintained is not practical in children. There may be little difference between deep sedation as defined by the American Academy of Paediatrics and uncontrolled anaesthesia. Ideal sedation conditions achieve depression of the nervous system, allowing the relevant procedures to occur, with preservation of the airway reflexes. In practice this is difficult to achieve.
- It is important not to confuse sedation with analgesia. Painful procedures may require topical anaesthetic cream, infiltration with local anaesthetics, and occasionally systemic opioids.
- Contraindications include children with airway problems, apnoeic episodes, respiratory disease, raised intracranial pressure, risk of pulmonary aspiration, and epilepsy.
- The most frequently used oral sedative drugs are chloral hydrate (50–100 mg/kg), triclofos (50–75 mg/kg), and to a lesser extent benzodiazepines, trimeprazine, and ketamine. Opioids are also used, in combination with other sedatives. (See paediatric drug guidelines for dosages.) (p. 815).
- Midazolam 0.5 mg/kg PO or in incremental doses of 0.1 mg/kg IV can produce useful conditions for sedation and has the addtional property of amnesia. Ketamine 1–2 mg/kg IV is indicated for short, painful procedures. Emergence delirium is less of a problem with children but a drying agent is often required.
- With appropriate planning, organization, and safety, nurse-led sedation services have been developed at several centres following strict protocols (see below). The children are fasted conventionally but allowed unrestricted clear fluids. A pulse oximeter is mandatory. Surprisingly young children can tolerate scans awake with encouragement, careful explanation, and parental presence.

Example of nurse-led oral sedation protocol

Age or weight	Sedation
<44 weeks	Nil. Swaddle and feed
<5 kg	Chloral hydrate 50 mg/kg 30 min prescan
<10 kg	Chloral hydrate 100 mg/kg 30 min prescan
10–20 kg	Temazepam 1 mg/kg (max. 20 mg) with droperidol 0.25 mg/kg (max. 5 mg) 1 h prescan

- If oral sedation is not effective consider an IV top-up:
  - diazemuls 0.1 mg/kg increments up to 1 mg/kg or
  - midazolam 0.2 mg/kg increments up to 0.8 mg/kg.
- For reversal of sedation use flumazenil 10–20 μg/kg IV and repeat if necessary.

Paediatric drug guidelines

Premedication

Atropine	10 µg/kg	IV	induction
	20 µg/kg	IM	30 min preop.
	40 µg/kg	PO	60 min preop.
Chloral hydrate	25–50 mg/kg	PO	60 min preop.
Clonidine	4 µg/kg	PO	90–120 min preop.
Droperidol	50–100 µg/kg	PO	60 min preop.
Midazolam	0.5 mg/kg	PO	30 min preop.
Morphine	200–250 µg/kg	IM	30 min preop.
Pethidine compound injection (Inj. Peth. Co.: 1 ml contains Pethidine 25 mg, Promethazine 6.25 mg. Chlorpromazine 6.25 mg)	0.06–0.08 ml/kg. Max. dose 1.5 ml	IM	45 min preop.
Temazepam	0.5–1.0 mg/kg	PO	60 min preop.
Triclofos	50–75 mg/kg	PO	45 min preop.
Trimeprazine	2 mg/kg	PO	90 min preop.

Induction

Etomidate	0.3 mg/kg	IV
Ketamine	2 mg/kg	IV
	5–7 mg/kg	IM
Propofol	2–3 mg/kg	IV
— if unpremedicated	3–5 mg/kg	IV
Thiopental	4–6 mg/kg	IV
— neonates	2–4 mg/kg	IV

Muscle relaxants

Atracurium	0.5 mg/kg
Cis-atracurium	0.2–0.4 mg/kg
Mivacurium	0.1–0.2 mg/kg
Pancuronium	0.1 mg/kg
Rocuronium	0.6 mg/kg
Suxamethonium	1–2 mg/kg
Vecuronium	0.1 mg/kg

Reversal

Atropine	20 μg/kg
Glycopyrrolate	10 μg/kg
Neostigmine	50 μg/kg

Robinul-Neostigmine is neostigmine methylsulphate 2.5 mg plus glycopyrronium bromide 500 μg in 1 ml of solution. Add ampoule to 4 ml normal saline, then reversal dose is 1 ml per 10 kg.

Intra-operative analgesia

Alfentanil	30–50 μg/kg as slow bolus, supplemental doses 15 μg/kg
	Infusion: 50–100 μg/kg as slow bolus, then 0.5–1 μg/kg/min
Fentanyl	2–5 μg/kg
	For cardiac surgery: up to 25 μg/kg
Morphine sulphate	50–200 μg/kg
Remifentanil	Infusion: 300 μg/kg in 50 ml of 5% dextrose
	Loading dose: 1–2 μg/kg
	Infusion: 0.1–2 μg/kg/min

Mild to moderate postoperative pain

Codeine phosphate	1–1.5 mg/kg	IM, PO, PR	6-hourly
Diclofenac	1 mg/kg (over 1 yr)	PO, PR	8-hourly
Ibuprofen	5–10 mg/kg (over 7 kg)	PO	8-hourly
Paracetamol	20 mg/kg	PO, PR	6-hourly
	Rectal loading dose (if >44 weeks postconception) 30–40 mg/kg	PR	Once
Oramorph	400 μg/kg	PO	4-hourly

Severe postoperative pain

Morphine	50–100 μg/kg IV incremental boluses or 200 μg/kg IM
Morphine infusion	1 mg/kg in 50 ml saline or 5% dextrose, i.e. 20 μg/kg/ml
	Rate: 1–2 ml/h (20–40 μg/kg/h)
Morphine NCA	1 mg/kg morphine in 50 ml saline or 5% dextrose
	Rate: 1 ml/h. Bolus: 1 ml. Lockout: 20 min
Morphine PCA	1 mg/ kg morphine in 50 ml saline or 5% dextrose
	Rate: 0.2 ml/h. Bolus: 1 ml. Lockout: 5 min

NB: Morphine infusions should be in a dedicated IVI or have an antireflux valve.

Antagonists

Naloxone	5–10 μg/kg IV incrementally		
Flumazenil	10–20 μg/kg IV, repeat if necessary		

Anti-emetics

Cyclizine	1 mg/kg	IV	8-hourly
Dexamethasone	0.15 mg/kg	IV	6-hourly
Droperidol	20–75 μg/kg	IV	Intra-operative only
Metoclopramide	0.15 mg/kg	IV, PO	8-hourly
Ondansetron	0.1–0.15 mg/kg	IV, PO	8-hourly
Prochlorperazine	0.25 mg/kg	IV, PO, PR	8-hourly

Regional analgesia doses

Caudal extradural blockade	Sacral: 0.5 mg/kg 0.25% bupivacaine
	Lumbar: 1 ml/kg 0.25% bupivacaine
	Thoracolumbar: 1.25 ml/kg 0.19% bupivacaine
Supplements to extend duration of block	Ketamine 0.5 mg/kg (preservative-free)
	Clonidine 1 μg/kg
	Diamorphine 30 μg/kg
	Morphine 50 μg/kg (preservative-free)
Lumbar epidural (intra-operative)	0.75 ml/kg of 0.25% bupivacaine (or 0.2% ropivacaine)
Epidural infusion	60 ml of 0.125% bupivacaine + 1 mg preservative-free morphine
	Rate: 0.1–0.4 ml/kg/h
Spinal block	0.1 ml/kg 0.5% 'heavy' bupivacaine + 0.06 ml for needle deadspace
Wound infiltration	1 ml/kg 0.25% bupivacaine

Paediatric quick reference guide

Age	Approx. weight (kg)	Body surface area (m²)	% Adult drug dose (approx.)	ETT size (mm)	ETT length (cm)	LMA size	Suxamethonium dose (mg) IV	Atropine dose (μg) IV
Term	3.5	0.23	12.5	3.5	9	1	7	35
1 month	4.2	0.26	14.5	3.5	10	1	8	40
3 months	6	0.33	15	3.5	10	1.5	12	60
6 months	7.5	0.38	22	3.5/4.0	11	1.5	15	75
1 year	10	0.47	25	4.0	12	1.5/2	20	100
2 years	12	0.53	30	4.5	13	2	24	120
3 years	14	0.61	33	4.5/5	13/14	2	28	140
5 years	18	0.73	40	5.0/5.5	14.5	2.5	36	180
7 years	22	0.86	50	6.0	15.5	2.5	44	220
10 years	30	1.10	60	6.5 cuffed	17	3	60	300
12 years	38	1.30	75	7.0 cuffed	18	3 or 4	75	380

Note: Weights are approximations only—patient should be weighed accurately.

Chapter 36
Anaesthetic emergencies

Andrew McIndoe

General principles

Anaesthetic emergencies may develop rapidly into life-threatening conditions. Although critical incidents frequently occur in the presence of a theatre team, the anaesthetist is likely to be the person present with the specialist knowledge and skills to deal with the problem. This can give rise to intense pressure. Critical incident protocols and drills have been designed to aid in the management of the more complex or common emergencies, and some are detailed below. However, a protocol-driven approach is heavily reliant upon recognition that a serious problem exists.

Communication

- Declare problems early to the rest of the theatre team before you lose control of the situation. Basic resuscitation measures should be on-going while you figure out the diagnosis.
- No matter whatever or whoever 'caused' the crisis, use objective and non-judgmental comments. Insults tend to provoke an aggressive or withdrawn response from the recipient and inhibit team function.
- To communicate effectively, your messages or commands must be:
  - ADDRESSED: Ask specifically named individuals, not 'someone', to perform tasks.
  - HEARD: Reduce background noise and distractions by turning off the radio, etc.
  - UNDERSTOOD: If you make a complex request, ask the recipient to repeat it back to you.
- If the cause of the problem is unknown, say so. Say what you don't know as well as what you do know. Encourage others to contribute.
- Reappraise the situation regularly. Update the rest of the team with new information. If you are still unsure about what to do, send for help–second person with a fresh approach may pick up on missed clues.

Invoke a team approach

- A team should have one clearly identified leader, who should make effective use of the mixture of skills and resources available within the rest of the team.
- A good team leader is able to step back from the situation to consider the whole picture. This can only be achieved by delegation of responsibility for tasks to other members of the team. It should then be possible to evolve and communicate a plan of action.
- A repeated and systematic ABC approach helps render the patient 'safe', buys thinking time, and increases the likelihood of detecting signs that may lead to a definitive diagnosis.
- Most members of an impromptu emergency team will need to adopt the role of 'team players'. A good team player is adaptable, assumes complete responsibility for delegated problems, and feels comfortable enough to advocate an opinion or feed back information to the rest of the team.

Basic life support (BLS)[1]

Adopt a SAFE approach:
- **S**hout for help.
- **A**pproach with care.
- **F**ree the patient from immediate danger.
- **E**valuate the patient's ABC.

Rescue breathing

- Each inflation should take about 1.5–2 s.
- Resistance will be greater if inflation is too quick and less air will get into the lungs.
- Ideal V_t = 400–500 ml in an adult, about the amount required to produce visible lifting of the chest.
- Wait 2–4 s for full expiration before giving another breath. Ten breaths will therefore take about 40–60 s.

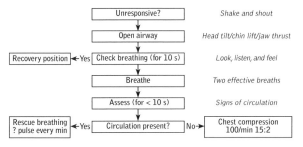

Fig 36.1 Basic life support for adults.

Chest compressions

- **Finding the right place:** Using your index and middle fingers, identify the lower rib margins. Keeping your fingers together, slide them upwards to the point where the ribs join the sternum. With your middle finger on this point, place your index finger on the sternum. Slide the heel of your other hand down the sternum until it reaches your index finger; this should be the middle of the lower half of the sternum. Place the heel of one hand there, with the other hand on top of the first. Interlock the fingers of both hands and lift them to ensure that pressure is not applied over the victim's ribs. Do not apply any pressure over the upper abdomen or bottom tip of the sternum.

....

1 UK Resuscitation Council Guidelines 2000. http://www.resus.org.uk

- **Aim to depress the sternum approximately 4–5 cm** and apply only enough pressure to achieve this.
- At all times the pressure should be firm, controlled and applied vertically. Erratic or violent action is dangerous.
- The recommended rate of compression is a rate and not the number of compressions which are to be given in a minute; this will depend upon interruptions for rescue breathing.
- About the same time should be spent in the compression phase as in the released phase.

Suspected cervical spine injury

- Despite the risk of spinal cord damage, untreated cardiorespiratory arrest will kill the patient.
- Potential secondary damage will be minimized by in-line immobilization of the cervical spine.
- Try to use a jaw thrust and/or a Guedel airway to open the airway rather than tilting the neck.
- Avoid placing the patient in the recovery position.

Advanced life support (ALS)

Adopt a SAFE approach
- **S**hout for help.
- **A**pproach with care.
- **F**ree the patient from immediate danger.
- **E**valuate the patient's ABC.

Defibrillation

- First cycle = 200 J, 200 J, 360 J. All subsequent shocks should be 360 J.
- Electrode polarity is unimportant. Use defibrillation pads to improve electrical contact. One paddle is placed below the right clavicle in the midclavicular line, the other over the lower left ribs in the mid/anterior line (outside the position of the normal cardiac apex), avoiding placement over the breast tissue in females. Transdermal patches should be removed to prevent arcing, and defibrillator pads/paddles should be placed 12–15 cm away from implanted pacemakers.
- For safety reasons, charge the defibrillator only when the paddles are in contact with the patient. Hold the oxygen mask away from the patient during actual defibrillation.
- VT and pulseless VT are the commonest causes of reversible cardiac arrest in adults. These are the most 'recoverable' rhythms and it is therefore always worthwhile persisting with CPR whilst they are present. However, successful resuscitation does depend on **early defibrillation**. Basic life support, IV access, and airway control should not delay delivery of shocks. There is no point in palpating for a pulse between shocks if the ECG rhythm still shows VF since it will only delay delivery of the next shock.

Ventilations

- Once the trachea is intubated, chest compressions should continue uninterrupted (except for pulse checks and defibrillation) at a rate of 100/min whilst ventilations are administered simultaneously at a rate of 12/min.
- A pause in chest compressions allows coronary perfusion pressure to fall substantially and is followed with a delay before the original perfusion pressure is restored after chest compressions are recommenced.
- Over 1 min you should have completed about six cycles of 15:2 compressions:breaths.

Bicarbonate

- Is best administered on the basis of ABGs. Currently it is recommended in the presence of severe acidosis (arterial pH <7.1, base excess < −10) as a dose of 50 mmol (50 ml of 8.4% sodium bicarbonate).
- If ABG analysis is impossible it may be reasonable to give bicarbonate after about 20 min of CPR.

Antiarrhythmics

- Amiodarone should be considered (150 mg IV over 10 min then 300 mg IV over 1 h) in cardiac arrest due to VF or pulseless VF after the third shock.

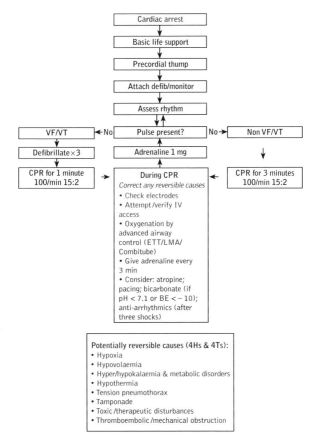

Fig 36.2 Advanced life support for adults.

- Consider lidocaine (lignocaine) as second-line treatment for VF/VT after 12 unsuccessful shocks (four loops). A starting dose of 50–200 mg (5–20 ml of 1% lidocaine (lignocaine)) is reasonable, followed by a maintenance dose of 2 mg/min.
- Bretylium is no longer recommended.

Management of periarrest arrhythmias[2,3]

General points

- Identify and eliminate the primary cause wherever possible.
- If a central line has been placed ensure the tip has not migrated from the SVC into the right atrium.
- Maximize myocardial oxygen delivery.
- Check for and correct electrolyte disturbances, especially K^+ (to >4 mmol/litre) and Mg^{2+} (to >0.7 mmol/litre).
- Check ABGs and correct acid–base imbalance.
- Antiarryhthmic agents may themselves cause hypotension and myocardial depression.
- Use of anticoagulants during the perioperative phase will have to be balanced against the risk of surgical bleeding.

2   UK Resuscitation Council Guidelines 2001. http://www.resus.org.uk
3   European Resuscitation Council Guidelines 2000. http://www.erc.edu

Severe bradycardia, despite anticholinergic treatment.

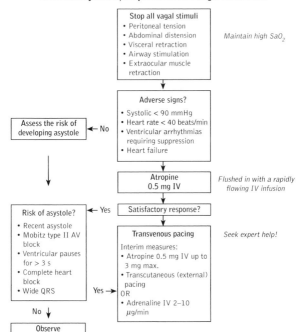

Note: a transvenous pacing wire can be passed relatively easily via an *in situ* Swan sheath/introducer.

Broad complex tachycardia.

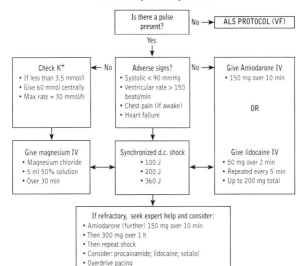

Notes:

• Broad complex tachycardia with adverse signs (systolic BP < 90 mmHg; VR > 150 beats/min; ischaemia) requires urgent **synchronized** d.c. shock.

• Secondary treatment is aimed at stabilizing sinus rhythm and preventing recurrence (antiarrhythmics and electrolyte correction).

• If the patient is not adversely affected by the tachydysrhythmia, correct electrolytes whilst giving antiarrhythmics

Narrow complex tachycardia.

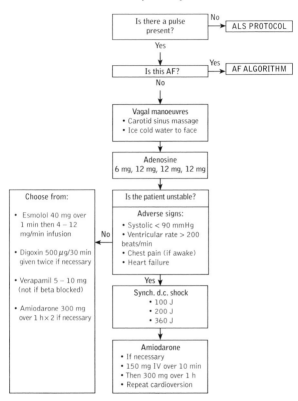

Notes:
- Narrow complex tachycardia with adverse signs (systolic BP < 90 mmHg; VR > 200 beats/min; ischaemia) requires urgent **synchronized** d.c. shock.
- Differentiating narrow from broad complex tachycardia can be difficult, especially at high ventricular rates. Vagal manoeuvres or amiodarone should slow AV conduction of an SVT but not a VT.
- Theophylline interacts with adenosine and tends to block its effect.
- Dipyridamole and carbimazole potentiate the effects of adenosine.
- Adenosine can be used with caution in WPW syndrome.
- Atrial fibrillation now has its own algorithm (see below).
- Verapamil should not be administered in the presence of beta blockade.
- Serum therapeutic range for digoxin = 0.8– 2.0 μg/litre.

Atrial fibrillation.

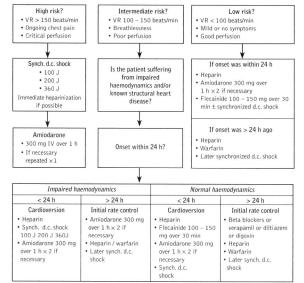

High risk?	Intermediate risk?	Low risk?
• VR > 150 beats/min • Ongoing chest pain • Critical perfusion	• VR 100 – 150 beats/min • Breathlessness • Poor perfusion	• VR < 100 beats/min • Mild or no symptoms • Good perfusion

Synch. d.c. shock
- 100 J
- 200 J
- 360 J

Immediate heparinization if possible

Is the patient suffering from impaired haemodynamics and/or known structural heart disease?

If onset was within 24 h
- Heparin
- Amiodarone 300 mg over 1 h ×2 if necessary
- Flecainide 100 – 150 mg over 30 min ± synchronized d.c. shock

Amiodarone
- 300 mg IV over 1 h
- If necessary repeated × 1

Onset within 24 h?

If onset was > 24 h ago
- Heparin
- Warfarin
- Later synchronized d.c. shock

Impaired haemodynamics		*Normal haemodynamics*	
< 24 h	> 24 h	< 24 h	> 24 h
Cardioversion	Initial rate control	Cardioversion	Initial rate control
• Heparin • Synch. d.c. shock 100 J 200 J 360J • Amiodarone 300 mg over 1 h ×2 if necessary	• Amiodarone 300 mg over 1 h × 2 if necessary • Heparin / warfarin • Later synch. d.c. shock	• Heparin • Flecainide 100 – 150 mg over 30 min • Amiodarone 300 mg over 1 h × 2 if necessary • Synch. d.c. shock	• Beta blockers or verapamil or diltiazem or digoxin • Heparin • Warfarin • Later synch. d.c. shock

Notes:

- At risk patients include those with pre-existing electrolyte disturbance, acidosis, ischaemic heart disease, mitral valve disease, thyrotoxicosis, undergoing cardiothoracic surgery, central line insertion.
- Check the site of a CVP line tip and withdraw from the right atrium if necessary.
- Check electrolytes and correct if necessary.
- Serum therapeutic range for digoxin = 0.8 – 2.0 μg/l.
- Do not administer verapamil to patients on beta blockers.

Paediatric advanced life support[4–6]

Adopt a SAFE approach:

- **S**hout for help.
- **A**pproach with care.
- **F**ree the patient from immediate danger.
- **E**valuate the patient's ABC.

Assess the airway and breathing first. Give two effective breaths (chest seen to rise and fall) before assessing the circulation. Check the carotid pulse in a child but use the brachial pulse in an infant.

The most common arrest scenario in children is bradycardia proceeding to asystole–a response to severe hypoxia and acidosis. Basic life support aimed at restoring early oxygenation should therefore be a priority of management. VF is relatively uncommon, but may complicate hypothermia, tricyclic poisoning, and those children with pre-existing cardiac disease.

- **Children over 8 years of age** should be given basic life support at the adult ratio of 15:2 (compressions:ventilations) aiming for 100 compressions per minute (five cycles).
- **Children under 8 years of age** should be given basic life support at a ratio of 5:1 (compressions:ventilations) aiming for 100 compressions per minute (20 cycles).
- Chest compressions should be started if a central pulse cannot be palpated or the child has a pulse rate <60 beats/min with poor perfusion.
- Where no vascular access is present, immediate intraosseous access (I. O.) is recommended (p. 781).

4 UK Resuscitation Council Guidelines 1998. http://www.resus.org.uk
5 European Resuscitation Council Guidelines 2000. http://www.erc.edu
6 Pediatric Advanced Life Support Manual. American Heart Foundation 1997.

Asystole or pulseless electrical activity (EMD).

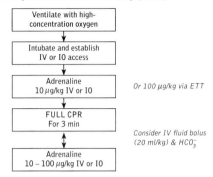

Notes: Consider the following:

- Hypoxia
- Hypovolaemia
- Hyper/hypokalaemia
- Hypothermia
- Tension pneumothorax
- Cardiac tamponade
- Toxin/drug overdose
- Metabolic disturbances
- Thromboemboli

Ventricular fibrillation or pulseless VT.

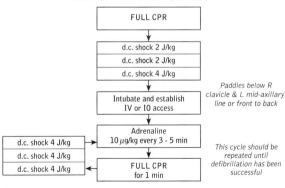

Notes:

- Consider hypokalaemia, hypothermia, and poisoning
- Anti-arrhythmic agents: 1st line = amiodarone 5 mg/kg IV
  2nd line = lidocaine (lignocaine) 1 mg/kg IV
  Torsade de points: magnesium sulphate 25 – 50 mg/kg

Estimated drug doses (see also p. 815)

Drug	Estimated dose
Adrenaline	Initial 10 μg/kg
	Subsequent 100 μg/kg
Aminophylline	5 mg/kg
Amiodarone	5 mg/kg
Atropine	10–20 μg/kg
Bicarbonate	1 mmol/kg
Calcium chloride	0.2 ml/kg of 10% solution slowly
Calcium gluconate	0.6 ml/kg of 10% solution
Cefotaxime	50 mg/kg
Cefuroxime	25 mg/kg
Dextrose (10%)	5 ml/kg
Diazepam	0.1 mg/kg IV
	0.5 mg/kg PR
Ketamine	2 mg/kg
Lidocaine (lignocaine)	1 mg/kg
Lorazepam	0.1 mg/kg recommended for status epilepticus (repeatable after 10 min)
Magnesium	25–50 mg/kg
Metronidazole	7.5 mg/kg
Naloxone	10–100 μg/kg
Neostigmine	50 μg/kg
Phenytoin	15 mg/kg (therapeutic range = 10–20 mg/litre (40–80 μmol/litre))
Salbutamol	2.5 mg nebulizer

Circulation

- Blood volume:
  - 75 ml/kg for children aged 1–10 years
  - 70 ml/kg for children aged >10 years.
- Fluid bolus 20 ml/kg.
- Fluid maintenance:
  4 ml/kg/h for first 10 kg body weight
  + 2 ml/kg/h for next 10 kg body weight
  + 1 ml/kg/h for each remaining kg body weight.

Severe hypotension in theatre

Consider	Patient factors:	Hypovolaemia
		Obstructed venous return
		Raised intrathoracic pressure including tension pneumothorax
		Anaphylaxis
		Embolus (gas/air/thrombus/cement/fat/amniotic fluid)
		Primary pump failure/tachydysrhythmia
		Systemic sepsis
	Technique:	Measurement error
		Excessive depth of anaesthesia
		High regional block (including unexpected central spread from peribulbar/interscalene etc.)
		Iatrogenic drug error including LA toxicity, barbiturates + porphyria
Action		100% oxygen; check surgery/blood loss; check ventilation; reduce volatile; lift legs (if feasible); IV fluid challenge; vasoconstrictors/inotropes.
Investigations		ECG; CXR; ABGs; cardiac enzymes

Risk factors

- Untreated or 'white coat' hypertension preoperatively (increased lability).
- Preoperative fluid deficit (dehydration, diarrhoea and vomiting, blood loss).
- Mediastinal/hepatic/renal surgery (blood loss and caval compression).
- Pre-existing myocardial disease/dysrhythmia.
- Multiple trauma.
- Sepsis.
- Carcinoid syndrome (bradykinin).

Differential diagnosis

- Measurement error: palpate the distal pulse manually whilst repeating an NIBP; check when pulsation returns against the monitor deflation figure. Invasive BP–check the transducer height.
- Suspect tension pneumothorax (particularly following central line insertion) if IPPV and trachea are shifted away from a hyperresonant lung field with diminished breath sounds. Neck veins may be engorged. Treat immediately by decompressing the pleural cavity with an **open** cannula placed in the second intercostal space in the midclavicular line.

- Suspect dehydration if the patient is thirsty, has a dry tongue, is producing dark concentrated urine, and has globally elevated blood cell, urea, creatinine, and electrolyte values.
- Suspect hypovolaemia if the patient has a heart rate >100 beats/ min, respiratory rate >20, capillary return >2 s, cool peripheries, collapsed veins, a narrow and peaked arterial line trace, or marked respiratory swing to either CVP or arterial line trace.
- Suspect cardiac failure if the patient has heart rate >100 beats/min, respiratory rate >20, engorged central veins, capillary return >2 s, cool peripheries, pulmonary oedema, worsening SaO_2 with fluid challenge.
- Suspect air or gas embolus if the patient had a pre-existing low CVP and open venous bed. Signs are variable but may include sudden fall in $ETCO_2$, fall in SaO_2, loss of palpable pulse, EMD, and subsequent rise in CVP.
- Suspect fat embolus or cement reaction in the presence of multiple bony injuries or long bone intramedullary surgery.
- Iatrogenic drug response: histamine releasing drugs, etc. or wrong dilution.
- High central neural blockade may be heralded by Horner's syndrome (small pupil, ptosis, stuffy nose, anhydrosis).
- Anaphylaxis–cardiovascular collapse 88%, erythema 45%, bronchospasm 36%, angio-oedema 24%, rash 13%, urticaria 8.5%.

Immediate management

ABC. ... Check what the surgeons are doing (caval compression/blood loss); prevent further losses by clamp or direct pressure. Administer high FiO_2. Maintenance of organ perfusion and oxygenation is more important than achieving blood pressure alone. BP = SVR × CO therefore improvement in cardiac output may help ameliorate low perfusion pressure:

- 'Optimize preload' (check initial CVP if already sited, change in CVP is more informative than actual CVP): Lifting the legs returns blood into the central venous compartment and also increases afterload. Give a fluid challenge of 10 ml/kg crystalloid/colloid using a pressure infusor. Assess response (BP/HR/CVP), and repeat if appropriate.
- Increase contractility: ephedrine 3–6 mg IV (mixed direct and indirect action); adrenaline 10 µg IV (beta$_{1,2}$ and alpha activity); consider calcium slowly IV (up to 10 ml of 10% calcium chloride).
- Systemic vasoconstriction (NB: alpha agonists increase perfusion pressure but may reduce cardiac output): methoxamine 1–2 mg IV, metaraminol 1–2 mg IV; phenylephrine 0.25–0.5 mg IV; adrenaline 10 µg IV.

Subsequent management

- Correct acidosis to improve the myocardial response to inotropes. Check ABGs and correct respiratory acidosis first. If a severe metabolic acidosis exists (arterial pH <7.1, base excess <−10) consider using bicarbonate 50 mmol (50 ml of 8.4% sodium bicarbonate).
- Maintenance infusion of vasoconstrictor (e.g adrenaline or noradrenaline) or inotrope (e.g dobutamine) if required.

Other considerations

Adrenaline 1 in 10 000 = 100 µg/ml. 1 in 10 dilution results in a 1 in 100 000 solution (10 µg/ml).

Severe hypertension in theatre

Consider	Inadequate depth of anaesthesia/analgesia
	Measurement error
	Hypoxia/hypercapnia
	Iatrogenic drug error
	Pre-eclampsia
	Raised intracranial pressure
	Thyroid storm
	Phaeochromocytoma
Action	Stop surgery until controlled; confirm readings; increase depth of anaesthesia; analgesia; vasodilators; beta blockade; alpha blockade
Investigations	ECG; cardiac enzymes; thyroid function tests; 24 h urinary catecholamine excretion.

Risk factors

- Untreated or 'white coat' hypertension pre-operatively (increased lability).
- Aortic surgery (cross clamp may greatly increase SVR); pregnancy-induced hypertension.
- Drugs: MAOIs (+ pethidine); ketamine; ergometrine.
- Family history of multiple endocrine neoplasia (type 2) syndrome, medullary thyroid carcinoma, Conn's syndrome.
- Acute head injury.

Differential diagnosis

- Hypoxia/hypercapnia: go through ABC and check for patient colour and SpO_2.
- Inadequate depth of anaesthesia: sniff test (smell gases); check volatile agent concentration; check TIVA pump, line, and IV cannula.
- Inadequate analgesia: if in doubt administer alfentanil 10–20 $\mu g/kg$ and observe the effect.
- Measurement error: palpate the distal pulse manually whilst repeating an NIBP; check when pulsation returns against the monitor deflation figure. Invasive BP–check the transducer height.
- Iatrogenic drug response: cocaine, wrong drug such as ephedrine, methoxamine, etc. or wrong dilution (remember surgical drugs, e.g. adrenaline with LA, Moffat's solution, phenylephrine).
- PET: if the patient is over 20 weeks pregnant, check for proteinurea, platelet count ± clotting studies, and LFTs.
- Cushing response = hypertension and reflex bradycardia (baroreceptor mediated) often in the presence of a blown pupil. This intracranially mediated response maintains cerebral perfusion in the presence of increasing ICP (see below).

- Thyroid storm causing elevated T4 and T3 levels.[7]
- Phaeochromocytoma causing elevated plasma noradrenaline levels. Adrenaline will also cause tachydysrhythmias.[8]

Immediate management

ABC…. Assuming this is not a physiological response to a correctable cause, the overall aim of symptomatic management is to prevent hypertensive stroke or subendocardial ischaemia/infarct. Apart from increasing the depth of anaesthesia and analgesia (systemic or regional), treatment options at cardiovascular effector/receptor level include:

- Vasodilators (may cause tachycardia): increase isoflurane concentration, this is most rapidly achieved by simultaneously increasing fresh gas flow. Hydralazine 5 mg slow IV every 15 min. GTN (50 mg/50 ml start at 3 ml/h and titrate to BP) or SNP. Magnesium sulphate 2–4 g slow IV (8–16 mmol) over 10 min, followed by infusion of 1 g/h.
- Beta blockade (particularly in the presence of increased heart rate or dysrhythmias): esmolol 25–100 mg then 50–200 μg/kg/min. (Note that esmolol is supplied as 10 mg/ml **and** 250 mg/ml solutions). Labetalol 5–10 mg IV prn (1–2 ml increments from a 100 mg/20 ml ampoule). Beta:alpha block ratio = 7:1.
- Alpha blockade (particularly in the presence of normal or decreased heart rate): phentolamine 1 mg IV prn (10 mg ampoule made up to 10 ml, in 1 ml increments).

Subsequent management

- For intense analgesia try remifentanil 0.25–0.5 μg/kg/min titrated to BP.
- Check for myocardial damage with an ECG, serial cardiac enzymes including CKMB and/or troponins.
- Thyroid function tests, 24 h urine collection for noradrenaline, adrenaline, and dopamine excretion.

Other considerations

Hypertension in the presence of raised intracranial pressure requires head CT and urgent neurosurgical intervention. Maintain MAP >80 mmHg, normocapnia, head up tilt, unobstructed SVC drainage, low airway pressures, and good oxygenation. Consider mannitol 0.5 g/kg. Bradycardia can be treated with anticholinergics.

7   Farling PA (2000). Thyroid disease. *British Journal of Anaesthesia*, **85**, 15–28.

8   Prys-Roberts C (2000). Phaeochromocytoma. *British Journal of Anaesthesia*, **85**, 44–57.

Severe hypoxia in theatre

Consider	Hypoxic gas mixture	Incorrect flowmeter settings
		Second gas effect (especially on extubation)
		Oxygen failure
		Anaesthetic machine error
	Failure to ventilate	Ventilatory depression or narcosis (NB: regional block after opioids)
		Paralysis but inadequate IPPV (NB: drug error)
		Disconnection
		Misplaced ETT (oesophageal or endobronchial)
		Obstruction to the airway, ETT, filter, mount, circuit, etc.
		Increased airway resistance (laryngospasm, bronchospasm, anaphylaxis)
		Decreased FRC (pneumothorax, raised intra-abdominal pressure, morbid obesity)
	Shunt	Atelectasis
		Airway secretions
		Decreased hypoxic pulmonary vasoconstriction (vasodilators or β_2 agonists)
		CCF with pulmonary oedema
		Aspiration of gastric contents
		Pre-existing pathology (e.g. VSD, ASD + decreased SVR with reversal of flow)
	Poor oxygen delivery	Systemic hypoperfusion (hypovolaemia, sepsis)
		Embolus (gas/air/thrombus/cement/fat/amniotic fluid)
		Local problems (cold limb, Raynaud's, sickle cell)
	Increased oxygen demand	Sepsis
		Malignant hyperthermia

Action	100% oxygen; check FiO$_2$; expose patient and check for central cyanosis; check ventilation bilaterally; hand ventilate on a simple system giving 3 to 4 large breaths initially to recruit alveoli; secure airway; endotracheal suction; initially remove any PEEP; give adrenaline if accompanied by poorly palpable pulses
Investigations	Capnography; chest radiograph; ABGs; CVP ± PCWP; echocardiography

Risk factors

- Reduced FRC (obesity, intestinal obstruction, pregnancy) reduces oxygen reserves.
- Failure to preoxygenate exacerbates any airway difficulties at induction.
- Laryngospasm can result in negative pressure pulmonary oedema.
- Head and neck surgery (shared access to the airway) increases the risk of undetected disconnection.
- History of congenital heart disease or detection of a heart murmer (L–R communication).
- Chronic lung disease.
- Sickle cell disease.
- Methaemoglobinaemia (interpreted as deoxyhaemoglobin by pulse oximeters).

Differential diagnosis

- FiO$_2$: use an oxygen analyser at all times.
- Ventilation: cross-check rise and fall of chest with auscultation over stomach and in both axillae, capnograph trace, measured expired tidal volume and airway pressure.
- Measurement error: does the patient appear cyanosed (beware in anaemia when 5 g/dl deoxyhaemoglobin may not be visible)?
- Aspiration/airway secretions: auscultate and aspirate using tracheal suction catheter ± litmus paper.
- Suspect tension pneumothorax (particularly following central line insertion) if IPPV and trachea are shifted away from a hyperresonant lung field with diminished breath sounds. Neck veins may be engorged. Treat immediately by decompressing the pleural cavity with an **open** cannula placed in the second intercostal space in the midclavicular line.
- Suspect hypovolaemia if the patient has a heart rate of >100 beats/ min, respiratory rate of >20/min, capillary return >2 s, cool peripheries, collapsed veins, a narrow and peaked arterial line trace, or marked respiratory swing to either CVP or arterial line trace.
- Suspect cardiac failure if the patient has a heart rate of >100 beats/ min, a respiratory rate of >20/min, engorged central veins, capillary return >2 s, cool peripheries, pulmonary oedema, worsening SaO$_2$ with fluid challenge.

- Suspect air or gas embolus if the patient had a pre-existing low CVP and open venous bed. Signs are variable but may include sudden decrease in $ETCO_2$, decrease in SaO_2, loss of palpable pulse, EMD, and subsequent rise in CVP.
- Suspect fat embolus or cement reaction in the presence of multiple bony injuries or long bone intramedullary surgery.
- Malignant hyperthermia: especially if accompanied by increased $ETCO_2$, respiratory rate, heart rate, and ectopics.
- Anaphylaxis–cardiovascular collapse 88%, erythema 45%, bronchospasm 36%, angio-oedema 24%, rash 13%, urticaria 8.5%.

Immediate management

ABC…. Expose the chest, all the breathing circuit, and all airway connections. Administer 100% O_2 by manual ventilation–at least three to four large breaths initially will help to recruit collapsed alveoli (and gives continuous tactile feedback about the state of the airway). If no improvement:

- Confirm FiO_2: If there is any doubt about inspired oxygen concentration from the anaesthetic machine, use a separate cylinder supply (as a last resort use room air via a self-inflating bag = 21% oxygen).
- Misplaced ETT? Cross-check the rise and fall of the chest with auscultation over the stomach and in both axillae and the capnograph trace.
- Ventilation problems: Simplify the breathing system until the problem is removed, i.e. switch to a bag rather than the ventilator, use a Bain circuit instead of the circle system, try a self-inflating bag, use a mask rather than ETT, etc.
- Diagnosis of the source of a leak or obstruction: This is not as important initially as oxygenation of the patient. Make the patient safe first then use a systematic approach. The fastest way to isolate the problem is probably by division. For instance, does breaking the circuit at the ETT connector leave the problem on the patient's side or the anaesthetic machine's side?
- Severe R–L shunt: Severe hypoxia occurs when blood starts flowing through a congenital heart defect in the presence of low SVR, thus bypassing the pulmonary circulation. The resultant hypoxaemia then exacerbates the problem by causing hypoxic pulmonary vasoconstriction which increases PVR and increases the tendency for blood to shunt across the cardiac defect. Treatment is therefore twofold:
  - Increase SVR by lifting the legs and giving adrenaline and IV fluid, especially in sepsis.
  - Minimize PVR by removing PEEP, avoiding high intrathoracic pressure, and maximizing FiO_2.
- Bronchospasm: Eliminate ETT obstruction by sounding ETT with a gum elastic bougie. Treat by increasing volatile agent concentration, IV salbutamol (250 µg) (see status asthmaticus, p. 848).

Other considerations

- In chronic bronchitis the bronchial circulation can shunt up to 10% of cardiac output.
- The foramen ovale remains patent in 20–30% of patients but is normally kept closed because left atrial pressure is usually higher than right atrial pressure. IPPV, PEEP, breatholding, CCF, thoracic surgery, or PE can reverse the pressure gradient and result in shunt.

Severe laryngospasm

Condition	Acute glottic closure by the vocal cords
Presentation	Crowing or absent inspiratory sounds and marked tracheal tug
Immediate action	Avoid painful stimuli; 100% oxygen; CPAP; jaw thrust; remove irritants from the airway; deepen anaesthesia
Follow-up action	Muscle relaxation if intractable
Also consider	Bronchospasm
	Laryngeal trauma/airway oedema (esp. if no leak with paediatric ETT)
	Recurrent laryngeal nerve damage
	Tracheomalacia
	Inhaled foreign body
	Epiglottitis or croup

Risk factors

- Barbiturate induction or light anaesthesia, especially in anxious patients
- Intense surgical stimulation: anal stretch; cervical dilatation; incision and drainage of abscesses.
- Extubation of a soiled airway.
- Thyroid surgery.
- Hypocalcaemia (neuromuscular irritability).
- Multiple crowns (inhaled foreign body).

Immediate management

- Remove the stimulus that precipitated the laryngospasm.
- Check that the airway is clear of obstruction or potential irritants.
- Give high concentration oxygen with the expiratory valve of the circuit closed and maintain a close seal by holding the mask with two hands if necessary to maintain CPAP. The degree of CPAP can be controlled by intermittently relaxing the airway seal at the level of the mask.
- If the laryngospasm has occurred at induction, it may be relieved by deepening anaesthesia using further increments of propofol (disadvantage: potential ventilatory depression) or by increasing the volatile agent concentration (disadvantage: irritation of the airway, less so with sevoflurane, more with isoflurane). Don't use nitrous oxide, it will decrease oxygen reserves.
- If the laryngospasm fails to improve remove any airways that may be stimulating the pharynx.
- Suxamethonium 0.25–0.5 mg/kg will relieve laryngospasm. If IV access is impossible, consider giving 2–4 mg/kg intramuscularly or sublingually.

Subsequent management

- Monitor for evidence of pulmonary oedema.
- CPAP may have inflated the stomach with gas so decompress it with an orogastric tube and recover the patient in the lateral position.

Other considerations

- The risk of laryngospasm may be reduced by co-induction with IV opioids, IV lidocaine (lignocaine), or by topical lidocaine (lignocaine) spray prior to laryngoscopy (don't use more than 4 mg/kg).
- Laryngospasm is caused by acute glottic closure of the vocal cords and is mediated by the superior laryngeal nerve. Blockade can be achieved by injecting 2 ml of LA 1 cm medial to the superior cornu of the hyoid through the thyrohyoid membrane prior to awake fibreoptic intubation.
- Unilateral recurrent laryngeal nerve trauma results in paralysis of one vocal cord and causes hoarseness, ineffective cough, and potential to aspirate. Bilateral vocal cord paralysis is more serious, leading to stridor on extubation–this may mimic laryngospasm but doesn't get better with standard airway manoeuvres. The patient will require reintubation and possibly tracheostomy.
- Tracheomalacia is likely to cause more stridor with marked negative inspiratory pressure so treat initially with CPAP. Reconstructive surgery may be necessary.

Air/gas embolism

Condition	Venous gas produces airlock in RV and obstructs pulmonary capillaries
Presentation	Decreased $ETCO_2$, decreased SaO_2, loss of palpable pulse, EMD, decreased CVP then increased CVP
Immediate action	Remove source of embolus; flood wound; compress drainage veins
Follow-up action	Increase venous pressure; turn off N_2O; left lateral head down tilt; CVS support
Investigations	Auscultation; Doppler; ECG; chest radiograph
Also consider	Breathing circuit disconnection (loss of $ETCO_2$ trace and decreased SaO_2)
	Pulseless cardiac arrest—other causes of EMD (4Ts and 4Hs) (see p. 826)
	Cement reaction
	Pulmonary embolism of thrombus
	Amniotic fluid embolus

Risk factors

- Patient: spontaneous ventilation (negative central venous pressure); patent foramen ovale (risk of paradoxical emboli).
- Anaesthesia: hypovolaemia; any open vascular access point; operation site higher than heart; pressurized infusions.
- Orthopaedic surgery: multiple trauma; long bone surgery, especially intramedullary nailing; hip surgery.
- General surgery: laparoscopic procedures; hysterectomy; neck surgery; vascular surgery.
- ENT surgery: middle ear procedures.
- Neurosurgery: posterior fossa operations in the sitting position (now almost historical).

Diagnosis

- 'At risk' patient, dramatic fall/loss of the $ETCO_2$ trace and fall in SaO_2.
- Awake patients complain of severe chest pain.
- Heart rate may rise.
- Sudden rise in CVP due to a fall in cardiac output and rise in PVR.
- Classically a 'millwheel' murmur can supposedly be heard.
- Doppler ultrasound is extremely sensitive (0.25 ml air!) but possibly unavailable as a diagnostic tool.
- EMD arrest may occur. ECG may show signs of acute ischaemia, e.g. ST segment depression >1 mm.

- It is claimed that symptoms/signs of air embolus appear following 0.5 ml/kg/min of intravascular gas.

Immediate management

ABC…. Eliminate breathing circuit disconnection; give 100% oxygen; check ECG trace and pulse.

- Prevent further gas/air from entering the circulation. Get the surgeon to apply compression to major drainage vessels and flood the wound with irrigation fluid or cover with damp pack, stop reaming, etc.
- Decompress any gas-pressurized system/cavity, e.g the abdomen during laparoscopy.
- Lower the operation site to below heart level.
- Turn off N_2O (it will expand any intravascular gas volume).
- Increase venous pressure with rapid IV infusion of fluids ± vasopressors.
- If EMD arrest occurs, start external cardiac massage and adopt advanced life support protocol for non-VF/VT cardiac arrest.
- Aspirate CVP line. Classic teaching is to the tip patient head down in the left lateral position to keep the bubble in the right atrium or apex of the right ventricle until it dissolves or can be aspirated via a central line advanced into the right atrium. In practice, if there is not already a CVP line *in situ* aspiration is likely to be difficult.
- Moderate CPAP has been advocated as a means of rapidly increasing intrathoracic and therefore central venous pressure in the event of gas embolus. Whilst this manoeuvre may limit the extent and progress of an air embolus, it must be borne in mind that 10% of patients may have a patent foramen ovale. Sustained rise in right atrial pressure may then lead to a right to left shunt and paradoxical air embolism to the cerebral circulation.

Subsequent management

- Ask the surgeon to apply bone wax to exposed bone edges.
- Correct any pre-existing hypovolaemia.
- Avoid nitrous oxide for the remainder of the anaesthetic, and maintain a high FiO_2.
- Perform a 12-lead ECG to look for ischaemia. Air in coronary arteries is suggestive of paradoxical air embolism.
- Consider hyperbaric therapy if available: increased ambient pressure (3–6 bar) will decrease the volume of gas emboli.

Other considerations

Carbon dioxide is the safest gas to use for laparoscopic insufflation. It is non-flammable and is more soluble than other agents. Should a gas embolus occur, it will dissolve over time. The priority of management should therefore be to limit the extent and central progress of the gas 'bubble' thereby minimizing its systemic cardiovascular effect.

Aspiration

Condition	Chemical pneumonitis; foreign body obstruction and atelectesis
Presentation	Tachypnoea; tachycardia; decreased lung compliance; decreased SaO_2
Immediate action	Minimize further aspiration; secure the airway; suction
Follow-up action	100% oxygen; consider CPAP; empty the stomach
Investigations	Chest radiograph; bronchoscopy
Also consider	Pulmonary oedema (see p. 850)
	Embolus
	ARDS

Risk factors

- Full stomach.
- Known reflux.
- Raised intragastric pressure (intestinal obstruction, pregnancy, laparoscopic surgery).
- Recent trauma.
- Perioperative opioids.
- Diabetes mellitus.
- Topically anaesthetized airway.

Diagnosis

- Clinical: auscultation may reveal a wheeze and crepitations; tracheal aspirate may be acidic (but a negative finding does not exclude aspiration).
- Chest radiograph: diffuse infiltrative pattern especially in right lower lobe distribution (but often not acutely).

Immediate management

- Avoidance of general anaesthesia in high-risk situations. Use of a rapid sequence technique when appropriate.
- Administer 100% oxygen and minimize the risk of further aspirate contaminating the airway.
- If the patient is awake or nearly awake, suction the oro/nasopharynx and place in the recovery position.
- If the patient is unconscious but breathing spontaneously, apply cricoid pressure. Avoid cricoid pressure if the patient is actively vomiting (risk of oesophageal rupture) and place patient in a left lateral head down position. Intubate if tracheal suction and ventilation are indicated.
- If the patient is unconscious and apnoeic intubate immediately and commence ventilation.

Treat as an inhaled foreign body: minimize positive pressure ventilation until the ETT and airway have been suctioned and all aspirates are clear.

ubsequent management

Empty the stomach with a large-bore nasogastric tube prior to attempting extubation.

Monitor respiratory function and arrange a chest radiograph. Look for evidence of oedema, collapse, or consolidation.

If SpO_2 remains at 90–95%, atelectasis can be improved with CPAP (10 cmH_2O) and chest physiotherapy.

If SpO_2 remains <90% despite 100% oxygen, there may be solid food material obstructing part of the bronchial tree. If the patient is intubated, consider using fibreoptic/rigid bronchoscopy or bronchial lavage using 0.9% saline to remove any large foreign bodies or semisolid material from the airway. Refer to ICU postoperatively.

ther considerations

Corticosteroids may modify the inflammatory response early after aspiration but don't alter the outcome, except by potentially interfering with the normal immune response.

Prophylactic antibiotics are not generally given routinely (unless infected material aspirated), but may be required to treat subsequent secondary infections.

If gastric aspirate has been buffered to pH 7, the resulting aspiration pneumonitis is less severe, volume for volume, than if it is highly acidic. However, solid food material can produce prolonged inflammation, even if the overall pH is neutral.

Blood, although undesirable, is generally well tolerated in the airway.

Status asthmaticus

Condition	Intractable bronchospasm
Presentation	Increased airway pressure; sloping expiratory capnograph trace
Immediate action	100% oxygen; salbutamol 250 µg IV/2.5 mg nebulizer; aminophylline 250 mg slow IV
Follow-up action	Hydrocortisone 200 mg
Investigations	Chest radiograph; ABGs
Also consider	Breathing circuit obstruction
	Kinked ETT/cuff herniation
	Endobronchial intubation/tube migration
	Foreign body in airway
	Anaphylaxis
	Pneumothorax

Risk factors

+ Asthma, particularly with previous acute admissions, especially to ICU and/or systemic steroid dependence.
+ Intercurrent respiratory tract infection.
+ Carinal irritation by ETT.

Diagnosis

+ Increased airway pressure, prolonged expiratory phase to capnograph trace.
+ Central trachea with bilaterally hyperexpanded and resonant lung fields expiratory wheeze (absent if severe).
+ Severe bronchospasm is a diagnosis of exclusion. The quickest method of ascertaining the source of the increased airway resistance is to break the breathing circuit distal to all connectors/filters and to try ventilating directly with a self-inflating bag. If the inflation pressure still feels too high the problem is due to airway/ETT obstruction or reduced compliance.
+ Eliminate ETT obstruction by 'sounding' the ETT with a graduated gum elastic bougie (note the distance it can be inserted down the ETT and compare it with the external tube markings).

Immediate management

ABC…. 100% oxygen.

+ Increase concentration of volatile agent–sevoflurane is the least irritant and is less likely to precipitate dysrhythmias in the presence of hypercapnia (halothane is most likely to).

- Salbutamol 250 μg intravenously or 2.5 mg by nebulizer Alternatively (as an immediate measure) administer two to six puffs of beta agonist inhaler into the airway by placing the device in the barrel of a 50 ml syringe. Attach the syringe by Luer lock to a 15 cm length of fine-bore infusion/capnograph tubing, which can then be fed directly down the ETT. The inhaler can be discharged by pressure applied via the syringe plunger. Use of the fine bore tubing decreases deposition of the drug on the ETT.

- Aminophylline 250 mg by slow intravenous injection (up to 5 mg/kg).

Subsequent management[9,10]

- If immediate treatment fails or is unavailable, consider ipratropium bromide (0.25 mg nebulizer), adrenaline IV boluses (10 μg = 0.1 ml of 1 in 10 000), ketamine (2 mg/kg IV), magnesium (2 g by slow IV).

- Hydrocortisone 200 mg IV.

- Check the drug chart and notes for possible drug allergies to agents already administered.

- Arrange a chest radiograph–check for pneumothorax and ETT tip position (withdraw if carinal).

- Check ABGs and electrolytes (prolonged use of beta$_2$ agonists causes hypokalaemia).

- Refer to ICU.

Other considerations

- Pulsus paradoxus is a systemic blood pressure deficit measured during the spontaneous ventilatory cycle. A paradox of greater than 10 mmHg (1.3 kPa) indicates severe asthma.

- Gas trapping: raised mean intrathoracic pressure may result from IPPV in the presence of severe bronchospasm. If the pulse pressure falls and neck veins appear distended, consider obstructed venous return and a dependent fall in cardiac output. Intermittently disconnect the ETT from the circuit and observe the (connected) capnograph trace for evidence of prolonged expiration and return of pulse pressure.

- Ventilator setting advice during this phase: 100% oxygen, initially by hand, may need high pressures, slow rate, prolonged expiration, do **not** worry about CO_2 levels provided that SpO_2 is alright. It may be necessary to accept a reduced respiratory ventilation rate to allow adequate expiration to occur (permissive hypercapnia).

9 Asthma: a changing perspective on management (1996). *Current anaesthesia and critical care*, vol. 7, pp. 260–5. Churchill Livingstone, Edinburgh.

10 British Thoracic Society *et al.* (1993) Guidelines on the management of asthma. *British Medical Journal*, **306**, pp. 776–82.

Pulmonary oedema

Condition	Increased hydrostatic pressure; increased vascular permeability; decreased plasma colloid osmotic pressure; negative interstitial pressure; obstructed lymphatic drainage
Presentation	Pink frothy sputum; increased heart rate, respiratory rate, CVP, and PCWP; decreased SaO_2
Immediate action	100% oxygen; decrease PCWP by posture
Follow-up action	Opioids; diuretics; vasodilators
Investigations	Chest radiograph; ECG; ABG; consider PA catheter studies
Also consider	Asthma
	MI
	ARDS
	Drug reaction
	Aspiration

Risk factors

- MI or pre-existing myocardial disease (pump failure).
- Drugs/toxins (fluid overload–especially in renal failure and the elderly, drug reaction, myocardial depression).
- Aspiration (chemical pneumonitis).
- Pre-existing lung disease or infection (increased capillary permeability).
- Malnutrition (low oncotic pressure); this is rare!
- Acute head injury or intracranial pathology (neurogenic).
- Severe laryngospasm or airway obstruction (negative intrathoracic pressure)[11].
- Severe hypertension; LVF; mitral stenosis (high pulmonary vascular hydrostatic pressure).
- Lateral decubitus position (unilateral).
- Impairment of lymphatic drainage (e.g malignancy).
- Rapid lung expansion (e.g. re-expansion of a pneumothorax).
- Following pneumonectomy.

Diagnosis

- Clinical: wheeze; pink frothy sputum; fine crackles; quiet bases; triple rhythm; increased JVP; liver engorgement.

11 Lang SA, Duncan PG, Shephard DAE, Hung CH (1990). Pulmonary oedema associated with airway obstruction. *Canadian Journal of Anaesthesia*, **37**, 210.

- Monitors: increased heart rate; increased respiratory rate; decreased SaO_2; increased airway pressure; increased CVP; increased PCWP (greater than 25–30 mmHg).
- Chest radiograph: basal shadowing; upper lobe diversion; bat's wing or stag horn appearance; hilar haze; bronchial cuffing, Kerley B lines; pleural effusions; septal/interlobar fluid lines.
- ECG: evidence of right heart strain; evidence of MI.

Immediate management

- ABC…then management depends upon the current state of the patient.
- If awake and breathing spontaneously: sit up to offload the pulmonary vasculature and improve FRC; high flow 100% oxygen via mask with reservoir bag; furosemide (frusemide) 50 mg IV; diamorphine 5 mg IV; consider using CPAP 5–10 mmHg and a vasodilator if hypertensive (e.g. GTN 0.5–1.5 mg sublingually, or 10 mg transcutaneous patch, beware of IV GTN administration in the absence of invasive BP monitoring).
- If anaesthetized and intubated: commence IPPV with PEEP (5–10 cmH$_2$O) in a 15° head up position to reduce atelectasis and improve FRC; aspirate free fluid from the trachea intermittently; drug therapy as above.

Subsequent management

- Optimize fluid therapy and maintain plasma colloid oncotic pressure on the basis of serial CVP measurements. If in doubt, measure PCWP via a PA catheter.
- Consider inotropic support with a beta agonist (e.g. dobutamine) or venesection (500 ml) if filling pressures remain high or signs of inadequate circulation persist.

Can't intubate … can't ventilate

Condition	Failure to oxygenate by ETT/facemask/LMA/COPA/Combitube
Presentation	1 in 10 000 anaesthetics
Immediate action	Summon help; 100% oxygen; CPAP; wake up if possible
Follow-up action	Needle cricothyrotomy
Also consider	Emergency tracheostomy;
	Fibreoptic intubation
	Blind nasal approach

Risk factors

• See 'failed intubation' risks (p. 874).

• Inexperienced anaesthetist.

• No preoxygenation (increases rate of arterial desaturation).

Immediate management

• Call for help, but retain your trained assistant.

• Attempt oxygenation even if it appears futile. Insert both an oral **and** nasopharyngeal airway. Lock on the emergency oxygen flush. Apply a close fitting facemask with two hands and lift/dislocate the mandible firmly forwards (jaw thrust). Although an assistant may help by bag squeezing, it may be easiest to attempt ventilation by allowing an intermittent leak around the mask.

• Consider using an LMA, Intubating LMA, Combitube, COPA. No single airway adjunct has clear advantages over others. This is not a time to experiment with unfamiliar devices so stick to whatever you feel comfortable with and abandon them early if they prove to be of no benefit.

• If the patient is making spontaneous effort and respiratory noise, maintain CPAP and 100% oxygen until the patient wakes.

Subsequent management

• Cricothyrotomy (see also p. 877): The decision to attempt transtracheal oxygenation is not an easy one to make. However, remember that it is likely to take over a minute to achieve access, and even then, ability to oxygenate will be severely limited. Speed is essential in order to prevent hypoxic cardiac arrest or brain damage.

• Extend the neck: You may find access easier if someone else does this for you and simultaneously fixes the skin by applying slight traction bilaterally to the soft tissues of the neck.

• Find the cricothyroid membrane (it lies between the superiorly notched thyroid cartilage and the cricoid cartilage; see diagram).

Attach a 20 ml syringe containing 10 ml of 0.9% saline to a large-bore needle or cannula (14–16G). Advance through the cricothyroid membrane in a slightly caudally inclined direction aspirating until air bubbles freely into the syringe.

If you have used a needle, hold it firmly in place. If you have used a cannula guard against kinking.

There are several ways of connecting a needle/cannula to a standard breathing circuit:

- Connect a 10 ml syringe, remove the plunger, and intubate the barrel with a cuffed ETT.
- Insert an ETT connector from a neonatal 3.5 mm ETT to the hub of the needle/cannula.
- Unscrew the capnograph tubing from the monitor, attach the Luer lock end to the hub of the needle/cannula. Take the other end and attach the sampling end (T-piece) to the common gas outlet. Use your thumb to intermittently occlude the other end of the T-piece.
- Use a Sanders injector or similar jetting device attached by Luer lock. **Beware**: high-pressure oxygen can cause a catastrophic surgical emphysema via a misplaced cannula. Check for rise **and** fall of the chest wall.[12]

Transtracheal oxygenation by needle/cannula is a temporary emergency measure. Full ventilation is unlikely to be possible. However, there should be flow of oxygen down the bronchial tree to the alveoli.

Call urgently for an ENT surgeon to perform an emergency tracheostomy. If possible, improve transtracheal access with a 'Minitrach' or similar device. There are several easy to use commercial kits that exist based around a Seldinger method of insertion. If the patient remains paralysed attempt fibreoptic/blind nasal intubation.

Consider transtracheal jet ventilation but stop ventilating immediately if surgical emphysema forms in the neck.

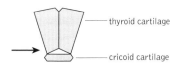

Fig 36.3 Cricothyroid membrane (arrow) between thyroid and circoid cartilages.

2 Benumof JL, Scheller MS (1989). The importance of transtracheal jet ventilation in the management of the difficult airway. *Anesthesiology*, **71**, 769.

Other considerations

- The best treatment is prevention, or at least anticipation of potential airway difficulties. Avoidance of muscle relaxants is prudent until one has determined that ventilation can be achieved manually. Thorough preoxygenation will ensure that the FRC contains approximately 2 litres of oxygen rather than 0.5 litre at induction. Have the kit and personnel required for the creation of a surgical airway close at hand if you anticipate difficulties intubating.

- If the problem is an inability to achieve a seal due to the presence of a beard, quickly apply a large transparent self-adhesive dressing over the whole of the lower face. Make a large hole in it for the mouth and nostrils, and re-apply the mask ± an airway.

- If the problem is an inability to pass a small enough ETT tube down a narrowed trachea (either the ETT is too short or a suitable size is unavailable), consider passing an airway exchange catheter. This is a robust guide that resembles a white but hollow gum elastic bougie. It comes with either Luer lock or 15 mm connector allowing oxygen to be passed through it into the distal airway whilst a more definitive airway is established either by rail-roading a larger tube over it or by surgical tracheostomy.[13]

- Commercially available transtracheal needles and injectors are now widely available.

- Check that your theatres have a well-stocked difficult/failed intubation trolley available at all times.

13 Padkin A, McIndoe A (2000). Use of the airway exchange catheter for the patient with a partially obstructed airway. *Anaesthesia*, 55, 87.

Malignant hyperthermia (see also p. 199)

Condition	Hypermetabolism due to increased skeletal muscle intracellular Ca^{2+}
Presentation	Increased $ETCO_2$; decreased SaO_2; increased heart rate; CVS instability; dysrhythmias; increased core temperature
Immediate action	Stop triggers (volatile agents + suxamethonium); hyperventilate with high-flow 100% oxygen; dantrolene 1–10 mg/kg
Follow-up action	Cool; correct DIC, acidosis, hyperkalaemia; promote diuresis (risk of acute renal failure)
Investigations	Clotting studies, ABGs, K^+; urine myoglobin; CK
Also consider	Rebreathing
	Sepsis
	Awareness
	Neuroleptic malignant syndrome
	Ecstacy
	Thyroid storm

Risk factors

- Family history.
- Exposure to suxamethonium or volatile agents (even if previous exposures were uneventful).
- Exertional heat stroke. Exercise-induced rhabdomyolisis, central core disease, scoliosis, hernias, strabismus surgery.

Diagnosis

- Sustained jaw rigidity after suxamethonium (masseter spasm).
- Unexplained tachycardia together with an unexpected rise in $ETCO_2$ (IPPV) or minute volume (SV).
- Falling SaO_2 despite increased FiO_2.
- Cardiovascular instability, dysrhythmias especially multiple ventricular ectopics, peaked T waves on ECG.
- Generalized rigidity.
- Core temperature rise of 2° C/h.

Immediate management[14,15]

- Check ABC. … Turn off all volatile agents, don't administer any further doses of suxamethonium.
- Hyperventilate with 100% oxygen using a high fresh gas flow to flush out volatile agent and expired CO_2.
- Tell the rest of the theatre team what the problem is. Ask for more help and obtain dantrolene immediately.
- Use a fresh breathing circuit ± a 'vapour-free' machine if it is easy to do so, but not if it results in rebreathing of expired CO_2, a low FiO_2, or delays administration of dantrolene.
- When available, give dantrolene 1 mg/kg IV (it comes in 20 mg ampoules so about four are required). Repeat. Usually about 2.5 mg/kg are required in total, but up to 10 mg/kg may be given.
- Stop surgery if feasible, otherwise maintain anaesthesia with TIVA (propofol).
- Reduce core temperature by: evaporation; ice to groins and axillae; cold fluids into intravenous lines, the bladder via urinary catheter, stomach via a nasogastric tube, or peritoneal cavity if open.
- Check ABGs and K^+, especially if dysrhythmias occur, and correct acidosis/ hyperkalaemia where appropriate.
- Surgical team—call for senior help to conclude the operation as quickly as is safely possible.

Subsequent management

- Place invasive BP and CVP monitoring lines.
- Send a clotting screen for DIC, and serum CK assay (up to 1000 times normal).
- Send a urine sample for myoglobin estimation secondary to muscle break-down.
- Monitor for acute renal failure and promote a diuresis with fluids and mannitol.
- Refer to the MH Investigation Unit[15] for *in vitro* muscle contracture tests (IVCTs).

Other considerations

- Dantrolene is formulated with 3 g mannitol per ampoule.
- Emptying several ampoules into a sterile dish and adding a large volume of sterile water may help mix dantrolene more rapidly.
- Follow-up involves muscle biopsy under LA and *in vitro* halothane, caffeine, ryanodine, and chlorocresol contracture tests.

14 Hopkins PM (2000). Malignant hyperthermia: advances in clinical management and diagnosis. *British Journal of Anaesthesia*, **85**, 118–28.

15 UK MH Investigation Unit, Academic Unit of Anaesthesia, Clinical Sciences Building, St James' University Hospital Trust, Leeds LS9 7TF, UK tel. 0113 206 5274. Emergency hotline 07947 609601.

Anaphylaxis

Condition	IgE mediated type B hypersensitivity reaction to an antigen resulting in histamine and serotonin release from mast cells and basophils
Presentation	Cardiovascular collapse; erythema; bronchospasm; oedema; rash
Immediate action	Remove trigger; 100% oxygen; elevate legs; adrenaline 50 µg; fluids
Follow-up action	Chlorpheniramine 10–20 mg; hydrocortisone 100–300 mg; ABGs
Investigations	Plasma tryptase; urinary methylhistamine
Also consider	Primary myocardial/cardiovascular problem
	Latex sensitivity
	Airway obstruction
	Asthma
	Tension pneumothorax

Risk factors

- Intravenous administration of the antigen.
- Note that cross-sensitivities with NSAIDs and muscle relaxants mean that previous exposure is not always necessary.
- True penicillin allergy is a reaction to the basic common structure present in most penicillins.

Diagnosis

- Cardiovascular collapse (88%).
- Erythema (45%).
- Bronchospasm (36%)
- Angio-oedema (24%)
- Rash (13%)
- Urticaria (8.5%)

Immediate management[16]

- Check ABC. … Stop the administration of any potential triggers, particularly intravenous agents. Muscle relaxants, antibiotics and NSAIDs are the most frequent triggers.
- Call for help.
- Maintain the airway and give 100% oxygen.

---

16 Working Party of the Association of Anaesthetists and the British Society of Allergy and Clinical Immunology (October 1995 and March 1999).

- Lay the patient flat with the legs elevated.
- Give adrenaline in 50 μg IV increments (0.5 ml 1:10 000 solution) at a rate of 100 μg/min until pulse pressure or bronchospasm improves. Alternatively, give adrenaline 0.5–1 mg IM (repeated after 10 min if necessary).
- Give intravenous fluid (colloid or suitable crystalloid).

Subsequent management

- Antihistamines: give chlorpheniramine (Piriton®) 10–20 mg by slow IV. Consider H_2 antagonists (ranitidine 50 mg slow IV).
- Corticosteroids: give hydrocortisone 100–300 mg IV.
- Catecholamine infusion as CVS instability may last several hours: Adrenaline 0.05–0.1 μg/kg/min (= 4 ml/h of 1:10 000 for a 70 kg adult) Noradrenaline 0.05–0.1 μg/kg/min = 4 ml/h of a solution of 4 mg made up to 40 ml in 5% dextrose for a 70 kg adult).
- Check ABGs for acidosis and consider bicarbonate 0.5–1.0 mmol/ kg (8.4% solution = 1 mmol/ml).
- Check for the presence of airway oedema by letting down the ETT cuff and confirming a leak prior to extubating.
- Consider bronchodilators (see status asthmaticus) for persistent bronchospasm.

Other considerations

- Investigations can wait until the patient has been stabilized. Take a 10 ml clotted blood sample 1 h after the start of the reaction to perform a tryptase assay. The specimen needs to be spun down and the serum stored at – 20 °C.
- The anaesthetist should follow up the investigation, report reactions to the Committee on Safety of Medicines (CSM), and arrange skin prick testing with immunologists (see p. 956 for follow-up management).

Arterial injection

Condition	Chemical endarteritis characterized by: arterial vasospasm and local release of noradrenaline; crystal deposition within the distal arteries (thiopental); subsequent thrombosis and distal ischaemic necrosis
Presentation	Intense burning pain on injection; distal blanching; blistering
Immediate action	Stop injection but leave the cannula in situ and administer 1% lidocaine (lignocaine) 5 ml and papaverine 40 mg, flush with heparinized saline
Follow-up action	Regional sympathetic blockade; anticoagulation
Investigations	Monitor anticoagulation
Also consider	Extravasation
	Dilution error of drug administered

Risk factors

- Antecubital lines: inadvertent cannulation of brachial artery or aberrant ulnar artery.
- Radial aspect of wrist: inadvertent cannulation of superficial branch of radial artery.
- Arterial injection is more likely to cause damage with stronger drug concentration (e.g. 5% thiopental).
- Cannula which has been inserted previously and only been flushed with saline (not painful) may present later.

Diagnosis

- Awake patients complain of intense burning pain on injection that may last for several hours.
- Blanching of the skin.
- Blistering.
- Within 2 h: oedema, hyperaesthesia, motor weakness.
- Later: signs of arterial thrombosis ± gangrene.

Immediate management

- Stop injecting!
- Principles of treatment are to dilute the irritant, reverse vasospasm, and prevent thrombosis.
- Keep the cannula *in situ*–you will need access to reverse local vasoconstriction within the distal arteriolar tree.
- If the drug administered was highly irritant, flush the vessel with isotonic saline or 'Hepsal'.
- Administer local anaesthetic down the cannula to reduce vasospasm and reduce pain (e.g. 10 ml 1% lidocaine (lignocaine)).

- Administer a vasodilator (e.g. papaverine 40 mg).
- Once the immediate reaction has subsided, if the hand is well perfused and pink, remove the cannula and apply sufficient pressure to the puncture site to minimize local haematoma formation.

Subsequent management

- Sympathetic blockade and anticoagulation to reduce the risk of thrombosis:
    - sympathectomy via stellate ganglion or brachial plexus block– probably most easily achieved via the axillary approach, or
    - guanethidine block: performed like a Bier's block (guanethidine 10–20 mg IV + heparin 500 units in 25–40 ml saline, cuff left inflated for 20 min), guanethidine blocks alpha adrenergic neurons and depletes noradrenaline stores. The effects can last for several weeks. Ask for assistance from consultants with a special interest in chronic pain since this block is also used to treat reflex sympathetic dystrophy.
- Heparinize after achieving sympathetic blockade to minimize the risk of late arterial thrombosis.

Other considerations

The nerve supply to the arm is C_5–T_1. Sympathetic nerve supply to the arm comes from T_1 via the sympathetic chain and the stellate ganglion (fusion of the inferior cervical ganglion and the first thoracic ganglion).

Unsuccessful reversal of neuromuscular blockade

Condition	Competitive antagonism at the nicotinic acetylcholine receptor of the neuromuscular junction
Presentation	Uncoordinated, jerky patient movements during the recovery phase. Inability to maintain an airway or inadequate spontaneous ventilation
Immediate action	Maintain and protect an airway and provide adequate ventilation
Follow-up action	Maintain anaesthesia if appropriate; correct the cause
Investigations	Nerve stimulator train-of-four, post-tetanic count (see below); double burst stimulation
Also consider	Non-functional peripheral nerve stimulator (check the battery charge)
	Volatile agent concentration (maintained by hypoventilation)
	Hyperventilation ($ETCO_2$ <4 kPa) or CO_2 narcosis (over about 9 kPa)
	Undiagnosed head injury (examine pupils)
	Cerebrovascular accident

Risk factors

- Recent dose of relaxant/backflow in IVI/drug error.
- Renal and hepatic impairment causing delayed elimination of relaxant in long cases (except atracurium).
- Perioperative administration of magnesium (especially above the therapeutic range 1.25–2.5 mmol/litre).
- Hypothermia.
- Acidosis and electrolyte imbalance.
- Co-administration of aminoglycoside antibiotics.
- Myasthenia gravis (reduced number of receptors).
- Low levels of plasma cholinesterase (pregnancy, renal and liver disorders, hypothyroidism) or competition with drugs that are also metabolized by plasma cholinesterase (etomidate, ester LAs, and methotrexate).
- Abnormal plasma cholinesterase (suxamethonium apnoea).
- Ecothiopate eyedrops for glaucoma (historical–now not available on general prescription).

Diagnosis

- Uncoordinated, jerky patient movements are suggestive of inadequate reversal of neuromuscular blockade. A sustained lift of the head from the pillow for 5 s is a good clinical indicator of adequate reversal.
- Train-of-four is classically measured as adductor pollicis twitches in response to supramaximal stimulation via two electrodes placed over the ulnar nerve. The train-of-four (TOF) ratio is force of the fourth twitch divided by the force of the first. In depolarizing blockade there are equal but reduced twitches in response to TOF therefore the ratio is 1. In non-depolarizing blockade the TOF ratio is <1. In terms of assessing reversal of neuromuscular blockade, return of a TOF ratio of at least 0.75 would normally be deemed adequate prior to extubation.
- Double burst stimulation is said to be more accurate as a means of quantifying TOF ratio. Two standardized 60 ms bursts of 50 Hz tetanic stimulation are given 0.75 s apart and the responses compared.
- Post-tetanic count is used to monitor deep relaxation, when the TOF will not show any twitches. Firstly establish that the peripheral nerve stimulator is actually working and has adequate battery charge. A 50 Hz tetanic stimulus is applied for 5 s followed by single stimuli at 1 Hz. Post-tetanic facilitation in the presence of non-depolarizing blockade allows a number of twitches to be seen. Reversal should be possible with a count of 10.

Immediate management

- ABC...then check for signs of awareness, assess anaesthetic depth, and check ETCO$_2$.
- If you have already given a dose of neostigmine ensure it was adequate (0.05 mg/kg) and that it did actually enter the circulation (check the intravenous line for backflow and the site of cannulation for swelling).
- Hypothermia, electrolyte imbalance, and acidosis will impair reversal and should be corrected.
- Aminoglycoside or Mg^{2+} induced poor reversal may improve with calcium gluconate (10 ml 10%) titrated IV.
- Poor/abnormal plasma cholinesterase levels can be partially normalized by giving fresh frozen plasma.

Subsequent management

- Wait patiently–this is not an emergency!
- Suspected myasthenia gravis should be confirmed postoperatively with a 'Tensilon' test.
- If the patient has suffered a period of awareness whilst paralysed, admit it, explain it, apologize, and ensure that the patient has access to professional counselling if required.

Other considerations

A dual (phase II) blockade occurs when large amounts of suxamethonium are used and the depolarizing block is gradually replaced by one of non-depolarizing characteristics (fade, etc.).

Section VI
Practical issues

Chapter 37
Airway assessment and management

Richard Telford

Airway assessment

Careful assessment of the airway is an essential component of every preoperative visit. Difficulty in airway management is the single most important cause of anaesthesia-related morbidity and mortality. It has been estimated that as many as 30% of deaths totally attributable to anaesthesia are associated with inadequate airway management.

The site and nature of the proposed surgery, the type of anaesthetic selected, and patient factors will determine a plan for airway management by the anaesthetist.

It may be obvious that a patient's airway will be difficult (e.g. masses, abscesses, anatomical abnormalities, etc.), but most catastrophes happen when unexpected difficulty occurs. Assessment of the airway involves taking a history, examination, and the use of a few simple bedside tests.

History

* Ask about previous anaesthetics and scrutinize previous anaesthetic records. Check for previous airway problems. If the patient was intubated there should be a comment about the best view obtained of the glottis as graded by Cormack and Lehane[1] (see p. 867, Fig. 37.1).

* When airway or intubation problems have been recorded, were they related to an acute event (e.g. trauma, airway disease process, pregnancy) or is the underlying problem still present?

* Is there a history of dental damage or severe sore throat with previous anaesthetics?

* Ascertain whether the patient has had previous head and neck surgery, radiotherapy to the head and neck, or has medical conditions that may predispose to difficult tracheal intubation–diabetes mellitus, acromegaly, rheumatoid arthritis, cervical arthropathy, morbid obesity, or obstructive sleep apnoea. Patients with Down's syndrome or degenerative cervical spine disease are at increased risk of atlantoaxial instability.

* An occasional patient may have written notification of previous airway problems.

Examination

* Look for neck masses, scars of previous head and neck surgery, burns, or the skin changes associated with radiotherapy.

* Adverse anatomical features include a small mouth, receding chin, high arched palate, large tongue, bull neck, morbid obesity, and large breasts.

* Look for protruding/awkwardly placed or loose teeth. Document the position of any caps or crowns and inform the patient of the risk of damage to these.

1 Cormack RS, Lehane J (1984). Difficult intubation in obstetrics. *Anaesthesia*, **39**, 1105–11.

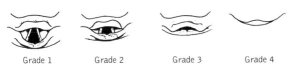

Fig 37.1 Cormack and Lehane classification of glottic visualization.

- Note the position of the larynx and trachea and the accessibility of the cricothyroid membrane.
- Look out for patients with beards (which may hide adverse anatomical features) or occipital hair buns (which may prevent extension at the craniocervical junction).
- If the nasal route is chosen for intubation remember to check the patency of the nasal passages and for any history of epistaxis.

Clinical tests

These are used in an attempt to predict difficult laryngoscopy (i.e. Cormack and Lehane grades 3 and 4), which occurs in approximately 1–2% of the surgical population. Ideally, these tests should have a high specificity (the ability to correctly identify normal patients as normal) and a high sensitivity (to detect true difficult intubations). No single test can be used to predict difficult laryngoscopy with certainty. Combining two or more tests improves the positive predictive value (the percentage of difficult laryngoscopies correctly predicted as difficult) and increases the specificity, but decreases the sensitivity.

Prediction of difficult laryngoscopy is imprecise. The tests described have high specificities (that is they are good at predicting when laryngoscopy will be easy). Since the same factors are involved in easy laryngoscopy and successful airway maintenance with a mask (extension at the craniocervical junction and mandibular protrusion), predicting easy laryngoscopy is also a prediction of successful control of the airway changes associated with induction of anaesthesia. If several of the tests are positive the clinician should have a high index of suspicion that direct laryngoscopy will be difficult and consider securing the airway before inducing anaesthesia.

Interincisor gap

- Ask the patient to open their mouth as wide as possible.
- Less than two finger breadths (3 cm) distance between the incisor teeth is associated with difficulty in conventional laryngoscopy.
- An interincisor gap of less than 3 cm reduced the prevalence of easy intubation from 95% to 62% in one large series.

Protrusion of the mandible

- Ask the patient to protrude their mandible. Look at the position of the lower teeth in relation to the upper teeth.[2] Classes B and C are associated with difficult laryngoscopy:
  - Class A: the lower incisors can be protruded anterior to the upper incisors.
  - Class B: the lower incisors can be brought 'edge to edge' with the upper incisors.
  - Class C: the lower incisors cannot be brought 'edge to edge'.

Mallampati test (with Samsoon and Young's modification)[3]

- Sit in front of the patient who should be sitting up with their head in the neutral position. Ask the patient to open their mouth maximally and protrude their tongue without phonating. Note which of the following structures are visible: (Fig. 37.2)
  - Class 1: faucial pillars (palatoglossal and palatopharyngeal folds), soft palate, and uvula visible.
  - Class 2: faucial pillars and soft palate visible. Uvula masked by base of tongue.
  - Class 3: only soft palate visible.
  - Class 4: soft palate not visible.
- Class 3 and 4 views are associated with difficulty. When used in isolation the Mallampati test correctly identifies about 50% of difficult intubations.

Flexion/extension at the craniocervical junction

This is best assessed by asking the patient to maximally flex their neck. The examiner's hand is then placed on the back of the patient's neck to prevent movement of the cervical spine and the patient is asked to nod their head. Alternatively a pen can be held against the forehead whilst maximally flexing

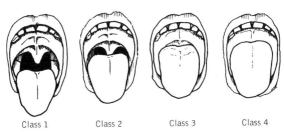

Class 1 Class 2 Class 3 Class 4

Fig 37.2 Mallampati test (Samsoon and Young modification)

2 Calder I (1992). Predicting difficult intubation. *Anaesthesia*, 47, 528–9.

3 Samsoon GLT, Young JRB (1987). Difficult tracheal intubation: a retrospective study. *Anaesthesia*, 42, 487–90.

and extending the neck. Greater than 90° of movement should be possible. Reduced movements are associated with difficult laryngoscopy.

The thyromental distance (Patil's test)[4]

The distance from the tip of the thyroid cartilage to the tip of the mandible, with the neck fully extended. This should be greater than 6.5 cm (three finger breadths) and estimates the potential space into which the tongue can be displaced on laryngoscopy. A distance of less than 6 cm is associated with difficult laryngoscopy and predicts 75% of difficult laryngoscopies.

The sternomental distance[5]

The distance from the upper border of the manubrium to the tip of the mandible with the neck fully extended. A distance of less than 12.5 cm is associated with difficult laryngoscopy in adults.

Other tests

- Radiographs of mandibular length and depth have been used to predict difficult intubation. These are time-consuming and are probably no better than the above clinical tests.

- With cervical spine disease (e.g. ankylosing spondylitis, rheumatoid arthritis, Klippel–Feil abnormality) flexion/extension views are useful to determine the stability of the odontoid peg, the mobility of the atlanto-axial–occipital complex and the presence of fracture dislocations. Patients with disease that involves the atlantoaxial-occipito complex have a higher prevalence of difficult laryngoscopy than those with disease below C2.[6]

- Adults with a partially obstructed airway may, if time allows, be investigated with CT scanning. The scan will show the site of the lesion, the dimensions of the trachea, the relationship of the lesion to the carina and in the case of malignancies, whether or not the tracheal wall has been invaded.[7]

Successful airway management is dependent on careful patient assessment. If there is a high likelihood that mask ventilation and/or direct laryngoscopy will be difficult, consideration should be given to securing the airway with the patient awake.

4 Patil VU, Stehling LC, Zauder HL (1983). Predicting the difficulty of intubation using an intubation guage. *Anesthesiology Review*, **10**, 32–3.

5 Savva D (1994). Prediction of difficult intubation. *British Journal of Anaesthesia*, **73**, 149–53.

6 Calder I. Calder J, Crockard HA (1995). Difficult direct laryngoscopy in patients with cervical spine disease. *Anaesthesia*, **50**, 756–63.

7 Mason RA, Fielder CP (1999). The obstructed airway in head and neck surgery. *Anaesthesia*, **54**, 625–8.

Management of the obstructed airway

Management of patients with an obstructed airway

Each patient should be assessed to identify the level and nature of the obstruction. Broadly these can be divided into:

- Oropharyngeal problems (trauma, tumour, infection).
- Lesions in and around the larynx (usually malignant or infective).
- Mid tracheal obstruction (often secondary to retrosternal goitres).
- Lower tracheal and bronchial obstruction (usually large mediastinal masses, e.g. lymphomas, thymomas, and carcinomas).

A careful history will identify those patients in whom obstruction is severe. Stridor at rest implies a reduction of airway diameter of at least 50%. In addition to noisy breathing, there may be a history of waking up at night in a panic and sleeping upright in a chair.

Upper airway obstruction

Upper airway obstruction can be divided into two groups:

- Intubation is likely to be straightforward (see airway assessment p. 866). These patients should have an inhalational induction (see p. 879) in the operating theatre with the ENT surgeon gowned with a tracheostomy tray and rigid ventilating bronchoscope close to hand. The patient may be intubated with a tracheal tube or with a rigid ventilating bronchoscope. If the patient is impossible to intubate a tracheostomy can be performed in the anaesthetized spontaneously breathing patient.
- Intubation is expected to be difficult or impossible (extensive tumour, fixed hemilarynx, or gross anatomical distortion). This may require preliminary tracheostomy under local anaesthetic. Helium may help ameliorate stridor whilst the tracheostomy is performed. Heliox (premixed helium/oxygen) contains only 21% oxygen. The oxygen content may be increased by adapting rotameters to fit the Heliox cylinder, or using a simple 'Y' connector and an oxygen cylinder.

Mid tracheal obstruction

- Usually there is a history over several months. If time allows a CT scan should be performed to show the site of the lesion, the dimensions of the trachea, the relationship of the lesion to the carina, and whether the tracheal wall is invaded.
- Remember that in these patients an emergency tracheostomy may not be an option since access to the trachea may be compromised by the presence of a large neck mass. In some patients, it may be possible to perform a tracheostomy but the tube may not be long enough to bypass the obstruction.
- The most common cause of mid tracheal obstruction is a retrosternal goitre. In the majority of cases visualization of the larynx is not difficult and tracheal intubation is easy. The site of compression is of sufficient distance above the carina to accommodate both the tracheal cuff and the bevel thus allowing conventional induction of anaesthesia.

- If there is concern that conventional intubation will be difficult, awake fibreoptic intubation may be the technique of choice. However, if the lumen of the trachea is very small passage of the fibreoptic scope and tube may be unpleasant for the patient (the 'cork in a bottle' phenomenon). An experienced operator is required.
- Some patients with very marked tracheal obstruction may be best managed with an inhalational induction and intubation with either a very small tracheal tube or a rigid bronchoscope.

Lower tracheal and bronchial obstruction

These are very difficult cases. Detailed discussion should take place and management be planned by experienced specialists. Sudden respiratory obstruction can occur at any stage of the anaesthetic. Induction of anaesthesia can alter the support of the bronchial tree so that collapse can occur with total respiratory obstruction:

- Obtain tissue diagnosis if possible under local anaesthesia.
- If superior vena caval obstruction is present, urgent 'blind' chemotherapy or radiotherapy may have to be considered, even in the absence of a histological diagnosis.
- The use of a rigid intubating bronchoscope to relieve the obstruction may be lifesaving.
- Transfer to a unit where facilities for extracorporeal oxygenation are available may be necessary in some cases.

Further reading

Goh MH, Liu XY, Goh YS (1999). Anterior mediastinal masses: an anaesthetic challenge. *Anaesthesia*, **54**, 670–4.

Mason RA, Fielder CP (1999). The obstructed airway in head and neck surgery. *Anaesthesia*, **54**, 625–8.

Management of the unexpected difficult airway (see also p. 852)

Despite careful assessment, unexpected airway problems can occur. Approximately 50% of airway difficulties will only become apparent after the induction of general anaesthesia. When a problem does arise, the first priority is to decide whether the problem lies with difficult airway maintenance, difficult intubation or both:

- If the main problem is intubation, but facemask ventilation is easy, a controlled stepwise approach can be followed.
- If the problem lies with facemask ventilation, then an airway emergency develops. Maintenance of patient oxygenation becomes the priority.

Failed mask ventilation

Is the problem due to:

- Failure to maintain upper airway patency (most common problem)?
- Laryngospasm?
- Laryngeal pathology?
- Lower airway pathology?

Failure to maintain airway patency

- 100% oxygen should be used whenever an airway problem appears to be developing.
- Triple-thrust manoeuvre–two hands are used to thrust the jaw forwards. An assistant should squeeze the anaesthetic bag.
- Oral and/or nasal airways may help.
- Ensure that head positioning is optimal–'sniffing the morning air', a single pillow under the head only, neck flexed, head extended.
- If still unable to ventilate by facemask insert a laryngeal mask airway (LMA) or Combitube.
- If cricoid pressure has been applied try releasing it carefully.
- Cricothyroidotomy.

Laryngospasm

- Apply 100% oxygen with the mask held tightly and the expiratory valve closed. Apply CPAP/PEEP and gently attempt manual ventilation. Avoid excessive pressure as this may distend the stomach.
- Deepening anaesthesia with an IV induction agent (particularly propofol) may reduce spasm, or consider a small dose of suxamethonium (0.25–0.5 mg/kg).
- As laryngospasm starts to 'break' anaesthesia should be deepened with a volatile agent or further doses of intravenous agent as appropriate.
- If laryngospasm is severe a full dose of suxamethonium (1.5 mg/kg) should be administered.
- If there is no venous access suxamethonium may be administered intramuscularly or into the tongue (3 mg/kg).

Laryngeal pathology

Unexpected laryngeal pathology causing problems with mask ventilation is a very rare scenario. Cricothyroidotomy may be lifesaving.

Lower airway pathology

- Acute severe bronchospasm may present as difficulty in mask ventilation. This may present de novo or may be part of an adverse drug reaction. The management of acute severe bronchospasm is discussed on p. 848.
- Very rarely lower airway pathology due to diagnosed or undiagnosed mediastinal masses may present as difficulty with ventilation at induction of anaesthesia. The use of a rigid bronchoscope to maintain airway patency may be lifesaving.

Failed intubation

Defined as difficulty in viewing the larynx, causing failure to intubate the trachea. Remember that patients do not die from failure to intubate but failure to oxygenate.

The clinical scenario determines the best management:

- If the patient has a full stomach and is undergoing a rapid sequence induction then it is best to institute a failed intubation drill early and wake the patient up. Rarely there are clinical situations (e.g. in obstetrics) where you may decide to proceed with surgery under mask anaesthesia.
- In an elective case, when the patient has received a full dose of a nondepolarizing muscle relaxant and mask ventilation is easy, it may be appropriate to try a full range of techniques (see Fig. 37.3).

Possible strategies in a case of difficult intubation

- Optimize the position of the head (flexion of the cervical spine with maximal extension at the craniocervical junction).
- Have different laryngoscope blades available. The McCoy blade with a flexing tip can be particularly helpful.
- Manipulation of the larynx by the assistant.
- Use a gum elastic bougie ('Eschmann tracheal tube introducer (reusable)', Sims Portex Ltd, New Portex House, Military Road, Hythe, Kent CT21 5BN, UK, tel: 01303 260551). This is probably the most useful piece of equipment for any unexpected difficult intubation. Keep the bougie well anterior to ensure it does not enter the oesophagus, and in the midline to avoid right or left pyriform fossae. 90° counter clockwise rotation of the tube aids successful railroading once the bougie is in position.
- Consider alternative intubating techniques (intubating LMA, Combitube, fibreoptic scope, retrograde methods).
- With abnormal anatomy the cords may be difficult to see. Pressure on the chest may produce a bubble at the laryngeal opening.

Diagnosis of misplacement

- Retain a high index of suspicion after a difficult intubation.
- Suspect oesophageal placement if you cannot confirm: normal breath sounds in both axillae and absent sounds over the stomach; rise **and** fall of chest; normal ETCO$_2$ trace; normal airway pressure cycle.
- The trachea is a rigid structure, the oesophagus is not. If negative pressure is applied to the ETT, failure to aspirate air (e.g. with a bladder syringe directly attached to the ETT) suggests oesophageal placement.
- Confirm ETT placement with a fibreoptic scope.
- Remember–**if in doubt, pull it out** and apply bag and mask ventilation.

The intubating laryngeal mask airway (ILMA)

- Intubation via the laryngeal mask airway may be performed blind, aided by a fibrescope, or aided via a variety of other methods (guidewire, bougie, lightwand).

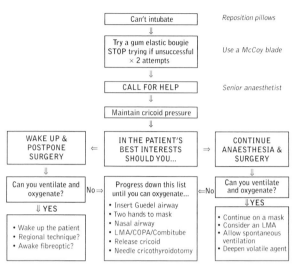

Fig 37.3 Failed intubation.

- The ILMA (Intavent) is a modification of the LMA designed to facilitate blind orotracheal intubation, fibreoptic intubation, or in very cooperative patients awake intubation.
- It features a rigid anatomically curved airway tube terminating in a standard 15 mm connector. It is fitted with a rigid metal handle.
- Unlike a standard laryngeal mask, it has a single epiglottic elevating bar replacing the two bars of a standard LMA. The caudal end of the bar is not fixed to the mask floor allowing it to elevate the epiglottis when an endotracheal tube is passed through the aperture.
- It comes in three sizes:
  - size 3 for a small adult or large child
  - size 4 for a normal adult
  - size 5 for a large adult.

All three sizes will accept a tube of up to 8 mm internal diameter.

- It is designed to be used with a straight silicone wire-reinforced cuffed endotracheal tube not exceeding 8 mm internal diameter capable of being passed through the ILMA including the pilot balloon and pilot balloon valve. The tube has an atraumatic tip to minimize the risk of pharyngeal trauma.
- The tube may be passed into the trachea blindly or under direct vision using a suitable fibreoptic scope.
- It is recommended that the ILMA is removed once the tube is passed into the trachea.

+ A stabilizing rod is available to keep the tracheal tube in place and slide the ILMA out of the mouth.

The Combitube

+ The Combitube™ (Sheridan Catheter Corporation) is an airway device that combines the functions of an oesophageal obturator airway and a conventional endotracheal airway.

+ It has two lumens–an oesophageal with an open proximal end and a blocked distal end with perforations at pharyngeal level and a tracheal with open proximal and distal ends.

+ It has two inflatable cuffs–a large proximal cuff (85 ml) inflated in the pharynx to seal off the oral and nasal cavities and a smaller distal cuff (10 ml) to seal off the proximal oesophagus or trachea.

+ The small size is recommended for general use.

+ Insertion:
  + With the head in the neutral position insert the Combitube blindly into the pharynx until the two black rings are level with the teeth. A laryngoscope may be helpful.
  + Inflate the large cuff (blue) with 85 ml of air. This may require considerable force. The Combitube may ride up like a laryngeal mask.
  + Inflate the distal cuff (white) with 10 ml of air.
  + In 98% of cases the Combitube will be inserted into the oesophagus. First attach the breathing system to the blue oesophageal lumen and confirm ventilation by auscultation and capnography.
  + In 2% of cases the Combitube will have entered the trachea. If there is no air entry on connecting the ventilation system to the blue lumen try the distal white lumen and confirm positioning by auscultation and capnography.

+ Contraindications:
  + Patients less than 5 feet (1.5 m) tall.
  + Those with intact gag reflexes.
  + Patients with oesophageal pathology–oesophageal perforation has been reported.
  + Patients who have ingested caustic substances.

Retrograde intubation

+ Many different methods have been described, all based on the technique of Waters.[8]
+ The airway is anaesthetized as described. (For awake intubation see p. 882).
+ A Tuohy needle is passed through the cricothyroid membrane. Correct positioning is confirmed by the aspiration of air.
+ A guidewire is passed via the Tuohy needle and retrieved from the nose or mouth.

---

8   Waters DJ (1963). Guided blind endotracheal intubation. *Anaesthesia*, **18**, 158–62.

- An introducer is passed over the guidewire–a 16G ureteric dilator fits over a 145 cm 0.038 in Amplatz Super Stiff guidewire and is a snug fit for a 6.0 mm flexometallic tube.
- The tube is passed over the guidewire and introducer until it arrests against the guidewire protruding through the posterior surface of the cricothyroid membrane.
- The guidewire and introducer are withdrawn from above whilst applying forward pressure on the tube.
- Correct tube placement is confirmed in the usual way.
- An alternative technique involves threading the guidewire through the suction port of the fibrescope and using the wire to guide the fibresope into the trachea.
- Cook (UK) make a commercially available retrograde intubation kit for use with endotracheal tubes of internal diameter 5 mm or larger.

Needle cricothyroidotomy   (see also p. 853)

In the can't intubate, can't ventilate scenario emergency tracheal access may be required. Needle cricothyroidotomy is quicker and easier than formal tracheostomy. It is performed percutaneously with either a large (less than 2 mm ID) intravenous cannula or with a larger (greater than 2 mm ID) specifically designed cannula.

Intravenous cannula

- A 14G cannula attached to a 10 ml syringe is inserted through the cricothyroid membrane in the midline at an angle of 30–45°.
- Air is aspirated to confirm placement and the catheter advanced into the trachea.
- Oxygen may be from a jet injector (flow rate through a 14G cannula 800 ml/s), a flow regulator at 15 litre/min (flow rate through a 14G cannula 400 ml/s), anaesthetic machine oxygen flush at 32 kPa (flow rate through a 14G cannula 200 ml/s), or anaesthetic bag at 60 cmH$_2$O (flow rate through a 14G cannula 80 ml/s).
- Complications include kinking, surgical emphysema, and problems with exhalation.

Formal cricothyroidotomy kit

- Examples are the Melker or Patil cricothyroidotomy sets (Cook UK Limited, Monroe House, Letchworth, Herts SG6 1LN, UK).
- A guidewire is passed into the trachea via a needle inserted into the cricothyroid membrane.
- A cannula is passed into the trachea over a dilator.
- Ventilation is via the anaesthetic circuit or a Sanders type injector–most cannulas have both standard (15 mm connector) and Luer lock connectors.
- Complications include pneumothorax, surgical emphysema, and bleeding.

  It is important to make sure there is no obstruction to expiration otherwise barotrauma may result.

Extubation of the patient who has been difficult to intubate

Following multiple attempts at intubation the airway may be oedematous and bloody. On occasions, an elective tracheostomy may be necessary.

- Optimize the patient's medical condition:
  - Aspirate secretions, administer bronchodilators.
  - Ensure normovolaemia. Attenuate the cardiovascular stress effects of extubation. Esmolol may be useful.
  - Minimize stomach contents if possible.
  - Can airway oedema be minimized? Position the patient head up. Consider the use of intravenous dexamethasone or nebulized adrenaline.
  - Ensure there is no residual muscular paralysis.
- Optimize position for extubation:
  - Consider sitting the patient up to maximize the FRC and minimize airway obstruction.
- Aids to extubation:
  - Consider extubation over a jet stylet (Cook airway exchange catheter), a nasogastric tube, or a fibreoptic scope through which oxygen can be supplied.
  - Consider a tongue stitch to pull the tongue forward if obstruction with the tongue is likely to be a problem
  - A nasal airway (or cut nasotracheal tube) may help prevent obstruction.
- Have a back up plan:
  - LMA
  - Combitube
  - cricothyroidotomy.

Further reading

Dyson A, Isaac PA, Pennant JH, Giesecke AH, Lipton JM (1990). Esmolol attenuates the cardiovascular responses to extubation. *Anaesthesia and Analgesia*, **71**, 675–8.
Hartley M, Vaughan RM (1993). Problems associated with extubation. *British Journal of Anaesthesia*, **71**, 561–8.

Inhalational induction

Common indications for inhalationl induction include:

* babies and young children
* needle phobic adults
* acute upper airway obstruction due to lesions in and around the larynx, e.g. acute epiglottitis, perilaryngeal tumours
* bronchopleural fistula
* no easily accessible veins.

If possible explain the procedure to the patient at the preoperative visit.

  Masks with integral teets are useful in babies who are still suckling. In older children use of a cupped hand around the fresh gas delivery tube is used. Halothane or sevoflurane are the induction agents of choice to permit smooth induction of anaesthesia. For patients with airway obstruction 100% oxygen is used, otherwise 50% nitrous oxide in oxygen is satisfactory. When using halothane the initial inspired concentration should be 1% and increased in 0.5% increments until surgical anaesthesia is established (small central pupils and a reduction in blood pressure). Sevoflurane can be introduced at 4–8%.

  In cooperative patients a single breath induction technique can be used. A 4 litre bag (or two 2 litre bags in series) is prefilled with halothane 5% or sevoflurane 8% in oxygen. The patient exhales fully and then takes a single vital capacity breath and is encouraged to breath hold for as long as possible. Smooth induction may be achieved within 30–60 s.

Difficulties with inhalational induction

* Slow induction of anaesthesia. Patients with stridor have low alveolar minute volumes. Induction of anaesthesia and deepening of the anaesthetic will be slow. Sevoflurane may fail to provide anaesthesia of sufficient depth to allow instrumentation of the airway. Adequate depth of anaesthesia is usually evidenced by a decrease in blood pressure and small central pupils. A change to halothane may be worthwhile.
* With stridor maintain CPAP during induction.
* Occasionally airway obstruction may be so severe that gas induction is not possible. Consider tracheostomy under local anaesthetic.
* Airway problems may occur in stage 2 of anaesthesia (excitation) immediately after the patient loses consciousness. Attempt chin lift and jaw thrust. Insertion of an oral airway can induce coughing and laryngospasm. Consider the use of a nasal airway in these circumstances.
* Laryngospasm (see p. 872).

Rapid sequence induction

Rapid sequence induction is employed in the patient with a full stomach who requires general anaesthesia. The concept is loss of consciousness followed by intubation in the presence of cricoid pressure, without facemask ventilation. If intubation fails the drugs should wear off rapidly and the patient restart spontaneous ventilation before hypoxia intervenes.

Meticulous assessment of the airway is mandatory preoperatively to look for likely difficulties with tracheal intubation. If preoperative evaluation suggests a problem with intubation, consider alternative techniques such as surgery under local or regional anaesthesia or awake fibreoptic intubation.

The anaesthetist must have a management plan should intubation fail (see p. 874).

Technique

- Check the anaesthetic machine, laryngoscopes, and tracheal tubes.
- The patient must be on a tipping trolley.
- Attach appropriate monitoring devices.
- Position the patient's head as if 'sniffing the morning air' (one pillow under the head, cervical spine flexed with extension at the craniocervical junction).
- At least one skilled assistant is needed to perform cricoid pressure.
- Suction apparatus is switched on and passed under the patient's pillow to the anaesthetist's right hand.
- Preoxygenate with 100% oxygen for 3–5 min (or four vital capacity breaths with high flow into the circuit in emergencies).
- Administer a sleep dose of intravenous induction agent (thiopental 2–5 mg/kg, etomidate 0.2–0.3 mg/kg, propofol 1–2 mg/kg) followed immediately by 1.5 mg/kg of suxamethonium.
- Apply cricoid pressure as soon as consciousness is lost.
- Intubate as soon as the patient relaxes.
- Maintain cricoid pressure until the tracheal cuff is inflated and correct placement of the tube is confirmed by capnography and auscultation of the lungs.

The main problem with rapid sequence induction is haemodynamic instability. Excessive doses of induction agent may result in circulatory collapse (especially if the patient is hypovolaemic), whereas an inadequate dose may result in tachycardia and hypertension.

Special considerations

- Thorough preoxygenation is essential. The mask must be close fitting and the reservoir bag moving. Any entrainment of air during preoxygenation negates the whole process. Start again.
- Inject drugs into a rapidly running saline infusion through a large cannula.
- In patients who will not tolerate preoxygenation (e.g. distressed children) consider gentle IPPV after injection of drugs.

- With patients in whom hypertension and tachycardia is undesirable (e.g. ischaemia/hypertension) consider alfentanil 10 μg/kg 1 min prior to induction and following preoxygenation. In the event of intubation failure this may be reversed with naloxone (400 μg IV).

Correct application of cricoid pressure

The technique of cricoid pressure to prevent regurgitated material entering the pharynx was described by Sellick.[9] This simple manoeuvre must be applied correctly as incorrect application can cause difficulties.

The cricoid cartilage is held between the thumb and middle finger and pressure is exerted mainly with the index finger. Some authors recommend a bimanual technique with the second hand behind the neck. A minimum force of 30 N is required. Correctly applied, cricoid pressure should allow facemask ventilation without risk of gastric distension, but airway obstruction is possible, particularly when applied with a poor technique.

9 Sellick BA (1961). Cricoid pressure to control regurgitation of stomach contents during induction of anaesthesia. *The Lancet*, **2**, 404–6.

Awake fibreoptic intubation

Indications for awake fibreoptic intubation

- Known or suspected difficult intubation.
- Known or suspected cervical cord injury.
- Morbid obesity.
- A patient with full stomach in whom a difficult intubation is anticipated.

Contraindications to awake fibreoptic intubation

- The uncooperative patient.
- Haemorrhage in the upper airway.
- Severe stridor secondary to perilaryngeal tumour.
- Allergy to local anaesthetics.

The degree of psychological and physical disturbance to a patient depends on the experience of the operator and their lightness of touch. The technique is easily mastered with practice. Pharyngeal and laryngeal reflexes are obtunded by local anaesthetic agents. With judicious sedation intubation can be achieved with little discomfort to the patient.

Equipment

- The fibreoptic scope must be sterilized appropriately beforehand.
- The light source must be checked and the fibrescope prefocused on printed material.
- The tip should be defogged with a commercial solution.
- The fibrescope should be lubricated along its length with a water-soluble lubricant.
- The suction port should be checked to ensure that it is patent and the connections are airtight.
- The patient should be monitored with ECG, non-invasive blood pressure measurement, and pulse oximetry.

Assistance

Skilled assistance from an operating department assistant or anaesthetic nurse is mandatory.

Preparation of the patient

- A comprehensive preoperative assessment of the patient's airway must be made. While the nature and site of the proposed surgery usually dictate the route for intubation, consider simple facts like nostril patency and limitation of mouth opening before making the decision.
- Explain the indication to the patient, emphasizing the primary consideration of safety.
- Administer an antisialogogue (intramuscular glycopyrrolate 200 μg 1 h prior to intubation). This improves the view by decreasing secretions and enhances the action of topical local anaesthetics.
- Apply monitoring and obtain intravenous access. Administer supplemental oxygen to all patients via a nasal catheter.

- Sedate the patient judiciously with a combination of narcotics and benzodiazepine. Narcotics give mild sedation, analgesia, and are antitussive. Fentanyl (25 μg increments to a maximum of 1 μg/kg) is suitable. Naloxone should be available to reverse narcotic-induced respiratory depression. Benzodiazepines produce amnesia and sedation–midazolam (0.5–1 mg increments) until sedated but maintaining verbal contact. Flumazenil should be available. Over-sedation is a common error and should be avoided at all costs.

Position of the patient

Sit the patient up with the operator in front. This prevents the tongue and pharynx collapsing backwards and obstructing the view. It also prevents any secretions pooling at the back of the oropharynx. It is, however, confusing for beginners who are used to viewing the anatomy from the head of the patient. Otherwise stand in the normal intubating position with the patient supine.

Nasal route

- The route of choice if available, but the passage of a nasal tube is always uncomfortable.

- Contraindications to the nasal route include bleeding diathesis, an anticoagulated patient, severe intranasal disease, basal skull fracture, or a CSF leak.

- Advantages include ideal positioning to see the larynx, no gagging, no biting, and less interference with the tongue.

- Local anaesthesia of the nose must be accompanied by vasoconstriction. Conventionally 10% cocaine solution is used, but some worry about coronary vasoconstriction. 4% lidocaine (lignocaine) 3 ml and 1% phenylephrine 1 ml is a useful alternative.

- Dilate the nostrils to the anticipated size of the endotracheal tube to be used with warmed nasal airways lubricated with lidocaine (lignocaine) jelly.

- The posterior third of the tongue and oropharynx should be anaesthetized with five to ten sprays from a metered dose 10% lidocaine (lignocaine) spray. Each spray contains 10 mg lidocaine (lignocaine). Alternatively 2 ml 4% lidocaine (lignocaine) can be sprayed onto the back of the pharynx via the nasal airway.

- Anaesthesia below the cords is accomplished by puncture of the cricothyroid membrane with a 22G cannula with the neck in extension. Correct positioning is confirmed by the ability to easily aspirate air. 2 ml 4% lidocaine (lignocaine) is injected at end expiration. Coughing spreads the local anaesthetic above and below the vocal cords. Absolute contraindications are a coagulopathy and local tumour. Relative contraindications are an unstable cervical spine, when neck extension is undesirable, and morbid obesity, when identification of the anatomical landmarks is difficult.

- Nebulized 4% lidocaine (lignocaine) 4 ml plus 1% phenylephrine 1 ml is a useful alternative. This is administered using a standard oxygen-driven nebulizer with a flow rate of 8 litre/min and the patient in the sitting position. The patient is asked to breathe through the nose and a standard facemask is used (it may still be necessary to anaesthetize the larynx and trachea via the suction port of the fibreoptic scope as described below). This method has the advantage of minimal patient disturbance and no requirement for identification of anatomical structures. It can be used in the patient with an unstable cervical spine.

- An alternative to a cricothyroid puncture is to inject lidocaine (lignocaine) via the suction port of the fibrescope. 4% lidocaine (lignocaine) 2 ml is sprayed onto the vocal cords and a further 2 ml is injected down the trachea once the tip of the fibrescope has been manoeuvred between the cords.

- Superior laryngeal nerve blocks are advocated by some, but in practice are not usually necessary. The superior laryngeal nerves convey sensation from the inferior aspect of the epiglottis and the laryngeal inlet above the vocal cords. They may be anaesthetized by applying pledgets soaked in 4% lidocaine (lignocaine) into each pyriform fossa with Krause's forceps for 2 min. Alternatively, in patients who have limited mouth opening, the nerves may be anaesthetized by injecting 2–3 ml of local anaesthetic bilaterally, deep to the thyrohyoid membrane, just above the thyroid cartilage at a point one-third of the distance between the midline and the tip of the superior cornu.

Oral route

- This route is more difficult because the fibrescope is not anatomically directed towards the glottis.

- An endoscopic oral airway or bite block should be used to protect the fibrescope. The endoscopic oral airway has the advantage of preventing dorsal displacement of the tongue and keeping the instrument in the midline. Such devices include the Berman airway (Vital Signs Inc.) and the Ovassapian airway (Kendall).

- The mouth can be anaesthetized with 10% lidocaine (lignocaine) spray to the tongue and oropharynx as described above. Alternatively nebulized 4% lidocaine (lignocaine) can be administered via a standard nebulizer mouthpiece with the nose occluded.

- Laryngeal and tracheobronchial anaesthesia is obtained with cricothyroid puncture, or instillation of lidocaine (lignocaine) through the suction port of the fibrescope as described above.

Passing the endotracheal tube

- Stand at the head or in front of the patient as a matter of personal preference. The control section of the fibrescope is held in the dominant hand with the thumb positioned on the angle control and the index finger on the suction port. The light source should be to the operator's left. If available a camera and monitor should be used. The fibrescope should be held fully extended with the other hand. A suitably sized, reinforced endotracheal tube should be mounted on the fibrescope. This can be prewarmed to soften it.

- If the nasal route is chosen the fibrescope is advanced 15 cm into the pharynx. If the oral route is used it should be advanced 8–10 cm.

- If in the midline the vocal cords will come into view as the tip is flexed slightly upwards.

- Rotation of the fibrescope about its long axis may be required to bring the tip into the midline.

- The first view after the fibrescope is advanced through the vocal cords will be the thyroid cartilage. The tip is straightened or returned to the neutral position and the instrument advanced until the tracheal cartilages and finally the carina is seen.
- The endotracheal tube is threaded over the fibrescope and into the trachea. The bevel should face backwards.
- Correct positioning above the carina is confirmed visually. The presence of carbon dioxide in the expired gas confirms tracheal placement. Avoid cuff inflation until the last moment as the increased resistance to breathing may panic some patients.

Difficulties

Can't get a good view

- Always think 'where am I, what am I looking at?'.
- The most common problem is that the tip of the fibrescope is in one of the pyriform fossae and not in the midline. Try rotating the scope to centralize the tip or pull back until recognizable structures appear. Dimming the lights to see where the tip of the fibrescope transilluminates tissues of the neck is sometimes useful. The light is visible, deviated laterally or invisible. If the light is invisible the tip of the scope is either not sufficiently far advanced or is in the oesophagus.
- Excess secretions may obscure anatomical landmarks. Try using the suction port or alternatively insufflate oxygen down it (2 litre/min). If this does not work remove the scope and try to clear secretions with a sucker or dry swab.
- If the tongue base is against the posterior pharyngeal wall ask the patient to protrude their tongue.

Problems with passage of the endotracheal tube

- Sometimes it is easy to intubate the trachea with the scope, but the endotracheal tube cannot be railroaded into the trachea.
- Protrusion of the tongue, maximum inspiratory efforts, tube rotation, changing the axis of the airway, and external laryngeal manipulation are all worth trying.
- It may be necessary to use a smaller endotracheal tube.

Awake intubation in the presence of a full stomach

- Patients at risk of aspiration of stomach contents must be approached with common sense. Clearly the nose, mouth, and oropharynx can safely be anaesthetized.
- Some anaesthetists worry that anaesthesia of the larynx and tracheobronchial tree may suppress protective airway reflexes to unacceptable levels. Others believe that a lightly sedated patient can respond to a threat to the airway from vomiting or regurgitation, and clear it by turning and coughing, retching, or swallowing repeatedly. There are published reports of the safety of awake intubation in the presence of a full stomach.[10]

---

10 Ovassapian A, Krejcie TC, Yelich SJ, Dykes MHM (1989). Awake fibreoptic intubation in the presence of a full stomach. *British Journal of Anaesthesia*, 62, 13–16.

Apnoeic oxygenation

Interruption of ventilation may precipitate catastrophic hypoxaemia. This can be delayed or prevented by the correct use of oxygen. A detailed understanding of the mechanisms pertinent to apnoeic oxygenation is vital.

Apnoea whilst breathing air

- Resting oxygen consumption is 250–300 ml/min in a typical adult.
- At the onset of apnoea the oxygen available to support vital organ function is almost entirely that stored in the alveoli (about 200 ml) and that combined with haemoglobin (about 800 ml).
- After 2 min, about half this store will be exhausted and the alveolar (P_AO_2) and arterial (PaO_2) partial pressures of oxygen will be less than 4 kPa.
- By contrast, because CO_2 is very soluble and well buffered in the body, the alveolar (P_ACO_2) and arterial ($PaCO_2$) partial pressures of carbon dioxide rise slowly such that at 2 min the $PaCO_2/P_ACO_2$ will be about 6.6 kPa.
- Within 4 min, hypoxaemia will cause cardiac arrest or severe brain injury whilst the change in $PaCO_2/P_ACO_2$ remains clinically unimportant.

Apnoea whilst breathing 100% oxygen

- After breathing 100% oxygen the only gases present in the alveoli are oxygen, carbon dioxide, and water vapour.
- Total alveolar pressure is 100 kPa (1 atmosphere). This comprises water vapour (6 kPa), carbon dioxide (5 kPa), and oxygen (89 kPa).
- After 2 min of apnoea $PaCO_2$ will have risen to about 6.6 kPa, and PaO_2/P_AO_2 decreased to 87.4 kPa.
- After 30 min of apnoea P_ACO_2 will have risen to about 15 kPa and PaO_2/P_AO_2 decreased only to 79 kPa.
- At the start of apnoea the oxygen stored in alveoli and blood is only about 2.4 litres. Over 30 min of apnoea oxygen consumption is 7–9 litres. The required oxygen enters the body from the breathing system by convective flow (see below).
- By 30 min there is a severe respiratory acidosis but without hypoxia. Buffering the pH change with intravenous trihydroxymethylaminomethane (THAM) will further extend survival. Sodium bicarbonate is ineffective, serving only to increase $PaCO_2$ during apnoea.
- This process of preventing hypoxaemia is known as apnoeic oxygenation.

Convective flow

- During ventilation, carbon dioxide enters alveoli at the same rate it is produced (about 250 ml/min). However, during apnoea most of the carbon dioxide produced is buffered within the body and only about 5 ml/min enters the alveoli.
- Oxygen continues to be absorbed from the alveoli at a rate of 250 ml/min, resulting in a net loss of volume and a fall in alveolar pressure.
- This pressure drop causes convective gas flow (not diffusion) through the conducting airways to the alveoli. Provided the patient's airway remains patent and connected to an oxygen supply then oxygen will be passively drawn down the airway at a rate of about 245 ml/min.

Airway obstruction

- Should the airway become obstructed then no gas will flow into the alveoli as oxygen is absorbed and lung volume will, therefore, decrease by 245 ml/min.

- The reduction in lung volume will lead to alveolar collapse (absorption atelectasis). This will cause intrapulmonary shunting and arterial hypoxaemia.

- By the time that one-third of alveolar volume is lost (2–3 min) the shunt fraction will have risen above 50% and hypoxaemia will be severe.

Air entrainment

- Should the patient be disconnected from the oxygen source whilst apnoeic, for example if the face mask is removed to permit laryngoscopy, then room air instead of oxygen is drawn down the trachea at the same rate of about 245 ml/min. In about 30 s nitrogen will start to enter the alveoli.

- Since the rate of extraction of oxygen from an alveolus is determined by its perfusion, air (with its nitrogen) is directed preferentially to the better-perfused (dependent) alveoli.

- Oxygen will be rapidly diluted in these alveoli and the time to significant hypoxaemia may now be as little as 2–3 min.

- This is still substantially better than if the patient had not been preoxygenated at all.

Practical application

These considerations explain why, with careful use of oxygen and attention to airway patency, it is often possible to allow for an extended period of apnoea without consequent hypoxaemia. In contrast, loss of airway control or failure to maintain oxygen supply may rapidly precipitate a hypoxaemic crisis.

Changes in alveolar gas composition during extended periods of apnoea

	Period of apnoea					
	0 min	2 min	4 min	15 min	30 min	60 min
After breathing air:						
P_AO_2 (kPa)	12	3.8	<0.5	–	–	–
P_ACO_2 (kPa)	5	6.6	7.2	–	–	–
After breathing 100% oxygen:						
P_AO_2 (kPa)	89	87.4	86.8	83.5	79	70
P_ACO_2 (kPa)	5	6.6	7.2	10.5	15	24

Chapter 38
Target-controlled infusion

Anne Troy and Gavin Kenny

Target-controlled infusion

Target-controlled infusion (TCI) allows the anaesthetist to achieve a target blood concentration of drug for a given patient. The system delivers the required amount of drug (optimized by factors such as the patient's weight, gender, and age) and maintains this calculated target value until changed by the anaesthetist. Propofol has been studied extensively and population pharmacokinetics have been incorporated into the Diprifusor system, the only commercially available TCI system.

Components of a TCI system

The infusion pump contains:

- A keyboard allowing entry of patient information and target values.
- A display showing the target and calculated blood concentration, the infusion rate, the amount of drug delivered, the effect site concentration (the estimated concentration at the effector site in the brain), and the estimated time required to reach a lower target concentration.
- Diprifusor has two different microprocessors from deliberately different manufacturers that work in parallel to calculate the propofol concentration in different ways. A warning occurs if the two values differ by more than a preset value.
- Diprifusor has an identification tag which enables the Diprifusor to recognize the drug and concentration in the prefilled syringe and also prevents reuse of syringes by disabling the magnetic pattern in the tag.

Basic pharmacokinetics

A three-compartment model has been used to describe the redistribution and elimination of propofol. Drug is delivered into the central compartment and then distributed throughout the body, governed by rate constants. For example, K_{eo} is the rate constant that determines the brain or effect site concentration. This constant allows the effect site concentration to be calculated and displayed. Once the target value, age, and weight of the patient are entered, the initial bolus is calculated according to the estimated volume of the central compartment (C_1), and then delivered. The system then infuses propofol at a series of rates that maintains the target value by compensating for the loss of drug from C_1 caused by redistribution and elimination. If the target value is increased, the system delivers a rapid infusion to achieve the new target, and then again infuses at the calculated rates required to compensate for drug loss from C_1. If a lower target is entered, the infusion stops until it has calculated that the patient's blood concentration has reached the new target value. The infusion then continues to maintain this new target.

How accurate are target-controlled infusions?

Measured blood concentrations tend to be higher than predicted during infusion. However, once the infusion is stopped this bias is close to zero. Pharmacodynamic variation is much greater then pharmacokinetic variation and the target concentration must therefore be titrated to achieve the required effect in any individual patient.

What numbers to use?

With inhalational agents the vaporizer is adjusted to the clinical situation, and the MAC value of a particular agent guides the anaesthetist. For propofol, the TCI system permits easy adjustment of the depth of anaesthesia. The EC_{50} (effective concentration required to prevent 50% of patients moving in response to a painful stimulus) has been found to be 6–7 µg/ml with oxygen-enriched air and 4–5 µg/ml with 67% nitrous oxide in ASA 1 and 2 patients.

Interindividual variations in pharmacokinetics and pharmacodynamics, as well as the interaction between drugs, account for the different responses between patients. The target should be titrated according to the clinical situation. At present, only adult pharmacokinetics are available for TCI propofol using the Diprifusor. Children require a different set of pharmacokinetic variables that have not yet been implemented in the commercial system. Diprifusor is not licensed for use in patients under 16 years of age.

Benzodiazepine premedication, nitrous oxide, and opioids all reduce propofol requirements.

Induction of anaesthesia

- Select a target concentration less than anticipated (4–6 µg/ml is the requirement in the majority of patients).
- Wait to allow time for the effect site concentration to increase towards the target blood concentration. Oxygen should be administered during the induction phase to ensure an adequate SpO_2.
- Increase the target concentration to achieve the desired level of anaesthesia for the procedure, the individual patient, and the balance of other agents such as analgesics.

Rapid induction of anaesthesia using TCI

- Choose a high target such as 6–8 µg/ml, but only in young, fit patients.
- Wait to allow the effect site concentration to rise towards the target concentration.
- Reduce the target value as propofol continues to be distributed to the tissues. The effect site concentration increases until blood and effect site reach equilibrium.
- There is no experience in rapid sequence induction of anaesthesia using TCI propofol.

TCI for high-risk patients

- Select a low target such as 1 µg/ml.
- Wait to allow for the effect site concentration to rise.
- Increase the target in small steps (0.5–1 µg/ml) until the desired effect is achieved.

Maintenance of anaesthesia

- 3–6 µg/ml is required in the majority of patients but the exact value will depend on the patient, premedication, analgesia, and the degree of surgical stimulation.
- Titrate to effect.

- The majority of patients will wake at 1–2 µg/ml.
- When patients are breathing spontaneously, the combination of respiratory rate and $ETCO_2$ is a good guide to the adequacy of anaesthesia. As the patient lightens, the respiratory rate will increase and the $ETCO_2$ will decrease.
- The use of moderate doses of opioid analgesics, especially in combination with nitrous oxide, will allow a lower target concentration of propofol to be used, perhaps lower by one-third.

Sedation only

Target concentrations of 0.5–2.5 µg/ml are required to produce good-quality sedation during surgery performed under local and regional anaesthesia.

Intravenous access

- Requires a secure access of an adequate size to allow the infusion pump to run at its maximum rate of 1200 ml/h (20G or larger).
- If drug and IV fluids are connected to the same IV cannula by means of a T-piece or three way tap:
  - Ensure that the fluids are running otherwise the drug may pass up the giving set and not to the patient.
  - To prevent reflux use a one-way valve fitted to the fluid infusion line
  - Minimize the use of extensions to reduce the dead-space from the point of administration of the drug, to delivery into the patient.
- Co-administration of drugs by the same giving set is not ideal as a change in the rate of one infusion can affect the other, especially if there is a significant dead-space after the common connection or T-piece.
- The most reliable method is to use a separate, dedicated access site.

Benefits of total intravenous anaesthesia

- Decreases the incidence of PONV.
- Can be used without nitrous oxide.
- Beneficial in laryngoscopy and bronchoscopy, where delivery of an inhalation agent may be difficult, and in thoracic surgery, where intravenous anaesthesia does not appear to inhibit the hypoxic vasoconstrictor reflex, in contrast with inhalational agents.
- Environmentally friendly.
- Safe to use in patients with a history of malignant hyperthermia.
- Postoperative benefit of recovery with minimal 'hangover' effects.

Disadvantages

- Cost.
- There is slow recovery in long operations if high targets are maintained.
- Unlike the inhalational agents, where their delivery is part of airway management, interruption to the delivery of propofol may take longer to recognize.
- The latest study of awareness in almost 12 000 patients showed no awareness in the IV group, only in the inhalational group. There is no difference in the variable pharmacodynamic response/interindividual variation between volatile and IV agents.

TCI remifentanil

Remifentanil has a rapid onset of action, a short elimination half-life, and a context-sensitive half-time of approximately 3 min, which does not change as the infusion time increases. It is often used in combination with propofol. The pharmacokinetics of remifentanil have been incorporated into several custom-built TCI systems, but at present these are only available for research.

Further reading

Davidson JAH, Macleod AD, Howie JC, White M, Kenny GNC (1993). Effective concentration 50 for propofol with and without 67% nitrous oxide. *Acta Anaesthesiologica Scandinavica*, **37**, 458–64.

Milne SE, Kenny GNC (1998). Future applications for TCI systems. *Anaesthesia*, **53** (Suppl. 1), 56–60.

Chapter 39
Perioperative antibiotic therapy

Marina Morgan

Prophylactic antibiotics

Effective antimicrobial prophylaxis should provide adequate bactericidal blood or tissue concentrations of relevant antibiotics during procedures where bacteria may be released or encountered. The timing of prophylaxis is crucial and is most commonly given at induction of anaesthesia, but may need repeating in lengthy operations or in those with extensive blood loss.

Endocarditis prophylaxis

Indicated for patients with heart valve lesions, septal defects, patent ductus, prosthetic valves, or previous endocarditis. (For full details consult the current BNF.)

Dental treatment

Endocarditis is most commonly due to α-haemolytic streptococci from the mouth, hence clindamycin or amoxicillin are used.

Condition	Prophylaxis (adult)
Structural heart lesion or prosthetic valve with no previous endocarditis	Amoxicillin 1 g IV at induction, then amoxicillin 500 mg PO 6 h later, or Amoxicillin 3 g PO 4 h before induction, then amoxicillin 3 g PO as soon as possible after the procedure
As above, and allergic to penicillin or had more than a single dose of penicillin in last month	Vancomycin 1g IV over at least 100 min then 120 mg gentamicin IV at induction or 15 min prior to procedure, or Clindamycin IV 300 mg over at least 10 min at induction, then IV or oral clindamycin 150 mg 6 h later
Previous endocarditis or prosthetic valve and GA	Amoxicillin 1 g IV plus gentamicin 120 mg IV at induction with amoxicillin 500 mg PO 6 h later

Genitourinary procedures

Condition	Prophylaxis
Heart valve lesions, septal defects, patent ductus or prosthetic valve, or patients who have had endocarditis	Amoxicillin 1 g IV plus gentamicin 120 mg IV at induction, with amoxicillin 500 mg PO 6 h later. If urine is infected, prophylaxis should also cover the infective organism
As above, and allergic to penicillin or received more than one dose of penicillin in the preceding month	Vancomycin 1 g IV over 100 min before induction then IV gentamicin 120 mg at induction or 15 min prior to procedure, or Teicoplanin 400 mg IV plus gentamicin 120 mg IV at induction or 15 min prior to procedure

Obstetrical, gynaecological, and gastrointestinal procedures

As for genitourinary procedures but prophylaxis is only needed for those who have prosthetic valves or have had endocarditis.

Points to note

Antibiotic prophylaxis is not routinely recommended for:

* dental surgery in patients with prosthetic joints
* simple dermatological procedures
* immunocompromised and transplant patients unless other indications for prophylaxis are present.

Splenectomy prophylaxis

Postsplenectomy, the incidence of serious sepsis (usually with encapsulated organisms, e.g. pneumococcus, meningococcus, haemophilus) is 0.5–1% per year.

Vaccinations	Pneumovax® one vial and
	Meningovax® (covers group A and C only) one vial and
	Hib (Haemophilus influenzae type B) one vial
	Give 2–4 weeks prior to elective splenectomy for optimal results, or within 48 h of emergency splenectomy
Antibiotics	Amoxicillin 250 mg once daily or
	Penicillin 250 mg twice daily (penicillin won't cover haemophilus) or
	Erythromycin 250 mg once daily

Antibiotic prophylaxis after splenectomy should be offered to:

* Children until they are 16 years of age.
* All asplenic/hyposplenic adults for 2 years.
* Lifelong if there is long-term immunosuppression.

Compliance is a problem, so advise patients that if they develop a respiratory tract infection, they should seek medical advice early and begin therapy aimed at covering pneumococcus, haemophilus, and meningococcus (e.g. co-amoxiclav). Malaria prophylaxis is particularly important if malarial areas are to be visited.

Animal bites or scratches in asplenic patients can cause septicaemia and high mortality with unusual organisms such as *Capnocytophaga canimorsus* (also sensitive to co-amoxiclav). Patients must be warned of the risks of even trivial bites and scratches, since infection with this organism is clinically indistinguishable from meningococcal septicaemia, and the mortality can be higher.

Prophylaxis for perioperative aspiration pneumonia

Generally there is a tendency to overtreat 'aspiration pneumonia', much of which is due to a chemical pneumonitis. The organisms likely to cause infection come from the oropharynx, mainly anaerobes, but may include Gram-negative aerobes including Pseudomonas spp. in patients that have been in hospital for some time. A logical approach to choosing antibiotic prophylaxis would include antimicrobials with antianaerobic activity. Suitable regimes include:

* Co-amoxiclav 1.2 g IV for three doses 8 h apart.
* Clarithromycin 500 mg IV for 2 doses 12 h apart.

- Where Gram negatives may be a problem use cefuroxime 750 mg IV three times a day ± metronidazole 500 mg IV three times a day.

Meningitis and prophylaxis for contacts

As a clinican you should not need to organize prophylaxis for contacts, this is decided upon and organized by the consultant in communicable disease control (CCDC). Staff do not need prophylaxis unless they have been spat upon/vomited over or given mouth-to-mouth resuscitation. Routine nursing procedures should not put staff at risk. Where indicated, the most effective (but unlicensed) prophylaxis for adult contacts of meningococcal infection is ciprofloxacin 500 mg stat PO. (See the BNF for alternative regimens.)

General surgery prophylaxis

Timing

- Give the first dose within 30 min of surgery and not more than 2 h before surgery, particularly with β-lactams.
- Normally one dose of antibiotics should suffice, lasting about 12 h from induction. Additional doses are necessary if the operation carries on for more than 4 h or if there is extensive blood loss (>one blood volume).

Definitions

'Clean' (Class 1) surgery

- 1–2% risk of infection, e.g. body surface surgery (no contamination from colonized or contaminated viscus or infected body cavity, hence normally no prophylaxis needed).
- The exception is prosthesis insertion (joint, vascular graft, stent, etc.) or neurosurgery where infection (although rare) can be devastating. Cover staphylococci—hence cefuroxime 1.5 g or co-amoxiclav 1.2 g IV commonly used. Arterial surgeons are increasingly using prostheses impregnated with rifampicin.
- Beware, patients with MRSA may need a glycopeptide, e.g. vancomycin—discuss with the microbiologist.

'Clean-contaminated' (Class 2) surgery

Less than 10% risk of infection, e.g. with an open viscus, but no spillage (e.g. cholecystectomy or routine appendicectomy).

'Contaminated' (Class 3) surgery

Rectal surgery has a high rate of infection (15–20%), so suggest gentamicin 3–5 mg/kg IV and metronidazole 500 mg IV, or cefuroxime 1.5 g IV and metronidazole 500 mg IV on induction.

'Dirty' surgery

- Already heavily contaminated wound/ pus/faecal contaminants, e.g. perforation/devitalized tissue.
- Needs maximal cover (see table).
- Will need more than simple prophylaxis, with antibiotics continued for several days as therapy.

Soiling risk	Operation	Bacterial prevalence	Antibiotics (usually single dose)
Clean Class 1	Head and neck	Oral streptococci, anaerobes, *Staphylococcus aureus*	Clindamycin 300 mg IV **or** Co-amoxiclav 1.2 g IV
	Hysterectomy	*Staphylococcus aureus*, anaerobes	Co-amoxiclav 1.2 g IV or Cefuroxime 1.5 g IV + metronidazole 1 g PR or 500 mg IV
	Cardiac surgery, vascular surgery needing inguinal incision, amputation, vascular prosthesis	*Staphylococcus aureus*, coagulase-negative staphylococci	Cefuroxime 1.5 g IV **or** Co-amoxiclav 1.2 g IV **or** Vancomycin 1 g IV (over 2 h) if penicillin allergic
	Urinary catheterization, instrumentation	Previously not catheterized, or uninfected urine	None necessary
		Change of catheter or recently catheterised	Gentamicin 80 mg IV **or** Cefuroxime 1.5 g IV **or** Ciprofloxacin 500 mg orally
	Prosthetic joint insertion	Staphylococci including coagulase-negative staphylococci	Cefuroxime 1.5 g IV at induction **or** Vancomycin 1 g IV over 2 h. (Some surgeons add vancomycin or gentamicin to cement for revision surgery in complicated cases.) Prophylaxis may be for one or three doses according to local protocols

Soiling risk	Operation	Bacterial prevalence	Antibiotics (usually single dose)
Clean-contaminated/ contaminated Class 2 and 3	ERCP (significant sepsis occurs in 0.5–1%)	Gram negatives, *Pseudomonas*, enterococci	Ciprofloxacin 750 mg PO stat (will not cover enterococci) **or** Piperacillin 2 g IV + gentamicin 160 mg IV stat
	Cholecystectomy		Gentamicin 160 mg IV stat **or** Cefuroxime 750 mg IV + metronidazole 500 mg IV
	'Routine' appendicectomy	Anaerobes	Metronidazole 1 g PR or 500 mg IV stat ± cefuroxime 750 mg IV stat
	Elective colorectal surgery	Coliforms, anaerobes, Pseudomonas, enterococci	Gentamicin 3–5 mg/kg IV stat at induction + metronidazole 500 mg IV **or** Cefuroxime 1.5 g IV + metronidazole 500 mg IV
'Dirty'	Often emergency, perforated viscus, peritonitis	Coliforms, anaerobes, Pseudomonas, enterococci	Gentamicin 3–5 mg/kg stat IV + cefotaxime 2 g IV + metronidazole 500 mg IV **or** Imipenem 0.5–1 g IV + metronidazole 500 mg IV. Continuation therapy needed

Choosing antibiotics

Consult your hospital formulary for local protocols. The following is intended only as a general guide:

- Review the need for IV antibiotics after 2 days' therapy.
- If a patient develops diarrhoea on any antibiotic, think of C. difficile infection. Discuss with the microbiologist.
- If the patient is not improved on current therapy, discuss with the microbiologist and consider changing.

Penicillin allergy

- How 'allergic' is the patient? What happens (e.g. diarrhoea is not an allergy). ?Anaphylaxis.
- Check old drug charts–they may well have had a penicillin in the past without problems. This further strengthens the case against the patient being genuinely penicillin allergic.
- If penicillin allergy is only a rash, cephalosporins may be used with care: there is 2–5% cross-sensitivity in practice.
- If there is a history of anaphylaxis with penicillin, avoid any β-lactam (i.e. no penicillins, cephalosporins, or carbapenems). Discuss alternatives with the microbiologist. Remember vancomycin has no Gram-negative cover whatever.

Antibiotics and indications

Signs	Organisms	Antibiotics	Comments	If penicillin allergic
No obvious focus in 'septic' patient who needs broad antibiotic cover until diagnosis is established	Anything!	Gentamicin 3–5 mg/kg stat IV + cefotaxime 2 g tds IV + metronidazole 500 mg tds IV **or** Gentamicin 3–5 mg/kg IV + imipenem 500 mg IV qds	Discuss with microbiologist. Note: may need vancomycin IV to cover MRSA, or antifungals if clinically indicated, e.g. colonized or on TPN	Gentamicin 3–5 mg/kg IV + ciprofloxacin 400 mg IV bd + metronidazole 500 mg IV tds
Pneumonia	New admission: *Streptococcus pneumoniae*, *Haemophilus influenzae*	Cefotaxime 2 g tds or benzylpenicillin 1.2 g IV qds + a quinolone with pneumococcal activity, e.g. levofloxacin 500 mg IV od–bd	If *Legionella* or 'atypical infection' suspected, macrolide/ quinolone	Clarithromycin 500 mg IV bd plus a quinolone with pneumococcal activity
	Old admission/ recent anaesthetic where Gram negatives can predominate	Gentamicin 3–5 mg/kg IV + cefotaxime 2 g tds IV **or** Gentamicin 3–5 mg/kg IV + imipenem 500 mg qds IV **or** Gentamicin 3–5 mg/kg IV + ceftazidime 1–2 g tds IV	Most potent anti-Gram-negative quinolone is ciprofloxacin, may be useful in converting from IV to oral but many hospital strains resistant	Gentamicin 3–5 mg/kg IV + ciprofloxacin 400 mg bd + ceftazidime 2 g IV tds

Signs	Organisms	Antibiotics	Comments	If penicillin allergic
	Aspiration pneumonia	Cefuroxime 750 mg tds IV + metronidazole 500 mg IV tds	Alcoholics may have Klebsiellae, resistant to ampicillin.	
Pressure sores, amputation	Anaerobes	Benzylpenicillin 1.2 g qds IV + metronidazole 500 mg IV tds		Clindamycin 300 mg qds IV + metronidazole 500 mg IV tds
Gut sepsis (faecal peritonitis)	Coliforms, *Pseudomonas*, anaerobes	Cefotaxime 2 g IV tds + gentamicin 3–5 mg/kg IV tds + metronidazole 500 mg tds **or** Imipenem 500 mg IV qds + metronidazole 500 mg IV tds		Gentamicin 3–5 mg/kg IV + ciprofloxacin 400 mg IV bd + metronidazole 500 mg IV tds

od = once daily; bd = twice daily; tds = thrice daily; qds = four times daily.

Chapter 40
Using muscle relaxants

John Saddler

Suxamethonium

Suxamethonium is the only depolarizing relaxant in clinical use today and is metabolized by plasma cholinesterase. Plasma cholinesterase (pseudocholinesterase/non-specific cholinesterase) is synthesized in the liver, has a half-life of 5 to 12 days, and metabolizes 70% of a 100 mg bolus of suxamethonium within 1 min. Other drugs metabolized by plasma cholinesterase include mivacurium, cocaine, and diamorphine. Reduced enzyme activity does not, however, appear to have any effect on metabolism of esmolol or remifentanil, both of which also contain ester links.

Enzyme structure is determined genetically by autosomal genes– over 95% of the population have normal genes, designated $E_1^u E_1^u$. The duration of action of suxamethonium will be prolonged if variant genes are present. The commonest of these is the atypical gene E_1^a, present in about 4% of the population. An individual who is heterozygous for the atypical gene ($E_1^u E_1^a$) may have a slightly prolonged neuromuscular block following a bolus of suxamethonium (up to 30 min), but if homozygous ($E_1^a E_1^a$) will remain paralysed for several hours (prevalence approximately 1 in 2500). Other rarer genes exist, e.g. the silent gene E_1^s and the fluoride-resistant gene E_1^f. The presence of these genes will also prolong neuromuscular block.

The activity of plasma cholinesterase can be measured using a spectrophotometric technique examining hydrolysis of benzoylcholine. Phenotype clarification is possible by adding different enzyme inhibitors (dibucaine, sodium fluoride, Ro-020683), which cause differential enzyme inhibition depending upon the enzyme phenotype present. Percentage inhibition with 10^{-5} M dibucaine corresponds to the dibucaine number. Patients with normal enzyme activity have a high dibucaine number, usually over 75. Patients heterozygous for the E_1^a gene have dibucaine numbers around 50, and homozygotes less than 30.

Reduced plasma cholinesterase activity can also occur for acquired reasons. In this case, enzyme structure itself is normal, but activity is reduced. This can occur in the following situations:

* Hepatic disease, carcinomatosis, and malnutrition, because less enzyme is synthesized.

* Administration of drugs which share the same metabolic pathway, and therefore compete with suxamethonium for the enzyme, e.g. esmolol, monoamine oxidase inhibitors, methotrexate.

* Presence of anticholinesterases (e.g. edrophonium, neostigmine, ecothiapate eye drops), which inhibit plasma cholinesterase as well as acetyl cholinesterase.

* Pregnancy, where the enzyme activity is reduced by 25%.

* Plasmapheresis and cardiopulmonary bypass.

Suxamethonium has a number of unwanted effects. These include:

* Postoperative muscle pains: more common in young muscular adults and most effectively reduced by precurarization–the prior use of a small dose of non-depolarizing relaxant, e.g. atracurium (5–10 mg). A larger dose of suxamethonium (1.5 mg/kg) is then required.

* Raised intra-ocular pressure: this is of no clinical significance in most patients, but may be important in poorly controlled glaucoma or penetrating eye injuries (p. 575).

- Hyperkalaemia: serum potassium increases by 0.5 mmol/litre in normal individuals. This may be significant with pre-existing elevated serum potassium. Patients with burns or certain neurological conditions, e.g. paraplegia, muscular dystrophy, and myotonia dystrophica, may develop severe hyperkalaemia following administration. Patients who have sustained significant burns or spinal cord injuries can be given suxamethonium, if necessary, within the first 48 h following injury. Thereafter there is an increasing risk of life-threatening hyperkalaemia, which reduces over the ensuing months. Many would consider it inadvisable to administer the drug until 12 months have elapsed after a burns injury and there may be a permanent risk of hyperkalaemia after upper motor neuron lesions.

- Bradycardias, particularly in children, or if repeated doses of the drug are given. Can be prevented or treated with antimuscarinic agents, e.g. atropine and glycopyrrolate.

- Malignant hyperthermia (see pp. 199, 855): suxamethonium is a potent trigger for this condition in predisposed individuals.

Further reading

Davis L, Britten JJ, Morgan M (1997). Cholinesterase: its significance in anaesthetic practice [review]. *Anaesthesia*, **52**, 244–60.

Non-depolarizing agents

Non-depolarizing muscle relaxants (NDMRs) are highly ionized with a relatively small volume of distribution. Structurally, they are either benzylisoquinolineums (e.g. atracurium and mivacurium) or aminosteroids (e. g. vecuronium and rocuronium). They can also be classified according to their duration of action:

* Short-acting compounds with a duration of action of up to 15 min (mivacurium).
* Medium-acting compounds which are effective for approximately 40 min (atracurium, vecuronium, rocuronium, cis-atracurium).
* Long-acting compounds which have a clinical effect for 60 min (pancuronium, d-tubocurarine).

Most volatile agents prolong the duration of action of NDMRs. Other drugs may do the same; these include the aminoglycoside antibiotics, calcium channel blockers, lithium, and magnesium. Neuromuscular block may also be prolonged by acidosis, hypokalaemia, hypocalcaemia, and hypothermia.

Choice of relaxant

Choice is based on individual preference, the length of procedure, and certain patient characteristics:

* Suxamethonium is still the drug of choice for rapid sequence induction.
* Many of the benzylisoquinolineums release histamine. The amount of histamine released is related to the speed of injection, so a slower injection will reduce this effect. Avoid these drugs in severely atopic or asthmatic individuals. Cis-atracurium, however, does not cause histamine release.
* Like suxamethonium, mivacurium is metabolized by plasma cholinesterase. Patients with reduced levels of this enzyme will exhibit prolonged paralysis.
* Cis-atracurium and atracurium are mainly broken down by Hoffman degradation, a process that is pH and temperature dependent. This metabolism is not affected by the presence of renal failure, so these relaxants are the agents of choice in patients with renal impairment.
* Rocuronium, at doses of 0.6 mg/kg or greater, gives satisfactory intubating conditions within 60 s. Its speed of onset is significantly faster than all other non-depolarizing relaxants.
* Mivacurium is the agent of choice for very short procedures, and does not need to be reversed routinely.

Neuromuscular monitoring

A peripheral nerve stimulator allows the degree of neuromuscular block to be assessed. These devices apply a supramaximal stimulus (strong enough to depolarize all axons) to a peripheral nerve using a current of 30–80 mA. Several peripheral nerves are suitable:

- Electrodes placed on the medial aspect of the wrist proximal to the hypothenar eminence stimulate the ulnar nerve. The response is assessed on the adductor pollicis muscle.
- The common peroneal nerve can be stimulated just inferior to the head of the fibula. Foot dorsiflexion is assessed.
- Facial muscles can be stimulated with electrodes placed in front of the hairline on the temple.

Peripheral nerve stimulators offer a number of modes of stimulation. Commonly used patterns include:

- Train-of-four (TOF) stimulus, where four supramaximal stimuli are applied over 2 s. If NDMR block is profound, no response will be elicited. As neuromuscular function starts to return, the first twitch reappears, then the second, the third, and finally the fourth. This phenomenon, where the second and subsequent twitches decrease in amplitude, is known as fade, and is a characteristic of partial non-depolarizing block. The train-of-four ratio (TOFR) is the ratio of amplitude of the fourth to the first response. Fully reversed patients have no fade and TOFRs of 1. Unfortunately, fade is difficult to assess clinically (visually or by tactile means) once the TOFR has reached 0.4. This may mean that full recovery of muscle function may not have occurred, despite four apparently identical twitches following a TOF stimulus.
- Double-burst stimulation (DBS) is a stronger stimulus, where two short bursts of 50 Hz tetanus are separated by 750 ms. DBS and TOF ratios correlate well, but fade is more accurately assessed with DBS, and an absence of fade is usually good evidence of reversal.
- Post-tetanic count can be used to assess deep relaxation when the TOF is zero. A 50 Hz tetanic stimulation is applied for 5 s followed by 1 Hz single twitches. Reversal should be possible at a post-tetanic count of 10 or greater.

These patterns of stimulation are usually assessed by visual or tactile means, but can be assessed more objectively using mechanomyography, electromyography, or accelerometers. It is sensible to apply the electrodes for nerve stimulation before the induction of anaesthesia, and to assess the effect of stimulation before muscle relaxants are administered, preferably after the patient is asleep. This enables the anaesthetist to place the electrodes in an optimal position, apply a supramaximal stimulus, and assess the onset of neuromuscular block once a relaxant has been given.

Different muscle groups throughout the body exhibit differing sensitivities to NDMRs. In general, muscles which are bulkier and closer to the central circulation, e.g. diaphragm and anterior abdominal wall muscles, exhibit a block that is less profound and wears off more rapidly. Smaller muscles at a greater distance from the heart, e.g the muscles of the arm and hand, are more sensitive and remain blocked for longer. If, therefore, peripheral muscles are assessed with a nerve stimulator, and no residual block is apparent, the central muscles, particularly the respiratory muscles, will be fully functional. The corollary of this is that patients may start to breathe or even cough when there is minimal response to peripheral nerve stimulation.

The depth of neuromuscular block required depends on the type of surgery. Certain operations may need profound paralysis, e.g. laparotomies or micro-surgery. An adequate non-depolarizing block can be maintained at around two TOF twitches or one DBS twitch. At this degree of relaxation, patients will be adequately relaxed but also reversible.

Neuromuscular reversal (see also p. 861)

- Clinical signs of reversal: a substantial degree of paralysis may be present with virtually normal tidal volumes, so the ability to breathe is not a good indicator of adequate reversal. The ability to demonstrate sustained muscle contraction is better, e.g. hand grip or head lift for 5 s.

- Nerve stimulator: an acceptable recovery from block occurs when the TOF ratio has reached 0.7 or greater. The absence of any detectable fade with double-burst stimulation indicates that the patient has reasonable recovery.

- At the completion of surgery, normal neuromuscular transmission can be facilitated by the use of anticholinesterase drugs. Neostigmine (50 µg/kg) has a clinical effect for approximately 30 min, whilst edrophonium (0.5–1 mg/kg) has a shorter onset (producing signs of recovery within 1 min), but has a much shorter duration of action. These drugs should be administered in conjunction with an anticholinergic (e.g. glycopyrrolate 10 µg/kg).

- Reversal agents should not be given until there is evidence of return of neuromuscular transmission, e.g. at least two TOF twitches, one DBS twitch or a post-tetanic count greater than 10. Clinically, this might include evidence of breathing or spontaneous muscle movement. Intense neuro-muscular block may not be reversible.

- Patients who are inadequately reversed exhibit jerky and uncoordinated muscle movements. If awake, they exhibit extreme anxiety. If residual block is confirmed by TOF or DB stimulation, one further dose of reversal agent may be administered. If the block persists, anaesthesia, intubation, and artificial ventilation should be undertaken and the cause sought.

Chapter 41
Blood transfusion

Richard Telford

General principles

Perioperative anaemia is frequent and is associated with increased morbidity and mortality, especially in patients with cardiovascular disease. In the past, treatment of anaemic patients would have involved transfusion of donor blood, but current attitudes have altered, leading to a radical change in transfusion practice. Although the risks of transmission of viral disease has been reduced significantly by more extensive testing and preparation it is still an important consideration.

Risk of viral transmission in blood in the United Kingdom

Infectious agent	Risk of transmission (per units transfused)
Hepatitis B and C	1 in 200 000
Human immunodeficiency virus (HIV)	<1 in 2000 000
New variant CJD	Not proven

In 1998 there were two proven cases of hepatitis B and one case of hepatitis C related to blood transfusion. In 1999 there was one case of hepatitis B and one case of hepatitis C related to blood transfusion. There have been no reported cases of HIV infection related to transfusion in the past 2 years.

Improvements in surgical technique in association with blood conservation methods such as intra-operative cell salvage are now standard practice, enabling many major operations to take place without transfusion.

Clinical guidelines for red cell transfusion

- Clinicians prescribing red cell transfusions should be aware of the risks and benefits.
- Patients should be given information about the risks and benefits wherever possible, and also be informed about possible alternatives (predonation, acute normovolaemic haemodilution, and cell salvage). Patients have the right to refuse blood transfusion.
- Establish the cause of any anaemia. Red cell transfusions should not be given where effective alternatives exist, e.g. treatment of iron deficiency, megaloblastic, and autoimmune haemolytic anaemia.
- There is no given level of haemoglobin at which transfusion of red cells is appropriate for all patients (transfusion trigger). Clinical judgement plays a vital role in the decision whether to transfuse or not (see below).
- In acute blood loss, crystalloids or colloids and not blood should be used for rapid acute volume replacement. The effects of anaemia need to be considered separately from those of hypovolaemia. In massive blood loss empirical decisions have to be taken; however, it is still important to define a patient's need for blood component and fluid replacement as specifically as possible to ensure that blood is prescribed rationally.
- The reason for blood transfusion should be documented in the patient's records.

In the United Kingdom blood is supplied as leucocyte depleted red cells to minimize the theoretical risk of transmission of new variant Creutzfeldt–Jacob disease (CJD). Most of the plasma has been removed and replaced by a supplement of saline, adenine, glucose, and mannitol (SAG-M). Most of the leucocytes have been removed by filtration (leucocyte count $<5 \times 10^6$ per unit). Leucocyte depleted blood is considered CMV safe and may be used as an alternative to CMV seronegative blood. Volume is in the range 190–420 ml; haematocrit is 50–70%; shelf life is 35 days (14 days if gamma irradiated). All red cell products are stored at 4 °C ± 2 °C. The present cost of a unit of red cells (December 2001) is £82.50.

Gamma irradiated blood should be used for:

+ Allogeneic bone marrow recipients from the time of conditioning therapy.

+ Allogeneic bone marrow donors.

+ Autologous stem cell or peripheral blood stem cell recipients (from 7 days before harvest).

+ Patients with Hodgkin's disease.

+ Patients treated with purine analogue drugs such as fludarabine.

+ Patients with congenital immunodeficiency states.

Indications for blood transfusion

Acute blood loss

- First attempt to classify the amount of circulating volume lost (see table):
  - Class I: <15% of circulating blood volume. Do not transfuse unless blood loss is superimposed on a pre-existing anaemia or if the patient is unable to compensate for this level of blood loss because of reduced cardiorespiratory reserve.
  - Class II: <30% of circulating blood volume. Will need resuscitation with crystalloids or colloids, requirement for blood transfusion unlikely unless patient has pre-existing anaemia, reduced cardiorespiratory reserve, or if blood loss continues.
  - Class III: <40% of circulating blood volume. Rapid volume replacement is required with crystalloids or colloids; blood transfusion will almost certainly be required.
  - Class IV: >40% of circulating blood volume. Rapid volume replacement including blood transfusion.
- Next consider the haemoglobin. Have in mind a target level at which to maintain the patient's haemoglobin:
  - Blood transfusion is not indicated when the haemoglobin level is >10 g/dl.
  - Transfusion is always indicated if the haemoglobin level is <7g/dl.
  - In patients who may tolerate anaemia poorly, e.g. patients over 65 and those with cardiovascular or respiratory disease, transfusions are always indicated if the haemoglobin level is <8 g/dl.
  - Patients whose haemoglobin levels are between 8 and 10 g/dl are in a grey area. Some will require a transfusion if they display symptoms of acute anaemia (fatigue, dizziness, shortness of breath, new or worsening angina).
  - Finally consider the risk of further bleeding from disordered haemostasis.
- Check the platelet count and perform a coagulation screen.
- Administer platelets and clotting factors according to guidelines (p. 920).

Perioperative transfusion

Apply the same target values as for acute blood loss. Consider iron supplements in patients whose haemoglobin levels are between 8 and 10 g/dl.

Anaemia in critical care

Apply the same target values as for acute blood loss. There is some evidence that excess transfusion may increase mortality in intensive care.[1]

1 Hebert PC, Wells G *et al.* (1999). A multicenter randomised controlled trial of transfusion requirements in critical care. *New England Journal of Medicine*, **340**, 409–17.

		Class I	Class II	Class III	Class IV
Blood loss	Percentage	<15	15–30	30–40	>40
	Volume (ml)	750	750–1500	1500–2000	>2000
Blood pressure (mmHg)	Systolic	Unchanged	Normal	Reduced	Very low
	Diastolic	Unchanged	Raised	Reduced	Very low/unrecordable
Pulse rate (beats/min)		<100	>100	>120	>140
Capillary refill		Normal	Slow (>2 s)	Slow (>2 s)	Undetectable
Respiratory rate (breaths/min)		14–20	20–30	30–40	>40
Urine output (ml/h)		>30	20–30	10–20	Negligible
Mental status		Slightly anxious	Mildly anxious	Anxious/confused	Confused/lethargic

Making requests for cross-matched red cells and 'group and save' serum

When requests for blood and platelets are made by telephone the patient's blood group and rhesus status must be known. If the patient's blood group is unknown serum must be sent for blood grouping. If a patient has been transfused more than 72 h previously a new sample must be sent to the laboratory in case new antibodies have developed following the transfusion.

Collecting blood samples from patients

- In adults a 7.5 ml EDTA sample is required. The patient's identity should be checked by:
  - Questioning the patient (name and date of birth).
  - Checking that the patient's details on the wristband match those on the request form and the answers given to the above questions.
- All sample tubes must be labelled with:
  - patient's surname
  - patient's forename
  - date of birth
  - patient identification number
  - ward/department
  - date sample collected.
- The sample and request form must be signed by the person collecting the sample.
- Preprinted labels must not be used for sample labelling.

'Group and save' or cross-match?[2]

- For either investigation the laboratory first determines the patients ABO and rhesus type and then the patient's serum is screened for IgG antibodies. The patient's serum is held in the laboratory, usually for 7 days.
- Once 'grouped and saved' (and provided that antibody screening was negative) blood units can be cross-matched against the patient's serum within about 20 min. This entails a further quick test to exclude ABO incompatibility for each unit.
- There should be a maximum surgical blood ordering schedule (MSBOS) which stipulates which operations require blood to be cross-matched.
- In an emergency the patient can be given group-specific blood or O rhesus negative, Kell negative blood ('universal donor' blood). The risk of a transfusion reaction is very small provided the patient does not have atypical antibodies. This must be balanced against the risk of the patient bleeding to death.

2 Murphy MF, Wallington TB *et al* (2001). British committee for standards in haematology, blood transfusion task force. Guidelines for the clinical use of red cell transfusions. *British Journal of Haematology*, 113, 24–31.

Blood conservation techniques

Preoperative autologous donation

Patients donate a unit of blood per week in the month prior to their operation. Eligibility depends on a number of guidelines summarized in a publication by the British Committee for Standards in Haematology.[3] Such a system is labour intensive and depends on good organization both of collection and storage of blood and coordination of operating lists with guaranteed operating dates. Cost-effectiveness is low mainly because of a high proportion of discarded units. Such systems are not widely used in the United Kingdom.

Preoperative use of erythropoetin

Erythropoetin is licensed in the European Union for use in patients donating autologous blood before surgery. It stimulates erythropoesis and permits more aggressive preoperative donation (up to 6 units in a 3-week period). It has also been used to increase the efficacy of acute normovolaemic haemodilution by increasing the preoperative haemoglobin. Its use has been described to permit major elective surgery (e.g. liver transplantation) in Jehovah's Witnesses without exposure to allogeneic blood. It remains, however, an expensive method of minimizing allogeneic blood transfusions.

Acute normovolaemic haemodilution

This involves the immediate preoperative collection of whole blood from the patient with simultaneous infusion of crystalloid or colloid to maintain normovolaemia. It is usually performed in the anaesthetic room. Venesection can be undertaken using a large-bore intravenous cannula or arterial line into citrated blood bags (available from the blood transfusion department). The volume of blood to be removed to achieve the desired haematocrit can be calculated using the following formula:

$$V \text{ (ml)} = \text{EBV} \times [(H_I - H_F)/H_{av}]$$

where EBV is the estimated blood volume (70 ml/kg), H_I is the initial haematocrit, H_F is the final haematocrit, and H_{AV} is the average haematocrit (mean of H_I and H_F).

Once collected, bags should be labelled and stored at room temperature for reinfusion once surgical blood loss has ceased. They must be reinfused to the patient within 6 h. Mathematical modelling has suggested that severe haemodilution (perioperative haematocrit less than 20%) accompanied by substantial blood losses would be required before the red cell volume saved becomes clinically important. Current United Kingdom guidelines state that acute normovolaemic haemodilution should be considered when the potential surgical blood loss is likely to exceed 20% of the blood volume. Patients should have a preoperative haemoglobin of more than 10 g/dl and not have severe myocardial disease(e.g. moderate to severe left ventricular impairment, unstable angina, severe aortic stenosis, or critical left main stem coronary artery disease).

3   British Committee for Standards in Haematology, Blood Transfusion Task Force (1993). Guidelines for autologous transfusion. *Transfusion Medicine*, 3, 307–16.

Acute normovolaemic haemodilution has several advantages over autologous blood donation. The blood procured by haemodilution requires no testing. The units are not removed from the operating theatre so that the possibility of an administrative error resulting in an ABO incompatible blood transfusion is virtually eliminated, as is the risk of bacterial contamination. Finally, blood obtained by haemodilution does not require substantial investment of time by the patient as it is obtained at the time of surgery.

Intra-operative cell salvage and reinfusion[4]

This involves the collection and reinfusion of autologous red cells lost during surgery. Most machines depend on a centrifugal principle using a collection bowl that spins and separates the red cells from plasma, white cells, and platelets. Shed blood is aspirated into a collection reservoir via heparinized tubing. The cells are separated by haemoconcentration and differential centrifugation and finally washed in 1–2 litres of normal saline. This removes circulating fibrin, debris, plasma, leucocytes, microaggregates, complement, platelets, free haemoglobin, circulating procoagulants, and most of the heparin. The end product of the process is packed red cells with a haematocrit of 50–60%. Salvaged red cells are superior to or at least equal to banked homologous blood in terms of red cell survival, pH, 2,3-diphosphoglycerate (2,3-DPG), and potassium levels. Cell washing devices can provide the equivalent of 10 units of bank blood per hour in cases of massive bleeding. The technique is applicable to open heart surgery, vascular surgery, total joint replacements, spinal surgery, liver transplantation, ruptured ectopic pregnancy, and some neurosurgical procedures. Some Jehovah's Witnesses may accept intraoperative cell salvage, provided the equipment is set up in continuity with the circulation. Specific consent must be obtained.

Cell salvage devices should not be used in the presence of contamination of the operative field since bacteria have been shown to survive the washing process. Malignant disease has been considered a contraindication because malignant cells can survive the collection process. Recent work suggests that the risk of dissemination of malignant disease is minimal. Blood containing fat or amniotic fluid should not be salvaged because of the risk of embolism and disseminated intravascular coagulation (DIC), although one group has advocated the use of cell salvage with leucocyte depletion filtration in life-threatening obstetric haemorrhage (e.g. at caesarean section). Topical clotting agents such as collagen, cellulose, and thrombin and topical antibiotics or cleansing agents used in the operative field should not be aspirated into a cell salvage machine. Complications have been reported in patients with sickle cell disease.

The high cost of the machinery and the need for trained operators are drawbacks. Once set up the disposable kits can process limitless units of packed red cells. Current disposable costs are very similar to the cost of one unit of leucodepleted red cells. A recent NHS circular 'Better blood transfusion'[5] recommended that by March 2000 all NHS Trusts where blood is transfused should have considered the introduction of perioperative cell salvage.

4 Napier JA, Bruce M, Chapman J *et al.* (1997). Guidelines for autologous transfusion II. Perioperative haemodilution and cell salvage. *British Journal of Anaesthesia*, **78**, 768–71.

5 Winyard G (1998). Better blood transfusion. *NHS Executive Clinical Effectiveness Circular*, appendix 1, SC 1998/2, 11 December 1998.

Postoperative recovery of blood

This involves the collection of blood from surgical drains followed by reinfusion, with or without processing. The blood recovered is dilute, partially haemolysed and defibrinated and may contain high concentrations of cytokines. Most experience has been gained in cardiac and orthopaedic surgery, especially total knee replacements. The safety and benefit of the use of unwashed blood remains questionable. Some groups have reported considerable savings in the use of bank blood.

Massive blood transfusion

Defined as the replacement of the patient's total blood volume with stored blood in less than 24 h. A dilutional coagulopathy occurs due to diminution of clotting factors and platelets. This presents clinically as oozing of blood from cut surfaces, wounds and venepuncture sites. Thrombocytopenia is the most likely cause of bleeding in massive transfusion. Regular platelet counts and tests of blood coagulation should be performed to assess the underlying trend and the adequacy of treatment. In critical situations give FFP and platelets empirically rather than wait for results. Stringent efforts should be made to maintain the patient's temperature since hypothermia impairs platelet function and clotting.

Complications of blood transfusion

- Mismatch: most commonly giving the wrong blood to the wrong patient. Stop the transfusion and return the blood to the blood bank. Take blood for FBC, clotting, and a serum sample. Signs and symptoms of a transfusion reaction will be present. These may range from mild reactions (fever sweating, tachycardia, and urticaria) to full-blown haemolytic reaction (back and chest pain, hypotension, oliguria, haemoglobinuria, and renal failure).
- Metabolic: with large volume rapid transfusions acidosis and hyperkalaemia can develop.
- Hypothermia: warm the blood. This may exacerbate coagulopathy of massive transfusion by further impairing platelet function.
- Dilutional caogulopathy.
- Infection: viral (HIV, hepatitis B and C, CMV), bacterial, parasitic (e.g. malaria).
- Transfusion associated graft versus host disease (TA-GVHD).
- Transfusion related acute lung injury (TRALI).

Guidelines for the use of fresh frozen plasma (see p. 141)

Fresh frozen plasma (FFP) is obtained from whole blood and rapidly frozen to a temperature that will maintain the activity of labile clotting factors. FFP is stored at $-30\,°C$ for up to 12 months. It is thawed at $37\,°C$ immediately before use. Each unit should contain normal levels of stable clotting factors, albumin, and immunoglobulin. Factor VIIIc levels are >0.7 IU/ml and fibrinogen 2–5 mg/ml. FFP must be ABO compatible. Premenopausal females who are Rh-D negative must receive Rh-D negative FFP.

- The usual starting dose is 10–15 ml/kg (equivalent to four packs of FFP for a 70 kg person) which raises the coagulation levels 12–15%.
- FFP takes 20 min to thaw, infusion should be started within 2 h of thawing and completed within 4 h of thawing.

Guidelines for platelet transfusion

A standard adult therapeutic dose (ATD) pack has platelets from six units of blood and contains $>240 \times 10^9$ platelets. One ATD should increase the platelet count by $20–40 \times 10^9$ in an adult. Platelets should be given through a *fresh* blood giving set or a special platelet giving set. Ideally they should be ABO and rhesus compatible. For invasive procedures (insertion of central lines) or surgery the platelet count should be maintained above 50×10^9 /litre.

Guidelines for the use of cryoprecipitate

Cryoprecipitate is prepared from a single donation. Each unit contains a volume of 20–40 ml. It is stored at –30 °C for up to 12 months and is thawed to 37 °C immediately before use. The concentration of fibrinogen is >140 mg/unit and factor VIIIc >70 IU/unit. ABO compatible units should be used, and treatment considered if the plasma fibrinogen is <0.8 g/litre. Ten units of cryoprecipitate should increase fibrinogen level by 1 g/litre.

Cost of blood components (2000/2001)

Product	Cost
Red cells (leucocyte depleted)	£82.50
Platelets (leucocyte depleted), one ATD	£156.60
Fresh frozen plasma (leucocyte depleted)	£19.47
Cryoprecipitate (leucocyte depleted)	£23.40

Chapter 42
Postoperative nausea and vomiting

David Conn

General principles

While rarely life-threatening, morbidity associated with postoperative nausea and vomiting may be the most unpleasant memory associated with a patient's hospital stay. Severe cases can lead to increased length of hospital stay, increased bleeding, incisional hernias, and aspiration pneumonia.

Frequency

Incidence is between 5% and 75% in published series. If no prophylaxis is used the incidence is probably around 20% for PONV within 6 h and 30% for PONV within 24 h. The best anti-emetic drug or anti-emetic strategy has a numbers needed to treat (NNT) of about 5. All treatments carry finite risks.

Physiology

The vomiting reflex can be activated by stimulation of the following pathways:

* abdominal vagal afferents
* area postrema including the nucleus tractus solitarius
* vestibular system.
* Other pathways may include those from cerebral hemispheres, visual, olfactory, and gustatory organs.

The chemical receptors involved in transduction of signals in the area of the vomiting centre and the area postrema include dopaminergic, cholinergic, histaminergic, serotinergic, and opioid. With so many pathways and different receptors, there is currently no perfect anti-emetic. Neurokinin-1 may represent the final common pathway for PONV and trials are under way examining drugs affecting this pathway.

Risk factors

All the risk factors below have been described as contributing to PONV:

Surgery

- Gynaecological, especially ovarian surgery.
- Bowel or gall-bladder surgery.
- Head and neck surgery, including tonsillectomy and adenoidectomy.
- Ophthalmic, especially squint surgery.
- Prolonged surgery.

Anaesthesia

- Induction with methohexitone, etomidate, or ketamine (compared with propofol or thiopental).
- Maintenance with N_2O. Avoidance reduces risk with an NNT of 5, but a number needed to harm (NNH) of 50—awareness.
- Use of intra-operative opioids increases the incidence of PONV. However, untreated pain is also emetogenic.
- Spinal anaesthesia—high blocks (above T5), hypotension, and the use of adrenaline in the local anaesthetic.
- Intra-operative dehydration—IV fluids reduce the incidence.
- Gastric dilatation from inexperienced 'bag and mask ventilation'.
- 'Motion' sickness due to fast or careless patient movement during emergence from anaesthesia.

Patient factors

- Previous history of PONV.
- Children more than adults.
- Women more than men, until after 70 years of age.
- Obesity may be a risk factor. May be due to a higher incidence of gastric reflux in this population.
- History of motion sickness.

Organizational

- Failure to audit and set up appropriate treatment protocols.
- Poor education of medical and nursing staff, leading to under-use of effective treatment.

Drugs and dosages

Some drugs have multiple actions, so the following classification is pragmatic.

Antidopaminergic agents
- Phenothiazines such as prochlorperazine (12.5 mg IM):
  - Active against the emetic effect of opioids.
  - Sedative and short acting. Extrapyramidal side-effects. Should not be administered intravenously.
- Butyrophenones such as droperidol (0.5–2.5mg IV—optimum dose 1–1.25mg):
  - Droperidol is effective when added to morphine for use in PCA pumps (2.5–5 mg/50 ml).
  - Can cause disturbing dysphoric, sedative, and extrapyramidal side-effects. This is less likely with lower doses.
- Substituted benzamides such as metoclopramide (10 mg IV, IM, or PO):
  - Said to be active against the emetic effect of opioids, but has a high incidence of extrapyramidal side-effects, especially in young women.
  - Popular, but evidence suggests that it is of little use in the postoperative period.

Avoid combinations of drugs with extrapyramidal side-effects, and avoid completely in patients with Parkinson's disease.

Antihistamines
Cyclizine (25–50 mg IM or slow IV):
- Commonly used for PONV after middle ear surgery.
- Sedation can be a problem. Intravenous injection may lead to tachycardia and hypotension with consequent myocardial ischaemia.
- Also has antimuscarinic effects.

Anticholinergics
Hyoscine hydrobromide ('scopolamine' 0.3–0.6 mg IM):
- Useful for the treatment of motion sickness, opioid-induced vomiting, and PONV.
- Sedation, confusion, and dry mouth may limit use.

Antiserotonergic (5HT$_3$ antagonists)
Ondansetron (1–8 mg PO, IV, IM), granisetron (1 mg PO, IV), tropisetron (5 mg PO, IV):
- Widely regarded as the anti-emetics with the lowest side effect profile. Particularly effective in chemotherapy-induced emesis.
- Evidence suggests that they are only slightly better than other anti-emetics for either prophylaxis or treatment of PONV.
- In paediatric practice where the extrapyramidal effects of the antidopaminergic drugs can be a serious problem, ondansetron (50–100 μg/kg by slow IV injection) is the drug of first choice. Side-effects include headache, constipation, and altered liver enzymes.

Other drugs

- Benzodiazepines have been shown to decrease anticipatory vomiting before chemotherapy.
- Cannabis is said to be effective in nausea and vomiting. Nabilone is a cannabis extract primarily used in chemotherapy-induced vomiting. The $5HT_3$ antagonists have superseded it.
- Dexamethasone (150 µg/kg in children or 8 mg in adults) is used for reducing sickness related to chemotherapy and has been shown to be useful in PONV. There are positive studies looking at the combination with ondansetron.
- Ginger root has been shown to be as effective as metoclopramide in patients having day case laparoscopy.
- Anti-NK1 drugs are the subject of current research and may represent the final common pathway in the stimulation of the vomiting reflex.

Combination therapy

There is increased interest in using combinations of anti-emetics to increase efficacy. The logical approach is to combine two drugs with different actions (and presumably side-effects).

Studies with the combination of dexamethasone and ondansetron, or ondansetron and droperidol showed clear improvements over monotherapy.

Non-pharmacological causes and treatments

- Perioperative fluid therapy leads to both decreased PONV and earlier oral fluid intake.
- Too early oral fluid intake, especially in children, may lead to increased PONV.
- Hypnosis over 4–6 days preoperatively will decrease PONV.
- Perioperative suggestion may decrease the incidence.
- Acupuncture may decrease the incidence–using the P6 point over the median nerve at the wrist, but only in the awake patient.

The vomiting patient

Have anti-emetics been given?

Has a reasonable dose been administered by a reasonable route?

Has a different anti-emetic been added?

Look for a treatable cause.

Too much or too little opioid analgesic?

Hypotension, e.g. spinal or epidural anaesthesia, bleeding.

Too early oral intake or inadequate intravenous intake?

Surgical complications, e.g. bowel obstruction.

Drugs, e.g. opioids, antibiotics, chemotherapy.

Psychological–fear, anxiety, previous bad experience.

Strategies for decreasing the impact of PONV

• Try to identify your 'at-risk' group and consider prophylactic anti-emetics.
• If a 'high-risk' patient is identified then consider combination anti-emetics, from different pharmacological groups.
• Treat PONV quickly when it occurs.
• Avoid strong analgesics, where possible, by providing good pain relief with local anaesthesia and simple analgesics.

Further reading

Fisher DM (1997).The big little problem of postoperative nausea and vomiting. *Anesthesiology*, **87**, 1271–3.

Strunin L, Rowbotham O, Miles (ed.) (1999). *The effective management of post-operative nausea and vomiting.* Aesculapius Medical Press,

Tramèr MR (2000). Systematic reviews in PONV therapy. In: Tramèr MR (ed.) *Evidence based resource in anaesthesia and analgesia.* BMJ Books, London.

Chapter 43
Perioperative arrhythmias

Juliet Lee

Perioperative arrhythmias

Arrhythmia detection and management

If the arrhythmia is causing haemodynamic instability, rapid recognition and treatment is required. However, most will respond to basic measures—sometimes even before identification of the exact rhythm abnormality is possible.

Practical interpretation of arrhythmias

This ideally is done with a paper printout of the ECG trace—preferably in a 12–lead format.

Determine

- What is the ventricular rate?
- Is the QRS complex of normal duration or widened?
- Is the QRS regular or irregular?
- Are P waves present and are they normally shaped?
- How is atrial activity related to ventricular activity?

Ventricular rate

- Calculate approximate ventricular rate (divide 300 by the number of large squares between each QRS complex).
- Tachyarrhythmias—rate greater than 100/min.
- Bradyarrhythmias—rate less than 60/min.

QRS complex

Arrhythmias may be due to impulses arising from:

- Atria—a supraventricular rhythm.
- AV node—a nodal or junctional rhythm.
- Ventricles—a ventricular rhythm.
- Supraventricular and nodal rhythms arise from a focus above the ventricles. Since the ventricles still depolarize via the normal His/Purkinje system the QRS complexes are of normal width (<0.1 s or two small squares) and are termed 'narrow complex rhythms'.
- Arrhythmias arising from the ventricles will be 'broad complex' with a QRS width of >0.1 s (two small squares). In the presence of bundle branch block a supraventricular rhythm may have broad complexes. This may be present on the 12–lead ECG or develop as a consequence of the arrhythmia—so called rate related aberrant conduction.

Regularity

The presence of an irregular rhythm will tend to suggest ectopic beats (atrial or ventricular), atrial fibrillation, atrial flutter with variable block, or second degree heart block with variable block.

P waves

The presence of P waves indicates atrial depolarization. Absent P waves associated with an irregular ventricular rhythm suggests atrial fibrillation, whilst a saw-toothed pattern is characteristic of atrial flutter.

Atrial/ventricular activity

Normally there will be one P wave per QRS complex. Any change in this ratio indicates a blockage to conduction at some point in the pathway from atria to the ventricles.

Action plan when faced with an abnormal rhythm on the ECG monitor

- Assess vital signs–A, B, C.
- Determine whether the arrhythmia is serious (cardiovascular compromise/symptoms in awake patient).

Is there a problem with the anaesthetic?

- Oxygenation–increase the inspired oxygen concentration?
- Ventilation adequate to prevent CO_2 build up?–check $ETCO_2$.
- Anaesthesia too light or too deep?–alter the inspired volatile agent concentration.
- Drug interaction/error?

Is there a problem with the surgery?

- Vagal stimulation from traction on the eye or peritoneum.
- Trigeminal stimulation from jaw.
- Loss of cardiac output–air/fat embolism.
- Unexpected blood loss.
- Injection of adrenaline.
- Mediastinal manipulation.

Classification of arrhythmias

Arrhythmias may be classified into narrow and broad complex for the purposes of rapid recognition and management.

Narrow complex rhythms:

- sinus arrhythmia
- sinus tachycardia
- sinus bradycardia
- junctional/AV nodal tachycardia
- atrial fibrillation
- atrial ectopics
- atrial tachycardia, atrial flutter.

Broad complex rhythms:

- ventricular ectopics
- ventricular tachycardia
- supraventricular tachycardia with aberrant conduction
- ventricular fibrillation.

Narrow complex rhythms

Sinus arrhythmia

This is irregular spacing of normal complexes associated with respiration. There is a constant P–R interval with beat-to-beat change in the R–R interval. It is a normal finding especially in young people.

Sinus tachycardia

Rate greater than 100/min in adults. Normal P–QRS–T complexes are evident. Causes include:

* inadequate depth of anaesthesia
* pain / surgical stimulation
* fever/sepsis
* hypovolaemia
* anaemia
* heart failure
* thyrotoxicosis
* drugs, e.g. atropine, ketamine, catecholamines.

   Management of sinus tachycardia involves correction of any underlying cause where possible. Beta-blockers may be useful if tachycardia causes myocardial ischaemia, but should be used with caution in patients with heart failure and avoided in asthma.

Sinus bradycardia

Rate less than 60/min in an adult. May be normal in athletic patients and may also be due to vagal stimulation during surgery. Other causes include:

* drugs, e.g. beta-blockers, digoxin, anticholinesterases, halothane, and suxamethonium
* myocardial infarction
* sick sinus syndrome
* raised intracranial pressure
* hypothyroidism
* hypothermia.

   It is often not necessary to correct this in a fit person, unless the rate is less than 40 beats/ minute, and/or there is haemodynamic comprise. However, consider

* Correcting the underlying cause, e.g. stop the surgical stimulus.
* Atropine up to 20 µg/kg or glycopyrrolate 10 µg/kg IV.
* Patients on beta-blockers may be resistant and an isoprenaline infusion occasionally may be required (0.5–10 µg/min). Alternatively glucagon (50–150 µg/kg IV in 5% glucose) can be used—this is an unlicensed indication and dose.

Arrhythmias due to re-entry (circus movement of electrical impulses)

These arrhythmias occur where there is an anatomical branching and rejoining of conduction pathways. Normally conduction would occur equally down both limbs, but if slowed in one limb the impulse can then spread backwards up the abnormal pathway. If it arrives at a time when the first pathway is no longer refractory, it can pass around the circuit repeatedly activating it. The classical example of this is the Wolf–Parkinson–White (WPW) syndrome where a relatively large accessory conduction pathway exists between atria and the ventricles. This is called a 'macro re-entry' circuit. Other macro re-entry circuits occur within the atrial and ventricular myocardium, and are responsible for atrial flutter, atrial fibrillation, and ventricular tachycardia. In AV nodal re-entrant tachycardia there are 'micro re-entry circuits' within the AV node itself.

Junctional/AV nodal tachycardia

'Supraventricular tachycardia' (SVT) applies to all tachyarrhythmias arising from above the ventricles. However, it is often used to describe junctional (AV nodal) tachycardias arising from micro re-entry circuits in or near the AV node, or from an accessory conduction pathway between atria and ventricles. The ECG appearance is of a narrow complex tachycardia (QRS <0.1 s or two small squares), with a rate of 150–200/min. A broad complex pattern may occur if antegrade conduction is down an accessory pathway. The typical features seen on 12-lead ECG taken during sinus rhythm are:

- a short P–R interval
- a slurred upstroke on the R wave (the delta wave)
- inverted T waves in V2–V5 are characteristic.

Junctional/AV nodal tachycardia is occasionally associated with severe circulatory disturbance and needs to be managed as an emergency if it occurs during anaesthesia:

- In the presence of hypotension, especially where the patient is anaesthetized in theatre, the first-line treatment is synchronized direct current cardioversion with 200 then 360 J.

- Carotid sinus massage rarely converts to sinus rhythm but may slow the rate and reveal the underlying rhythm. It is helpful in differentiating it from atrial flutter and fast atrial fibrillation.

- Adenosine—this slows conduction and is especially useful for terminating re-entry SVT of the Wolf–Parkinson–White type. Give 6 mg IV rapidly, followed by a saline flush. Further doses of 12 mg may be given at 2 min intervals if there is no response to the first dose. The effects of adenosine last only 10–15 s. It should be avoided in asthma.

- Verapamil, beta-blockers, or other drugs such as amiodarone or flecainide may control the rate or convert to sinus rhythm.

- Verapamil 5–10 mg IV slowly over 2 min. A further 5 mg may be given after 10 min if required. This may cause a siginificant fall in blood pressure. Administration together with beta-blockers may cause severe hypotension and asystole.

- Beta-blockers, e.g. propranolol 1 mg over 1 min repeated if necessary at 2 min intervals (maximum 5 mg), sotalol 100 mg over 10 min repeated 6-hourly if necessary. Esmolol is a relatively cardioselective beta-blocker with a very short duration of action and may be given by intravenous infusion at 50–200 µg/kg/min.

- Digoxin should be avoided—it facilitates conduction through the AV accessory pathway in Wolf–Parkinson–White syndrome and may worsen the tachycardia. Atrial fibrillation in the presence of an accessory pathway may allow very rapid conduction which can degenerate to ventricular fibrillation.

Atrial fibrillation[1]

One of the commonest arrhythmias encountered in anaesthetic practice. There is chaotic and uncoordinated atrial depolarization, an absence of P waves on the ECG with an irregular baseline, and a completely irregular ventricular rate. Transmission of atrial activity to the ventricles via the AV node depends on the refractory period of the conducting tissue. In the absence of drug treatment or disease which slows conduction, the ventricular response rate will normally be rapid, i.e. 120–200/min.

Causes of atrial fibrillation (AF) include:

* ischaemia
* myocardial disease/pericardial disease/mediastinitis
* mitral valve disease
* sepsis
* electrolyte disturbance (especially hypokalaemia or hypomagnesaemia)
* thyrotoxicosis
* thoracic surgery.

Since contraction of the atria contributes up to 30% of the normal ventricular filling, the onset of AF may result in a significant fall in cardiac output. Fast AF may precipitate cardiac failure and myocardial ischaemia. Systemic thromboembolism may occur if blood clots in the fibrillating atria and subsequently embolizes into the circulation. There is a 4% risk per year of an embolic cerebrovascular event at the age of 75.

Treatment of AF aims to restore sinus rhythm where possible. Where this is not possible, the aim is control of the ventricular rate to <100/min and the prevention of embolic complications. In acute AF restoration of sinus rhythm is often possible, whereas in longstanding AF control of the ventricular rate is the usual aim of therapy. Ideally the ventricular rate should be controlled by appropriate therapy preoperatively. However, more rapid control of the rate in theatre is occasionally required.

Management of AF depends on whether the AF is paroxysmal or persistent. For paroxysmal AF occurring in theatre or onset within the last 48 h:

* Correct precipitating factors where possible, especially electrolyte disturbances.
* Synchronized d.c. cardioversion. If AF has been present for more than 24 h there is a risk of arterial embolization unless the patient is anticoagulated first. Shock at 200 J, then 360 J.
* Digoxin can be used to slow the ventricular rate in the presence of a normal plasma potassium concentration. An intravenous loading dose of 500 µg in 100 ml of normal saline over 20 min may be given and repeated at intervals of 4–8 h if necessary, to a total of 1–1.5 mg. This is contraindicated if the patient is already taking digoxin when lower doses are required. There is no evidence that it is useful for converting AF to sinus rhythm or maintaining it once established.

1 Nathanson MH, Gajraj NM (1998). Perioperative management of atrial fibrillation. *Anaesthesia*, 53, 665–76.

- Amiodarone may also be used to slow the ventricular rate. It does not restore sinus rhythm, but will help to sustain it once regained. It is especially useful in paroxysmal atrial fibrillation associated with critical illness, and where digoxin or beta-blockers cannot be used. A loading dose of 300 mg IV via a central vein is given over an hour and then followed by 900 mg over 23 h.

- Flecainide 50–100 mg slowly IV is the best drug for converting to sinus rhythm. It should be used with caution in the presence of LV dysfunction and ventricular arrhythmias.

- Verapamil 5–10 mg IV over 2 min can be used to control ventricular rate, where there is no impairment of left ventricular function or coronary artery disease. It should be avoided if left ventricular function is poor, if there is evidence of ischaemia, or if the patient is beta-blocked.

- Beta-blockers (e.g. esmolol or propranolol as above) are sometimes used to control the ventricular rate but may precipitate heart failure in the presence of an impaired myocardium, thyrotoxicosis, or calcium channel blockers.

With persistent AF, if the ventricular rate is above 100/min, it should be slowed to allow adequate time for ventricular filling and myocardial perfusion during diastole. Management strategies are:

- Digitalization–if the patient is not already fully loaded with digoxin. This should usually be done over 1–2 days preoperatively. Occasionally rapid IV digitalization is required where the surgery is urgent. Beware signs of digoxin toxicity, i.e. nausea, anorexia, headache, visual disturbances, and arrhythmias, especially ventricular ectopics and atrial tachycardia with 2:1 block. Determination of adequate digitalization preoperatively, can usually be determined from the ventricular rate at rest, which should be 60–90 beats/ min. Digoxin levels can be measured, and may be helpful where there is doubt. However, unwanted effects depend on both plasma levels and on the sensitivity of the conducting system or myocardium which is often increased in heart disease. Therapeutic levels should be 1–2 ng/ml.

- Beta-blockers or verapamil.

- Amiodarone (verapamil, nifedipine, and amiodarone when co-administered with digoxin can increase digoxin levels).

When AF has been present for more than 24 h anticoagulation is necessary before d.c. cardioversion to prevent embolization. Usually patients should be warfarinized for 3 weeks prior to elective d.c. cardioversion. An INR >2 is satisfactory. Warfarin should be continued for 4 weeks afterwards. Occasionally when a patient develops AF with haemodynamic compromise, d.c. cardioversion must be considered even where anticoagulation is contraindicated (e.g. recent surgery).

Atrial ectopics

These are very common and invariably benign. An abnormal P wave is followed by a normal QRS complex. The P wave is not always easily visible on the ECG trace. The term ectopic indicates that depolarization originated in an abnormal place, i.e. not the SA node, hence the abnormal shape. If such a focus depolarizes early the beat produced is called an extrasystole or premature atrial contraction and may be followed by a compensatory pause. If the underlying SA node rate is slow, a focus in the atria sometimes takes over and the rhythm is described as atrial escape, as it occurs after a small delay. Extrasystoles and escape beats have the same QRS appearance on the ECG, but extrasystoles occur early and escape beats occur late.

Causes of atrial ectopics are varied:

- They often occur in normal hearts.
- They may occur with any heart disease.
- Ischaemia, hypoxia.
- Light anaesthesia.
- Sepsis.
- Shock.
- Anaesthetic drugs are common causes.

Management involves:

- Correction of any underlying cause.
- Specific treatment of atrial ectopics is unneccesary unless runs of atrial tachycardia occur–see above.

Atrial flutter and atrial tachycardia

An ectopic focus depolarizes anywhere within the atria. The atria contract faster than 150/min and P waves can be seen superimposed on the T waves of the preceding beats. In atrial flutter there is no flat baseline between P waves and the typical 'saw-tooth' pattern of flutter waves is be seen. Atrial tachycardia is uncommon in adults. Atrial tachycardia and flutter may occur with any kind of block, e.g. 2:1, 3:1 etc.

Atrial tachycardia is typically a paroxysmal arrhythmia presenting with intermittent tachycardia/palpitations and may be precipitated by anaesthesia and surgery. It is associated in particular with rheumatic valvular disease as well as ischaemic and hypertensive heart disease and can be seen in with mitral valve prolapse. It may precede the onset of permanent atrial fibrillation. Atrial tachycardia with 2:1 block is characteristic of digitalis toxicity.

Management is as follows:

- This arrhythmia is very sensitive to synchronized direct current cardioversion–there is a success rate of nearly 100%. Therefore, in the anaesthetized patient with any degree of cardiovascular compromise, this should be the first line of treatment.
- Carotid sinus massage and adenosine will slow AV conduction and reveal the underlying rhythm and block where there is any doubt.
- Other drug treatment is as for atrial fibrillation–see above.

Sick sinus syndrome (bradycardia–tachycardia syndrome)

This is a clinical term which describes a combination of spontaneous, often repetitive depression of sinoatrial activity sometimes with sinoatrial block and with or without depression of atrioventricular nodal activity. There are often also episodes of supraventricular tachydysrhythmias (atrial tachycardia, atrial flutter, and fibrillation). Causes include congenital, ischaemic, rheumatic, and hypertensive heart disease, and it may be either asymptomatic or present with dizziness or heart failure (from bradycardia) or with palpitations. It is an indication for prophylactic preoperative pacing—see below.

Broad complex rhythms

Ventricular ectopic beats

Depolarization spreads from a focus in the ventricles by an abnormal, and therefore slow, pathway so the QRS complex is wide and abnormal. The T wave is also abnormal in shape. In the absence of structural heart disease, these are usually benign. They may be related to associated abnormalities especially hypokalaemia. They are common during dental procedures and anal stretch particularly in combination with halothane, raised CO_2, light anaesthesia, or inadequate analgesia. In fit young patients under anaesthesia, they are of little significance and respond readily to manipulation of the anaesthetic. Small doses of intravenous beta-blockers are usually effective in this situation.

They may occasionally herald the onset of runs of ventricular tachycardia. However, the value of prophylactic treatment of ectopics is questionable and in general the risk of causing further arrhythmias outweighs any advantages. Management involves:

- Correction of any contributing causes—ensuring adequate oxygenation, normocarbia, and analgesia.
- If the underlying sinus rate is slow (<50/min), then the 'ectopics' may actually be ventricular escape beats. In this situation increasing the rate using IV atropine or glycopyrrolate may be effective.

Ventricular tachycardia

In this rhythm a focus in the ventricular muscle depolarizes at high frequency. Excitation spreads through the ventricles by an abnormal pathway and therefore the QRS complexes are wide and abnormal. The appearance is characterized by wide QRS complexes which may be slightly irregular or vary in shape. P waves may be seen if there is AV dissociation.

This is a serious, potentially life-threatening arrhythmia. It may be triggered intra-operatively by:

- hypoxia
- hypotension
- fluid overload
- electrolyte imbalance (low K^+, Mg^+, etc.)
- myocardial ischaemia
- injection of adrenaline, or other catecholamines.

Management of VT is as follows:

- Synchronized d.c. cardioversion (200 J then 360 J) is the first-line treatment if the patient is haemodynamically unstable. This is safe and effective. It will restore sinus rhythm in virtually 100% of cases. If the VT is pulseless or very rapid, synchronization is unnecessary. Otherwise synchronization is used to avoid a 'shock on T' phenomenon, which may initiate VF. If the patient lapses back into VT, drugs such as lidocaine (lignocaine) or amiodarone may be given to sustain sinus rhythm.
- Lidocaine (lignocaine) given as a 100 mg bolus restores sinus rhythm in 30–40% of cases and may be followed by a maintenance infusion of 4 mg/min for 30 min, then 2 mg/min for 2 h, and then 1 mg/min.

- Verapamil is ineffective in VT and may worsen hypotension or precipitate cardiac failure.
- Other drugs which may be used if lidocaine (lignocaine) fails include:
  - Amiodarone 300 mg IV via central venous catheter over 1 h followed by 900 mg over 23 h.
  - Procainamide 100 mg IV over 5 min followed by one or two further boluses before commencing infusion at 3 mg/min.
  - Sotalol 100 mg IV over 5 min, has been shown to be better than lidocaine (lignocaine) for acute termination of VT.
- Overdrive pacing can be used to suppress VT by increasing the heart rate.

Acute management of broad complex tachycardia

1. If in doubt as to nature of rhythm assume it is a ventricular rather than a supraventricular tachycardia (98% will be, especially if there is a history of ischaemic heart disease).
2. In the presence of hypotension/cardiovascular compromise—synchronized d.c. shock with 200 J, then 360 J.
3. Perform a 12-lead ECG–if possible both before and after correction, as this will help with retrospective diagnosis.
4. If the patient is not acutely compromised, adenosine 6 mg, followed if necessary by 12 mg rapidly IV and flushed through, will be both diagnostic and curative if it is a supraventricular tachycardia.

Supraventricular tachycardia with aberrant conduction

When there is abnormal conduction from the atria to the ventricles, a supraventricular tachycardia (SVT) may be broad complex as discussed above. This may occur, for example, if there is a bundle branch block. Sometimes the bundle branch block may be due to ischaemia and only appear at high heart rates (rate related aberrant conduction). SVTs may be due to an abnormal or accessory pathway (as in the Wolf–Parkinson–White syndrome), but the complex will be of normal width if conduction in the accessory pathway is retrograde (i.e. it is the normal pathway that initiates the QRS complex), but broad complex if conduction is anterograde in the accessory pathway. Adenosine may be used diagnostically to slow AV conduction and will often reveal the underlying rhythm if it arises from above the ventricles. In the case of SVT it may also result in conversion to sinus rhythm. In practice, however, all broad complex tachycardias should be treated as ventricular tachycardia if there is any doubt.

Ventricular fibrillation (see page 826)

This results in cardiac arrest. There is chaotic and disorganized contraction of ventricular muscle and no QRS complexes can be identified on the ECG. Management involves immediate direct current cardioversion as per established resuscitation protocol (200 J, 200 J, thereafter 360 J).

Conduction abnormalities/heart block

(see p. 30)

Management of intra-operative heart block is as follows:
- Atropine is rarely effective.
- If hypotension is profound then an isoprenaline infusion can be used to temporize: 1–10 μg/min (dilute 0.2 mg in 500 ml of 5% glucose or saline and titrate to effect (2–20 ml/min if 70 kg)).
- Transcutaneous pacing is rarely practical in theatre because of difficulty siting the posterior pad. Oesophageal pacing is effective–the electrode is passed into the oesophagus like a nasogastric tube and connected to the pulse generator. The position can be adjusted until there is ventricular capture.
- Transvenous pacing is both more reliable, effective and relatively easy. A Swan Ganz sheath of adequate size to pass the wire is inserted into the internal jugular or subclavian vein (this can be done while other equipment is being collected). A balloon tipped pacing wire is then inserted to the 20 cm mark. The balloon is inflated and a pulse generator connected at 5 V. It can then be advanced, atrial capture is often seen followed by ventricular capture. When this happens the balloon is deflated and a further 5 cm of catheter inserted. If the 50 cm mark is reached the catheter is coiling up or not entering the heart. Deflate the balloon, withdraw to the 20 cm mark and try again.

Inoculation injuries

There are probably in excess of one million inoculation injuries per annum in United Kingdom healthcare workers (HCWs). There are three main routes of exposure to blood-borne viruses (BBV) in health care settings:

- percutaneous injury—needles/bites/scalpels
- blood contact with broken skin—cuts/abrasions, etc.
- blood contact with mucus membranes—mouth/eyes, etc.

The commonest cause of transmission of infection to health care workers is by blood-to-blood contact by a 'sharps injury', usually a needle. The highest-risk needle injuries are with large bore, hollow needles, and the least risk is with solid/suturing needles. Risk of transmission by contamination of broken skin or mucous membranes with infected blood is small. Seroconversion rate is highest following hollow needlestick injury, and can roughly be quantified as below:

Human immunodeficiency virus (HIV)	0.3% chance (0.03% with mucocutaneous splash)
Hepatitis B virus (HBV)	>30% if source patient is 'e' antigen positive and 'victim' is not immune*
Hepatitis C virus (HCV)	3%

* This transmission rate has declined greatly in recent years due to the widespread vaccination of health care workers against hepatitis B, which provides protection in up to 90% of recipients.

Prevention of infection with blood-borne viruses

- Ensure you are effectively vaccinated against HBV. Some 10% of people fail to respond adequately to a primary course of vaccine, so response must be checked. If after two, and certainly if three or four more boosters have still not achieved acceptable levels of immunity, regard yourself as susceptible. You would therefore need hepatitis B immunoglobulin should you be the victim of an injury from a hepatitis B infectious patient.
- Treat all patients as infection risks—principle of 'universal precautions':
  - Wash hands between each patient contact, and both before and after wearing gloves.
  - Change gloves between patients.
  - Cover existing cuts, scratches, and skin abrasions with waterproof dressing.
  - Wear gloves when contact with blood or blood-stained body fluids is anticipated.
  - Where blood spillage may be extensive (as in haematemesis, trauma, etc.) also wear impermeable gowns or aprons, and eye protection.
  - Never resheath needles.
  - Dispose of sharps in the appropriate container, and do not overfill.
  - If you spill blood or bloodstained fluids inform the person in charge of the department straightaway so that surfaces and floors can be decontaminated appropriately.

In the event of exposure

- Immediately wash the wound/ area liberally with soap and water, but without scrubbing.
- Encourage free bleeding of a puncture wound. Irrigate eyes if necessary.
- Follow your local hospital policy, and report the exposure promptly to the occupational health department/ medical microbiologist/ genitourinary medicine physician—as appropriate. Out of hours, most hospitals have a 24 h advice line giving the name of whom to contact for advice.
- Complete the appropriate incident forms—a chore but medicolegally in your best interests.
- Perform a risk assessment of the incident (see below).
- Most hospitals now have protocols where the 'donor' is counselled, routinely requested for consent and blood tested for hepatitis B, C, and HIV. Blood can only be tested with informed consent.

Risk assessment of an inoculation injury

By convention we refer to the 'victim' or 'recipient' (often a health care worker) and the 'donor' or 'source' (usually a patient).

Assessment of the injury

- Blood in contact with intact skin (negligible to very low risk).
- Blood in contact with a mucous membrane (very low risk)—(HIV transmission <0.03%).
- 'Needlestick' with solid blade (high risk).
- 'Needlestick' with suture needle—half the risk of a hollow needle.
- 'Needlestick' with hollow needle (HIV transmission approx 0.3%).
- Deep wounds—high risk.
- Combinations, e.g. gloves plus suture needle, lower risk than gloves plus hollow needle.

Assessment of the risk of carriage of BBV by the 'donor'

- Lowest risk if a regular blood donor—each time automatically tested for HBV/HCV/HIV.
- High-risk lifestyle:
  - Male–male sex, sex with prostitutes, casual sex abroad, multiple partners.
  - IV drug abuse.
  - Blood transfusion/blood products abroad.
  - Recently living in a country with a high incidence of HIV infection, e.g. sub-Saharan Africa. The annual occupational risk of HCWs acquiring HIV infection in Tanzania has recently been calculated as 0.27%.
  - Far East: high carriage rate of hepatitis B, mostly perinatally acquired.
- About 1% of Western HCW are estimated to be HCV positive.
- History of jaundice.
- History of blood transfusions, especially abroad.
- Known HIV positive: will probably be on retroviral treatment, so 'normal' postexposure prophylaxis (PEP) may be inadequate if the virus has developed resistance. Consult a GU physician for advice.

Assessment of victim's susceptibility

- Hepatitis B immunization status—?seroconversion with adequate levels of antibody ever demonstrated (if yes, just needs a booster dose of hepatitis B vaccine).
- Never been vaccinated against hepatitis B—a 'truly susceptible' victim (may need hepatitis B immunoglobulin, available from the local Public Health Laboratory) as well as rapid hepatitis vaccination course.
- Recognized 'non-responder' to vaccine—discuss with occupational health, usually hepatitis B immunoglobulin administered within 3 days of the injury.

Conclusion

There is no 'scoring system'. A balancing of the above factors should give you a reasonable evaluation of the necessity for post exposure prophylaxis (PEP) for hepatitis B or HIV. There is no PEP for hepatitis C. Individuals also differ in their reactions to having an inoculation injury. Weigh up the risks and benefits of having PEP based on perception of the risks of infection whilst acknowledging the final decision is up to the individual.

Testing the donor/source

Few laboratories provide results within 2 h, so the first dose(s) of any HIV PEP will have to be given on the basis of a risk assessment. The donor must be counselled and asked to consent for testing of HIV, hepatitis B and hepatitis C. Most hospitals provide a consent form for completion. 10 ml clotted blood samples from the donor and the victim should be sent to the laboratory clearly marked with the reasons for sending and cross-referenced. Victim blood is stored as a baseline in case of later seroconversion to any BBV.

If the donor refuses or is unable to give permission, blood cannot be taken or tested for any BBV. A relative's permission will not suffice. A judgement as to the next course of action has to be made, usually by a combination of the occupational health physician/microbiologist/clinician in charge of the patient. The pragmatic approach is to perform a risk assessment, taking the most pessimistic scenario, then balance the perceived risk of infection against the potential side-effects of PEP.

Inoculation injury forms/accident forms should be completed, and the incident documented in the patient's notes.

Counselling the donor/source patient for HIV testing

Explain

- The reason for requesting testing—victim may be offered prophylaxis.
- The same viruses will be tested for as with routine blood donation.
- Advantages for the donor:
  - if positive, treatment can be started sooner and more effectively
  - sexual partners can be protected.
- Potential disadvantages of testing for the donor:
  - possible adverse psychological impact if positive
  - possible adverse effects on family/relationships
  - may be difficulties obtaining insurance if positive, though a negative test should not affect insurance applications.

- Confidentiality will be maintained (GPs will not be informed of the result without the patient's consent although it may be necessary to inform the victim of the donor status if prophylaxis is envisaged).

Postexposure prophylaxis (PEP) regimens

- Should be as soon as possible where justified/indicated.
- Ideally for HIV exposure prophylaxis should be administered within 2 h, hence an adequate risk assessment is essential as testing would be unlikely to be completed in that time.

Hepatitis B PEP

- If there is a history of successful immunization give a booster dose of hepatitis B vaccine only.
- If the victim is completely susceptible give a 'rapid' hepatitis B vaccination course (e.g. 0, 1, 2, and 12 months) plus hepatitis B immunoglobulin (HBIG).

HIV PEP

- No antiviral has yet been licensed for postexposure prophylaxis.
- Consult your local protocol, but generally a combination of three drugs:
  - lamivudine (3TC) 150 mg twice daily (Epivir®), nelfinavir 750 mg three times a day (Viracept®), and zidovudine ('AZT' Retrovir®) 200 mg three times a day **or**
  - lamivudine (3TC) 150 mg twice daily (Epivir®), indinavir 800 mg three times a day, and zidovudine ('AZT' Retrovir®) 200 mg three times a day.
- Not to be undertaken lightly as there are often unpleasant side-effects and interactions with other drugs. If in doubt, it is probably better to start the PEP, and reconsider continuing when test results are available and the stress of the event has lessened somewhat. About 50% of people given PEP fail to complete it due to side-effects. These vary from severe nausea to bone marrow suppression.
- There have been almost 300 reported seroconversions to HIV following inoculation injury world wide, with 10 failures of PEP, four cases of combination drug failure, at least one due to drug resistance.
- The full course of PEP for HIV is 4 weeks.

Hepatitis C PEP
Nothing has yet been proven effective.

Follow-up blood testing
Nearly all HIV seroconversions are within 6 months of the injury, hence a negative blood test at 6 months is reassuring. Hepatitis C antibodies can, rarely, take up to 1 year to develop. Hepatitis B seroconversion takes about 6 weeks if no HBV vaccine or immunoglobulin is given.

The infected doctor

BBV may also be transmitted from health workers to patients. Any HCW performing exposure-prone procedures has a duty of care to inform their employer and take professional and occupational health advice. HCV was recently transmitted to five patients by an infected anaesthetic assistant, probably via an unhealed wound on his hand. No anaesthetist has yet been shown to have transmitted HIV to their patients.

Further reading

Department of Health (1998). Guidance for clinical health care workers: protection against infection with blood-borne viruses: Recommendations of the Expert Advisory Group on AIDS and the Advisory Group on Hepatitis. UK Health Departments.

Department of Health (2000). HIV post exposure prophylaxis. Guidance from the UK Chief Medical Officers' Expert Advisory Group on AIDs.

Hawkins DA (2000). Postexposure to HIV prophylaxis. *Current Opinion in Infectious Diseases*, **13**, 53–7.

Parkin J, Murphy M, Anderson *et al.* (2000). Tolerability and side-effects of post-exposure prophylaxis for HIV infection. *The Lancet*, **355**, 722.

Chapter 45
Nerve injuries
Gavin Werrett

Nerve injury

Nerve injury is an important source of patient morbidity and professional liability:

+ True incidence is unknown due to significant under-reporting. Many of the data presented below are from the ASA Closed Claims Project Database (1975–95).[1]

+ Nerve injury is the second most common claim in the entire database (16% of total). Specific nerve injuries: ulnar nerve (28%), brachial plexus (20%), lumbosacral root (16%), and spinal cord (13%). Less commonly affected nerves were sciatic, median, radial, and femoral nerves.

+ Recently claims for ulnar nerve injury have been decreasing; the current leading cause of claims for nerve damage is spinal cord injury.

+ Many cases of perioperative nerve damage have no identifiable mechanism (only 9% of ulnar injuries have an identifiable mechanism). However, the mechanism for spinal cord injury is determined in 48% of claims and a regional anaesthetic has been administered in 68% of cases of spinal cord injury.

Aetiology

+ Direct trauma by needles, sutures, and instruments.
+ Injection of neurotoxic material.
+ Mechanical factors such as stretch and compression.
+ Ischaemia is likely to be contributory to all these causes.

Classification

The degree of damage will determine the level of intervention required and the likely recovery:

+ Neuropraxia–myelin damaged, axon intact. Recovery in weeks to months. Good prognosis.
+ Axonotmesis–axonal disruption. Prognosis and recovery variable.
+ Neurotmesis–nerve completely severed. Surgery may be required. Prognosis poor.

Predisposing factors

+ Patients with pre-existing generalized peripheral neuropathy are at increased risk of trauma/ischaemia. Document carefully any pre-existing deficit preoperatively.

+ Surgery itself and subsequent positioning may predispose to specific nerve injury.

+ Anaesthetic factors include direct needle damage during regional anaesthesia. This can be decreased with good anatomical knowledge and careful technique. Optimum needle design is not entirely clear but short bevelled needles certainly cause less nerve fascicle perforation and are currently

1 Cheney FW *et al.* (1999). Nerve injury associated with anaesthesia—a closed claims analysis. *Anaesthesiology*, **90**, 1062–9.

popular. Eliciting paraesthesia should be discouraged and severe pain on injection is an indication to stop injection immediately (likely intraneural or intrafascicular injection). Such phenomena add weight to the argument for 'awake' blocks. Minimize tourniquet times and always use pneumatic tourniquets. Solutions of local anaesthetics with preservatives should not be used for spinal or epidural blocks.

- Systemic factors include: hypothermia, hypotension, hypoxia, and electrolyte disturbances, e.g. uraemia, diabetes mellitus, vitamin B_{12}, and folate deficiency.

Symptoms[2]

- Symptoms can occur within a day but may not present for 2–3 weeks.
- The intensity and duration of symptoms vary with severity of injury–from numbness and mild paraesthesia lasting a few weeks to persistent painful paraesthesia, sensory loss, motor loss lasting years and developing into reflex sympathetic dystrophy.

Ulnar neuropathy

- More common in males (3:1).
- Increased at extremes of weight and with prolonged hospital stay. Uncommon in young patients.
- Prospective studies indicate a frequency of 1 in 200 to 1 in 350 patients acutely, but clinically significant lesions are much less common at 3 months.
- 85% of cases occur in association with GA, 15% occur after regional block (6% after spinal) indicating the unclear aetiology.
- Injuries occur at the superficial condylar groove of the elbow. Men appear to have less fat at this site and a narrower tunnel possibly explaining the sex distribution.
- Recent work suggests that there is less ulnar nerve compression with the arm in supination. Abduction of the neutral arm is beneficial to the ulnar nerve, but this must be offset against possible stretch at the brachial plexus.[3]
- Additional padding was explicitly stated to have been used in 27% of closed claims!
- In 62% the onset was 'delayed' (i.e. more than 1 day postoperatively).
- Abnormal nerve conduction is common in the contralateral, unaffected arm indicating subclinical neuropathy that may have become symptomatic in the perioperative period.

Brachial plexus injury

- Causal factors include excessive stretch (arm abduction with lateral rotation of the head to the opposite side), compression (upward movement of the clavicle and sternal retraction) and associated regional block (only 16% of closed claims for brachial plexus injury).

2 Sawyer RJ *et al.* (2000). Peripheral nerve injuries associated with anaesthesia. *Anaesthesia*, 55, 980–91.

3 Prielipp RC et al. (1999). Ulnar nerve pressure. *Anaesthesiology*, 91, 345–54.

- Pain or paraesthesia on injection was noted in 50% of claims associated with a regional technique.
- The long thoracic nerve was damaged in 13% of closed claims for brachial plexus injury (causing winging of the scapula). The mechanism was unknown.
- Lesions affecting the upper roots are more common.

Lumbosacral root injury (radiculopathy)

- Over 90% occur in association with a regional technique (55% spinal, 37% epidural).
- Parasthesia or pain during needle insertion or injection of drug are suggestive of damage. Postoperative radicular pain may persist in up to 0.2% of cases but will almost always resolve in weeks/months.
- Multiple unsuccessful attempts increase the likelihood of damage.
- Persisting paraesthesia, with or without motor symptoms, is the most common complaint.

Spinal cord injury

- 58% of cases were associated with regional anaesthesia in the closed claims data.
- A definitive pathogenesis was implicated in about 50% of the cases—much higher than with other causes of nerve damage.
- The commonest mechanisms were epidural haematoma, chemical injury, anterior spinal artery syndrome, and meningitis respectively.
- Lumbar epidural was the commonest regional technique implicated, four times more frequently than subarachnoid block and eight times more than thoracic epidural (related partly to frequency of block attempted).
- Injury was more common in blocks performed for chronic pain management and in the presence of systemic anticoagulation (fractionated heparin (LMWH) introduced to the United States in 1993).
- Significant delays in the diagnosis of cord or nerve compression were noted. Persistent weakness or numbness was often presumed to be secondary to epidural infusions. Investigate all suspected lesions after appropriate history and examination with MRI if possible, especially if anticoagulated.
- The true incidence of major neurological injury post spinal/ epidural is very hard to estimate. Scott suggested an incidence of 1 in 100 000 for permanent disability in an obstetric population.[4] Epidural haematoma in the presence of LMWH may be as high as 1 in 1000 to 1 in 10 000, but other estimate the risk to be nearer 1 in 150 000 to 1 in 220 000 (following epidural and spinal respectively).[5] Epidural abscess is less common but should be suspected in long-term epidural catheters, the immunocompromised and the anticoagulated.

....

4 Scott DB, Hibbard BM (1990). Serious non-fatal complications associated with extradural block in obstetric practice. *British Journal of Anaesthesia*, **64**, 537–41.

5 Horlocker TT et al. (1998). Spinal and epidural blockade and perioperative low molecular weight heparin: Smooth sailing on the Titanic (Editorial). Anesthesia and *Analgesia*, **86**, 1153–6.

- Anterior spinal artery syndrome typically causes a lower limb spastic paralysis below the level of the lesion, flaccid paralysis at the level of the lesion, variable sensory loss, and sphincter impairment. It can be associated with GA or regional anaesthesia and is usually related to prolonged hypotension. Aortic cross-clamping, thrombosis, embolus, dissecting AAA, polyarteritis nodosa, SLE, and vertebral surgery are all non-anaesthesia related causes.

- Arachnoiditis is a rare cause of paraplegia with no effective treatment. It typically presents as a gradual, progressive weakness and sensory loss beginning days to months after spinal anaesthetic, sometimes leading to complete paraplegia or death. Causes include meningitis, haemorrhage, spinal surgery, and secondary to substances introduced into the spinal or epidural space, e.g. preservatives, accidental administration of the wrong drug, etc.

- Transient neurological symptoms (TNS) is defined as back pain or dysaesthesia radiating bilaterally to the legs or buttocks after total recovery from spinal anaesthesia and beginning within 24 h. Usually no objective neurological signs can be demonstrated. Pain is usually moderate and may be relieved by NSAIDs. Symptoms usually resolve over a few days. Clinical significance is uncertain and the data are very inconsistent but it appears to occur more frequently following the use of spinal 5% hyperbaric lidocaine (lignocaine)/adrenaline. Some studies also suggest a high incidence following spinal plain lidocaine (lignocaine).

- Cauda equina syndrome (CES) is characterized by lower back pain, saddle anaesthesia, sphincter impairment, and motor or sensory symptoms below the knees. A series of CES was reported in association with the use of spinal microcatheters (28G) and 5% hyperbaric lidocaine (lignocaine). This was presumed secondary to pooling of hyperbaric local anaesthetic, leading to a subsequent ban in the United States on spinal catheters thinner than 24G by the Food and Drug Administration in 1992.

Prevention

- Awareness of complications and common causes of injury is crucial (e.g. careful positioning).
- Thorough history, examination, and documentation of preoperative nerve lesions.
- Careful anaesthetic records of all aspects of regional techniques (including type of needle, paraesthesia, agent used, etc.).
- Consider performing blocks awake or lightly sedated (not practical in children).
- Avoid regional techniques in an unwilling patient.
- Always stop injecting if there is pain or paraesthesia.

Diagnosis and treatment

- Neurophysiological tests such as EMG and nerve conduction studies coupled with MRI can often diagnose specific sites of a lesion, which may indicate cause and possible culpability.
- Treatment and prognosis will depend on the severity of the lesion, and is best left to neurologists and neurosurgeons.
- Spinal cord compression or the cauda equina syndrome require urgent neurosurgical referral and decompression.

- Drugs useful for neuropathic pain include tricyclic antidepressants (amitriptyline up to 150 mg/day, starting at 25 mg nocte) or anti-epileptics (carbamzepine 100 mg once or twice daily increased to 200 mg four times a day or gabapentin, better tolerated, 300 mg once daily increased to 600 mg three times a day).

Further reading

Wheatley RG, Schug SA and Watson D (2001). Safety and efficacy of postoperative epidural analgesia. *British Journal of Anaesthesia,* **87**(1), 47–61.

	Epidural abscess	Epidural haematoma	Anterior spinal artery syndrome
Age	Any	90% over 50 years	Elderly
History	Infection, immunocompromised	Abnormal clotting	Atheroma, peripheral vascular disease, low BP
Onset	1–3 days	Hours	Sudden
General symptoms	Unwell, fever, backache, meningism	Sharp pain, radicular	None
Scan	Compression	Compression	Normal
CSF	Infected	Normal	Normal
Blood	WBC raised, CRP raised	Coagulation abnormal	Normal

Chapter 46
Anaphylaxis follow-up

Paul Harvey

Anaphylaxis follow-up

(For immediate management of acute anaphylaxis see p. 857.)

Anaesthetists bypass the body's primary defence systems when giving intravenous drugs. Potentially noxious chemicals are presented rapidly to sensitive cells such as polymorphs, platelets, and especially mast cells. Degranulation, whether immune or non-immune, releases inflammatory mediators, such as histamine, prostaglandins, and leucotrienes.

Apparent 'anaesthetic adverse drug reactions' (AADR) may also be due to non-drug mechanisms such as:

- Underlying disease or pathology, e.g. asthma, systemic mastocytosis, malignant hyperthermia.
- Adverse pharmacological effect related to genetic status, e.g. angio-oedema.
- Machine or operator error.
- A vasovagal episode.

Drug involved reactions may be:

- True allergic reactions: type 1 anaphylaxis (IgE mediated) or type 3 immune complex (IgG mediated).
- Pseudoallergic or anaphylactoid reactions: direct histamine release by active agent or indirect release by complement activation.

Clinically, anaphylactic reactions may be indistinguishable from anaphylactoid responses in that the end point, mast cell degranulation, is the same. However, life-threatening reactions are more likely to be immune mediated and this implies previous exposure to the triggering agent. Neuromuscular blocking agents are responsible for 60–75% of serious AADR, more than half of which occur on first contact with the drug. However, the quaternary ammonium group found in muscle relaxants is widely present in other drugs, foods, cosmetics, and hair care products. This could explain why anaphylaxis to muscle relaxants is five to ten times more common in females. Benzylisoquinolones (atracurium, *cis*-atracurium, mivacurium) and suxamethonium are responsible for a greater number of AADR than aminosteroids (pancuronium, vecuronium, rocuronium).

Antibiotic sensitivity

Penicillin reactions are frequently IgE mediated but seldom as severe as AADR. The incidence of cross-reactivity to cephalosporins in patients with penicillin allergy is probably about 8%. Even then, cross-reactivity is often incomplete and cephalosporins can be given to most patients. If, however, there is a history of a severe penicillin reaction, neither cephalosporins nor imipenem should be used. The antigenic stimulus is usually the β-lactam group.

Aggregate (immune complex or type 3) anaphylaxis

An aggregate is a drug–antibody complex, which activates complement by the classical pathway, leading to mediator release. Aggregates are formed when large particles (e.g. colloid solutions) are infused, or by rapid bolus injection of a drug into a small vein. Thiopental can act in this way by precipitating plasma proteins.

Incidence

The incidence of AADR in the United Kingdom is unknown. In France, suspected anaphylactic reactions have been estimated to occur in 1 in 3500 anaesthetics with true anaphylaxis in approximately 1 in 6000.

Presentation of anaphylactoid or anaphylactic reactions

- Isolated cutaneous erythema is commonly seen following intravenous thiopental or atracurium. This may be the first clinical feature in severe reactions, but if no further histaminoid manifestations occur investigation is unwarranted.
- Timing is important. Onset is usually rapid following an intravenous drug bolus. A gradual onset would be expected if, for example, gelatin infusion, latex sensitivity, or a diclofenac suppository were responsible. While reactions to gelatin may be anaphylactoid, it is now recognized that it can also produce a slower-onset type 1 response. Latex and diclofenac reactions will depend on the rate of mucosal absorption.
- Cardiovascular collapse occurs in 88%, bronchospasm in 36%, and angio-oedema in 24% of AADR. Cutaneous signs will occur in approximately 50% of AADR.

Investigation of reactions

Serum tryptase evaluation

Tryptase is a neutral protease released from secretory granules of mast cells during degranulation. In vivo half-life is 3 h (compared with 3 min for histamine) and it is stable in isolated plasma or serum. Since it is not present in red or white cells, it is not affected by haemolysis. 10 ml clotted venous blood should be taken within 30–120 min of the onset of a suspected reaction. Serum should be separated and stored at minus 20 °C for onward transmission to an appropriate laboratory. This need not be outside working hours. As an alternative, a urine sample taken up to 4 h after the event can demonstrate degranulation by raised levels of urinary n-methyl histamine.

Basal plasma tryptase concentration is usually less than 1 ng/ml. Levels up to 15 ng/ml are seen both in pseudoallergy, i.e.non-specific or anaphylactoid reactions, and mild anaphylaxis. A higher value is more likely to indicate an IgE response.

RAST/CAP tests

Radioallergosorbent tests (RAST) for antigen-specific IgE antibodies have now been largely superseded by the CAP system (Pharmacia). Unfortunately these tests are currently helpful only in confirming suxamethonium and latex allergy and have a low sensitivity (a negative result still requires skin testing).

Skin testing

The diagnosis of AADR depends on skin-prick (SPT) or intradermal (IDT) testing. In proven muscle relaxant anaphylaxis, no laboratory test has been shown to compare for specificity and sensitivity. Skin testing will probably be diagnostic in anaphylaxis, but not in anaphylactoid reactions. The patient should be referred to an immunologist or to an anaesthetist with experience in the interpretation of these tests.

- Tests should not take place for a minimum of 4 weeks post-event to allow regeneration of IgE.

- Use SPT in preference to IDT. With some drugs, such as atracurium and suxamethonium, it is relatively easy to produce a false positive result with IDT.

- Neuromuscular blocking agents, local anaesthetics, and thiopental usually cause anaphylaxis and skin testing is likely to be positive.

- Narcotics and NSAIDs normally cause anaphylactoid reactions and positive skin testing, due to direct histamine release, will be misleading.

- Gelatin/dextran solutions and latex may produce immune or non-immune reactions and skin testing should always be performed.

- As a rule the patient should be tested to all drugs given before the episode. Remember antibiotics, latex, and lidocaine (lignocaine), if mixed with propofol.

- Negative control with normal saline (to exclude dermographia) must always be included. While morphine or codeine phosphate can be used for a positive control, greater consistency occurs with commercially available histamine solutions (Alk-Abello (UK), 2 Teal Gate, Hungerford RG17 0YT, UK). The latter demonstrates normal skin response and the weal and flare gives a reference for reactions to test drugs.

- Testing should be performed in hospital on an outpatient basis. Rarely, resuscitation skills and equipment may be required. A recovery ward is ideal, HDU unnecessary.

- The patient should not have received antihistamine therapy within the last 5 days but steroid therapy probably does not affect the validity of skin testing.

- Dark-skinned patients will show a weal if allergic and any flare is usually visible if the volar aspect of the forearm is used.

- Apply a drop of undiluted solution to the degreased forearm skin and make a single vertical prick through it with a solid shouldered lance. Alternatively, a hollow 25G needle can be used.

- Blot any excess fluid after 5 min. Avoid cross-contamination and carefully identify individual skin pricks.

- Interpret at 15 min.

- A weal more than 2 mm wider than the saline control is likely to be a positive result with SPT, especially if accompanied by any surrounding flare.

- Repeat any positive test with 1:10 dilution to reduce the chance of a false positive.

- After a positive SPT, test other drugs in the same pharmacological group. Sensitivity to other muscle relaxants occurs in up to 60% of patients who have already reacted to one relaxant.

After testing

- The patient must know the importance and implications of the diagnosis. The address of MedicAlert (12 Bridge Wharf, 156 Caledonian Road, London N1 9UU, UK) should be provided. A warning bracelet can be supplied at the patient's own expense. There is a small annual retention fee payable to remain on an internationally accessible register.

- Ensure the patient's hospital notes are appropriately marked and the referring physician and general practitioner informed.

- Report reaction to the Medicines Control Agency ('yellow card system'). Failure to do this perpetuates the under-reporting of AADR.

Future anaesthesia

- Avoid all untested drugs in the same group as that which caused the original problem.

- Do not use intravenous 'test' doses–these are unreliable and, if true allergy exists, are unsafe.

- If in doubt over induction agents use an inhalational induction. There are no reports of anaphylaxis to inhalational anaesthetics.

- If the reaction was to a muscle relaxant, give a relaxant-free anaesthetic if possible. In a long-term follow-up of patients with severe reaction to neuromuscular blocking agents Thacker and Davis[1] found 3 of 40 later anaesthetics using muscle relaxants produced probable anaphylactic reactions.

- If a relaxant must be used, ideally test to your chosen drug by SPT preoperatively.

- In proven muscle relaxant allergy, premedicate with H_1 and H_2 receptor antagonists (eg promethazine 50 mg and ranitidine 150 mg PO), plus 24 h of preoperative steroid therapy if time permits.

Further reading

The Association of Anaesthetists of Great Britain and Ireland and The British Society of Allergy and Clinical Immunology (1995). Suspected anaphylactic reactions associated with anaesthesia.

Fisher MM, Bowey CJ (1997). Intradermal compared with prick testing in the diagnosis of anaesthetic allergy. *British Journal of Anaesthesia*, **79**, 59–63.

Fisher MM, Merefield D, Baldo B (1999). Failure to prevent an anaphylactic reaction to a second neuromuscular blocking drug during anaesthesia. *British Journal of Anaesthesia*, **82**, 770–3.

Fisher MM, Bowey CJ (1997). Alleged allergy to local anaesthetics. *Anaesthesia and Intensive Care*, **25**, 611–14.

1 Thacker MA, Davis FM (1999). Subsequent general anaesthesia in patients with a history of previous anaphylactoid/anaphylactic reaction to muscle relaxant. *Anaesthesia and Intensive Care*, **27**, 190–3.

Death on the table

All anaesthetists experience a patient dying on the operating table or in the recovery room at some time in their careers. In most cases death is expected and the cause is understood. Usually, the patient's relatives and theatre staff will have been informed about the high risk of mortality and are therefore prepared for the event. However, when death is unexpected, the experience can be shattering for all concerned. Added to this is the stress of potential litigation.

Guidelines help to ensure that the legal requirements following a death on the table are fulfilled and may reduce the trauma of the situation for all concerned. The Coroner or equivalent (Procurator Fiscal in Scotland) must be notified of all deaths that occur during anaesthesia, or within 30 days of an operation.

- Dealing with the patient. All lines and tubes must be left in place. The patient should be transferred to a quiet area where the relatives are able to view the body.

- Dealing with the relatives. Care must be taken to break the news to the relatives in a sympathetic and considerate way. This should be done by senior staff adopting a team approach involving the surgeon, anaesthetist, nurse, and other professionals as necessary (e.g. interpreter, chaplain, social worker). One member of the team should take the lead and be the principal communicator. It is highly inadvisable to let the surgeon see the relatives alone as misunderstandings can occur. The initial interview should convey brief facts about the case in order to allow the relatives to take in the bad news. A nurse or carer should stay with the family to comfort them and offer practical help as required. After a suitable interval, the team should return and provide further details as appropriate and answer the family's questions. Any queries should be answered as fully and accurately as possible as omissions may lead to doubt and speculation.

- Notifications. The supervizing consultant must be contacted, if not already present. The patient's family doctor and the Coroner should be informed of the death by telephone at the earliest opportunity.

Unexpected death

When death is unexpected, the cause of death may not be known at the time. The event needs to be accurately documented and in addition to the procedures outlined above, the following must be addressed:

- Equipment. The anaesthetic machine and drug ampoules used should be isolated and checked by a senior colleague, preferably someone unconnected with the original incident. An accurate record of these checks must be kept for future reference. Drug checks should include the identity, doses used, expiry dates, and batch numbers. The drug ampoules and syringes should also be kept.

- The anaesthetist. The help of a senior colleague (consultant on call or the clinical director) as mentor to provide guidance and support is invaluable in these cases. The mentor can help with the initial telephone notifications and later with the composition and editing of reports. The mentor should also liaise with the anaesthetist's family, if appropriate, and offer them further support as necessary. The rest of the operating list should be delayed until another anaesthetist and surgeon are found to take over. The anaesthetist involved with the case needs to ensure that the medical record is complete and accurate. All entries in the patient's notes should be dated and signed. The facts of the case should be clearly documented on an incident form (or equivalent) and copies of this should be forwarded to the clinical director and medical director, so that any immediate action required may be instigated. A copy should also be retained for forwarding to the anaesthetist's medical defence organization, if required, at a later date.

Preparing for legal proceedings

If legal proceedings do ensue, it may be a long time after the event. The medical records will assume utmost importance and form the basis of the case. Anything not recorded in the notes may be assumed not to have been done. The records should be completed within a few hours of the event and must not be altered in any way. An electronically recorded printout alone is insufficient. The record needs to show the reasoning behind the action taken and some indication of the working diagnosis. In preparation for any subsequent court action the anaesthetist may find it helpful to record a detailed account of the case within a few days of the death. This private record should include all the preoperative discussions with the patient and the perioperative events, noting the personnel and times involved. The document should be used as an aide-mémoire for the anaesthetist and kept in a personal file. The anaesthetist's medical defence organization should be consulted for help and further advice.

The theatre team

An unexpected death on the table is upsetting for all members of the theatre team. It may be necessary to organize a debriefing session to help the staff understand the event and come to terms with it. Such group counselling may also serve to reduce post-event psychological trauma.

Further reading

Bacon AK (1989). Death on the table. *Anaesthesia*, **44**, 245–8.

Bacon AK (1990). Major anaesthetic mishaps–handling the aftermath. *Current Anaesthesia and Critical Care*, **1**, 253–7.

Chapter 48
Dealing with a complaint
Babinder Sandhar

Dealing with a complaint

Most doctors receive complaints, the majority of which can be resolved without legal proceedings. Patients are more likely to proceed to a legal claim if there is inadequate information or concern about the difficulty initially. The average acute hospital will investigate 120–160 formal complaints per 1000 doctors every year but very few are followed by a legal claim and fewer still by a trial.

Background

In the United Kingdom Crown Indemnity was introduced in 1990 and it is the Trust or Health Authority, therefore, which is sued and is liable for the payment of costs and damages, not the individual doctor. The actions of the doctor are considered separately, if required, by the clinical director or medical director. Crown Indemnity does not cover work performed outside the NHS contract (e.g. private practice, 'Good Samaritan' deeds) and separate medical defence insurance should be arranged for this. Legal claims arising from this work result in the named doctor being sued and must be handled by the relevant defence organization. The defence organization will also provide support for doctors who become the subject of disciplinary proceedings.

Local resolution

Complaints should be resolved quickly and to the satisfaction of all involved. The aim is to answer the complaint, offer an apology if that is appropriate, amend faulty procedures or practices (for the benefit of others), and to clarify if the complaint is groundless.

Verbal complaints

- Speak to the patient. Discuss the matters causing concern as soon as you hear of any problem. Give the patient a full, clear explanation of the facts and try to resolve any difficulty.

- Speak to a senior colleague. Do not feel that you must handle the problem on your own. Consider asking a senior consultant or the clinical director to see the patient with you. The patient may value the advice of a senior doctor. You may value the reassurance of a senior colleague.

- Apologies. Saying sorry is not an admission of liability. Patients will appreciate the concern you express about the difficulties experienced. However, do not apologize for the actions of others without giving them the opportunity to comment.

- Documentation. Always make a detailed entry in the patient's notes of any dissatisfaction expressed to you and the action taken to try and resolve it.

Formal written complaints

Trusts have a legal obligation to comply with national guidelines when dealing with formal complaints.[1] These have to be acknowledged within 2 working

---

1 Department of Health (1995). Acting on complaints. *Health Sevices Circular.*

days and investigated immediately. The Chief Executive is required to issue a formal response within 20 days or provide a letter explaining the delay. Complaints are investigated by copying the correspondence to all the relevant clinical staff and clinical directors. The information provided by the staff involved in the patient's care is used to produce a report explaining the course of events and any necessary action taken. When replying:

* Speak to a senior consultant/clinical director. Senior colleagues who have been in a similar position in the past can help to clarify the issues with you.
* Inform your medical defence organization who will provide advice and support.
* Record keeping. Keep a full account of the details of the incident for future reference, should the case be pursued. This will act as a personal aide-mémoire.
* Leave a forwarding address. A legal claim may be made many months after the event.

Independent review

Any patient not satisfied with the report produced by the Trust, can request an independent review, but this will only proceed if it is thought to be appropriate. The purpose of the review is to investigate how the complaint has been handled, not to investigate the circumstances of the complaint. If this fails to resolve the situation, the case can be referred to the ombudsman (Health Service Commissioner). These procedures do not apply if a legal claim is being investigated.

Legal proceedings

Adults usually have 3 years from the date of an incident to make a legal claim and children have until their 21st birthday. There are various stages of a claim once legal proceedings have been issued. The Trust's legal team will need to work with you and your clinical director to produce a statement of your involvement in the patient's care.

Preparing a statement

This should include the following:
* Full name and qualifications.
* Grade and position held (including duration).
* Full names and positions of others involved (patients, relatives, staff).
* Date(s) and time(s) of all the relevant matters.
* Brief summary of the background details (e.g. patient's medical history).
* Full and detailed description of the matters involved.
* Date and time that your statement was made, and your signature on every page.
* Copies of any supporting documents referred to in the statement (initialled by you).
  The statement should accord with the following points:
* Accuracy. There should be no exaggeration, understatement, or inconsistencies. Check the details with the patient's notes.
* Facts. Keep to the facts, particularly those which determined your decision-making, and avoid value judgements.

- Avoid hearsay. Try to avoid including details which you have not witnessed yourself. If reference has to be made to such information, record the name and position of the person providing it to you, when it was provided and how.

- Be concise. State the essential details in a logical sequence and avoid generalizations.

- Relevance. Include only the details required to understand the situation fully.

- Avoid jargon. Give layman's explanations of any clinical terms used and avoid abbreviations.

Discuss the statement with your clinical director. Make changes as necessary to ensure a clear factual account. Only sign the statement when you are completely happy with the text. Always keep a copy of the final signed version for your own reference. The Trust's legal team should provide advice on the legal process to be followed and discuss the management of the claim with you.

Remember good record keeping will help to support your case. Poor records give the impression of poor care. The medical records are the only proof of what occurred and anything not written down may be assumed to have not happened. Any later additions to the notes should be signed and dated with an explanation of the reasons why the entry was not made earlier.

Awareness

Complaints of awareness must be pursued promptly. It is important to confirm what the patient may have heard or felt and document this accurately. If possible, an explanation of the events and causes, if any, should be given. The patient needs reassurance that steps can be taken to reduce the risk of awareness during subsequent anaesthetics. Post-traumatic stress disorder can develop and it is important that these patients are offered counselling.

In any service it is recognized that mishaps will occur and mechanisms need to be in place to identify and rectify the causes. There is increasing awareness of the role of 'systems failure' in these cases, as there is usually a series of mistakes involved which result in the adverse incident. The adoption of a 'no blame' culture enables open, honest reporting of failures, which allows appropriate changes to be made thereby improving patient safety.

Section VII
Acute pain

Chapter 49
Acute pain

Julie Murdoch and David Conn

General principles

The management of pain is important, not just for humanitarian reasons, but also to improve recovery and reduce postoperative complications. Pain is a subjective sensation. Its perception is modulated by many factors, which can make assessment difficult.

Basic principles

- Assess pain appropriately (see below).
- Know a small number of drugs and techniques well.
- Prescribe analgesics regularly rather than 'as required'.
- Administer analgesics pre-emptively where pain is expected.
- Use a multimodal approach, i.e. paracetamol plus NSAID plus opioid and local anaesthetic, when there are no contraindications.
- Plan your technique preoperatively and discuss this with the patient, especially with PCA.
- Ensure that staff caring for the patient have the knowledge and skills required to manage postoperative pain.
- Non-pharmacological techniques, such as relaxation techniques, education, and positioning, are important in helping to reduce pain and may reduce the dose of drugs required.
- Unexpected pain or increasing pain should be investigated.

Pain assessment

- Patients should be encouraged to report pain and be educated about the importance of adequate pain relief to their postoperative recovery.
- Believe the patient's report of pain.
- Pain should be assessed regularly, at least every 4 h. The effects of analgesia should be assessed within 1 h of administration. Assessment should be more frequent with the advanced drug administration techniques, e.g. epidural and PCA opioids.
- Simple scoring scales can be used to assess the severity of pain. These scores should be documented on the standard observation chart or a separate pain chart. Changes in treatment can be documented on the pain chart or in the nursing care plan/medical notes.
- The patient should be asked to score their pain on movement or deep inspiration, not just at rest.
- Pain scoring scales include:
  - The verbal rating scale–the patient is asked to score their pain as none, mild, moderate, or severe: 0 = no pain, 1 = mild pain, 2 = moderate pain, 3 = severe pain.
  - Numerical rating scale–patient is asked to score their pain between 0 and 10, where 0 = no pain and 10 = worst pain ever.
  - Visual analogue scale–this is a 10 cm line with 'no pain' at one end and 'worst pain ever' at the other end. The patient is asked to place a mark on the scale to denote the severity of their pain. The line is then measured by the observer to give a score of 0–10 or 0–100.

- Pain scoring scales give only part of the assessment. They tell us how severe the patient perceives their pain to be. Assessment should also include site and description of pain and current pharmacological and non-pharmacological management interventions.
- Sedation is often scored at the same time, 0 = awake, 1 = dozing intermittently, 2 = mostly sleeping, 3 = difficult to awaken.

Analgesic drug therapy

Paracetamol

- A good analgesic.
- Well tolerated by the majority of patients.
- Prescribe regularly rather than 'as required'.

NSAIDs

- Effective analgesic as well as anti-inflammatory action.
- May be adequate as the sole analgesic after minor surgery.
- Reduces opioid consumption. May reduce side-effects of opioids due to opioid sparing effect but there is limited evidence to support this.
- The quality of analgesia is often enhanced if administered concomitantly with an opioid.
- NSAIDs increase bleeding time and may increase blood loss. It is suggested that NSAIDs should not be given prior to surgery if there is a significant risk of intra-operative bleeding.
- All NSAIDs exert a similar mode of action—do not prescribe more than one NSAID to be administered simultaneously, with the exception of low-dose aspirin.

Contraindications to NSAID therapy[1]

- History of gastrointestinal ulceration or bleeding.
- Renal impairment.
- Oliguria and hypovolaemia postoperatively.
- Renal transplantation.
- Circulatory failure (hypotension and/or cardiac failure).
- Pre-eclamptic toxaemia, eclampsia, and uncontrolled hypertension.
- Asthmatics who have a history of sensitivity to aspirin.
- Severe liver dysfunction.
- Coagulopathies.

Use NSAIDs with caution in:

- Patients over 65, as subclinical renal impairment is likely.
- Diabetics, who may have nephropathy and/or renal vascular disease.
- Patients with widespread vascular disease.
- Cardiac disease, hepatobiliary disease, major vascular surgery (highest incidence of acute renal failure).
- Patients taking ACE inhibitors, cyclosporin, potassium-sparing diuretics, beta-blockers, methotrexate.
- Loop diuretic therapy.
- Warfarin therapy.

---

1 Royal College of Anaesthetists (1998). Guidelines for the use of non-steroidal anti-inflammatory drugs in the perioperative period. *Royal College of Anaesthetists, London*

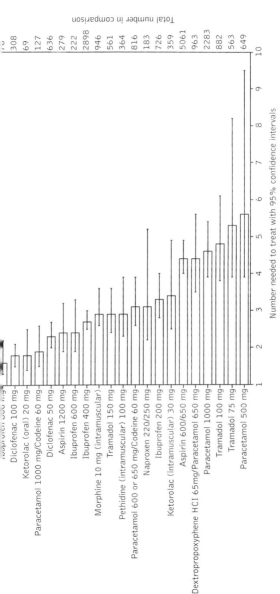

Total number in comparison

	308
Diclofenac 100 mg	69
Ketorolac (oral) 20 mg	127
Paracetamol 1000 mg/Codeine 60 mg	636
Diclofenac 50 mg	279
Aspirin 1200 mg	222
Ibuprofen 600 mg	2898
Ibuprofen 400 mg	946
Morphine 10 mg (intramuscular)	561
Tramadol 150 mg	364
Pethidine (intramuscular) 100 mg	816
Paracetamol 600 or 650 mg/Codeine 60 mg	183
Naproxen 220/250 mg	726
Ibuprofen 200 mg	359
Ketorolac (intramuscular) 30 mg	5061
Aspirin 600/650 mg	963
Dextropropoxyphene HCl 65mg/Paracetamol 650 mg	2283
Paracetamol 1000 mg	882
Tramadol 100 mg	563
Tramadol 75 mg	649
Paracetamol 500 mg	

Number needed to treat with 95% confidence intervals

Fig 49.1 Meta-analysis 'league table' of oral and intramuscular analgesics (courtesy of Pain Research Unit, Oxford; for more information see www.ebandolier.com).

Points to remember with NSAIDs

- Any deterioration in renal function, e.g. increase in plasma urea, creatinine, potassium or symptoms of gastric upset are indications for discontinuing NSAID therapy.
- The addition of omeprazole, misoprostol or H_2 antagonists may offer some protection against GI effects.
- NSAIDs are routinely administered jointly with epidural analgesia, although there are currently no published recommendations for safe use with epidural analgesia.
- Ibuprofen has the safest side-effect profile in lower doses, i.e. 400 mg three times a day. It exhibits an analgesic effect at this dose but little or no anti-inflammatory effect.
- Diclofenac has a safer side-effect profile than piroxicam, indometacin, and ketorolac and can be given by the rectal route. Intramuscular diclofenac should be avoided as it is painful on injection and can cause sterile abscesses. If administered IM it must be given by deep intramuscular injection into the ventrogluteal area only.
- Some NSAIDs can be administered intravenously if the oral and rectal routes are unavailable. Drugs such as ketorolac and tenoxicam should be prescribed for a maximum of 48 h owing to their higher side-effect profiles. The starting dose of ketorolac is 10 mg but this can be increased to 30 mg if necessary (maximum 90 mg in 24 h).
- Piroxicam can be administered once daily as a buccal preparation. Again, prescribe for a maximum of 48 h and then review.
- Indometacin may be preferred by some orthopaedic surgeons owing to its effect on bone formation following joint replacement. The drug is generally prescribed for short-term use only.
- Dexketoprofen is said to be safe to administer orally on an empty stomach.
- The new COX-2 specific inhibitors, e.g. rofecoxib and celecoxib, exhibit less effect on the gastrointestinal tract and platelet function and are analgesically as potent as other NSAIDs. They are contraindicated in patients with aspirin-sensitive asthma and renal impairment. They are currently unlicensed for postoperative pain.

Opioids

Weak opioids

- Commonly prescribed for moderate pain.
- Best used in combination with paracetamol.
- Cause side-effects such as nausea and constipation without the benefit of potent analgesia offered by the strong opioids.
- Dextropropoxyphene is not suggested for the treatment of pain in older adults—Coproxamol has little analgesic benefit over paracetamol and can cause confusion, possibly due to the metabolite norpropoxyphene.
- Codeine is thought to be a prodrug for morphine—there is some evidence to suggest that up to 10% of Caucasians cannot metabolize codeine to morphine.
- Some pain specialists recommend the use of tramadol or smaller doses of morphine as alternatives to the prescription of weak opioids.

Strong opioids

- The commonly used strong opioids for postoperative pain are all μ receptor agonists.
- All μ receptor agonists exhibit a similar side-effect profile in equianalgesic doses, although individual patients may tolerate one opioid better than another.
- Partial agonists, e.g. buprenorphine, and agonist/antagonist drugs, e.g. pentazocine (Fortral), have limited use in acute pain management.
- True allergic reactions are rare.
- Age may be a better determinant of dose needed than weight, although individual requirements can vary up to tenfold. It is suggested that smaller doses are used in patients over 70 years of age.
- The correct dose is 'enough for analgesia without unwanted side-effects'.

Morphine

- The 'gold' standard. It is cheap, widely used, and can be administered by a variety of routes.
- Has an active metabolite (morphine-6-glucuronide). There is a risk of accumulation in patients with renal impairment. These patients require closer monitoring for oversedation and respiratory depression, particularly if they are to receive regular morphine over a period of days, e.g. regular oramorph or continuous IV infusion.
- A history of asthma is not an absolute contraindication to using morphine. Do not give to those who are actively wheezy.
- Dosing of oral morphine should be two to three times that of an intramuscular dose.

Diamorphine

- Lipid soluble and rapidly hydrolysed to morphine.
- Twice as potent as morphine.
- Commonly used in the United Kingdom via the epidural and spinal routes.
- Not licensed for medical use in the United States.

Pethidine

- There is little or no evidence to suggest that pethidine is superior to morphine for pancreatic or colicky pain.
- Shorter-acting than morphine.
- Has a toxic metabolite–norpethidine. Norpethidine has a long half-life (15–20 h) and can accumulate, particularly in patients with renal impairment. Norpethidine is neurotoxic and can result in grand mal seizures. Cases are becoming more common since the advent of PCA where patients can self-administer large doses.
- As a guideline: maximum doses for a healthy adult: 1000 mg in first 24 h, 700 mg for each subsequent 24 h. These doses need to be reduced for patients with renal impairment.
- Exhibits some local anaesthetic activity.
- Can be effective as a small intravenous bolus (10–25 mg) in treating post-anaesthetic shivering.
- Can be used for those patients with a true morphine allergy.

Fentanyl

* A very potent opioid used primarily for intra-operative analgesia.
* Useful drug for PCA (intravenous route) if the patient is unable to have morphine.
* Fentanyl patches should not be used for the treatment of acute pain. They take up to 12 h to exhibit an effect and can take even longer to stop working once removed.
* If the patient has a fentanyl patch in situ prior to theatre, consider leaving the patch in place and providing supplementary postoperative analgesia with fentanyl PCA.

Alfentanil and remifentanil

* Ultra short-acting potent opioids used for intra-operative analgesia.
* Limited use in the postoperative period.

Oxycodone

* Licenced for use in February 2000.
* A popular analgesic in the United States for several decades.
* Only available in the United Kingdom as the oral preparation.
* Oxycodone 10 mg orally is equivalent to morphine 20 mg orally.
* It has around 60% oral bioavailability, which is better than that of other strong opioids.
* Oxycontin (sustained release preparation) may have a place in postoperative pain management. It has a biphasic release and absorption pattern following oral administration, which results in analgesia within 1 h that is sustained for 12 h. The starting dose is 10 mg twice daily for opioid naïve patients.
* Oxycodone may provide an alternative to the short-term use of weak opioids postoperatively.

Methadone

* Usually given via the oral route but can be administered IM or IV.
* Exhibits a long and variable half-life with a risk of accumulation.
* Do not use unless familiar with the drug and doses.
* Patients already on methadone should have the dose converted to morphine (see p. 988).

Hydromorphone

* Used for many years in the United States where it is available in oral and parenteral forms.
* Recently licensed in the United Kingdom, but only for the oral route.
* Via the oral route, hydromorphone is five to ten times as potent as morphine.

Tramadol

* Weak μ receptor agonist. Also exhibits an effect via noradrenergic and serotinergic pathways.
* Analgesic efficacy around one-tenth that of morphine.

- Maximum dose is currently stated at 600 mg in 24 h.
- There is some anecdotal evidence to suggest that larger doses (up to 1800 mg orally) can be given with continuing analgesic efficacy, but with an increased risk of convulsions.
- Can be used effectively in PCA.
- Contraindicated in patients with a history of epilepsy.
- A useful drug to remember for those patients intolerant to the side-effects of opioids, e.g. elderly trauma.
- A useful analgesic alternative to the weak opioids.

Entonox

- 50% nitrous oxide and 50% oxygen.
- Potent analgesic that depends on self-administration by a cooperative patient. It is ideal for acute pain of short duration, being quick acting and short-lived once administration ceases.
- Entonox can be used for procedures such as dressing changes, removal of drains, catheterization, application of traction, etc.
- Contraindications include pneumothorax, decompression sickness, intoxication, bowel obstruction, maxillofacial injuries, severe bullous emphysema, and head injury.
- Self-administration safeguards the patient from overdose.

Clonidine

- Prolongs the action of local anaesthetic when used in combination for regional techniques.
- Dose 1 μg/kg.
- Observed side-effects include sedation, bradycardia, and hypotension.
- Useful in paediatric surgery to enhance caudal anaesthesia.

Non-pharmacological techniques

- May reduce the need for drugs.
- Simple techniques include positioning the patient appropriately, applying traction, and the use of heat and cold therapy.
- Education and information assist in reducing patient anxiety. Reduced levels of anxiety are associated with reduced pain perception.
- Complementary techniques such as TENS, acupuncture, and hypnotherapy are currently used rarely in acute pain.

Routes of analgesic delivery

Oral

* The simplest route available.
* The oral bioavailability of most opioids is limited due to first-pass metabolism.
* The oral route is not suggested immediately following major surgery due to potential delays in gastric emptying. Initially analgesia is delayed. There is also a danger of overdose should accumulated doses be absorbed once gastric motility returns.

Intermittent subcutaneous or intramuscular injection

* The traditional administration route, often on an 'as required' basis (4- to 6-hourly). In many cases this results in grossly inadequate analgesic levels.
* This route is effective and safe if it is administered more regularly according to an algorithm (see Fig. 49.2).
* Morphine can be administered SC. Pethidine has to be administered IM.
* If morphine is to be given SC consider inserting an indwelling cannula over the deltoid muscle—this reduces the need for repeated injections and reduces the risk of sharps injuries. IM cannulas can also be inserted.

Intravenous bolus

* For the management of severe, acute pain.
* It gives the quickest onset and repeated doses can be titrated against effect.
* The suggested dose for morphine is 1–3 mg increments every 3–5 min, dependent on the age and medical condition of the patient.
* Morphine can take up to 15 min to exhibit its full effects.
* Close supervision of the patient is required. More caution is required for those patients with renal impairment.
* This method of administration is not appropriate for continuing pain management at ward level. If the intravenous route is required for maintenance of analgesia, consider PCA.

Intranasal bolus

Efficacy and speed of action are similar to that of IM injection and it is well tolerated by children. It offers an alternative method of administration for areas such as the emergency department and paediatric units.

Patient-controlled analgesia (PCA)

PCA can give high-quality analgesia, but can fail miserably if not applied appropriately. The success of PCA is dependent on several factors:

* Patient suitability and preoperative education. If the patient is unable to utilize their PCA postoperatively, analgesia will be inadequate–the need for appropriate selection and education cannot be overstressed.
* Education of staff in the concepts of PCA and the utilization of equipment.
* Appropriate monitoring of the patient for effect and side-effects. PCA charts are generally used, which assess respiratory rate, level of sedation, pain score, and pump observations.

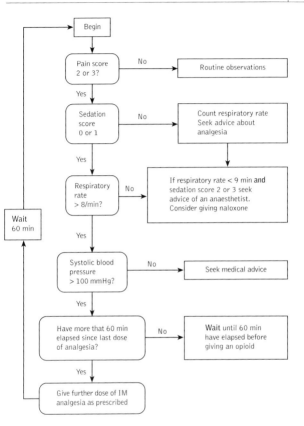

Fig 49.2 Algorithm for IM opioid administration (Reproduced by kind permission of *Anaesthesia*)[2]. See page 972–3 for pain and sedation scores.

- Morphine is the drug of choice for IV PCA. Prefilled syringes are commercially available or can be provided by the pharmacy department. If other drugs are used, the syringes have to be drawn up by nursing staff.

1 Harmer M, Davies KA (1998). The effect of education, assessment and a standardised prescription on postoperative pain management. *Anaesthesia*, 53, 424–30.

Standard PCA regimes

Drug	Concentration	Bolus dose	Lock-out time
Morphine	1 mg/ml	1–2 mg	5 min
Fentanyl	10 μg/ml	10–20 μg	5 min
Pethidine	10 mg/ml	10–20 mg	5 min
Tramadol	10 mg/ml	10–20 mg	5 min
Diamorphine	0.5 mg/ml	0.5–1 mg	5 min

- In general, background infusions are not used. Exceptions to this include children (under 50 kg) and patients who have been taking regular doses of strong opioid, e.g. MST, methadone. The background rate for children is calculated according to weight, the rate for those patients taking MST or methadone is calculated according to their preoperative dose of drug (p. 988). The suggested regime for children is:
  - 1 mg/kg of morphine made to 50 ml with normal saline = 20 μg/kg/ml.
  - Bolus dose = 20 μg/kg (1 ml).
  - Lock-out = 5 min.
  - Background infusion = 4 μg/kg/h (0.2 ml/h).
- The patient must have adequate analgesia prior to commencing PCA. This is obtained by the IV administration of bolus doses of opioid perioperatively.
- PCA can be utilized for most surgery where moderate to severe postoperative pain is expected.
- Epidural analgesia is usually superior to intravenous PCA for the management of pain following major abdominal surgery and lower limb amputation, but carries with it the increased risk of nerve or cord damage.
- Consider commencing PCA preoperatively in patients awaiting surgery, e.g. orthopaedic trauma.
- Consider the need for supplementary oxygen therapy at least for the first postoperative night.
  PCA is generally administered via the intravenous route. Several other routes are available:
- Patient controlled epidural analgesia (PCEA) (p. 726).
- Subcutaneous—may be of use in those patients with difficult intravenous access. The bolus dose is higher with a longer lock-out time to account for drug absorption via this route. It is suggested that the dose duration is also lengthened to prevent pain on injection, e.g morphine 2 mg bolus with 10–15 min lock-out and 3 min dose duration.
- Intranasal—the few studies to date have tended to use fentanyl as the opioid of choice. The efficacy is similar to that of IV PCA, with similar bolus dose and lock-out time. More work is needed to fully evaluate this method of administration.

Trouble-shooting PCA

* Breakthrough pain:
    * If pain is severe the patient will require additional intravenous bolus doses to achieve satisfactory analgesia prior to any changes to the PCA regime.
    * Add in regular paracetamol and NSAIDs if these are not contraindicated.
    * Increase the bolus dose of the infusion.
* Nausea and vomiting—the patient must be prescribed appropriate anti-emetic medication.
* Anti-emetic can be added to the PCA, e.g. ondansetron 4 mg, droperidol 2.5 mg or cyclizine 50–100 mg per 50 ml. If the patient uses large doses from the PCA they may then receive large doses of anti-emetic, with resultant side-effects. An alternative is to prescribe the anti emetic separately and regularly:
    * The aetiology of postoperative nausea and vomiting is multifactorial; consider other causes (p. 924).
    * Extend the dose duration—this can be altered on the pump programme.
    * Change the opioid if nausea and vomiting continue despite anti-emetic therapy.
* Sedation and decreased respiratory rate—ensure the patient has appropriate monitoring by nursing staff. Prescribe naloxone alongside the PCA prescription. Consider decreasing the bolus dose and/or increasing the lock-out time should the patient become sedated.
* Patient compliance—preoperative education of the patient is essential. This needs to be reinforced by nursing staff postoperatively. If the patient is unable to utilize the PCA effectively, consider changing to either a continuous intravenous infusion or intermittent IM/SC injection.
* Pump malfunction—the PCA monitoring chart should include pump observations for drug delivery. Syringe download from PCA pumps (pump delivers an excessive dose in a short period of time) can be avoided by:
    * using an antisiphon valve within the administration set
    * ensuring that the pump is positioned no higher than 80 cm above the patient's heart level.
* Inadvertant bolus of drug: PCA should not be administered into the same line as intravenous fluids due to potential risk of the infusion pumping back into the hydration fluids should the cannula become blocked. It is advised that a non-return valve is used within the IV fluid line or the PCA is infused via a dedicated cannula.
* Norpethidine toxicity—this is a potential problem when using pethidine PCA. Be aware of the amount of pethidine that the patient is using. If large doses are used, consider changing to a different opioid.

Continuous intravenous infusion

* Can provide an alternative to PCA in patients unable to use PCA effectively.
* Close monitoring of the patient is important to detect respiratory depression or over-sedation.
* Pain control may be superior to PCA especially for major surgery.
* Supplementary oxygen should be administered.
* IV boluses are used to achieve analgesia and then an infusion is started.
* Elderly patients and those with renal impairment are most at risk of overdose.
* A suitable regime consists of morphine 0–3.5 mg/h, with nurse administered top-ups of up to 1 h's infusion dose every 20 min as required. Top-ups should only be administered by suitably trained staff due to risk of side-effects.
* No additional opioids should be prescribed whilst receiving continuous infusion.

Epidural

* The epidural route has become increasingly common over the past 10 years.
* Safe to use at ward level, but this is dependent on adequate monitoring and on nursing staff who have received specific training in caring for patients with epidural infusions.
* Used mainly for the management of pain during childbirth and following major abdominal, thoracic, orthopaedic, and vascular surgery.
* Opioids exhibit around 10 times the potency when administered via the epidural route as opposed to the intravenous route.
* A combination of local anaesthetic and opioid is usually administered (see table). The two drugs act synergistically resulting in superior analgesia and improved side-effect profile.
* Anticoagulation or coagulopathy (INR >1.5) is a contraindication to central blockade. DVT prophylaxis is considered safe if the following times are permitted to elapse prior to epidural insertion and removal:
  * Low molecular weight heparin, e.g. fragmin 12 h.
  * Unfractionated heparin, e.g. minihep 4 h.
  * Heparin infusion—turn infusion off for at least 2 h (and check APTR).
* Other contraindications include hypovolaemia, local infection/ septicaemia, and lack of patient consent.
* Epidural abscesses and haematomas are rare. Do not delay further investigation should either of these sequelae be suspected— permanent nerve damage can occur within 8 h of initial symptoms (see below).
* In addition to its analgesic effects, the utilisation of epidural analgesia may decrease the incidence of DVT following orthopaedic surgery and improve circulation following vascular surgery.
* Ideally, pumps should be designated for epidural use only to reduce the risk of pump errors and to allow for the setting of higher occlusion pressures.
* Prescribe supplementary oxygen for at least the first postoperative night.
* Typical doses for single injection use would be fentanyl 1 µg/kg or diamorphine 2.5 mg.

Standard epidural regimes

Drug	Dose	Rate
Bupivacaine	0.25%	2–10 ml/h
Bupivacaine and diamorphine	0.1–0.167%, 50–100 μg/ml	0–8 ml/h
Bupivacaine and fentanyl	0.1–0.167%, 3–5 μg/ml	0–12 ml/h

Trouble-shooting epidurals

- Breakthrough pain—mild or moderate breakthrough pain can be treated by increasing the infusion rate and adding in paracetamol and an NSAID. Severe pain occurs if the infusion rate has been reduced too quickly, the catheter has migrated out of the epidural space, the epidural has been sited too low, or if the local anaesthetic action is uneven. In the event of severe pain:

  - Check all connections and the epidural site. It is useful if the amount of catheter to skin is recorded on the anaesthetic chart following insertion. This helps diagnose catheter migration. If it is obvious that the catheter has migrated out of the epidural space consider reinsertion or an alternative method of analgesia such as PCA.

  - Check the level of local anaesthetic block—the patient's response to cold gives the best indication of sensory loss. If the block is one-sided or 'patchy', pull back the catheter 1–2 cm if this is possible.

  - Administer a bolus dose of local anaesthetic ± opioid. Ensure that there is patent IV access for the administration of fluids and/or ephedrine. The administration of a bolus dose will achieve analgesia in a short period of time and assist in defining the efficacy of the epidural. If the patient is haemodynamically unstable, consider alternative methods of analgesia or transferring the patient to an area where there is more monitoring available, e.g. HDU.

- Side effects related to the opioid content include:

  - Sedation and respiratory depression—delayed respiratory depression can occur due to rostral spread within the CSF and is more common with increasingly hydrophilic agents (morphine >diamorphine >fentanyl). Contributing factors include increasing patient age and the use of other CNS depressant drugs, e.g. cyclizine, chlorpheniramine. Naloxone should be considered if the respiratory rate is less than 8/min or the patient is over sedated.

  - Nausea and vomiting—ensure appropriate anti-emetic medication is prescribed.

  - Pruritis—this can be troublesome in around 10% of patients. Consider treating with naloxone IV (50–100 μg) followed by 300 μg via IV infusion over 8 h. Antihistamine medication may help but can also increase sedation.

  - Urinary retention—catheterization is suggested. Small doses of naloxone may also reverse urinary retention.

  - If the patient has continued side-effects related to the opioid, consider removing from the infusion and using local anaesthetic alone, e.g. bupivacaine 0.25% at a higher infusion rate (2–10 ml/h). Additional analgesia can be administered via PCA or IM/SC injection. It may take up to 24 h for the epidural opioid to be metabolized and side-effects may be increased with the addition of parenteral opioids. Monitoring for respiratory depression and over-sedation should continue hourly.

* Side-effects related to the local anaesthetic content include:
  * Decreased sensation and mobility—this may affect patient mobility, particularly following lumbar epidural blockade. Nursing staff must be aware of the potential for epidurals to affect patient mobility and the increase risk of pressure area breakdown.
  * Hypotension—although local anaesthetics are known to cause hypotension, nursing and junior medical staff must be made aware of other reasons for hypotension, e.g. hypovolaemia and bleeding. If a patient requires a bolus dose to improve analgesia staff must monitor the blood pressure every 5 min for at least 20 min. The patient must have patent intravenous access to allow for the infusion of fluids and drugs should they become hypotensive.
  * High level of local anaesthetic block—nursing staff should monitor the degree of local anaesthetic blockade. This is simple, using ice in a glove to ascertain decreased perception of cold. The infusion must be stopped and the anaesthetist informed should the block be nipple level (T4) or higher.
* Epidural haematoma—early symptoms include increasing back or nerve root pain, back tenderness, and neurological symptoms due to nerve or spinal cord compression. The patient requires urgent CT/MRI scan and neurosurgical assessment.
* Epidural abscess—symptoms as for epidural haematoma but the patient may also exhibit signs of fever and meningism. Investigation and treatment is the same as for epidural haematoma plus the administration of suitable antibiotics.

Spinal

* Intrathecal opioids have approximately 10 times the potency of epidural opioids (i.e. 100 times the potency of an intravenous dose).
* Usually administered as a single dose intra-operatively. Analgesia can last up to 24 h.
* Supplementary analgesia, in the form of paracetamol and NSAIDs, should be prescribed.
* Can result in a high incidence of nausea and vomiting, and delayed respiratory depression (particularly with morphine).
* Opioids can be administered via alternative routes in the postoperative period but staff must be aware of the increased potential for side-effects due to the long-acting nature of spinal opioids.
* Typical doses for single injection would be fentanyl 10–15 µg, diamorphine 0.1–0.2 mg, morphine 0.1–0.3 mg. (NB: preservative-free preparation of morphine should be used).

Monitoring patients on regular opioid therapy

The importance of appropriate monitoring by ward staff cannot be over-stressed:

- Patients having epidural and PCA opioids should have pain and side-effects monitored as part of hospital policy.
- Ward staff must be made aware of the potential for overdose even in patients receiving oral opioids.
- Observations should include pain score, level of sedation, respiratory rate, pump observations, and presence of nausea and vomiting. For epidurals, the level of sensory block and the presence of pruritus should also be included.
- The frequency of observations is dependent on the condition of the patient and the mode of administration:
  - Patients with epidural/PCA continuous opioid infusion should be monitored at least hourly for 24 h.
  - Patients receiving IM/SC/oral opioid should be monitored 30–60 min following a dose.
  - All patients should be monitored at least 4-hourly for the first 24 h following surgery.
  - Patients should be monitored every 15 min for at least an hour following the administration of naloxone.

Local anaesthetic and regional techniques

- Regional techniques are now common in the management of perioperative pain. Suggested techniques are mentioned under the relevant surgery.
- The use of local anaesthetic blockade continued into the postoperative period may reduce wind-up and central sensitization, thereby reducing the incidence of chronic pain.
- The analgesic effects of regional blockade occasionally wear off rapidly. Ensure that suitable additional analgesia is prescribed.

Acute pain relief in opioid-dependent patients

Patients taking opioids on a regular basis who present for surgery need careful consideration.

General principles

- Each case needs to be planned individually, and having decided on an analgesic regime, frequent reassessment, particularly in the first 24 h, is essential to fine-tune the prescription.
- Involve the hospital's acute pain team as soon as possible.
- Try to use a balanced analgesic approach including regular paracetamol plus NSAIDs.
- Try and confirm regularly taken opioid doses from an independent source, e.g. GP, local pharmacist, drug rehabilitation unit.
- Monitor the patient carefully with hourly observations for the first 24 h and beyond if necessary. Large doses of opioids are often needed. Complications are rare but unreliable histories, illicit use, and variable tolerance to side-effects are possible.

Drug abuser taking unknown quantities of street opioids

These patients need acute pain relief like anyone else and withdrawal of drugs should never be attempted perioperatively. Tolerance to opioids is invariably present and dosing requirements are unpredictable:

- Check all drugs abused—types, frequency, last dose taken?
- If patient is a registered addict contact community team/counsellor for help and information.
- Particular problems in these patients include fear of withdrawal or that opioids will be denied, unrealistic expectations about analgesia, and continued illicit use in hospital.
- Reports of high pain scores. Do not rely solely on pain scores to guide therapy but combine with other objective findings such as pulse, blood pressure, respiratory rate, and the ability to breathe deeply, vocalize, cough, ambulate, etc. Remember to treat anxiety as well as pain.

Reformed drug abuser

There is no evidence that using opioids for pain relief precipitates a relapse into drug abuse. However, because of their past problems these patients often ask to avoid IV opioids. Use a regional technique or the PO/SC route whenever possible. The reformed drug abuser on a methadone maintenance programme will display opioid tolerance and may have the same fears regarding analgesia as current drug abusers.

Patients with chronic pain

These patients take a variety of opioids. When they present for 'pain-relieving procedures' (e.g. patient with carcinoma of the pancreas admitted for thoracoscopic sympathectomy) opioid requirements will be reduced postoperatively and may be weaned over a few days depending on the outcome of the procedure.

Perioperative analgesia

Never attempt to withdraw opioids perioperatively—the aim is to provide adequate, controlled doses of opioid for analgesia. Morphine is the best opioid to use. Pethidine is less useful as it can cause fits in large doses.

When planning the analgesic regime provide the following:

- A basal amount of opioid to replace the patient's regularly taken drug. This may be given as methadone (if the patient is already on it and can take oral preparations) or using parenteral morphine. This component will be needed until discharge.

- Regular analgesic dose of morphine. Base this on what the patient takes daily (see conversion factors below). Give a dose equivalent to 150–200% of the usual daily opioid consumption either by 4-hourly SC injections through a cannula or by IV infusion. Reassess whether this is too much or too little at regular intervals. As pain improves, reduce this dose regularly over a few days.

- Extra rescue doses of analgesia should be available for breakthrough pain. Base the dose on about 50% of the regular analgesia dose being given. Reduce this as pain improves.

Conversion factors

- Oral morphine (mg):parenteral morphine (mg) = 2:1. For example, morphine 20 mg PO = morphine 10 mg SC/IM.
- Oral methadone (mg):parenteral morphine (mg) = 1:1. For example, methadone 20 mg PO = morphine 20 mg SC/IM.

Conversion of oral opioids (mg) to oral morphine (mg)	
Buprenorphine	× 60
Codeine	× 0.08
Dextropropoxyphene HCl	× 0.1
Dextropropoxyphene napsylate	× 0.06
DF118	× 0.1
Pethidine	× 0.125
Tramadol	× 0.25

Routes of administration

- In theatre or recovery IV boluses of morphine should be given until the patient is comfortable. Start with 5 mg every 2–3 min and titrate to acceptable pain relief.
- Intermittent SC morphine. Drug addicts have a lot of faith in this regime. Use an indwelling SC cannula. An idea of the dose required can be gauged from the amount of morphine required in theatre or in recovery. Introduce an automatic reduction in the dose on a daily basis depending on the expected degree and duration of pain.
- Continuous IV infusion: effective but open to abuse especially if the infusion pump is not locked. Add calculated acute pain dose onto background (basal) infusion. Requires frequent reassessment and possibly additional boluses until the correct infusion rate is established on which rescue doses

are unnecessary. The rate should be reduced when appropriate until the basal rate is reached. When the oral route is available this should be converted into an oral opioid regime.

- PCA: a relatively difficult technique to use as a degree of control is lost. Often results in excessive use of opioids and problems weaning the patient from the PCA.

Regional/local techniques in opioid-dependent patients

Although often recommended as techniques of choice in these patients they are associated with problems:

- Success with regional/local techniques depends on patient confidence and this is often lacking, particularly if the technique is not 100% successful at relieving pain.
- Any residual pain or discomfort is treated as a complete failure and the intensity of the pain exaggerated by accompanying anxiety, etc.
- If the regional/local technique uses opioid then stop all other methods of opioid administration. The regional opioid should prevent withdrawal, but patients should be monitored in case it occurs.
- If withdrawal occurs it may be better to abandon the regional technique and convert to systemic opioids in sufficient quantities to treat the pain and prevent continuing withdrawal.

Automatic dose reduction

The principles should be discussed with the patient. Emphasize:

- This is not a subversive way of giving no pain relief but a method to allow assessment of the patient's pain and behaviour.
- The analgesia prescribed is constantly reviewed by the medical team and alterations will be made if suitable control of pain is not achieved. An increase in the amount of opioid required in the first 24 h is not unusual and should be done if the initial estimate is too small.
- The chart is kept at the nurses' desk and actual doses are not discussed with the patient.
- Aim to reduce dose over 5–7 days.

Withdrawal

The severity of withdrawal is not necessarily related to the quantity of drug consumed. Symptoms and signs include yawning, sweating, lacrimation, rhinorrhoea, anxiety, chills, piloerection, tachycardia, hypertension, nausea, vomiting, diarrhoea, and abdominal pain/ cramps. Untreated heroin withdrawal peaks 36–72 h after the last dose and subsides after 5 days. Methadone withdrawal peaks at 4–6 days, subsiding at 10–12 days.

Methadone

Methadone is an opioid used in drug rehabilitation programmes to prevent withdrawal. Its pharmacokinetic profile means it is less of a 'hit' than the short-acting opioids and therefore less addictive, allowing gradual withdrawal and rehabilitation. Its long duration of action means it is administered once a day. It is therefore an excellent choice for basal opioid prescription. It should not be given IV and should not be used on a PRN basis (toxic accumulation is possible).

Special considerations

- Pericyazine 2.5–5 mg 8-hourly is useful to manage excessive anxiety/distress which is often a significant component of the pain in these patients.
- People abusing drugs other than opioids should be treated as normal, cross-sensitivity is unusual although sedative effects can be additive.
- In patients taking opioids on a long-term basis having continuing severe postoperative pain, despite an escalating morphine prescription, the addition of tramadol 50–100 mg PO/IM four times a day may be helpful.
- In addicts who are on unknown doses of opioids, oral methadone will assist with opioid management. Seek advice from local drug abuse experts for regime.
- Patients using fentanyl patches. With minor/day-case procedures continue using a fentanyl patch and give other analgesics as normal. For more severe pain:
  - remove the fentanyl patch
  - use fentanyl perioperatively
  - use fentanyl PCA postoperatively with background infusion equivalent to the patch delivery and boluses of fentanyl (10–20 µg) with a 5 min lock-out.

Conversion factors

Fentanyl patch strength (µg/h)	Oral morphine equivalent (mg/day)
25	<135
50	135–224
75	225–314
100	315–404

Section VIII
Regional anaesthesia

Chapter 50
Regional anaesthesia
Barry Nicholls

General principles and complications

Used correctly regional anaesthesia can provide prolonged postoperative analgesia or a safer alternative to general anaesthesia. Detailed knowledge of anatomy, technique, and possible complications is important for correct placement. Experience avoids the 'two frightened people on either end of a needle' scenario!

Patient selection

Patient refusal and local sepsis are the only absolute contraindications to regional anaesthesia; therapeutic anticoagulation (prosthetic valves, etc.) needs to be assessed on an individual basis.

- All procedures should be discussed with the patient before arriving in the anaesthetic room.
- Informed verbal and/or written consent, documented in the notes, should be obtained.
- Potential complications should be discussed with the patient and recorded in the notes/anaesthetic record. Relevant complications are likely to be those with an incidence >1% in the operator's hands.
- Consider the appropriateness of the technique. Supraclavicular block in a respiratory cripple or sciatic/femoral nerve block with bupivacaine for day case knee arthroscopy may not be suitable.

Complications following regional anaesthesia

- Cardiac arrest 6–7 per 10 000 following spinal, 1 per 10 000 for all other techniques.
- Transient neurological sequelae 6–7 per 10 000 following spinal, 1–2 per 10 000 for all other techniques (see also p. 948).
- Permanent neurological damage (neurological dysfunction lasting longer than 3 months) 1–2 per 10 000 following spinal anaesthesia, <1 per 10 000 for peripheral nerve blocks (see also p. 948).
- Postoperative neurological dysfunction is strongly associated with paraesthesia on needle placement or pain on injection.
- Local anaesthetic toxicity.

Regional anaesthesia awake or asleep?

- Anaesthetized or heavily sedated patients are unable to respond to paraesthesiae or intraneural injection, which may precede neurological trauma and damage. However, regional analgesia performed in such patients has never been demonstrated to produce an increased incidence of neurological sequelae.
- Paediatric regional anaesthesia is almost exclusively performed following a general anaesthetic. Of over 24 000 central and peripheral blocks in paediatric patients, the complication rate was 1.5/1000 (all associated with central blocks) with no permanent neurological damage.
- The majority of regional techniques can be performed on an awake or lightly sedated adult patients with minimal discomfort.

- Continuing verbal contact with patients has distinct advantages in the likelihood of inadvertent paraesthesia, intravenous, intrathecal, or intraneural injection, both for recognition and management.
- In a case of neurological injury following operation, clarification of the cause (anaesthetic/surgical) is facilitated if documentation of no paraesthesia, pain, or bleeding was present when performing the block.
- On balance therefore, perform blocks on awake patients whenever possible. Judicious doses of analgesics/sedatives (fentanyl 50–100 µg ± midazolam 1–2 mg) will improve patient tolerance.

Anticoagulation and regional anaesthesia

Bleeding and compression neuropraxia is a potential complication of regional anaesthesia in patients who are anticoagulated or with clotting abnormalities. Peripheral nerve blockade may still be used where compression can be achieved or bleeding is unlikely (superficial nerves). More proximal/perivascular techniques are best avoided.

Anticoagulation and central neuraxial blocks

- Full oral anticoagulation with warfarin or standard heparin (SH) is an absolute contraindication to central neuraxial blockade, and a relative contraindication to peripheral nerve blockade.

- Partial anticoagulation with low molecular weight heparin (LMWH) or low-dose warfarin (INR <1.5) is a relative contraindication to central neural blockade and each patient should be assessed individually, with respect to risk/benefit.

- Minihep (low-dose standard heparin 5000 units twice daily SC) is not associated with an increased risk of spinal/epidural haematoma. Wait for 4 h after a dose before performing epidural/spinal injection. Minihep should not be given until 1 h following spinal/epidural injection. These guidelines also apply for removal of epidural or spinal catheters.

- LMWH (<40 mg enoxaparin): allow 12 h interval between LMWH administration and epidural/spinal injection. Avoid any further dose for 4 h post block. This also applies for removal of epidural or spinal catheters.

- NSAIDs (including aspirin) do not increase the risk of epidural/ spinal haematoma.

- Intra-operative anticoagulation using 5000 units IV heparin following epidural/spinal injection appears safe, but careful postoperative observations are recommended. Bloody tap or blood in the epidural catheter is controversial. Some teams delay surgery for 12 h, others (if preoperative coagulation is normal) delay an IV bolus of heparin for 1 h.

- Fibrinolytic and thrombolytic drugs (streptokinase, TPA-tissue plasminogen activator): avoid neuraxial blocks for at least 24 h—if <24 h check PT, APTT, and fibrinogen levels.

- Thrombocytopenia: epidurals are relatively contraindicated below platelet counts of 100 000 and a single intrathecal injection below 50 000.

- An epidural haematoma should be suspected in patients who complain of severe back pain a few hours/days following any central neuraxial block or with any prolonged or abnormal neurological deficit. An immediate MRI scan and neurosurgical referral are indicated.

Nerve identification

Location of a nerve or plexus can be achieved by:

- loss of resistance (epidural, paravertebral)
- measured advancement of the needle (peribulbar, intercostal)
- relation to arterial pulsation/transfixion (femoral, brachial plexus)
- paraesthesia
- percutaneous electrical stimulation.

Peripheral nerve stimulation

- This is the commonest method used to identify nerves percutaneously.
- Allows accurate localization of important peripheral nerves. Aids location but does not necessarily protect them from damage.
- Indicates motor supply of the nerve.
- Patient cooperation is desirable but not essential—sedation or GA are possible, but the patient should not be paralysed.
- Possible reduced potential for nerve damage as there is no direct physical contact.
- Usually comfortable for the patient.

Using a peripheral nerve stimulator (PNS)

- Connect the stimulating needle to the negative lead (black) and ground electrode or ECG pad to positive lead (red).
- 'Negative to Needle, Positive to Patient'.
- Keep the ECG pad at least 20 cm from the site of injection. Start with current of 1–2 mA and 1–2 Hz. This causes stimulation of type A motor fibres in mixed nerves, without sensory stimulation.
- Insert the insulated needle. At all times move the needle slowly and gently, watching for signs of stimulation.
- When stimulation is achieved try to optimize the position of the needle to obtain good motor response without paraesthesiae, with a stimulating current of 0.2–0.5 mA.
- Inject 1 ml solution; the motor response should disappear (the nerve is displaced by solution). Inject the full volume after careful aspiration, fractionating the dose if it is greater than 5 ml. If the motor response does not disappear with the initial 1 ml suspect misplacement. Reposition before further injection.
- If there is any pain or increased resistance to injection, stop immediately, consider intraneural positioning of the needle or reposition the needle.

Needle design

- Long bevelled (10–14°) needles are easier to pass through tissues, but have less feel. Intraneurally they will cut a small number of fibres.
- Short bevelled (18–45°) needles have more resistance and may give more feedback to the operator. Intraneurally they may damage (not cut) fibres.
- Pencil-point needles split fibres if used intraneurally and have side injection ports to minimize intraneural injection.

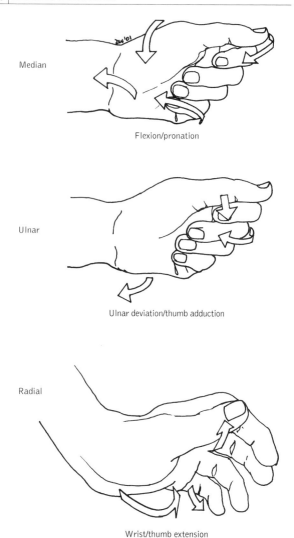

Median

Flexion/pronation

Ulnar

Ulnar deviation/thumb adduction

Radial

Wrist/thumb extension

Fig 50.1 Motor response of medial/ulnar/radial nerves to stimulation.

Motor response elicited with peripheral nerve stimulation

Nerve stimulated	Response
Median*	Finger and wrist flexion and pronation of the wrist. Thumb opposition
Ulnar*	Adduction of thumb, flexion ring and little finger, supination. Ulnar deviation
Radial*	Wrist and finger extension. Thumb abduction
Musculocutaneous	Elbow flexion (biceps, brachialis, coracobrachialis)
Femoral	Quadriceps contraction—patella twitch
Sciatic-tibial	Plantar flexion of foot and inversion—flexion of toes
Sciatic-peroneal	Dorsiflexion of foot and eversion—extension of the toes
Cervical roots	Contraction of scalenus medius C3, scalenus anterior C4, deltoid C5
Cervical trunks	Shoulder surgery: C5–C6 deltoid and biceps contraction. Humerus and forearm surgery: forearm or hand movement, especially extension
Cervical cords	Lateral cord: elbow flexion (musculocutaneous). Medial cord: forearm flexors, finger and wrist flexion. Posterior cord: (predominately radial nerve) wrist, fingers, and thumb extension
Lumbar plexus	Quadriceps contraction L2–L3

* Pure ulnar/radial/median nerve stimulation can only be achieved at the axilla or below. Cords/trunk stimulation gives a less defined motor response.

- There is no conclusive evidence to support increased nerve damage with any particular needle design.
- Insulated needles concentrate current density at the tip of the needle improving accuracy, but they are not essential for nerve localization.
- Uninsulated needles are adequate for superficial nerves/plexuses. With deeper nerves and plexuses excessive superficial muscle contraction may confuse identification.

Injection of local anaesthetic

- All injections must be pain free.
- Aspiration at the start and after every 5 ml will reduce the likelihood of intravascular injection.
- There should be no resistance to injection—do not use the heel of the hand to inject.
- With larger volumes, use multiple smaller syringes to give the same feel.

Characteristics of different local anaesthetic drugs

	pK_a	Relative lipid solubility	Relative potency	Protein binding (%)	Onset	Duration
Procaine	8.9	1	1	6	Slow	Short
Amethocaine	8.5	200	8	75	Slow	Long
Lidocaine (lignocaine)	7.7	150	2	65	Fast	Medium
Prilocaine	7.7	50	2	55	Fast	Medium
Etidocaine	7.7	5000	6	96	Fast	Long
Mepivacaine	7.6	50	2	78	Fast	Medium
Ropivacaine	8.1	400	6	94	Medium	Long
Bupivacaine	8.1	1000	8	95	Medium	Long
Levobupivacaine	8.1	1000	8	95	Medium	Long

* Potency is related to lipid solubility
* The duration of action is related to protein binding at the site of action and factors which affect removal of drug from the site, e.g. blood supply.
* The speed of onset/latency depends on the local availability of unionized free base. This can be improved by increasing the concentration of local anaesthetic or increasing the pH of the local anaesthetic/tissues. It is also dependent on the pKa of drug and the pH of the solution (a high pKa is associated with slow onset in normal pH settings, e.g. bupivacaine).

Choice of agent

* If rapid onset peripheral blockade for surgery is needed use lidocaine (lignocaine) 1–2% or prilocaine 1–2%. These agents diffuse more readily than bupivacaine (high protein binding capacity).
* If postoperative analgesia only is required use bupivacaine 0.25–0.5%, for its extended duration of action.
* In high-volume plexus anaesthesia or multiple blocks consider the use of levobupivacaine or ropivacaine (reduced toxicity).
* Continuous infusion—consider the use of less toxic drugs, i.e. ropivacaine and levobupivacaine. The addition of fentanyl or clonidine may augment blockade.

Mixtures of local anaesthetics

* Usually a mixture of short-acting LA (lidocaine (lignocaine)/prilocaine) with long-acting agents (bupivacaine/levobupivacaine/ ropivacaine).

Drug	Characteristics
Lidocaine (lignocaine)	Short-acting amide. Moderate vasodilatation. Cerebral irritation before cardiac depression. Duration enhanced and peak plasma levels reduced by adrenaline
Prilocaine	Short-acting amide. No vasodilatation. Rapid metabolism and low toxicity. Metabolized to o-toluidine causing methaemoglobinaemia (care in obstetrics/anaemia)
Bupivacaine	Long-acting amide. Racemic mixture of R and S enantiomers. Profound cardiotoxicity in higher doses
L-bupivacaine (levobupivacaine)	S-enantiomer of bupivacaine. Enhanced vasoconstriction. Reduced intensity and duration of motor block with less cardiotoxicity than bupivacaine
Ropivacaine	Long-acting amide. Reduced intensity and duration of motor block. Less cardiotoxic than bupivacaine or levobupivacaine
Amethocaine	Long-acting ester. Rapid absorption from mucous membranes or transdermal route. Relatively toxic
Benzocaine	Short-acting ester. Low potency. Used as lozenges
Cocaine	Short-acting ester. Slow onset, profound vasoconstriction. Limited local anaesthetic use, toxic

- The aim is to obtain rapid onset with the addition of extended anaesthesia and analgesia into the postoperative period.
- In practice, an agent of intermediate onset and duration is usually produced.
- Toxicity is cumulative—therefore the total dose of each individual drug should be reduced.
- There are no adverse pharmacological interactions.

Topical local anaesthetics

EMLA (eutectic mixture of local anaesthetic)

- Contains lidocaine (lignocaine) 2.5% + prilocaine 2.5%, arlatone (emulsifier), carbopol (thickener), distilled water and sodium hydroxide.
- Application 1–5 h before venepuncture.
- Side-effects are blanching and vasoconstriction.
- Avoid on broken skin/mucous membranes and in infants under 1 year.

Ametop (topical amethocaine gel)

- Contains amethocaine 4%, xanthan gum, methyl and propyl-p-hydroxy-benzoate, water, and saline.
- Application 30–45 min before venepuncture.
- Side-effects are erythema, oedema, and pruritus.
- Remove paste after 1 h.
- Not recommended in babies under 1 month.

Adjuvant drugs and additives

Bicarbonate
- Added to increase the pH of a solution—increases unionized LA.
- May increase the speed of onset.
- Risk of precipitation if there is >1 ml 8.4% NaHCO$_3$ in 10 ml LA.

Adrenaline
- Decreases vascular reabsorption, increasing the duration by making more drug available.
- Reduces peak plasma levels (lidocaine (lignocaine), mepivacaine).
- Is of reduced benefit with a long-acting LA.
- Less effective in epidurals.
- Effective concentration 5 μg/ml adrenaline. Add 0.1 mg of adrenaline (1 ml of 1:10 000) to 20 ml of LA.
- The total dose of adrenaline should not exceed 200 μg. This should be reduced by 50% during halothane anaesthesia.
- Avoid the use of adrenaline in digital nerve and penile blocks.

Felypressin
- Synthetic derivative of vasopressin.
- Promotes constriction of all smooth muscle.
- Available with prilocaine 3%.

Clonidine
- Prolongs the duration of sensory and motor block.
- Induces post block analgesia.
- Acts on spinal α2 adrenergic receptors.
- Effective in epidural/caudal/spinal anaesthesia.
- Epidural/intrathecal use is limited by hypotension and sedation.
- Dose: for caudal blocks 1 μg/kg; for peripheral blocks 0.3 μg/kg.

Ketamine
- An NMDA receptor agonist with weak local anaesthetic properties.
- Used in paediatric caudal blocks (0.5 mg/kg preservative free)— extends analgesia.
- Use a preservative free preparation only—standard preparations of ketamine must be avoided.

Opioids
- Proven synergism with epidural/intrathecal LA.
- All opioids have been used. Of debatable benefit in peripheral blocks.
- Intra-articular morphine 2–5 mg in knee surgery is used in combination with LA by some anaesthetists.

Hyaluronidase
- Used in peribulbar and retrobulbar blocks of the eye to enhance LA spread.
- Dose 5–30 units/ml.

Local anaesthetic toxicity

Local anaesthetic toxicity is related to high plasma levels of local anaesthetic found in:

* drug overdose
* direct intravascular injection
* rapid absorption/injection into a highly vascular area, e.g. intercostal
* continuous infusion of local anaesthetic
* cumulative effect of multiple injections or continuous infusion.

Recommended maximum doses as quoted by manufacturers' data sheets are a guide only. Equally important are:

* The site of injection with relation to vascularity and absorption.
* Metabolic status: acidosis, hypoxia, and hypercarbia all potentiate the negative inotropic/chronotropic effects of local anaesthetics.
* Whenever possible, keep within the maximum dosing recommendations, aspirate carefully before injection, and divide large-volume injections into smaller aliquots.

Maximum recommended doses of common agents

Agent	Maximum recommended doses	Maximum recommended doses with vasoconstrictor
Bupivacaine	2 mg/kg	2 mg/kg
Levobupivacaine	2 mg/kg (insufficient information)	
Ropivacaine	3 mg/kg (insufficient information)	
Lidcaine (lignocaine)	3 mg/kg	6 mg/kg
Prilocaine	6 mg/kg	8 mg/kg
Cocaine	3 mg/kg	

Treatment

* Stop injection or infusion as appropriate.
* ABC: 'Airway, Breathing, Circulation'.
* Mild symptoms may be best treated by oxygen, plus judicious doses of midazolam (1–4 mg) to increase the convulsant threshold.
* For moderate to severe toxicity, cardiovascular collapse is normally preceded by convulsions and is related to drug overdose in the presence of hypoxia.
* The first priority is, therefore, to prevent convulsions and maintain oxygenation.
* If the conscious level is deteriorating or there are convulsions intubate (use thiopental/suxamethonium for preference as this will decrease/stop con-

Symptoms and signs of toxicity

Mild toxicity	Tingling around the mouth
	Metallic taste
	Tinnitus
	Visual disturbance
	Slurred speech
Moderate toxicity	Altered conscious state
	Convulsions
	Coma
Potentially fatal toxicity	Respiratory arrest
	Cardiac arrhythmias
	Cardiovascular collapse

vulsions, but propofol or midazolam are suitable alternatives) and ventilate with 100% oxygen.

• If cardiovascular collapse ensues begin CPR (p. 825).

Methaemoglobinaemia

• Oxidation of haemoglobin to methaemoglobin by o-toluidine. Methaemoglobin has a reduced oxygen carrying capacity resulting in cyanosis.

• o-toluidine is formed by metabolism of prilocaine in the liver.

• Methaemoglobinaemia occurs with high doses of prilocaine (>600 mg).

• Avoid prilocaine in pregnancy and anaemia.

• Treatment: methylthioninium chloride (methylene blue) 1 mg/kg IV.

Head and neck blocks

- Cutaneous innervation of the face is from divisions of the trigeminal nerve (cranial nerve V).
- Muscles of facial expression are supplied by the divisions of the facial nerve (cranial nerve VII).
- Cutaneous innervation of the neck and posterior scalp is from the superficial branches of the cervical plexus (C1–C4).
- Innervation of the muscles of the neck is from the deep cervical plexus (C1–C4).

Facial blocks

For complete facial anaesthesia all branches of the trigeminal nerve and the greater auricular branch of the cervical plexus need to be blocked. The cutaneous sensory branches of the trigeminal nerve are:

- V_I ophthalmic–lacrimal, supraorbital, supratrochlear, infratrochlear, and external nasal.
- V_{II} maxillary—infraorbital, zygomaticofacial, and zygomaticotemporal.
- V_{III} mandibular—auriculotemporal, buccal, and mental.

Supraorbital nerve block

- Landmarks: supraorbital notch.
- Technique:
  - Palpate the supraorbital notch on the supraorbital rim, in line with the medial limbus of the iris.

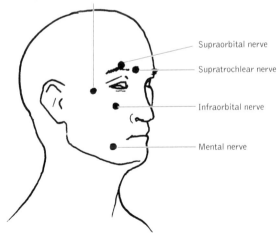

Fig 50.2 Facial blocks.

- Inject along the supraorbital rim from lateral to medial.
- Advance as far medial as the nasal bones using a 2.5 cm 27G needle.
- This will also block supratrochlear nerve, which emerges medial to supraorbital notch.
- Infiltrate approximately 3 ml in total—anaesthetizes forehead skin.

Infraorbital nerve block

- Landmarks: infraorbital foramen.
- Technique:
  - Locate the foramen, approximately 5 mm below the infraorbital rim, in line with the medial limbus of the iris. The foramen faces downwards and medially.
  - The injection point is just lateral to the alar groove (the uppermost point of the naso-labial fold).
  - Advance upward towards the infraorbital foramen.
  - Infiltrate approximately 2 ml—anaesthetizes the side of the nose (including ala and columella), lower eyelid, medial part of cheek, and upper lip.

External nasal nerve block

Terminal branch of the anterior ethmoidal nerve.

- Landmarks: base of the nasal bones.
- Technique:
  - Palpate the nasal midline to feel the lower edge of the nasal bones using the finger and thumb on either side of the nose.
  - Infiltrate 2 ml approximately 6–10 mm from the midline– anaesthetizes the nasal cartilage and tip.

Zygomaticotemporal/zygomaticofacial nerve block

- Landmarks: lateral orbital rim and lateral canthus.
- Technique (Zygomaticotemporal):
  - The nerve exits a foramen on the posterior concave surface of the lateral orbital rim, approximately 1 cm below the level of the lateral canthus.
  - Insert the needle at this point and infiltrate 2 ml—anaesthetizes the skin surrounding the temple, extending beyond the hairline.
- Technique (Zygomaticofacial):
  - The nerve exits a foramen on the anterior surface of the zygoma, just lateral to the infraorbital rim.
  - From the same insertion point as above infiltrate 2 ml local anaesthetic towards the prominence of the zygoma.
  - This nerve is usually blocked at the same time as the zygomatico-temporal—anaesthetizes the prominence (lateral part) of the cheek.

Mental nerve block

- Landmarks: mental foramen.
- Technique:
  - Palpate the mental foramen, approximately in line with the first lower premolar.
  - The supraorbital, infraorbital, and mental foramina are vertically aligned.

- Retract the lower lip, place the needle tip of a 2.5 cm 27G needle in the buccal sulcus near the base of the tooth and inject 1–2 ml. This anaesthetizes the lower lip.
- To block the skin overlying the chin, direct the needle to pass anterior to and beyond the lower border of the mandible but not quite out of the skin, injecting 2–3 ml.

Great auricular nerve block

The largest ascending branch of cervical plexus C2/3.

- Landmarks: sternomastoid muscle.
- Technique:
  - The greater auricular nerve lies on the fascial surface of the sterno-mastoid, 6.5 cm below the external auditory meatus (the approximate length of your little finger from tip to web space).
  - Infiltrate 2–3 ml at this insertion point; this anaesthetizes the lower part of the ear, the postauricular skin, and the skin over the angle of the jaw.

Mandibular nerve block

- Landmarks: coronoid notch.
- Technique:
  - The nerve lies 1 cm posterior to the pterygoid plate.
  - Palpate the coronoid notch; this is the notch between the condyle and coronoid process of the mandible.
  - This is felt below the zygomatic arch and 2.5 cm anterior to the tragus.
  - Mark the middle of the notch 'U' with a marker pen.
  - Insert a 22G spinal needle at 90° in both planes to contact with the posterior edge of the lateral pterygoid plate at approximately 3 cm depth. Infiltrate 4–5 ml.
  - Local anaesthetic will diffuse around the pterygoid plate to block the mandibular nerve; this anaesthetizes the bulk of the cheek, also blocking the masseter muscle, teeth and gums of the mandible, and the floor of mouth.
  - Blockade of all branches of the mandibular division of the trigeminal nerve can be achieved with blockade of the mandibular nerve.

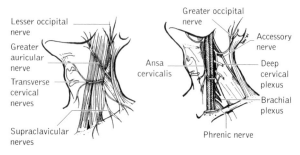

Fig 50.3 Superficial and deep cervical plexus.

Cervical plexus anatomy

- C1 has no cutaneous sensory branch.
- C1–C3 gives meningeal branches to the posterior cranial fossa.
- C1–C4 anterior primary rami form the cervical plexus, anterior to the scalenus medius but deep to the sternomastoid and the internal jugular vein.
- Supplies the ear, anterior neck, and 'cape area' (anterior and posterior aspect of shoulder and upper chest wall).
- Complete sensory analgesia of the anterior neck can be achieved with blockade of superficial branches of the cervical plexus (lesser occipital, greater auricular, transverse cervical, and supraclavicular nerves).
- Deep cervical plexus segmentally supplies the deep muscles of the neck and diaphragm.
- Motor and sensory connection to the diaphragm (phrenic nerve).

Greater/lesser occipital nerve blockade

Greater/lesser occipital nerve blockade is indicated for operations on the occipital scalp.

- Landmarks: greater occipital protuberance, mastoid process, posterior occipital artery.
- Technique:
  - Draw a line joining the occipital protuberance to the mastoid process.
  - Palpate the posterior occipital artery; the greater occipital nerve accompanies the artery.
  - Inject 5 ml of solution.
  - Infiltrate from this point along the line to the mastoid process with 5 ml solution to block the lesser occipital nerve.

Superficial cervical plexus block

Superficial cervical plexus block is indicated for carotid endarterectomy (with or without a deep cervical plexus block), neck and thyroid surgery, and ear and mastoid procedures (including a greater occipital nerve block).

- Landmarks: Posterior border of sternomastoid, cricoid cartilage.
- Technique:
  - Position the patient with their head turned slightly to the opposite side.
  - Draw a line from the cricoid to the posterior border of the sternomastoid and mark it (ask the patient to lift their head off the pillow to find the posterior border of the sternomastoid).
  - Insert a 22G needle perpendicular to the skin.
  - A click or pop is felt as the needle passes through the cervical fascia.
  - Inject 10 ml local anaesthetic solution at this point or fan the injection cranially and caudally along the posterior border of the muscle.

Deep cervical block

Indications are as for superficial cervical plexus block.

- Landmarks: mastoid process, Chassaignac tubercle (transverse process C6).
- Technique:
  - Draw a line connecting the tip of the mastoid process and the Chassaignac tubercle; draw a second line parallel but 1 cm posterior to the first.
  - The C2 transverse process lies 1–2 cm (one finger's breadth) caudad to the mastoid process, C3/4 transverse processes lie at 1.5 cm intervals along the second line.
  - After raising a skin weal a 22G 50 mm needle is inserted perpendicular to the skin, with a slight caudad angulation to contact bone (the transverse process).
  - Either paraesthesiae (nerve root) or bony contact is acceptable as there is free communication between paravertebral spaces. 4 ml of solution is injected at each level.
  - Paraesthesiae can be elicited by walking in an anteroposterior direction off the anterior tubercle of the transverse process.
  - Alternatively: single injection at C4 level using a peripheral nerve stimulator (Winnie). The junction of the interscalene groove and the superior border thyroid cartilage is at C4 level. Stimulate the scalenus anterior C4, scalenus medius C3 and inject 10–15 ml.
- Complications:
  - Inadvertent injection into the dural cuff (epidural/intrathecal).
  - Injection into the vertebral artery.
  - Phrenic nerve block, brachial plexus block.
- Clinical tips:
  - Avoid in patients with contralateral phrenic nerve palsy.
  - Do not perform bilateral deep cervical plexus blocks; there is the danger of bilateral recurrent laryngeal or phrenic nerve palsy.

Upper limb blocks

Brachial plexus anatomy

- Formed from anterior primary rami of C5–C8 and T1 nerves which emerge from the intervertebral foramina and form:
  - Roots between scalene muscles.
  - Trunks: (C5–6) upper, (C7) middle, (C8, T1) lower, are in the lower part of the posterior triangle of the neck, between the sternomastoid and trapezius muscles, above the middle third of the clavicle posterior to the subclavian artery.
  - Divisions: each trunk divides into anterior and posterior divisions behind the clavicle.
  - Cords: formed at the outer border of the first rib; they enter the axilla with the axillary artery, lying in their true anatomical relationship medial, lateral, and posterior to the second part of the artery behind the insertion of the pectoralis minor.
  - Branches of the cords are formed around the third part of the axillary artery within the axilla. A fascial sheath accompanies the brachial plexus from the scalene muscles down to the mid point of the upper arm, although the musculocutaneous and the radial nerves leave the sheath before then.
- The site of injection within the fascial sheath affects the spread of local anaesthetic.
- An interscalene block commonly misses the lower roots C8, T1 (ulnar sparing).
- Supraclavicular/infraclavicular: at this level there are only three components, the cords ('hour glass' shape of the sheath), allowing predictable spread and rapid onset.
- Axillary injection (single shot) commonly misses the radial nerve and the musculocutaneous nerve.

Interscalene brachial plexus block (classical Winnie)

Indications for this block are shoulder, humerus, or elbow surgery.

- Landmarks: cricoid cartilage, posterior border of sternomastoid, external jugular vein, interscalene groove.
- Technique:
  - The patient should be supine, with one small pillow under their head and neck.
  - The head should be turned comfortably to the opposite side.
  - At the level of the cricoid cartilage draw a line laterally to intersect the posterior border of the sternomastoid; this usually corresponds to where the external jugular vein crosses.
  - Palpate the scalenus anterior underneath the lateral border of the sternomastoid. Moving the fingers laterally, palpate the interscalene groove, between the scalenus anterior and medius.
  - To aid palpation ask the patient to their lift head gently off the pillow (contracting the sternomastoid) or sniff (contracting scalene muscles).

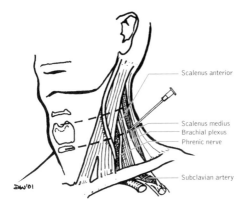

Fig 50.4 Interscalene approach to the brachial plexus.

- Stand to the side of patient or at their head, raise a weal and insert a 22G 25 mm/50 mm needle of choice perpendicular to the skin in all directions with a slight caudal direction.
- On entering the fascial sheath a pop may be elicited; advance until paraesthesia or specific motor stimulation is achieved (peripheral nerve stimulation).
- After careful aspiration inject 10–20 ml for postoperative analgesia or 20–40 ml for complete brachial plexus block.
- Complications:
  - Horner's syndrome if the stellate ganglion is affected (10–25%).
  - Vessel puncture (external/internal jugular, common carotid, vertebral).
  - Intrathecal/epidural injection.
  - Phrenic nerve block in all cases (100%).
  - Recurrent laryngeal nerve palsy causing a hoarse voice (5–10%).
- Clinical tips:
  - Take care in patients with COPD, and do not use in patients with contralateral phrenic nerve palsy.
  - In view of potential complications always perform this block on awake or lightly sedated patients.
  - The plexus is very superficial in thin people (1–2 cm deep). In all patients, the plexus should be identifiable using a 25 mm needle.
  - Avoid in obese patients with short necks, as landmarks can be impossible to locate.
  - If unable to locate the interscalene groove, consider a higher approach at the level of the thyroid cartilage or a lower approach (subclavian perivascular).
  - Digital compression above the injection site whilst injecting will aid caudal spread.

- Look for fullness in the posterior triangle on injection—if there is no swelling the injection is too deep, if there is cutaneous swelling it is too superficial.
- Use a short bevelled needle to aid 'feel'.
- Phrenic nerve stimulation indicates that the needle is too anterior (on scalenus anterior); levator scapulae stimulation indicates that the needle is too posterior (dorsal scapuler nerve).
- Do not use for surgery of the hand.
- Catheter insertion: after entering the interscalene sheath bring the hub of the needle towards the neck. Advance slightly, maintaining stimulation, and insert the catheter after distending the space with local anaesthetic.

Subclavian perivascular (supraclavicular) block (SPV)

This block is indicated for humerus, elbow, or hand surgery.
- Landmarks: interscalene groove, subclavian artery.
- Technique:
  - Position the patient lying flat, with their head turned 30° only to the opposite side.
  - Palpate the interscalene groove (as described for the interscalene approach).
  - Follow the interscalene groove caudally until the subclavian artery is felt above the clavicle (50% of patients).
  - With a finger on the subclavian artery insert a 22G 50 mm needle into the posterior part of the groove, and posterior to the subclavian artery.
  - Keeping the hub of the needle against the neck (this ensures that the needle direction is parallel to the long axis of the interscalene groove), direct the needle parallel to the floor and directly caudad; aim for the ipsilateral nipple or great toe.

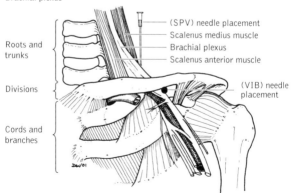

Brachial plexus

Roots and trunks

Divisions

Cords and branches

(SPV) needle placement
Scalenus medius muscle
Brachial plexus
Scalenus anterior muscle

(VIB) needle placement

Fig 50.5 Subclavian perivascular (SPV) and vertical infraclavicular (VIB) approaches to the brachial plexus.

- As the needle enters the fascial sheath a distinct 'pop' will be felt; advance slowly until paraesthesia or a specific motor response is elicited (peripheral nerve stimulator).
- The first rib may be encountered. If so 'walk' the needle anteroposteriorly on the rib until the plexus is encountered.
- Inject 40 ml in increments.
- Complications:
  - Subclavian artery puncture (20%).
  - Pneumothorax (0.1%).
- Clinical tips:
  - Best avoided if the subclavian artery cannot be palpated.
  - Can use a Doppler probe to locate the artery.
  - There should be absolutely no medial direction to the needle (risk of pneumothorax). Keep the hub of the needle against the side of the neck.
  - If the artery is punctured change to a more posterior direction.
  - If using a peripheral nerve stimulator aim for muscle contract below the elbow (flexion/extension of the wrist or fingers).
  - May miss the ulnar component: this is not the best block for hand surgery.

Vertical infraclavicular block (VIB)

Landmarks: suprasternal notch, anterior process of the acromion.

Technique:

- Position the patient supine without a pillow, with the arm to be blocked resting on the upper abdomen.
- Mark a point midway on a line joining the suprasternal notch and the anterior prominence of the acromion.
- Following the spine of the scapula anteriorly or the clavicle laterally you can locate the anterior prominence of the acromion.
- Palpate the subclavian artery above the clavicle; your mark should be just lateral to this.
- Using a 22G 50 mm insulated needle insert below but not touching the clavicle, and advance vertically posteriorly at right angles to the bed.
- Insert slowly using a peripheral nerve stimulator until stimulation of the posterior cord (extension of the wrist and fingers) is elicited.
- After careful aspiration inject 40–50 ml in increments.
- Complications:
  - Vessel puncture–subclavian artery, subclavian vein, cephalic vein (15%).
  - Pneumothorax (<0.5%).
  - Horner's syndrome (<5%).
- Clinical tips:
  - Confirm the lateral landmark by externally rotating the humerus—if you are on the acromion there will be no movement.
  - Flexion of the elbow or forearm motor responses (musculocutaneous) indicate the lateral cord and may result in inadequate block.
  - Ensure an absolute vertical direction of injection for safety—it avoids pneumothorax.

* If there is subclavian puncture the position is too medial—move laterally.
* If there is pectoral muscle contraction the position is too medial.
* This block is contraindicated in anticoagulated patients.

Axillary brachial plexus

Accompanying the axillary artery and vein in the brachial plexus sheath are:

* The medial cutaneous nerve of the arm (C8, T1).
* The medial cutaneous nerve of the forearm (C8, T1).
* The median nerve (C5–C8, T1).
* The ulnar nerve (C7–C8, T1).
* The radial nerve (C5–C8, T1).

Outside the axillary sheath are:

* The musculocutaneous nerve (C5–C7) to the biceps and brachialis (motor) and sensory to the skin on the radial border of the forearm from the elbow to the wrist.
* The intercostobrachial nerve (T2), supplying the skin of the axilla and the medial side of the upper arm.

Axillary plexus block

This block is indicated for elbow, forearm, and hand surgery.

Landmark: axillary artery, insertion of pectoralis major muscle.

Technique:

* The patient should be supine with their arm abducted, with their elbow flexed.
* Palpate the axillary artery in the axilla and mark its position.
* Draw a line down from the anterior axillary crease (insertion of the pectoralis major) crossing the axillary artery.
* At this point raise a weal, and fixing the artery against the humerus with the index and middle fingers insert a 22G 50 mm needle angled slightly proximally to pass either above or below the artery to contact either median or ulnar nerve respectively.

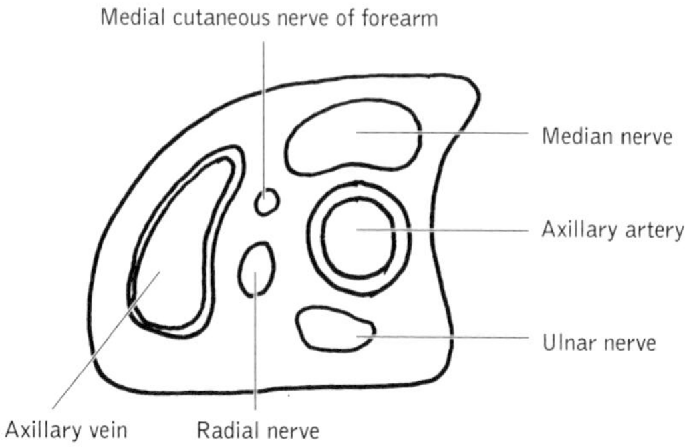

Fig 50.6 Relationship of the axillary artery and nerves in the axilla.

- A perceptible click or pop is felt on entering the fascial sheath, and paraesthesia or specific motor responses can be elicited.
- Inject 40–50 ml of solution in increments. Four different techniques can be employed: transarterial—injecting 20 ml of solution both anterior and posterior to the artery; multiple injections—finding each of the four nerves separately, the success of the block being increased when each successive nerve is identified; single loss of resistance using a short bevelled needle—fascial click, injecting after either through the needle or after insertion of a cannula; infiltration—fanwise injection of 15 ml of solution each side of the artery.
- Complications: vessel puncture–axillary artery or vein.
- Clinical tips:
  - The fascial sheath may be multicompartmental causing unreliable spread.
  - Remember 'M&M are tops'—musculocutaneous and median nerves are above the artery (ulnar below, radial behind).
  - The musculocutaneous nerve lies outside the sheath and needs to be blocked separately by injection of 10 ml into the body of coracobrachialis (using a peripheral nerve stimulator, direct the needle towards the head of the humerus: the motor response is flexion of the elbow 'hitching a ride').
  - The intercostobrachial nerve is blocked by infiltrating subcutaneously across the base of the axilla.
  - Decide on the area of operation and target the primary nerve if using a single injection technique.

Mid humeral block

All four peripheral nerves can be separately identified and blocked from the same point of entry. This block is indicated for elbow, forearm, and hand surgery.

- Landmarks: brachial artery, humeral canal.
- Technique:
  - The patient should be supine with their arm abducted and forearm supinated.
  - The brachial artery is palpated and marked at the junction of the upper and middle third of the humerus (humeral canal).
  - Draw a line from the insertion of the deltoid to cross the brachial artery at this point. Mark and raise a weal.
  - Insert a 22G 50 mm insulated needle above the artery in a proximal direction to elicit a motor response from the median nerve—flexion of the fingers.
  - Return to the skin, and then angle the needle 25° above the artery aiming at the superior border of the humerus to pass between the coracobrachialis and the biceps to elicit elbow flexion: this is the musculocutaneous nerve of the forearm.
  - Return to the skin, redirect the needle inferior to the artery to elicit an ulnar motor response—thumb adduction, wrist flexion.
  - Return to the skin, move the insertion point inferiorly (skin traction) and direct the needle to contact the inferior border of the humerus, pass-

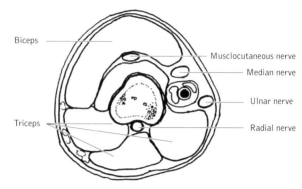

Fig 50.7 Mid humeral block.

ing under the humerus to elicit a radial motor response—extension of finger and thumb.

+ Inject 6–10 ml on each nerve.
+ The medial cutaneous nerve of the arm and forearm can be blocked by subcutaneous infiltration over the brachial artery at this level (5 ml).
+ Complications: vessel puncture of the brachial artery.
+ Clinical tip: depending on site of the operation, different concentrations of solution can be used for each nerve, allowing varying durations of anaesthesia and postoperative analgesia.

Elbow blocks

Elbow blocks are indicated for surgery on the forearm and hand.

+ Landmarks: flexion crease of the elbow, brachial artery, biceps tendon, medial and lateral epicondyles.

In all cases the arm should be slightly abducted with the elbow slightly flexed, the forearm supinated.

+ Median nerve technique:
  + The median nerve is medial and deep to the brachial artery, partially covered by the biceps muscle tendon.
  + The brachial artery is palpated and a 22G 50 mm needle is inserted medial to it, 1–2 cm above the elbow flexion crease at 45° to the skin.
  + A click may be felt as the needle pierces the deep fascia, and paraesthesia or a motor response elicited.
  + 5–8 ml of solution is injected.
  + On withdrawal of needle another 5–8 ml of solution is deposited subcutaneously along the medial border of the biceps tendon to block the medial cutaneous nerve of forearm
+ Radial nerve technique:
  + Palpate the intermuscular groove between the biceps and brachioradialis.

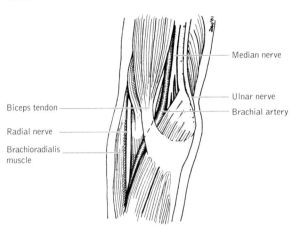

Fig 50.8 Elbow block (medial, radial, and ulnar) (ante-cubital fossa right arm).

- Insert a 22G 50 mm needle 2 cm above the flexion crease in this groove, towards the lateral epicondyle, elicit paraesthesia or a specific motor response.
- Inject 5–8 ml of solution.
- On withdrawal of the needle, inject 5–8 ml of solution subcutaneously along the lateral border of the biceps tendon to block the lateral cutaneous nerve of the forearm.
- Ulnar nerve technique:
  - The patient should be supine with their arm across their body and their elbow flexed to 90°.
  - The ulnar sulcus is palpated and a 22G 50 mm needle is inserted 1–2 cm proximal to the medial epicondyle in line with the ulnar sulcus, at 45° to the skin, directed proximally.
  - Paraesthesia or a specific motor response is elicited and 5 ml of solution injected.
  - Caution—do not inject into the medial epicondyle sulcus as this may cause pressure-induced neuropraxia.
  - Subcutaneous infiltration of 5 ml between the olecranon and lateral epicondyle of the humerus will block the posterior cutaneous nerve of the forearm.
- Clinical tips:
  - Elbow blocks can be useful for augmenting patchy axillary or supra/infraclavicular techniques.
  - If surgery is limited to cutaneous distribution of one nerve, individual nerves can be targeted.

Wrist blocks

The arm is abducted and the forearm supinated. This block is indicated for hand surgery.

- Median nerve technique:
  - Insert a 25G 25 mm needle between the tendons of the palmaris longus and flexor carpi radialis at the level of the proximal palmar crease.
  - Resistance is felt as the needle passes through the flexor retinaculum. 3–5 ml of solution can be deposited here or paraesthesia sought.
  - On withdrawal of the needle, subcutaneously infiltrate 2–3 ml to block the palmar cutaneous branch. Alternatively, an injection can be placed three fingerbreadths proximal to the skin crease to catch the palmar branch.
- Ulnar nerve technique:
  - Insert a 25G 25 mm needle medial to the ulnar artery, lateral to the tendon of the flexor carpi ulnaris at the level of the proximal ulnar crease, directed towards the ulnar styloid.

  or

  - Insert a 25G 25 mm needle on the medial aspect of the wrist underneath the tendon of the flexor carpi ulnaris.

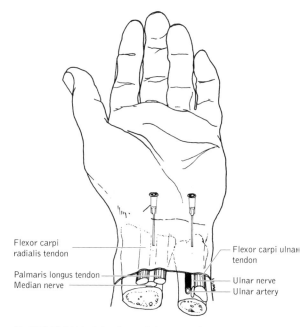

Flexor carpi radialis tendon
Palmaris longus tendon
Median nerve
Flexor carpi ulnaris tendon
Ulnar nerve
Ulnar artery

Fig 50.9 Wrist block (median and ulnar nerves).

- At a depth of approximately 1 cm paraesthesia will be elicited; slowly inject 3 ml of solution.
- Subcutaneous infiltration around the ulnar aspect of the wrist will block the dorsal cutaneous branch.
- Radial nerve technique:
  - The arm is abducted and the forearm slightly pronated.
  - The radial nerve is entirely sensory and cutaneous at this level. A field block of the terminal branches is achieved by infiltration of 5–8 ml of solution from the radial styloid over the posterior aspect of the wrist to the mid point of the dorsum of the wrist.
- Clinical tips:
  - If surgery is limited to cutaneous distribution of one nerve, individual nerves can be targeted.
  - Wrist blocks can be used in conjunction with wrist tourniquets for hand surgery.

Digital nerve block

- Technique:
  - Palpate the metacarpophalangeal joint and insert a 25G 25 mm needle perpendicular to the skin just distal to the joint. Advance the needle towards the palmar surface, injecting 3 ml on each side of the phalanx.
  - Insert a 25G 25 mm needle into the web space to a depth of 2 cm, injecting 5 ml of solution into each space; massage the space to aid spread.
  - Avoid adrenaline-containing solutions.

Intravenous regional anaesthesia (IVRA)–Bier's block

- Technique:
  - Apply a double cuff tourniquet (or single cuff) to either the wrist or the upper arm.
  - Select a suitable vein and insert a 22G IV cannula, below the cuff.
  - Insert a 22G IV cannula into the other hand as a safety needle.
  - Elevate or use an Eschmark bandage to ensanguinate the arm. Inflate cuffs to 100 mmHg above systole blood pressure, checking for absence of radial pulse. Deflate the distal cuff.
  - Inject a dilute solution of local anaesthetic, e.g. prilocaine 0.5%, 40 ml for a small arm, 50 ml for a medium arm, or 60 ml for a large arm. (Lidocaine (lignocaine) 0.5% maximum dose 250 mg).
  - Wait 5–10 min for the block to take effect, then inflate the distal cuff and deflate the proximal cuff.
  - The minimum time to cuff deflation is 15 min with prilocaine or 20 min with lidocaine (lignocaine).
- Complications: Accidental deflation of the cuff causes intravenous injection of a large volume of dilute local anaesthetic solution.
- Clinical tips:
  - Useful for cutaneous anaesthesia but often not adequate for bony surgery.
  - Use only for short procedures, less than 30 min.

- For short distal procedures, gripping the forearm during injection ensures that most local anaesthetic is retained distally. No analgesia is provided higher up the arm, however.
- Can use lidocaine (lignocaine) 0.5%: limit to 250 mg in adult.
- Never use bupivacaine.

Lower limb blocks

Anatomy of the lumbar plexus

The lumbar plexus lies within the psoas muscle, formed from the ventral rami of L1–L3 and the major part of the L4 nerve. It gives rise to the:

- iliohypogastric nerve (L1)
- ilioinguinal nerve (L1)
- genitofemoral nerve (L1–L2)
- lateral femoral cutaneous nerve (L2–L3)
- femoral nerve (L2–L4)
- obturator nerve (L2–L4).

Lumbar plexus block (posterior approach or 'psoas compartment' block)

This block is indicated for hip, knee, and femoral shaft surgery. In combination with sciatic nerve block it can be used for all operations on the knee, ankle, and foot including the use of tourniquet.

- Landmarks: posterior superior iliac spine (PSIS), line joining the iliac crests (Tuffier's line)—intercristine line.
- Technique:
    - Position the patient laterally, operative side uppermost, and draw a line parallel to the spinous processes, passing through the PSIS.
    - Mark the point where the intercristine line crosses.
    - Using insert a 22G 100 mm insulated needle perpendicular to the skin with a slight caudad angle. Insert until either the transverse process of L4 is encountered (if there is bony contact redirect the needle to pass beneath the transverse process) or quadriceps stimulation is encountered —approximately 8–10 cm.
    - Reduce stimulation to 0.2–0.4 mA and inject 30–40 ml of solution.
    - Alternatively, use the loss of resistance technique. 'Walk' a standard Tuohy needle along the caudad border of the L4 transverse process and inject after there is a loss of resistance at 0.5–1 cm.

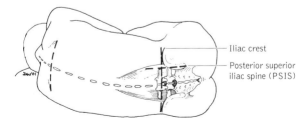

Iliac crest

Posterior superior iliac spine (PSIS)

Fig 50.10 Posterior approach to the lumbar plexus (psoas compartment block).

- Complications:
  - Vascular injection—injection should be slow, with repeated aspiration.
  - Epidural—intrathecal injection or spread.
- Clinical tips:
  - Avoid medial angulation as paravertebral space/epidural/intrathecal injection may occur.
  - If bone is encountered deeper than the initial stimulation (body of the vertebra) consider paravertebral placement of the needle.
  - Useful for intra/postoperative analgesia in surgery for a fractured femoral neck.

Femoral nerve block (anterior approach to lumbar plexus)

This block is indicated for surgery to the anterior thigh, knee, or femur.

- Technique:
  - Palpate the femoral artery at the level of the inguinal ligament.
  - Mark a point 1 cm lateral to the pulsation and 1–2 cm distal to the ligament.
  - Insert a 22G 50 cm needle at 45° to the skin in a cephalad direction. Two distinct 'pops' may be felt as the needle passes through fascia lata and iliopectineal fascia.
  - Paraesthesia in the knee or stimulation of quadratus femoris—'dancing patella'—indicates correct location of the needle. Inject 10–30 ml of solution.
- Clinical tips:
  - Sartorius stimulation is either from direct muscle contact or anterior division of the nerve—not acceptable for a good effect.
  - The nerve divides into multiple branches at or below inguinal ligament.
  - Commonly called a 3:1 block (femoral, lateral cutaneous nerve of thigh, obturator) when using high volume and distal pressure to aid cephalad spread. This is an unreliable method for obturator nerve block.
- Complications: vascular injection.

Obturator nerve block

This block is indicated for adductor spasm and knee surgery (optional).

- Landmarks: insertion of adductor tendons.
- Technique:
  - Position the patient supine with the leg placed in a 'figure of four' position.
  - Identify the insertion of the adductor magnus and brevis into the pubis.
  - At a point between the tendons, 1 cm inferior to the pubis, insert a 22G 80 mm insulated needle in the horizontal plane aiming at the ipsilateral anterior superior iliac spine.
  - At a depth of 5–6 cm resistance of the obturator membrane may be felt. Following a 'pop' either inject 5–15 ml or elicit a motor response (adductor stimulation).

Lateral cutaneous nerve of the thigh

Block of this nerve is indicated for analgesia of lateral femoral incisions (hip

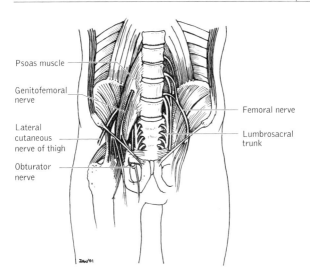

Fig 50.11 Lumbar plexus.

surgery and surgery for fractured neck of femur). It is commonly blocked by a femoral nerve block or femoral 3:1 block.

- Landmarks: anterior superior iliac spine, inguinal ligament.
- Technique:
  - At a point 2 cm medial and 2 cm inferior to the anterior superior iliac spine, below the inguinal ligament.
  - Insert a 22G 25–50 cm short-bevelled needle perpendicular to the skin. 10 ml of solution is injected beneath the fascia lata.

Subcostal nerve (lateral cutaneous branch of the T12 intercostal nerve)

This nerve is blocked in conjunction with the lumbar plexus for hip surgery (posterior approach).

- Landmarks: anterior superior iliac spine, iliac crest
- Technique: using 22G 80 mm needle make a subcutaneous infiltration backwards from the anterior superior iliac spine along the iliac crest using 8–10 ml of solution.

Anatomy of the sacral plexus

The sacral plexus is formed from the lumbosacral trunk (L4–L5), the ventral rami of S1–S3 and part of S4. The plexus lies on piriformis muscle on the anterior surface of the sacrum, covered by the parietal pelvic fascia. It gives several branches to the pelvis but only two nerves emerge from the pelvis to supply the leg:

- the posterior cutaneous nerve of the thigh (S1–S3)
- the sciatic nerve (L4–L5, S1–S3).

Sciatic nerve block (posterior approach–Labat)

This block is indicated for ankle and foot surgery. In combination with femoral nerve block it can be used for all surgery on the knee and lower leg.

- Technique:
  - Put the patient in Sim's position (recovery position with operative side uppermost) and arrange the knee, greater trochanter, and posterior superior iliac spine (PSIS) in a line.
  - Draw a line connecting the PSIS and greater trochanter. At its mid point, drop a perpendicular line to intersect another line joining the greater trochanter and the sacral hiatus.
  - Insert a 22G 100 mm needle perpendicular to the skin to a depth of 8–10 cm, and elicit either paraesthesia or motor stimulation—eversion (peroneal) or plantar flexion (tibial). Inject 10–20 ml of solution.
  - Three other approaches to the sciatic nerve have been described: the inferior approach (Raj), the lateral approach (Ichiangi), and the anterior approach (Beck).
- Clinical tips:
  - Only the classical posterior approach guarantees block of the posterior cutaneous nerve of the thigh.
  - If the nerve cannot be immediately identified, 'walk' the needle along the perpendicular joining the two lines (the sciatic nerve must cross this perpendicularly at some point).
  - The onset of the block is slow and may take up to 60 min.
  - The tibial and peroneal components may divide anywhere from the sciatic notch to the popliteal fossa; peroneal stimulation alone doesn't ensure tibial anaesthesia. Aim for inversion and dorsiflexion.
  - At the level of the greater trochanter the sciatic nerve bears a more constant relationship to the ischial tubercle being 1–2 cm lateral.
  - In approximately 25% of patients it is impossible or difficult to block the sciatic nerve by the alternative anterior approach. The nerve lies underneath the femur (external rotation of femur may help).

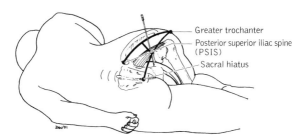

Fig 50.12 Posterior (Labat) approach to the sciatic nerve.

Anatomy of the nerve supply of the lower leg and foot

Below the knee the sciatic nerve supplies all motor and sensory innervation except for a cutaneous strip following the long saphenous vein to the medial border of the foot (long saphenous nerve–terminal branch of the femoral nerve). The sciatic nerve divides usually at the upper angle of popliteal fossa into:

- The tibial nerve (L4–L5, S1–S3), branching into the sural nerve and the tibial nerve.
- The common peroneal nerve (L4–L5, S1–S2), dividing into the superficial peroneal nerve and the deep peroneal nerve.

Popliteal block (posterior approach)

The popliteal fossa is diamond-shaped area bounded inferiorly by the medial and lateral heads of the gastrocnemius and superiorly by the long head of biceps femoris and the superimposed heads of the semimembranosus and semitendinosus. The posterior skin crease of the knee marks the widest point of the fossa, and with the knee slightly flexed, the popliteal artery can be palpated in the middle of the fossa. This block is indicated for ankle and foot surgery.

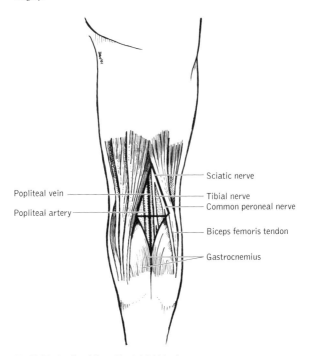

Fig 50.13 Popliteal fossa block (right leg).

- ◆ Landmarks: popliteal skin crease, popliteal artery.
- ◆ Technique:
  - ◆ With the patient prone flex the knee, marking the popliteal crease, and palpate the popliteal artery.
  - ◆ Mark a point 4 cm proximal to the popliteal skin crease and 1 cm lateral to the artery.
  - ◆ Insert a 22G 50/80 mm needle (depending on the size of the patient) at this point, directing the needle proximally at an angle of 45° to the skin.
  - ◆ Stimulation of the sciatic or tibial branch will be achieved at a variable depth of 2–4 cm.
  - ◆ Injection of 15 ml of solution will achieve blockade of the sciatic nerve, but to guarantee blockade of both branches inject 30–40 ml.
- ◆ Clinical tips:
  - ◆ As the sciatic nerve may well branch high within the popliteal fossa it may be necessary to identify it higher within the popliteal fossa or block the common peroneal and tibial nerve individually.
  - ◆ The tibial nerve follows the popliteal artery and can be located as above. Directing the needle in a more superolateral direction may be necessary to identify the peroneal nerve.
  - ◆ If the popliteal artery cannot be palpated, mark the popliteal crease and drop a line from the apex of the fossa to the middle of the crease; this marks the popliteal artery.

Intra-articular block

This block is indicated for knee arthroscopy.
- ◆ Landmarks: medial border of the patella.
- ◆ Technique:
  - ◆ Fully extend the knee.
  - ◆ Identify the gap between the medial border of the patella and the femur.
  - ◆ Insert a 22G 50 mm needle into the knee joint.
  - ◆ Inject 30 ml of local anaesthetic.
  - ◆ Inject portal sites with local anaesthetic.
- ◆ Clinical tips:
  - ◆ Sterile technique is of the utmost importance when injecting into a major joint.
  - ◆ Addition of morphine 2–5 mg may improve postoperative analgesia.
  - ◆ Adrenaline-containing solutions have the advantage of minimizing bleeding into the joint.

Saphenous nerve block

This is indicated in combination with sciatic nerve block for ankle and foot surgery.
- ◆ Landmarks: tibial tuberosity, medial tibial condyle.
- ◆ Technique:
  - ◆ The patient should be supine, with their leg externally rotated.
  - ◆ Identify the tibial tuberosity and inject 10–15 ml subcutaneously from the tibial tuberosity towards the medial tibial condyle.

Ankle and foot blocks

To ensure anaesthesia of the foot requires the following nerves to be blocked at the ankle:

Deep peroneal nerve

- Technique:
  - 3 cm distal to the inter-malleolar line palpate the extensor hallucis longus tendon (dorsiflexion of the big toe); lateral to this is the dorsalis pedis artery.
  - Insert a 23G 25 mm needle just lateral to the artery, until bony contact is made; withdraw slightly injecting 2 ml.

Superficial peroneal nerves

- Landmarks: injection point is the same as for the deep peroneal nerve.
- Technique: after performing blockade of the deep peroneal nerve infiltrate subcutaneously laterally and medially to the plantar junction of the foot with 10 ml of local anaesthetic. This blocks the medial and lateral cutaneous branches.

Tibial nerve

- Technique:
  - Draw a line from the medial malleolus to the posterior inferior calcaneum.
  - Palpate the posterior tibial artery.

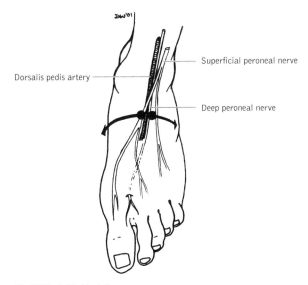

Superficial peroneal nerve

Dorsalis pedis artery

Deep peroneal nerve

Fig 50.14 Ankle block I.

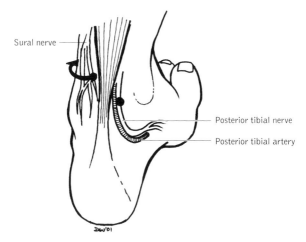

Sural nerve

Posterior tibial nerve

Posterior tibial artery

Fig 50.15 Ankle block II.

- Insert a 22G 50 mm needle just behind the artery, advancing until either stimulation or paraesthesia is elicited. If bone is encountered, withdraw slightly injecting 6–10 ml.

Sural nerve
- Landmarks: lateral malleolus, Achilles tendon.
- Technique: using a 22G 50 mm needle, inject 5 ml subcutaneously between the lateral malleolus and the lateral border of the Achilles tendon.

Digital nerves
- Metatarsal approach: 22G 50 mm needle at mid metatarsal level, 6 ml.
- Digital approach: a 22G 50 mm needle distal to the metatarsophalangeal joint, 3–6 ml.
- Web space: a 23G 25 mm needle in the web space, 6 ml.
- Avoid adrenaline-containing solutions.

Trunk blocks

Anatomy of the nerve supply to the thorax and abdomen

- The muscles and skin of the chest and abdomen are supplied by the spinal nerves of T2–T12 with a contribution of L1 in the inguinal region. These mixed spinal nerves emerge from the intervertebral foramen into the paravertebral space dividing into posterior and ventral rami.
- The posterior rami supply the deep muscle and skin over the dorsum of the trunk.
- The ventral rami form the intercostal nerves, which pass into the neurovascular plane between the internal intercostal and transversus muscles.
- A lateral cutaneous branch is given off before the costal angle, piercing the intercostal muscles and overlying muscles in the mid-axillary line.
- The intercostal nerves end as an anterior cutaneous nerve.

Thoracic paravertebral block

- This block has many indications:
  - thoracic surgery—postoperative pain control
  - breast surgery
  - fractured ribs—pain control
  - open cholecystectomy—postoperative pain control
  - renal surgery.
- Landmarks: spinous processes of the thoracic vertebrae.
- Technique:
  - The patient should be sitting or lying with the operative side up.
  - Palpate the cephalad aspect of the spinal process and make a mark 2.5–3 cm laterally.
  - Insert a 22G 80 mm needle perpendicular to the skin to contact the transverse process of the vertebra below.
  - Withdraw the needle, reinserting it to pass cephalad to the transverse process, advancing until loss of resistance or paraesthesia is elicited (usually 1–1.5 cm).
  - Inject 5 ml per level or 15 ml to obtain spread in 3–5 segments.
  - To insert a catheter use a 16G Tuohy needle until there is loss of resistance to air/saline.
- Complications:
  - Intravascular injection of local anaesthetic.
  - Epidural or intrathecal injection.
  - Pneumothorax.

Intercostal nerve block

Indications as for thoracic paravertebral block.
- Technique:
  - The patient should be prone or lateral with the operative side up.
  - Feel for the posterior angle of the rib at the posterior axillary line; place the index and middle fingers either side of the rib.

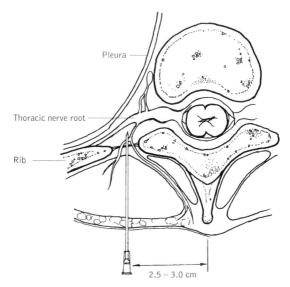

Fig 50.16 Thoracic paravertebral block.

- Insert a 22G 50 mm needle perpendicular to the skin, to touch the lower border of the rib.
- Pass the needle beneath the rib, insert 3–4 mm. A click or loss of resistance or paraesthesia may be felt–inject 3–5 ml.
- For catheter insertion use 16G Tuohy needle with an oblique angulation parallel to the rib until there is loss of resistance to air/saline.
- Complications:
  - Intravascular injection.
  - Bleeding.
  - Pneumothorax.
  - Local anaesthetic drug toxicity.
- Clinical tips:
  - It is important to be able to feel the rib.
  - Multiple levels increase the risk of pneumothorax.
  - Bilateral block best achieved with the patient prone.

Interpleural block

- This block is indicated for:
  - fractured ribs
  - breast surgery
  - unilateral upper abdominal surgery—open cholecystectomy
  - chronic pancreatic pain.

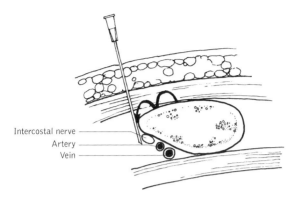

Fig 50.17 Intercostal nerve block.

- Landmarks: posterior angle of the sixth rib.
- Technique:
  - Position the patient laterally with the operative side uppermost.
  - Use a 16G Tuohy needle with a one-way or self-sealing valve connected to a bag of IV saline (Arrow catheter sheath adaptor).
  - Introduce the needle at 45° to the sixth rib to touch upper border.
  - Connect the infusion to the side arm of the sheath adaptor and turn it on.
  - Advance the needle over the top of the rib (avoiding the neurovascular compartment) until there is free flow of saline (the space between parietal and visceral pleura is entered).
  - Thread an epidural catheter through the self-sealing valve of the adaptor, 8–10 cm into the space, and secure.
  - Inject 20 ml solution.
- Complications: pneumothorax.
- Clinical tips:
  - Using a closed system ensures that no air is introduced into the space from outside.
  - Always go above the rib, avoiding the neurovascular bundle.
  - Effect is due to spread into the paravertebral gutter, blocking sympathetic as well as somatic nerves.
  - Keep the saline infusion no more than 10 cm above the height of the needle hub to avoid false loss of resistance.

Inguinal field block

Iliohypogastric, ilioinguinal and genitofemoral nerves, plus branches from overlapping intercostal nerves, supply the inguinal region. This block is indicated for inguinal hernia surgery.

- Technique:
  - At a point 2 cm (two fingers' breadth) medial to the anterior superior iliac spine insert a 22G 50 mm short bevelled needle perpendicular to the skin.
  - A pop is felt as the needle passes through the aponeurosis of the external oblique muscle. Inject 8 ml blocking the iliohypogastric nerve.
  - Redirect the needle deeper to pass through the internal oblique muscle, injecting 8 ml between the internal oblique and the transversus abdominis to block the ilioinguinal nerve.
  - Further fan-wise subcutaneous infiltration superficial to the aponeurosis will block the cutaneous supply from the lower intercostal and subcostal nerves.
  - Palpate the deep inguinal ring (1–1.5 cm above the mid point of the inguinal ligament). Insert a needle into the inguinal canal injecting 5 ml to block the genital branch of the genitofemoral nerve. This can only reliably be done at the time of surgery.
  - Subcutaneous infiltration at the medial end of incision or fan wise from the pubic tubercle will block contralateral innervation.
- Complications:
  - Intravascular injection.
  - Intraperitoneal injection.
  - Femoral nerve block.

Penile block

This is indicated for circumcision.
- Landmarks: symphysis pubis.
- Technique:

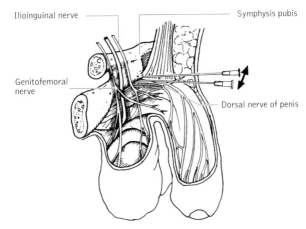

Fig 50.18 Penile block.

- Palpate the symphysis pubis above the root of the penis.
- Insert a 22G 25–50 mm needle to touch the inferior border of the pubis and advance 1–2 cm until loss of resistance is felt.
- The needle will be deep to the superficial fascia of the penis (Buck's fascia), inject 5–10 ml blocking both dorsal nerves.
- Complete the block by injecting subcutaneously around the root of the penis blocking ilioinguinal and gentiofemoral contributions.
- Complications: intravascular injection, bleeding.
- Clinical tips:
  - Never use adrenaline-containing solutions.
  - It is often prudent to perform two injections, one either side of the midline, to avoid the dorsal artery of the penis.
  - The nerve supply to the penis and scrotum is primarily via the dorsal nerve of the penis and posterior scrotal branches of the pudendal nerve (S2–S4), with additional branches from the ilioinguinal, genitofemoral, and posterior cutaneous nerve of the thigh.

Central neuraxial blocks

Spinal and epidural anatomy

- The spinal cord terminates at L1–L2 adults, L3 infants.
- The line joining the iliac crests–intercristine line (Tuffier's line)—is at the L3/4 interspace.
- The subarachnoid space ends at S2 in adults and lower in children (care with paediatric caudal block, use cannula rather than needle).
- The subarachnoid space extends laterally along the nerve roots to the dorsal root ganglia.
- There is a capillary interval (potential space) between the dura and the arachnoid mater (subdural space). This space is widest and most easily accessible in the cervical region.

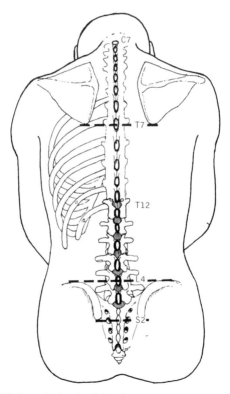

Fig 50.19 Boney landmarks of the spine.

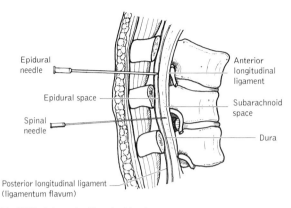

Fig 50.20 Subarachnoid and epidural spaces.

- The epidural (extradural) space lies between the walls of the vertebral canal and the spinal dura mater. It is a potential low-pressure space, occupied by areolar tissue, loose fat, and the internal vertebral venous plexus.
- The ligamentum flavum is thin in the cervical region reaching maximal thickness in the lumbar region (2–5 mm).

Spinal block

- Indications for spinal block are:
  - Lower abdominal surgery (caesarean section, inguinal hernia).
  - Lower limb surgery.
  - Perineal surgery.
  - Analgesia for upper abdominal surgery (in combination with GA), less commonly as sole anaesthesia for upper abdominal surgery.
- Landmarks: spinous processes of the lumbar vertebrae and the line joining the iliac crests (Tuffier's line).
- Technique:
  - The patient should be sitting or lying on their side.
  - Mark a line joining the iliac crests.
  - Identify the spinous processes at the level of this line.
  - The nearest interspace at this level is L3/4 (there is significant variation).
  - After raising a subcutaneous wheal, insert a 22–29G needle of your choice:
    - Midline: at the level of the interspace, insert a needle in the midline (coronal plane). With 15° cephalad angulation, advance until a click or pop is felt, at an approximate depth of 4–6 cm.
    - Paramedian: 1–2 cm lateral to the upper border of the spinous process. Insert a needle perpendicular to the skin to contact the lamina of the vertebra. Withdraw slightly, reinserting the needle 15° medially and 30° cephalad to pass over the lamina through the

intralamina space. Advance until a click or pop is felt (the dura is pierced).
  + After free flow of CSF inject the desired volume, check for free flow of CSF after injection.
+ Needle design:
  + Quincke (cutting) end hole—insertion parallel to dural fibres.
  + Whittaker/Sprotte (splitting)—side hole, 'pencil point'.
  + Use 25–29G depending on personal preference. Use 22G in an elderly patient with a difficult back.

Continuous spinal anaesthesia (CSA)—spinal catheters

+ Better control over level, intensity, and duration of block.
+ Possibly less hypotension due to incremental dosing and reduced total dose.
+ Trend to larger catheters, e.g. 20G epidural, 22–24G 'catheter-over-needle'.
+ Low incidence of post dural puncture headache in older patients (1–6%).
+ This block is indicated for lower abdominal, hip, and knee surgery.
+ Technique:
  + Make a dural puncture using your needle of choice (18G Tuohy, manufacturer's specific kit).
  + The level and technique are not critical.
  + Insert a catheter 3 cm into CSF and attach a bacterial filter.
  + Inject 1–1.5 ml (0.5% plain bupivacaine). Wait 15 min and test the block.
  + Inject a further 0.5–1.0 ml as necessary or when the level of block decreases by two segments.
+ Complications: post dural puncture headache (see p. 707).

Local anaesthetic drugs for spinal anaesthesia

+ There is no commercially marketed short-acting intrathecal preparation licensed for spinal anaesthesia within the United Kingdom. Manufacturers

Suggested doses for spinal anaesthesia

Block height	Volume of solution
Heavy bupivacaine 0.5%:	
T6–T10	2.5–3 ml
T11–L1	2.5 ml
L2–L5	2.0 ml
S1–S5 (saddle block)	1.0–1.5 ml (sitting position)
Plain bupivacaine 0.5% (or levobupivacaine 0.5%):	
T6–T10	Unreliable
T11–L1	2.5–3 ml
L2–L5	2.5 ml
S1–S5	Not possible to achieve saddle block

advise against the use of lidocaine (lignocaine) due to risks of cauda equina syndrome and transient radicular irritation or transient neurological symptoms.

- Transient neurological symptoms: back pain or dysaesthesia radiating into buttocks and legs. Begins within 24 h of procedure. Usually self-resolving in 3–5 days. No neurological sequelae (see also p. 951).

- Ropivacaine does not have a product licence for intrathecal use.
- Bupivacaine plain or heavy can be used (usually 0.5%).
- 'Heavy' is hyperbaric and contains 8% dextrose.
- 'Plain' bupivacaine is isobaric at body temperature.
- Due to spread in the intrathecal space, heavy solutions can be used to achieve a higher block. Plain solutions will usually produce a lower block height (T12–L1) with consequently less hypotension, under normal conditions.

Clinical tips

- Ideally injection should be at the L3/4 interspace; if there is difficulty go down not up as the level of termination of the conus is variable (L5–S1 Taylor's approach).
- Accurate surface identification of the L3/4 interspace is difficult– 70% of clinicians mark higher.
- A sitting position increases CSF pressure and hence improves CSF flow with fine needles. Also easier to find the midline in obese patients.
- Lateral position offers familiarity of practice and possibility of sedation.
- Often problems are due to too short an introducer and a flexible needle– can use a sterile 19G (white) needle as a longer introducer for most 25G spinal needles.
- The midline approach is conceptually easier, but osteophytes and calcification of the interspinous ligament in the elderly increase the difficulty.
- In the lateral/ paramedian approach the lamina acts as a depth gauge; the intralamina space is preserved in elderly patients.
- Low-dose bupivacaine/levobupivacaine 6–8 mg ± fentanyl 10–25 μg is possible for day case spinal anaesthesia.
- The use of lidocaine (lignocaine) is not recommended due to transient neurological symptoms (see above). Consider prilocaine 2% (60 mg) if the procedure is short.

Contraindications to spinal anaesthesia

- Relative contraindications:
  - Aortic stenosis/mitral stenosis (profound hypotension—sympathetic block).
  - Previous back surgery (technical difficulty).
  - Neurological disease (medicolegal).
  - Systemic sepsis (increased incidence of epidural abscess, meningitis).
- Absolute contraindications:
  - Local sepsis.
  - Patient refusal.
  - Full therapeutic anticoagulation.

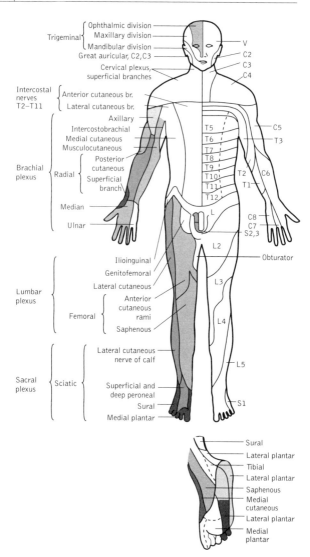

Fig 50.21 Dermatomes. With kind permission of Oxford University Press.

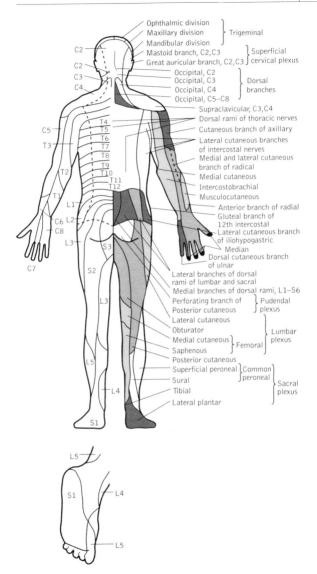

Fig 50.22 Dermatomes. With kind permission of Oxford University Press.

Epidural block

See p. 701 and p. 984.

Caudal block

See p. 789.
* Adult dose 20–25 ml bupivacaine (0.125–0.5%) plain.
* Use a 21G (green) needle or 20G intravenous cannula.
* Urinary retention is more common in adults.

Drug formulary

Appendix 1

For paediatric formulary see also p. 815.

Drug	Description and perioperative indications	Cautions and contraindications	Side-effects	IV dose (paediatric)	IV dose (adult)
Acetazolamide (Diamox®)	Carbonic anhydrase inhibitor used for acute reduction of intraocular pressure. Weak diuretic	Extravasation causes necrosis		2–7 mg/kg tds	500 mg bd
Adenosine	Endogenous nucleoside with antiarrhythmic activity. Slows conduction through AV node. Treatment of acute paroxysmal SVT (including WPW) or differentiation of SVT from VT. Duration 10 s	Second or third degree heart block. Asthma. Reduce dose in heart transplant or dipyridamole treatment	Flushing, dyspnoea, headache — all transient.	0.05 mg/kg, increasing by 0.05 mg/kg to max. 0.3 mg/kg	6 mg fast IV bolus, increasing to 12 mg at 2 min intervals as necessary
Adrenaline	Endogenous catecholamine with alpha and beta action: 1. Treatment of anaphylaxis 2. Bronchodilator 3. Positive inotrope 4. Given by nebulizer for croup 5. Prolongation of local anaesthetic action. 1:1,000 contains 1 mg/ml, 1:10 000 contains 100 μg/ml,	Arrhythmias especially with halothane. Caution in elderly. Via central catheter whenever possible	Hypertension, tachycardia, anxiety, hyperglycaemia, arrhythmias. Reduces uterine blood flow	1–3: IV/IM 0.1 ml/kg of 1:10 000 (10 μg/kg). Intraosseous /ET 0.1 ml/kg of 1:1000 (100 μg/kg). Infusion 0.05 –1 μg/kg/min.	1–3: IV/IM/ET 1 ml aliquots of 1:10 000 up to 5–10 ml (0.5–1 mg). Infusion 2–20 μg/min (0.04–0.4 μg/kg/min). 4: Nebulization 5 ml 1:1000. 5: Maximum dose for infiltration 2 μg/kg

IV = intravenous. IM = intramuscular. SC = subcutaneous. PO = per os (oral). SL = sublingual. ET = endotracheal. od = once daily. bd = twice daily. tds = three times daily. qds = four times daily. NR = not recommended. Doses are intravenous and dilutions in 0.9% saline unless otherwise stated.

Drug	Description and perioperative indications	Cautions and contraindications	Side-effects	IV dose (paediatric)	IV dose (adult)
	1:200 000 contains 5 μg/ml			4: Nebulization 0.5 ml/kg (up to 5 ml) 1:1000. 5. Maximum dose for infiltration 2 μg/kg	
Alfentanil	Short-acting, potent, opioid analgesic. Duration 10 min		Respiratory depression, bradycardia, hypotension	15–50 μg/kg over 5 min, then 0.5–1 μg/kg/min	250–750 μg (5–10 μg/kg). Attenuation of CVS response to intubation: 10–20 μg/kg
Aminophylline	Methylxanthine bronchodilator used in prevention and treatment of asthma. Converted to theophylline, a phosphodiesterase inhibitor. Serum levels 10–20 mg/litre (55–110 μmol/litre)	Caution in patients already receiving oral or IV theophyllines. Where serum level known aminophylline 0.6 mg/kg should increase level by 1 mg/litre	Palpitations, tachycardia, tachypnoea, seizures, nausea	5 mg/kg over 30 min, then 0.5–1 mg/kg/h	5 mg/kg over 30 min, then 0.5 mg/kg/h infusion
Amiodarone	Mixed class 1C and III antiarrhythmic useful in treatment of supraventricular and ventricular arrhythmias	Via central catheter. Sinoatrial heart block, thyroid dysfunction and pregnancy	Commonly causes thyroid dysfunction and reversible corneal deposits	25 μg/kg/min for 4 h, then 5–15 μg/kg/min	5 mg/kg over 1–2 h. Maximum 1.2 g in 24 h

IV = intravenous. IM = intramuscular. SC = subcutaneous. PO = per os (oral). SL = sublingual. ET = endotracheal. od = once daily. bd = twice daily. tds = three times daily. qds = four times daily. NR = not recommended. Doses are intravenous and dilutions in 0.9% saline unless otherwise stated.

Drug	Description and perioperative indications	Cautions and contraindications	Side-effects	IV dose (paediatric)	IV dose (adult)
Ampicillin	Broad spectrum penicillin antibiotic	History of allergy	Nausea, diarrhoea, rash	10–25 mg/kg qds	0.5–1 g qds
Amoxicillin	Broad spectrum penicillin antibiotic	History of allergy	Nausea, diarrhoea, rash	10–25 mg/kg tds. 50 mg/kg qds in severe infections	0.5–1 g qds
Aprotinin (Trasylol®)	Inhibits plasmin (responsible for fibrin dissolution) and reduces blood loss in major cardiac surgery		Hypersensitivity and phlebitis	0.05 mg/kg every 5 min—max. four doses	2000 000units (200 ml) over 30 min, then infusion of 500 000units (50 ml) per hour
Atenolol	Cardioselective beta-blocker. Long acting	Asthma, heart failure, AV block, verapamil treatment	Bradycardia, hypotension and decreased contractility	0.05 mg/kg every 5 min—max. four doses	5–10 mg over 10 min. PO: 50 mg od
Atracurium	Benzylisoquinolinium non-depolarizing muscle relaxant. Undergoes temperature- and pH-dependent Hoffman elimination (to laudanosine), plus non-specific enzymatic ester hydrolysis. Useful in severe renal or hepatic disease. Duration 20–35 min	Neuromuscular block potentiated by aminoglycosides, loop diuretics, magnesium, lithium, hypothermia, hypokalaemia, acidosis, prior use of suxamethonium, volatile anaesthetic agents. Store at 2–8 °C.	Mild histamine release and rash common with higher doses. Flush with saline before and after	Intubation: 0.3–0.6 mg/kg. Maintenance: 0.1–0.2 mg/kg. Infusion: 0.3–0.6 mg/kg/h, monitor neuromuscular blockade	Intubation: 0.3–0.6 mg/kg. Maintenance: 0.1–0.2 mg/kg. Infusion: 0.3–0.6 mg/kg/h, monitor neuromuscular blockade

IV = intravenous. IM = intramuscular. SC = subcutaneous. PO = per os (oral). SL = sublingual. ET = endotracheal. od = once daily. bd = twice daily. tds = three times daily. qds = four times daily. NR = not recommended. Doses are intravenous and dilutions in 0.9% saline unless otherwise stated.

Drug	Description and perioperative indications	Cautions and contraindications	Side-effects	IV dose (paediatric)	IV dose (adult)
Atropine	Muscarinic acetylcholine antagonist. Vagal blockade at AV and sinus node increases heart rate (transient decrease at low doses due to weak agonist effect). Tertiary amine therefore crosses blood–brain barrier	Obstructive uropathy and cardiovascular disease	Decreases secretions, and lower oesophageal sphincter tone, relaxes bronchial smooth muscle. Confusion in elderly	IV: 10–20 μg/kg. Control of muscarinic effects of neostigmine: 10–20 μg/kg. IM/SC: 10–30 μg/kg. PO: 40 μg/kg	300–600 μg. Control of muscarinic effects of neostigmine: 600–1200 μg.
Benzatropine	Antimuscarinic used in acute treatment of drug induced dystonic reactions (except tardive dyskinesia)	Glaucoma, gastrointestinal obstruction	Urinary retention, dry mouth, blurred vision	>3 years 0.02 mg/kg repeated after 15 min	IV/IM: 1–2 mg repeated if necessary
Benzylpenicillin	Broad spectrum antibiotic	History of allergy	Nausea, diarrhoea, rash	25 mg/kg qds. 50 mg/kg qds for severe infections	300–600mg qds. Higher doses may also be used (up to 2.4g qds)

IV = intravenous. IM = intramuscular. SC = subcutaneous. PO = per os (oral). SL = sublingual. ET = endotracheal. od = once daily. bd = twice daily. tds = three times daily. qds = four times daily. NR = not recommended. Doses are intravenous and dilutions in 0.9% saline unless otherwise stated.

Drug	Description and perioperative indications	Cautions and contraindications	Side-effects	IV dose (paediatric)	IV dose (adult)
Bicarbonate (sodium)	Alkaline salt used for correction of acidosis and to enhance onset of action of local anaesthetics. 8.4% = 1000 mmol/litre. Dose (mmol) in acidosis: weight (kg) x base deficit x 0.3	Precipitation with calcium containing solutions, increased CO_2 production, necrosis on extravasation. Via central catheter if possible	Alkalosis, hypokalaemia, hypernatraemia	1 ml/kg 8.4% solution (1 mmol/kg)	Dependent on degree of acidosis. Resuscitation: 50 ml of 8.4% then recheck blood gases. Bicarbonation of LA: 1 ml 8.4% to 20 ml bupivacaine. 1 ml 8.4% to 10 ml lidocaine (lignocaine)/ prilocaine
Bretylium	Treatment of resistant ventricular arrhythmias in resuscitation situation only. Class III antiarrhythmic	Phaeochromocytoma. Avoid sympathomimetic amines. May exacerbate arrhythmias due to cardiac glycosides	Severe hypotension, transient hypertension, dizziness, nausea	5–10 mg/kg over 10–30 min (dilute to 10 mg/ml in saline or dextrose), then 5–30 µg/kg/min	5–10 mg/kg over 10 min (dilute to 10 mg/ml in saline or dextrose)

IV = intravenous. IM = intramuscular. SC = subcutaneous. PO = per os (oral). SL = sublingual. ET = endotracheal. od = once daily. bd = twice daily. tds = three times daily. qds = four times daily. NR = not recommended. Doses are intravenous and dilutions in 0.9% saline unless otherwise stated.

Drug	Description and perioperative indications	Cautions and contraindications	Side-effects	IV dose (paediatric)	IV dose (adult)
Bupivacaine	Amide type local anaesthetic used for infiltration, epidural, and spinal anaesthesia. Slower onset than lidocaine (lignocaine). Duration 200–400 min (slightly prolonged by adrenaline)	Greater cardiotoxicity than other local agents. Do not use for IVRA. Adrenaline-containing solutions contain preservative	Toxicity: tongue/circumoral numbness, restlessness, tinnitus, seizures, cardiac arrest	Infiltration/epidural: maximum dose dependent upon injection site —2 mg/kg/4 h recommended	0.25–0.75% solution. Infiltration/epidural: maximum dose dependent upon injection site— 2 mg/kg/4 h. (2 mg/kg with adrenaline). 0.75% solution contraindicated in pregnancy
Buprenorphine (Temgesic®)	Opioid with both agonist and antagonist actions. Duration 6 h	May precipitate withdrawal in opioid addicts. Only partially reversed by naloxone	Nausea, respiratory depression, constipation	>6 months. Slow IV/IM: 3–6 µg/kg qds. SL: 3–6 µg/kg tds	Slow IV/IM: 300–600 µg qds. SL: 200–400 µg qds
Caffeine	Mild stimulant effective in the treatment of post dural puncture headache. Intravenous preparation available as caffeine sodium benzoate			SCBU: 5 mg/kg qds. Prevention of postop. apnoea: 10 mg/kg	IV/PO: 300–500 mg

IV = intravenous. IM = intramuscular. SC = subcutaneous. PO = per os (oral). SL = sublingual. ET = endotracheal. od = once daily. bd = twice daily. tds = three times daily. qds = four times daily. NR = not recommended. Doses are intravenous and dilutions in 0.9% saline unless otherwise stated.

Drug	Description and perioperative indications	Cautions and contraindications	Side-effects	IV dose (paediatric)	IV dose (adult)
Calcium chloride	Electrolyte replacement, positive inotrope, hyperkalaemia, hypermagnesaemia. Calcium chloride 10% contains Ca^{2+} 680 $\mu mol/ml$	Necrosis on extravasation. Incompatible with bicarbonate	Arrhythmias, hypertension, hypercalcaemia	0.1–0.2 ml/kg 10% solution	2–5 ml 10% solution (10 mg/kg, 0.07 mmol/kg)
Calcium gluconate	As calcium chloride. Calcium gluconate 10% contains Ca^{2+} 220 $\mu mol/ml$	Less phlebitis than calcium chloride	As calcium chloride	0.3–0.5 ml/kg 10% solution (max. 20 ml)	6–15 ml of 10% solution (30 mg/kg, 0.07 mmol/kg)
Cefotaxime	Third-generation cephalosporin broad spectrum antibiotic	Penicillin sensitivity		25 mg/kg tds. 50 mg/kg qds in severe infections	1 g bd (up to 12 g daily in divided doses in severe infections)
Cefuroxime	Second-generation cephalosporin broad spectrum antibiotic	10% cross-sensitivity with penicillin allergy		20–30 mg/kg tds	750 mg–1.5 g tds
Celecoxib (Celebrex®)	NSAID with selective inhibition of cyclo-oxygenase II (Cox II) enzyme. May therefore have reduced gastrointestinal side-effects	Hypersensitivity to sulphonamides or aspirin, asthma, severe renal impairment, peptic ulceration			PO: 100–200 mg bd

IV = intravenous. IM = intramuscular. SC = subcutaneous. PO = per os (oral). SL = sublingual. ET = endotracheal. od = once daily. bd = twice daily. tds = three times daily. qds = four times daily. NR = not recommended. Doses are intravenous and dilutions in 0.9% saline unless otherwise stated.

Drug	Description and perioperative indications	Cautions and contraindications	Side-effects	IV dose (paediatric)	IV dose (adult)
Cetirizine (Zirtek®)	Non-sedative antihistamine. Relief of allergy, urticaria	Prostatic hypertrophy, urinary retention, glaucoma, porphyria	Dry mouth	PO: 0.2 mg/kg up to 10 mg	PO: 10 mg od
Chloral hydrate	Formerly a popular hypnotic in children	Avoid prolonged use. Caution in elderly, gastritis, and porphyria	Gastric irritation, ataxia	PO: 25–50 mg/kg as single dose for sedation (up to 1 g)	PO: 0.5–1 g nocte
Chlorphenamine (chlorpheniramine) (Piriton®)	Sedative antihistamine. Relief of allergy, urticaria, anaphylaxis	Prostatic hypertrophy, urinary retention, glaucoma, porphyria	Drowsiness, dry mouth	<1 year NR. PO: 0.1 mg/kg up to 4 mg qds	Slow IV/IM/SC: 10–20 mg. PO: 4 mg 4-hourly
Chlorpromazine	Phenothiazine, antipsychotic. Mild alpha blocking action. Potent antiemetic and used for chronic hiccups	Hypotension	Extrapyramidal and anticholinergic symptoms, sedation, hypotension	0.1–1 mg/kg over 20 min	Up to 25 mg (at 1 mg/min diluted in saline to 1 mg/ml). Deep IM: 25–50 mg 6–8-hourly
Cimetidine	Competitive H₂ histamine receptor antagonist. Reduction of gastric acid		Hypotension and arrhythmias on rapid IV administration. Confusion in elderly	IV/PO: 10–15 mg/kg qds	200 mg over 2 min (diluted in saline) qds. PO: 400 mg bd

IV = intravenous. IM = intramuscular. SC = subcutaneous. PO = per os (oral). SL = sublingual. ET = endotracheal. od = once daily. bd = twice daily. tds = three times daily. qds = four times daily. NR = not recommended. Doses are intravenous and dilutions in 0.9% saline unless otherwise stated.

Drug	Description and perioperative indications	Cautions and contraindications	Side-effects	IV dose (paediatric)	IV dose (adult)
Cisatracurium	Single isomer of atracurium with greater potency, longer duration of action and less histamine release. Duration 55 min	Neuromuscular block potentiated by aminoglycosides, loop diuretics, magnesium, lithium, hypothermia, hypokalaemia, acidosis, prior use of suxamethonium, volatile anaesthetic agents. Store at 2–8 °C	Enhanced effect in myasthenia gravis, effects antagonized by anticholinesterases, e.g. neostigmine. Monitor response with peripheral nerve stimulator	>2 years. Intubation: 100 μg/kg. Maintenance: 20 μg/kg every 0–30 min Infusion: 0.06–0.18 mg/kg/hr	Intubation: 150 μg/kg. Maintenance: 30 μg/kg every 20–30 min. Infusion: 0.06–0.18 mg/kg/h
Citrate (sodium)	Non-particulate antacid oral premedication. Aspiration prophylaxis				PO: 30 ml 0.3 M solution
Clomethiazole (Heminevrin)	Hypnotic sedative used in alcohol withdrawal and status epilepticus.	Caution in elderly.	Nasal congestion, confusion, phlebitis, hypotension, coma.	1–2 ml/kg (8–16 mg/kg) over 15 min, then 0.5–1 ml/kg/hr (4–8mg/kg/hr)	3–7.5 ml/min (24–60 mg/min) as 0.8% solution, then reduced to 0.5–1 ml/min (4–8 mg/min) PO: 1–2 capsules at night

IV = intravenous. IM = intramuscular. SC = subcutaneous. PO = per os (oral). SL = sublingual. ET = endotracheal. od = once daily. bd = twice daily. tds = three times daily. qds = four times daily. NR = not recommended. Doses are intravenous and dilutions in 0.9% saline unless otherwise stated.

Drug	Description and perioperative indications	Cautions and contraindications	Side-effects	IV dose (paediatric)	IV dose (adult)
Clonidine	Selective α_2 agonist. Reduces requirement for opioids and volatile anaesthetics. Enhances epidural analgesia	Rebound hypertension on acute withdrawal of chronic therapy	Hypotension, sedation	3–5 μg/kg slowly. PO premed: 4 μg/kg. Caudal: 1 μg/kg	2–4 μg/kg over 5 min. Epidural: 150–500 μg (2–10 μg/kg) in 10 ml saline
Co-amoxiclav (Augmentin®)	Mixture of amoxicillin and clavulanic acid. 1.2 g contains 1 g amoxicillin.	See amoxicillin	See amoxicillin	25–50 mg/kg qds	600 mg–1.2 g tds (qds in severe infections)
Cocaine	Ester type local anaesthetic and potent vasoconstrictor. Topical anaesthesia of mucous membranes (nasal passages). Duration 30–120 min	Topical use only. Caution with other sympathomimetic agents, halothane, and in cholinesterase deficiency. Porphyria	Hypertension, arrhythmias, euphoria	1–3 mg/kg topical	4–10% solution. Maximum topical dose 1.5 mg/kg
Co-codamol 8/500	Combination oral analgesic containing codeine 8 mg and paracetamol 500 mg	See paracetamol		N R	PO: 1–2 tablets qds (maximum 8 tablets per day)
Co-codamol 30/500	Combination oral analgesic containing codeine 30 mg and paracetamol 500 mg	See paracetamol. When no strength is specified co-codamol 8/500 is dispensed		N R	PO: 1–2 tablets qds (maximum 8 tablets per day)

IV = intravenous. IM = intramuscular. SC = subcutaneous. PO = per os (oral). SL = sublingual. ET = endotracheal. od = once daily. bd = twice daily. tds = three times daily. qds = four times daily. NR = not recommended. Doses are intravenous and dilutions in 0.9% saline unless otherwise stated.

Drug	Description and perioperative indications	Cautions and contraindications	Side-effects	IV dose (paediatric)	IV dose (adult)
Co-codaprin	Combination oral analgesic containing codeine 8 mg and aspirin 400 mg	As NSAIDs		NR	PO: 1–2 tablets qds (maximum 8 tablets per day)
Codeine phosphate	Opioid used for mild to moderate pain		Nausea, vomiting, dysphoria, drowsiness	PO/IM/PR: 1–1.5 mg/kg 6-hourly	PO/IM: 30–60 mg 4-hourly
Co-dydramol	Combination oral analgesic containing dihydrocodeine 10 mg and paracetamol 500 mg	See paracetamol		NR	PO: 1–2 tablets qds (maximum 8 tablets per day)
Co-proxamol	Combination oral analgesic containing dextropropoxyphene 32.5 mg and paracetamol 325 mg	See paracetamol		NR	PO: 1–2 tablets qds (maximum 8 tablets per day)
Cyclizine	Antihistamine antiemetic agent. Antiemetic effect probably due to antimuscarinic activity	Caution in severe heart failure	Drowsiness, dry mouth, blurred vision, tachycardia	IV/IM: 1 mg/kg up to 50 mg	IV/IM/PO: 50 mg tds
Dalteparin (Fragmin®)	Low molecular weight heparin used in prevention of venous thromboembolism	Once daily dosing. APTT monitoring not usually required			SC prophylaxis: 2500 units od (5000 units in high risk)

IV = intravenous. IM = intramuscular. SC = subcutaneous. PO = per os (oral). SL = sublingual. ET = endotracheal. od = once daily. bd = twice daily. tds = three times daily. qds = four times daily. NR = not recommended. Doses are intravenous and dilutions in 0.9% saline unless otherwise stated.

Drug	Description and perioperative indications	Cautions and contraindications	Side-effects	IV dose (paediatric)	IV dose (adult)
Dantrolene	Direct-acting skeletal muscle relaxant used in treatment of malignant hyperpyrexia and neuroleptic malignant syndrome. 20 mg/vial—reconstitute in 50 ml water	Avoid combination with calcium channel blockers as may cause hyperkalaemia and cardiovascular collapse	Skeletal muscle weakness	1 mg/kg repeated every 5 min to a maximum of 10 mg/kg	1 mg/kg repeated every 5 min to a maximum of 10 mg/kg
Desmopressin (DDAVP®)	Synthetic analogue of vasopressin (ADH) with longer duration of action and reduced pressor effect. Used for neurogenic diabetes insipidus and haemophilia (enhances factor VIII activity)	Caution in hypertension and CVS disease	Hypertension, angina, abdominal pain, flushing, hyponatraemia	IV/IM/SC: 0.4 μg/day. Intranasal: 5–20 μg/day. PO: 100–200 μg tds	IV/IM/SC: 1–4 μg/day. Intranasal: 10–40 μg/day. PO: 100–200 μg tds. Haemophilia: 0.3 μg/kg (in 50 ml saline over 30 min IV)
Dexamethasone	Prednisolone derivative corticosteroid. Less sodium retention than hydrocortisone. Cerebral oedema, oedema prevention in certain operations	Interacts with anticholinesterase agents to increase weakness in myasthenia gravis	See prednisolone	IV/IM/SC: 200–400 μg/kg bd. Cerebral oedema: 100 μg/kg qds. Croup: 250 μg/kg, then 125 μg/kg qds for 24 h	IV/IM/SC: 4–8 mg. Cerebral oedema: 4 mg qds. (Dexamethasone 0.75 mg = prednisolone 5 mg)

IV = intravenous. IM = intramuscular. SC = subcutaneous. PO = per os (oral). SL = sublingual. ET = endotracheal. od = once daily. bd = twice daily. tds = three times daily. qds = four times daily. NR = not recommended. Doses are intravenous and dilutions in 0.9% saline unless otherwise stated.

Drug	Description and perioperative indications	Cautions and contraindications	Side-effects	IV dose (paediatric)	IV dose (adult)
Diamorphine	Potent opioid analgesic	Spinal/epidural use associated with risk of respiratory depression, pruritus, nausea	Histamine release, hypotension, bronchospasm, nausea, vomiting, pruritus, dysphoria	IV/SC: 50 μg/kg then 15 μg/kg/h. Epidural: 2–3 mg in 60 ml 0.125% bupivacaine at 0.1–0.4 ml/kg/h	IV/IM/SC: 2.5–5 mg 4hrly Epidural: 2.5 mg diluted in 10 ml local anaesthetic/saline, then 0.1–0.5 mg/hr Spinal: 0.25–0.5 mg
Diazepam	Long-acting benzodiazepine. Sedation or termination of status epilepticus	Thrombophlebitis: emulsion (Diazemuls®) less irritant to veins	Sedation, circulatory depression	0.2–0.3 mg/kg. Rectal: 0.5 mg/kg as Stesolid® or may use IV preparation	2–10 mg, repeat if required
Diclofenac sodium (Voltarol®)	Potent NSAID analgesic for mild to moderate pain	Hypersensitivity to aspirin, asthma, severe renal impairment, peptic ulceration	Gastrointestinal upset or bleeding, bronchospasm, tinnitus, fluid retention, platelet inhibition	PO/PR: 1 mg/kg tds. Maximum 3 mg/kg/day (> 1 yr)	PO/PR: 25–50 mg tds (or 100 mg 18-hourly). Maximum 150 mg/day

IV = intravenous. IM = intramuscular. SC = subcutaneous. PO = per os (oral). SL = sublingual. ET = endotracheal. od = once daily. bd = twice daily. tds = three times daily. qds = four times daily. NR = not recommended. Doses are intravenous and dilutions in 0.9% saline unless otherwise stated.

Drug	Description and perioperative indications	Cautions and contraindications	Side-effects	IV dose (paediatric)	IV dose (adult)
Digoxin	Cardiac glycoside. Weak inotrope and control of ventricular response in supraventricular arrhythmia. Therapeutic levels 0.5–2 µg/litre	Reduce dose in elderly. Enhanced effect/toxicity in hypokalaemia. Avoid cardioversion in toxicity	Anorexia, nausea, fatigue, arrhythmias	Rapid IV/PO loading: 15 µg/kg stat, then 5 µg/kg qds, then PO: 4 µg/kg bd	Rapid IV loading: 250–500 µg administered over 30 min, repeated dependent on response. Maximum 1mg/24 h. PO loading: 1–1.5 mg in divided doses over 24 h. PO maintenance: 125–250 µg/day
Dihydrocodeine tartrate	Opioid used for mild to moderate pain		Nausea, vomiting, dysphoria, drowsiness	PO/IM/PR: 1–1.5 mg/kg 6-hourly	PO/IM/: 30–60 mg 4-hourly
Dobutamine	β₁ adrenergic agonist, positive inotrope and chronotrope. Cardiac failure	Arrhythmias and hypertension. Phlebitis, but can be administered peripherally	Tachycardia. Decreased peripheral and pulmonary vascular resistance	Infusion: 2–20 µg/kg/min	Infusion: 2.5–10 µg/kg/min
Domperidone	Anti-emetic acting on chemoreceptor trigger zone	Renal impairment. Not recommended for PONV prophylaxis	Raised prolactin. Rarely acute dystonic reactions	PO: 200–400 µg/kg 4-hourly	PO: 10–20 mg 4-hourly. PR: 30–60 mg 4-hourly

IV = intravenous. IM = intramuscular. SC = subcutaneous. PO = per os (oral). SL = sublingual. ET = endotracheal. od = once daily. bd = twice daily. tds = three times daily. qds = four times daily. NR = not recommended. Doses are intravenous and dilutions in 0.9% saline unless otherwise stated.

Drug	Description and perioperative indications	Cautions and contraindications	Side-effects	IV dose (paediatric)	IV dose (adult)
Dopamine	Naturally occurring catecholamine with α, β_1 and dopaminergic activity. Inotropic agent	Via central catheter. Phaeochromocytoma (due to noradrenaline release)		Infusion: 2–20 μg/kg/min	Infusion: 2–10 μg/kg/min
Dopexamine	Catecholamine with β_2 and dopaminergic activity. Inotropic agent	Via central catheter. Phaeochromocytoma		Infusion: 0.5–6 μg/kg/min	Infusion: 0.5–6 μg/kg/min
Doxacurium	Long-acting non-depolarizing muscle relaxant. Onset and duration similar to pancuronium. Little histamine release	Neuromuscular block potentiated by aminoglycosides, loop diuretics, magnesium, lithium, hypothermia, hypokalaemia, acidosis, prior use of suxamethonium, volatile anaesthetic agents	Enhanced effect in myasthenia gravis, effects antagonized by anticholinesterases, e.g. neostigmine. Monitor response with peripheral nerve stimulator		Intubation: 50–80 μg/kg. Maintenance: 5–40 μg/kg
Doxapram	Respiratory stimulant acting through carotid chemoreceptors and medulla. Duration 12 min	Epilepsy, airway obstruction, acute asthma, severe CVS disease	Risk of arrhythmia. Hypertension	1 mg/kg slowly. Infusion: 0.5–1 mg/kg/h for 1 h	1–1.5 mg/kg over >30 s. Infusion: 2–4 mg/min

IV = intravenous. IM = intramuscular. SC = subcutaneous. PO = per os (oral). SL = sublingual. ET = endotracheal. od = once daily. bd = twice daily. tds = three times daily. qds = four times daily. NR = not recommended. Doses are intravenous and dilutions in 0.9% saline unless otherwise stated.

Drug	Description and perioperative indications	Cautions and contraindications	Side-effects	IV dose (paediatric)	IV dose (adult)
Droperidol	Butyrophenone related to haloperidol. Neuroleptic anaesthesia and potent antiemetic. Duration 4hr.	Alpha adrenergic blocker. Parkinson's disease.	Vasodilatation, hypotension. Dystonic reactions.	Antiemetic: 25–75 µg/kg	Antiemetic: 0.5–2.5 mg Neuroleptic anaesthesia: 0.2 mg/kg with fentanyl 4 µg/kg
Edrophonium (Tensilon®)	Anticholinesterase used in diagnostic assessment of myasthenia gravis	Once daily dosing and APTT monitoring not usually required	Bradycardia, AV block	20 µg/kg test dose, then 80 µg/kg	1 mg slow IV every 2–4 min. Maximum 10 mg
EMLA	Eutectic mixture of 2.5% lidocaine (lignocaine) and 2.5% prilocaine. Topical anaesthesia	Absorption of anaesthetic depends on surface area and duration of application. Avoid use on abrasions or mucous membranes	Methaemoglobin-aemia in high doses	NR <1 year	Apply under occlusive dressing 1–5 h before procedure (maximum 60 g)
Enoxaparin (Clexane®)	Low molecular weight heparin used in prevention of venous thromboembolism	Once daily dosing and APTT monitoring not usually required		SC prophylaxis: 0.4–0.8 mg/kg od	SC prophylaxis: 20 mg (2000 units) od (40 mg if high risk)
Enoximone	Selective phosphodiesterase inhibitor used in cardiac failure with increased filling pressures. Inodilator	Stenotic valvular disease, cardiomyopathy	Arrhythmias, hypotension, nausea	Infusion: 5–20 µg/kg/min	Infusion: 90 µg/kg/min for 10–30 min, then 5–20 µg/kg/min (maximum 24 µg/kg/day)

IV = intravenous. IM = intramuscular. SC = subcutaneous. PO = per os (oral). SL = sublingual. ET = endotracheal. od = once daily. bd = twice daily. tds = three times daily. qds = four times daily. NR = not recommended. Doses are intravenous and dilutions in 0.9% saline unless otherwise stated.

Drug	Description and perioperative indications	Cautions and contraindications	Side-effects	IV dose (paediatric)	IV dose (adult)
Ephedrine	Direct and indirect sympathomimetic (α and β adrenergic action). Vasopressor, safe in pregnancy. Duration 10–60 min	Caution in elderly, hypertension and CVS disease. Tachyphylaxis. Avoid with MAOI	Increases heart rate and blood pressure		3–6 mg repeated (dilute 30 mg in 10 ml saline, 1 ml increments). IM: 30 mg
Ergometrine	Ergot alkaloid used to control uterine hypotony or bleeding. Syntometrine® = ergometrine 500 µg/ml and oxytocin 5 units/ml	Severe cardiac disease or hypertension	Vasoconstriction, hypertension, vomiting		IM: 1 ml as Syntometrine®. Not recommended IV
Erythromycin	Macrolides antibiotic with spectrum similar to penicillin	Arrhythmias with cisapride, terfenadrine, astemizole	Nausea, diarrhoea	10–25 mg/kg qds over 15–60 min	500 mg–1 g qds over 15–60 min
Esmolol	Short-acting cardioselective beta-blocker. Metabolized by red cell esterases. Treatment of supraventricular tachycardia or intra-operative hypertension	Asthma, heart failure, AV block, verapamil treatment	Hypotension, bradycardia	SVT: 0.5 mg/kg over 1 min, then 50–200 µg/kg/min	SVT: 0.5 mg/kg over 1 min, then 50–200 µg/kg/min. Hypertension: 25–100 mg, then 50–300 µg/kg/min
Etamsylate	Reduces capillary bleeding, possibly by enhancing platelet adhesion	Porphyria	Nausea, headache, rash	PO: 12.5 mg/kg qds	PO: 500 mg qds

IV = intravenous. IM = intramuscular. SC = subcutaneous. PO = per os (oral). SL = sublingual. ET = endotracheal. od = once daily. bd = twice daily. tds = three times daily. qds = four times daily. NR = not recommended. Doses are intravenous and dilutions in 0.9% saline unless otherwise stated.

Drug	Description and perioperative indications	Cautions and contraindications	Side-effects	IV dose (paediatric)	IV dose (adult)
Ethanol	Useful sedative/hypnotic. Has been tried as an intravenous induction agent in doses of up to 44 g!	Administered as dehydrated absolute alcohol BP	Diuretic effect		2 g (2 ml) diluted to 5–10% solution in saline or dextrose, repeated as necessary
Etomidate	IV induction agent. Cardiostable in therapeutic doses	Pain on injection	Nausea and vomiting. Myoclonic movements	0.1–0.4 mg/kg	0.1–0.4 mg/kg
Fentanyl	Synthetic phenylpiperidine derivative opioid analgesic. High lipid solubility and cardiostability. Duration 30–60 min	Reduce dose in elderly. Delayed respiratory depression and pruritus if epidural/spinal	Circulatory and ventilatory depression. High doses may produce muscle rigidity	1–5 μg/kg, up to 25 μg/kg if postop. ventilation. Infusion: 2–4 μg/kg/h	1–5 μg/kg (up to 50 μg/kg). Epidural: 50–100 μg (diluted in 10 ml saline/local anaesthetic). Spinal: 5–20 μg
Flucloxacillin	Penicillinase-resistant antibiotic active against staphylococci	Hypotension on rapid IV administration	Thrombophlebitis	10–25 mg/kg qds	500 mg–1 g qds slow IV
Flumazenil	Benzodiazepine receptor antagonist. Duration 45–90 min	Benzodiazepine dependence (acute withdrawal), resedation if long-acting benzodiazepine	Arrhythmia, seizures	5 μg/kg, then repeat up to 40 μg/kg. Infusion: 2–10 μg/kg/h	200 μg then 100 μg at 60 s intervals (up to maximum 1 mg). Infusion: 100–400 μg/h

IV = intravenous. IM = intramuscular. SC = subcutaneous. PO = per os (oral). SL = sublingual. ET = endotracheal. od = once daily. bd = twice daily. tds = three times daily. qds = four times daily. NR = not recommended. Doses are intravenous and dilutions in 0.9% saline unless otherwise stated.

Drug	Description and perioperative indications	Cautions and contraindications	Side-effects	IV dose (paediatric)	IV dose (adult)
Furosemide (frusemide)	Loop diuretic used in treatment of hypertension, congestive cardiac failure, renal failure, fluid overload		Hypotension, tinnitus, ototoxicity, hypokalaemia and hyperglycaemia	0.5–1.5 mg/kg bd	10–40 mg slowly.
Gallamine	Long-acting non-depolarizing neuromuscular blocker	Impaired renal function (renal excretion)	Tachycardia	1–2 mg/kg	Intubation: 1–1.5 mg/kg. Maintenance: 0.1–0.75 mg/kg
Gentamicin	Aminoglycoside antibiotic active against Gram-negative bacteria. Peak level <10 mg/litre. Trough level <2 mg/litre	Impairs neuromuscular transmission—avoid in myasthenia	Ototoxicity and nephrotoxicity	2 mg/kg tds (administered over 5 min) or 5 mg/kg/day as a single dose (administered over 5 min)	0.6–1.6 mg/kg tds or 2–5 mg/kg/day as a single dose (administered over 5 min)
Glucagon	Polypeptide hormone used in treatment of hypoglycaemia and overdose of beta-blocker	Glucose must be administered as soon as possible	Hypertension, hypotension, nausea, vomiting	<25 kg 0.5 unit (0.5 mg). >25 kg 1 unit	SC/IM/IV: 1 unit (1mg). Beta-blocker overdose unresponsive to atropine: 50–150 μg/kg in glucose 5%

IV = intravenous. IM = intramuscular. SC = subcutaneous. PO = per os (oral). SL = sublingual. ET = endotracheal. od = once daily. bd = twice daily. tds = three times daily. qds = four times daily. NR = not recommended. Doses are intravenous and dilutions in 0.9% saline unless otherwise stated.

Drug	Description and perioperative indications	Cautions and contraindications	Side-effects	IV dose (paediatric)	IV dose (adult)
Glucose	Treatment of hypoglycaemia in unconscious patient	50% solution irritant therefore flush after administration		1 ml/kg of 50% solution	25–50 g (50–100 ml 50% solution). Can use more dilute solutions
Glyceryl trinitrate	Organic nitrate vasodilator. Controlled hypotension, angina, congestive cardiac failure	Remove patches before defibrillation to avoid electrical arcing	Tachycardia, hypotension, headache, nausea, flushing, methaemoglobinaemia	12–60 μg/kg/h starting dose up to 300 μg/kg/h	Infusion: 0.5–10 mg/h. SL tabs: 0.3–1 mg prn. SL spray: 400 μg prn. Patch: 5–10 mg/24 h
Glycopyrrolate	Quaternary ammonium anticholinergic agent. Bradycardia, blockade of muscarinic effects of anticholinesterases, antisialogogue	Caution in glaucoma, cardiovascular disease. Unlike atropine does not cross blood–brain barrier	Paradoxical bradycardia in small doses. Reduces lower oesophageal sphincter tone	4–8 μg/kg. Control of muscarinic effects of neostigmine: 10–15 μg/kg	200–400 μg. Control of muscarinic effects of neostigmine: 10–15 μg/kg
Haloperidol	Butyrophenone derivative antipsychotic	Neuroleptic malignant syndrome	Extrapyramidal reactions	N R	IM: 2–5 mg (not recommended IV)

IV = intravenous. IM = intramuscular. SC = subcutaneous. PO = per os (oral). SL = sublingual. ET = endotracheal. od = once daily. bd = twice daily. tds = three times daily. qds = four times daily. NR = not recommended. Doses are intravenous and dilutions in 0.9% saline unless otherwise stated.

Drug	Description and perioperative indications	Cautions and contraindications	Side-effects	IV dose (paediatric)	IV dose (adult)
Heparin	Endogenous mucopolysaccharide used for anticoagulation. Half-life 1–3 h. 100 units = 1 mg	Monitor activated partial thromboplastin time (APTT). Reversed with protamine	Haemorrhage	Low dose: 50–75 units/kg IV then 10–15 units/kg/h. Full dose: 200 units/kg IV then 15–30 units/kg/h	Low dose SC: 5000 units bd. Full dose IV: 5000 units, then per 24 h infusion 24 000–48 000 units
Hyaluronidase	Enzyme used to enhance permeation of injected fluids or local anaesthetics. Treatment of extravasation of drugs	Not for intravenous administration	Occasional severe allergy	Local anaesthetic: 25–50 units/ml	Ophthalmology: 10–30 units/ml local anaesthetic agent. Extravasation: 1500 units in 1 ml saline infiltrated to affected area
Hydralazine	Direct-acting arteriolar vasodilator used to control arterial pressure. Duration 2–4 h	Higher doses required in rapid acetylators	Increased heart rate, cardiac output, stroke volume	0.1–0.5 mg/kg	5 mg every 5 min to a maximum of 20 mg

IV = intravenous. IM = intramuscular. SC = subcutaneous. PO = per os (oral). SL = sublingual. ET = endotracheal. od = once daily. bd = twice daily. tds = three times daily. qds = four times daily. NR = not recommended. Doses are intravenous and dilutions in 0.9% saline unless otherwise stated.

Drug	Description and perioperative indications	Cautions and contraindications	Side-effects	IV dose (paediatric)	IV dose (adult)
Hydrocortisone	Endogenous steroid with anti-inflammatory and potent mineralocorticoid action (steroid of choice in replacement therapy). Treatment of allergy		Hyperglycaemia, hypertension, psychic disturbance, muscle weakness, fluid retention	4 mg/kg then 2–4 mg/kg qds	IV/IM: 50–200 mg qds. HPA suppression and surgery: 25 mg at induction then 25 mg qds (see p. 98) (hydrocortisone 20 mg = prednisolone 5 mg)
Hydromorphone hydrochloride	Opioid used for moderate to severe pain		Nausea, vomiting, dysphoria, drowsiness		PO: 2–4 mg 4-hourly increased as necessary. PO slow release: 4 mg bd
Hyoscine hydrobromide (Scopolamine)	Antimuscarinic sedative antiemetic agent used as premedication. Reduces secretions and provides some amnesia	See atropine. Avoid in elderly — delerium.	See atropine. Sedation.	IV/IM/SC: 10 µg/kg	IV/IM/SC: 200–600 µg. PO: 300 µg qds
Hyoscine butylbromide (Buscopan)	Antimuscarinic agent used as an antispasmodic	See atropine	See atropine		IV/IM: 20 mg slowly repeated if necessary

IV = intravenous. IM = intramuscular. SC = subcutaneous. PO = per os (oral). SL = sublingual. ET = endotracheal. od = once daily. bd = twice daily. tds = three times daily. qds = four times daily. NR = not recommended. Doses are intravenous and dilutions in 0.9% saline unless otherwise stated.

Drug	Description and perioperative indications	Cautions and contraindications	Side-effects	IV dose (paediatric)	IV dose (adult)
Ibuprofen	NSAID analgesic for mild to moderate pain. Best side-effect profile of NSAIDs	Hypersensitivity to aspirin, asthma, severe renal impairment, peptic ulceration	Gastrointestinal upset or bleeding, bronchospasm, tinnitus, fluid retention, platelet inhibition	PO: 5–10 mg/kg tds (>7 kg)	PO: 400 mg qds
Imipenem	Carbapenem broad spectrum antibiotic. Administered with cilastatin to reduce renal metabolism	Caution in renal failure	Nausea, vomiting, diarrhoea, convulsions, thrombophlebitis	>3 months 10 mg/kg over 30 min qds (25 mg/kg severe infections)	Slow IV (1 h): 500 mg–1 g qds. Surgical prophylaxis: 1 g at induction, repeated after 3 h
Indometacin	NSAID analgesic for moderate pain. High incidence of side-effects. Also used for neonatal ductus arteriosus closure	Hypersensitivity to aspirin, asthma, severe renal impairment, peptic ulceration	Gastrointestinal upset or bleeding, bronchospasm, tinnitus, fluid retention, platelet inhibition	Ductus closure: 100–200 µg/kg, three doses	PO: 50–100 mg bd. PR: 100 mg bd
Insulin (Actrapid®)	Human soluble pancreatic hormone facilitating intra-cellular transport of glucose and anabolism. Diabetes mellitus, ketoacidosis, and hyperkalaemia	Monitor blood glucose and serum potassium. Store at 2–8 °C	Hypoglycaemia, hypokalaemia	Ketoacidosis: 0.1–0.2 units/kg then 0.1 units/kg/h	Ketoacidosis: 10–20 units then 5–10 units/h. Sliding scale (p. 74). Hyperkalaemia (p. 101)

IV = intravenous. IM = intramuscular. SC = subcutaneous. PO = per os (oral). SL = sublingual. ET = endotracheal. od = once daily. bd = twice daily. tds = three times daily. qds = four times daily. NR = not recommended. Doses are intravenous and dilutions in 0.9% saline unless otherwise stated.

Drug	Description and perioperative indications	Cautions and contraindications	Side-effects	IV dose (paediatric)	IV dose (adult)
Isoprenaline	Synthetic catecholamine with potent beta adrenergic agonist activity. Emergency treatment of heart block or bradycardia unresponsive to atropine and beta-blocker overdose	Ischaemic heart disease, hyperthyroidism, diabetes mellitus	Tachycardia, arrhythmias, sweating, tremor	Infusion: $0.1-2\ \mu g/kg/min$	Infusion: $0.5-10\ \mu g/min$. (2 mg in 500 ml 5% dextrose at $7-150$ ml/h or 1 mg in 50 ml at $1.5-30$ ml/h)
Ketamine	Phencyclidine derivative producing dissociative anaesthesia. Induction/ maintenance of anaesthesia in high-risk or hypovolaemic patients	Emergence delirium reduced by benzodiazepines. Caution in hypertension. Control excess salivation with antimuscarinic agent	Bronchodilation. Increased ICP, blood pressure, uterine tone, salivation. Respiratory depression if given rapidly	Induction: $1-3$ mg/kg IV, $5-10$ mg/kg IM. Infusion: $1-3$ mg/kg/h	Induction: $1-3$ mg/kg IV, $5-10$ mg/kg IM. Infusion: $1-3$ mg/kg/h (analgesia only 0.2 mg/kg/h). Caudal: 0.5 mg/kg diluted in saline/local anaesthetic (preservative free only)
Ketorolac	NSAID analgesic for mild to moderate pain	Hypersensitivity to aspirin, asthma, severe renal impairment, peptic ulceration	Gastrointestinal upset or bleeding, bronchospasm, tinnitus, fluid retention, platelet inhibition	Slow IV/IM: 0.5 mg/kg up to 30 mg qds	Slow IV/IM: 10 mg then $10-30$ mg every $4-6$ h (maximum daily dose 90 mg -60 mg in elderly)

IV = intravenous. IM = intramuscular. SC = subcutaneous. PO = per os (oral). SL = sublingual. ET = endotracheal. od = once daily. bd = twice daily. tds = three times daily. qds = four times daily. NR = not recommended. Doses are intravenous and dilutions in 0.9% saline unless otherwise stated.

Drug	Description and perioperative indications	Cautions and contraindications	Side-effects	IV dose (paediatric)	IV dose (adult)
Labetalol	Combined α (mild) and β adrenergic receptor antagonist. Blood pressure control without reflex tachycardia. Duration 2–4 h	Asthma, heart failure, AV block, verapamil treatment	Hypotension, bradycardia, bronchospasm	0.2 mg/kg boluses up to 1 mg/kg. Infusion: 1–3 mg/kg/h	5 mg increments up to 100 mg. Infusion: 20–160 mg/h
Lansoprazole (Zoton®)	Proton pump inhibitor. Reduction of gastric acid secretion		Headache, diarrhoea	PO: 0.3–0.6 mg/kg od	PO: 15–30 mg od
Levobupivacaine	Levorotatory enantiomer of bupivacaine with reduced cardiotoxicity	See bupivacaine	See bupivacaine	See bupivacaine	See bupivacaine
Lidocaine (lignocaine)	Amide type local anaesthetic: 1. Treatment of ventricular arrhythmias. 2. Reduction of pressor response to intubation. 3. Local anaesthetic — rapid onset, duration 30–90 min (prolonged by adrenaline)	Adrenaline-containing solutions contain preservative	Toxicity: tongue/ circumoral numbness, restlessness, tinnitus, seizures, cardiac arrest	1. Antiarrhythmic: 1 mg/kg then 10–50 µg/kg/min. 2. Attenuation of pressor response: 1.5 mg/kg 3. Local anaesthesia: 0.5–2% solution. Maximum dose dependent upon injection site— 3 mg/kg/4 h (6 mg/kg with adrenaline)	1. Antiarrhythmic: 1 mg/kg then 1–4 mg/min. 2. Attenuation of pressor response: 1.5 mg/kg. 3. Local anaesthesia: 0.5–2% solution. Maximum dose dependent upon injection site— 3 mg/kg/4 h (6 mg/kg with adrenaline)

IV = intravenous. IM = intramuscular. SC = subcutaneous. PO = per os (oral). SL = sublingual. ET = endotracheal. od = once daily. bd = twice daily. tds = three times daily. qds = four times daily. NR = not recommended. Doses are intravenous and dilutions in 0.9% saline unless otherwise stated

Drug	Description and perioperative indications	Cautions and contraindications	Side-effects	IV dose (paediatric)	IV dose (adult)
Loratidine (Clarityn®)	Non-sedative antihistamine. Relief of allergy, urticaria	Prostatic hypertrophy, urinary retention, glaucoma, porphyria	Dry mouth	<2 years NR. PO: 0.2 mg/kg up to 10 mg od	PO: 10 mg od
Lorazepam	Benzodiazepine: 1. Sedation or premedication. 2. Status epilepticus. Duration 6–10 h	Decreased requirement for anaesthetic agents	Respiratory depression in combination with opioids. Amnesia		1. PO: 2–4 mg 1–2 h preop. 2. IV: 2–4 mg
Lormetazepam	Benzodiazepine hypnotic sedative premed.	Decreased requirement for anaesthetic agents	Respiratory depression in combination with opioids. Amnesia		0.5–1.5 mg 1–2 h preop. (elderly 0.5 mg)
Magnesium sulphate	Essential mineral used to treat: 1. Hypomagnesaemia 2. Arrhythmias 3. Eclamptic seizures. Magnesium sulphate 50% = 500 mg/ml = 2 mmol Mg^{2+}/ml. Normal plasma level Mg^{2+} 1.5–2.2 mEq/litre	Potentiates muscle relaxants. Monitoring of serum level essential during treatment. Heart block	CNS depression, hypotension	1. Hypomagnesaemia: 0.2 ml/kg 50% solution over 20 min	1. Hypomagnesaemia: 10–15 mg/kg over 20 min, then 1 g/h. 2. Arrhythmias: 2 g over 10 min. 3. Eclampsia: 4 g over 10 min then 1 g/h for 24 h

IV = intravenous. IM = intramuscular. SC = subcutaneous. PO = per os (oral). SL = sublingual. ET = endotracheal. od = once daily. bd = twice daily. tds = three times daily. qds = four times daily. NR = not recommended. Doses are intravenous and dilutions in 0.9% saline unless otherwise stated.

Drug	Description and perioperative indications	Cautions and contraindications	Side-effects	IV dose (paediatric)	IV dose (adult)
Mannitol	Osmotic diuretic used for renal protection and reduction of intracranial pressure. 20% solution = 20 g/100 ml	Extracellular volume expansion especially in severe renal or cardiovascular disease		0.25–0.5 g/kg	0.25–1 g/kg (typically 0.5 g/kg of 20% solution)
Metaraminol (Aramine®)	Potent direct acting α adrenergic sympathomimetic. Treatment of hypotension. Duration 20–60 min	MAOIs, pregnancy. Caution in elderly and hypertensives. Extravasation can cause necrosis	Hypertension, reflex bradycardia, arrhythmias, decreased renal and placental perfusion	10 μg/kg then 0.1–1 μg/kg/min	0.5–2 mg. Dilute 10 mg in 20 ml saline and give 0.5–1 ml increments (increase dilution in elderly)
Methohexitone	Short-acting barbiturate induction agent useful for E.C.T. Duration 5–10 min. 1% solution = 10 mg/ml	Porphyria. Premedication reduces excitation at induction	Excitatory phenomenon, hypotension, respiratory depression, hiccups	1–2 mg/kg	1–1.5 mg/kg. Infusion: 50–150 μg/kg/min
Methoxamine (Vasoxine®)	Potent direct-acting α₁ adrenergic sympathomimetic. Treatment of hypotension. Duration 15–60 min	MAOIs, pregnancy. Caution in elderly and hypertensives. Extravasation can cause necrosis	Hypertension, reflex bradycardia, arrhythmias, decreased renal and placental perfusion	10 μg/kg increment	1–2 mg. Dilute 20 mg in 20 ml saline and give 0.5–1 ml increments (increase dilution in elderly)

IV = intravenous. IM = intramuscular. SC = subcutaneous. PO = per os (oral). SL = sublingual. ET = endotracheal. od = once daily. bd = twice daily. tds = three times daily. qds = four times daily. NR = not recommended. Doses are intravenous and dilutions in 0.9% saline unless otherwise stated.

Drug	Description and perioperative indications	Cautions and contraindications	Side-effects	IV dose (paediatric)	IV dose (adult)
Methylthio-ninium chloride (methylene blue)	1. Treatment of methaemoglobinaemia. 2. Ureteric identification during surgery (renally excreted). 3. Identification of parathyroid glands during surgery	G-6-PD deficiency. Blue colouration causes acute changes in pulse oximetry readings	Tachycardia, nausea, stains skin	1–4 mg/kg slow IV	1–2 mg/kg slow IV
Metoclopramide	Dopaminergic anti-emetic which increases gastric emptying and lower oesophageal sphincter tone	Hypertension in phaeochromocytoma. Inhibits plasma cholinesterase	Extrapyramidal/dystonic reactions (treat with benztropine or procyclidine)	PO/IM/IV: 0.15 mg/kg up to 10 mg tds	PO/IM/IV: 10 mg tds
Metoprolol	Cardioselective beta-blocker	Asthma, heart failure, AV block, verapamil treatment	Causes bradycardia, hypotension and decreased cardiac contractility	0.1 mg/kg up to 5 mg over 10 min	1–5 mg over 10 min
Metronidazole	Antibiotic with activity against anaerobic bacteria	Disulfiram (Antabuse®) like effect		7.5 mg/kg tds. PR: 125–500 mg tds	500 mg tds. PR: 1 g tds

IV = intravenous. IM = intramuscular. SC = subcutaneous. PO = per os (oral). SL = sublingual. ET = endotracheal. od = once daily. bd = twice daily. tds = three times daily. qds = four times daily. NR = not recommended. Doses are intravenous and dilutions in 0.9% saline unless otherwise stated.

Drug	Description and perioperative indications	Cautions and contraindications	Side-effects	IV dose (paediatric)	IV dose (adult)
Midazolam	Short-acting benzodiazepine. Sedative, anxiolytic, amnesic, anticonvulsant. Duration 20–60 min. Oral administration of IV preparation effective though larger dose required	Reduce dose in elderly (very sensitive).	Hypotension, respiratory depression, apnoea	0.1–0.2mg/kg. PO: 0.5 mg/kg (use IV preparation in orange juice). Intranasal: 0.2–0.3 mg/kg (use 5 mg/ml IV preparation)	Sedation: 0.5–5 mg, titrate to effect. PO: 0.5 mg/kg (use IV preparation in orange juice). IM: 2.5–10 mg
Milrinone	Selective phosphodiesterase inhibitor used in cardiac failure with increased filling pressures. Inodilator used after cardiac surgery	Stenotic valvular disease, cardiomyopathy	Arrhythmias, hypotension, nausea	50 μg/kg over 10 min, then 0.375– 0.75 μg/kg/min. Maximum 1.13 mg/kg/day	50 μg/kg over 10 min, then 0.375– 0.75 μg/kg/min. Maximum 1.13 mg/kg/day
Mivacurium	Short-acting non-depolarizing muscle relaxant. Metabolized by plasma cholinesterase. Duration 6–16 min (often variable). Enhanced duration if low plasma cholinesterase. May be antagonized by neostigmine—but not usually necessary	Neuromuscular block potentiated by aminoglycosides, loop diuretics, magnesium, lithium, hypothermia, hypokalaemia, acidosis, prior use of suxamethonium, volatile anaesthetic agents	Enhanced effect in myasthenia gravis, effects antagonized by anticholinesterases, e.g. neostigmine. Monitor response with peripheral nerve stimulator. Some histamine release. Avoid in asthma	Intubation: 0.15–0.2 mg/kg. Maintenance: 0.1 mg/kg. Infusion: 10–15 μg/kg/min	Intubation: 0.07–0.25 mg/kg (doses of 0.07, 0.15, 0.2, and 0.25 mg/kg produce block for 13, 16, 20, and 23 min respectively). Maintenance: 0.1 mg/kg. Infusion: 0.3–0.6 μg/kg/h

IV = intravenous. IM = intramuscular. SC = subcutaneous. PO = per os (oral). SL = sublingual. ET = endotracheal. od = once daily. bd = twice daily. tds = three times daily. qds = four times daily. NR = not recommended. Doses are intravenous and dilutions in 0.9% saline unless otherwise stated.

Drug	Description and perioperative indications	Cautions and contraindications	Side effects	IV dose (paediatric)	IV dose (adult)
Morphine	Opioid analgesic	Prolonged risk of respiratory depression, pruritus, nausea when used via spinal/epidural	Histamine release, hypotension, bronchospasm, nausea, vomiting, pruritus, dysphoria	PO: 0.2–0.4 mg/kg 4-hourly. IV/SC: 0.1–0.2 mg/kg 4-hourly (infants 0.1–0.15 mg/kg 4-hourly). Infusion: 10–40 μg/kg/h (lower range in neonates)	IV: 2.5–10 mg. IM/SC: 5–10 mg 4-hourly. PO: 10–30 mg 4-hourly. PCA: 1 mg 5 min lockout. Infusion: 1–3.5 mg/h. Epidural: 2–5 mg preservative free. Spinal: 0.1–1 mg preservative free
Naloxone	Pure opioid antagonist. Can be used in low doses to reverse pruritus associated with epidural opiates and as depot IM injection in newborn of mothers given opioids	Beware renarcotization if reversing long-acting opioid. Caution in opioid addicts—may precipitate acute withdrawal		5–10 μg/kg. Infusion: 5–20 μg/kg/h. IM depot in newborn: 200 μg. Pruritus: 0.5 μg/kg	200–400 μg titrated to desired effect. Treatment of opioid/epidural pruritus: 100 μg bolus plus 300 μg added to IV fluids
Naproxen	NSAID analgesic for mild to moderate pain	Hypersensitivity to aspirin, asthma, severe renal impairment, peptic ulceration	Gastrointestinal upset or bleeding, bronchospasm, tinnitus, fluid retention, platelet inhibition	>5 years. PO: 5 mg/kg bd (>5 years)	PO: 500 mg bd

IV = intravenous. IM = intramuscular. SC = subcutaneous. PO = per os (oral). SL = sublingual. ET = endotracheal. od = once daily. bd = twice daily. tds = three times daily. qds = four times daily. NR = not recommended. Doses are intravenous and dilutions in 0.9% saline unless otherwise stated.

Drug	Description and perioperative indications	Cautions and contraindications	Side-effects	IV dose (paediatric)	IV dose (adult)
Neostigmine	Anticholinesterase used for: 1. Reversal of non-depolarizing muscle relaxant. 2. Treatment of myasthenia gravis. Duration 60 min IV (2–4 h PO)	Administer with antimuscarinic agent	Bradycardia, excessive salivation (muscarinic effects)	50 μg/kg with atropine 20 μg/kg or glycopyrrolate 10 μg/kg	1. 50–70 μg/kg (maximum 5 mg) with atropine 10–20 μg/kg or glycopyrrolate 10–15 μg/kg. 2. PO: 15–30 mg at suitable intervals
Neostigmine and glycopyrrolate	Combination of neostigmine methylsulphate (2.5 mg) and glycopyrrolate (500 μg) per 1 ml	See neostigmine.	See neostigmine.	0.02 ml/kg (dilute 1 ml with 4 ml saline, give 0.1 ml/kg)	1–2 ml over 30 s
Nimodipine	Calcium channel blocker used to prevent vascular spasm after subarachnoid haemorrhage	Via central catheter, Cerebral oedema, raised intracranial pressure, grapefruit juice	Hypotension, flushing, headache	Infusion: 0.1–1 μg/kg/min	PO: 60 mg 4-hourly (maximum 360 mg/day). Infusion: 0.5 mg/h increasing over 2 h to 2 mg/h
Nitroprusside (sodium—SNP)	Nitric oxide generating potent peripheral vasodilator. Controlled hypotension	Protect solution from light. Metabolism yields cyanide which is then converted to thiocyanate	Methaemoglobin-aemia, hypotension, tachycardia. Cyanide causes tachycardia, sweating, acidosis	Infusion: 0.3–1.5 μg/kg/min	Infusion: 0.3–1.5 μg/kg/min. Maximum dose: 3.5 mg/kg

IV = intravenous. IM = intramuscular. SC = subcutaneous. PO = per os (oral). SL = sublingual. ET = endotracheal. od = once daily. bd = twice daily. tds = three

Drug	Description and perioperative indications	Cautions and contraindications	Side-effects	IV dose (paediatric)	IV dose (adult)
Noradrenaline	Potent catecholamine α adrenergic agonist. Vasoconstriction	Via central catheter only. Potentiated by MAOI and tricyclic antidepressants	Reflex bradycardia, arrhythmia, hypertension	Infusion: $0.1–1$ $\mu g/kg/min$	Infusion: $2–20$ $\mu g/min$ ($0.04–0.4$ $\mu g/kg/min$)
Octreotide	Somatostatin analogue used in treatment of carcinoid, acromegaly, and variceal bleeding (unlicensed use)	Pituitary tumour expansion, reduced need for anti-diabetic treatments	GI disturbance, gallstones, hyper- and hypoglycaemia	SC: 1 $\mu g/kg$ od/bd	SC: 50 μg od tds increased up to 200 μg tds. IV: 50 μg diluted in saline (ECG monitoring)
Omeprazole (Losec®)	Proton pump inhibitor. Reduction in gastric acid secretion		Headache, diarrhoea	PO: 0.4–0.8 mg/kg up to 40 mg od	PO: 20–40 mg od. Premedication PO: 40 mg evening before and morning of surgery
Ondansetron	Serotonin (5-HT3) receptor antagonist anti-emetic		Hypotension, headache, flushing	>2 years. Slow IV: 100 $\mu g/kg$ (maximum 4 mg) qds	Slow IV/IM: 4 mg qds
Oxybuprocaine (Benoxinate®)	Local anaesthetic. Topical anaesthesia to cornea				0.4% solution. 0.5 ml eye drops

IV = intravenous. IM = intramuscular. SC = subcutaneous. PO = per os (oral). SL = sublingual. ET = endotracheal. od = once daily. bd = twice daily. tds = three times daily. qds = four times daily. NR = not recommended. Doses are intravenous and dilutions in 0.9% saline unless otherwise stated.

Drug	Description and perioperative indications	Cautions and contraindications	Side-effects	IV dose (paediatric)	IV dose (adult)
Oxycodone	Opioid used for moderate pain, often used in palliative care		Nausea, vomiting, dysphoria, drowsiness		PO: Oxynorm® 5 mg 4–6-hourly increased up to 400 mg/day as required. Oxycontin® 10 mg bd, increased up to 400 mg/day as required
Oxytocin (Syntocinon®)	Nonapeptide hormone which stimulates uterine contraction. Induction of labour and prevention of postpartum haemorrhage		Vasodilatation, hypotension, flushing, tachycardia		Postpartum slow IV: 5 units, followed by infusion if required (5–20 units in 500 ml dextrose at 0.02–0.04 units/min)
Pancuronium	Long-acting aminosteroid non-depolarizing muscle relaxant. Little histamine release. Duration 45–65 min	Increased heart rate and blood pressure due to vagolysis and sympathetic stimulation. Neuromuscular block potentiated by aminoglycosides, loop diuretics, magnesium, lithium, hypothermia, hypokalaemia, acidosis, prior use of suxamethonium, volatile anaesthetic agents	Enhanced effect in myasthenia gravis, effects antagonized by anticholin-esterases, e.g. neostigmine. Monitor response with peripheral nerve stimulator	Intubation: 0.08–0.15 mg/kg. Maintenance: 0.01–0.05 mg/kg	Intubation: 0.04–0.1 mg/kg. Maintenance: 0.01–0.05 mg/kg

IV = intravenous. IM = intramuscular. SC = subcutaneous. PO = per os (oral). SL = sublingual. ET = endotracheal. od = once daily. bd = twice daily. tds = three

Drug	Description and perioperative indications	Cautions and contraindications	Side-effects	IV dose (paediatric)	IV dose (adult)
Pantoprazole	Proton pump inhibitor used to inhibit gastric acid secretion	Liver disease, pregnancy	Headache, diarrhoea, pruritus, bronchospasm		Slow IV: (10–15 min): 40 mg od. PO: 40 mg od
Paracetamol	Mild to moderate analgesic and antipyretic		Liver damage in overdose	PO: 20 mg/kg then 15 mg/kg 4-hourly. PR: 30 mg/kg then 20 mg/kg 6-hourly. Maximum 90 mg/kg/day (neonates 60 mg/kg/day)	PO: 0.5–1 g qds
Paraldehyde	Status epilepticus			Deep IM: 0.2 ml/kg. PR: 0.3 ml/kg	Deep IM: 5–10 ml. PR: 10–20 ml
Pethidine	Synthetic opioid: 1. Analgesia (agent of choice in asthma). 2. Postoperative shivering	Seizures possible in high dosage—maximum daily dose 1 g/day (20 mg/kg/day). MAOI	Respiratory depression, hypotension, dysphoria	IV/IM/SC: 0.5–1 mg/kg. Infusion: 5 mg/kg in 50 ml 5% dextrose at 1–3 ml/h (100–300 µg/kg/h)	IM/SC: 25–100 mg 3-hourly. IV: 25–50 mg. Epidural: 50–100 mg in 10 ml saline or local anaesthetic. PCA: 10 mg/5 min lockout. Shivering: 10–25 mg IV

IV = intravenous. IM = intramuscular. SC = subcutaneous. PO = per os (oral). SL = sublingual. ET = endotracheal. od = once daily. bd = twice daily. tds = three times daily. qds = four times daily. NR = not recommended. Doses are intravenous and dilutions in 0.9% saline unless otherwise stated.

Drug	Description and perioperative indications	Cautions and contraindications	Side-effects	IV dose (paediatric)	IV dose (adult)
Phentolamine (Rogitine®)	α_1 and α_2 adrenergic antagonist. Peripheral vasodilatation and controlled hypotension. Treatment of extravasation. Duration 10 min	Treat excessive hypotension with noradrenaline or methoxamine (not adrenaline/ephedrine due to β effects)	Hypotension, tachycardia, flushing	0.1 mg/kg then 5–50 µg/kg/min	2–5 mg. (10 mg in 10 ml saline, 1 ml aliquots)
Phenylephrine	Selective direct-acting α adrenergic agonist. Peripheral vasoconstriction and treatment of hypotension. Duration 20 min	MAOI. Caution in elderly or cardiovascular disease	Reflex bradycardia, arrhythmias	2–10 µg/kg then 1–5 µg/kg/min	0.1–0.5mg increments. (10 mg in 20 ml saline, 1 ml aliquots.) IM: 2–5 mg. Infusion: 30–60 µg/min
Phenytoin	Anticonvulsant and treatment of digoxin toxicity. Serum levels 10–20 mg/litre (40–80 µmol/litre)	Avoid in AV heart block and pregnancy. Monitor ECG	Hypotension, AV conduction defects, ataxia	Loading dose: 15 mg/kg over 1 h.	Loading dose: 15 mg/kg over 1 h (dilute to 10 mg/ml in saline)
Piperacurium	Piperazinium derivative long-acting non depolarizing muscle relaxant. Duration 45–120 min	Neuromuscular block potentiated by aminoglycosides, loop diuretics, magnesium, lithium, hypothermia, hypokalaemia, acidosis, prior use of suxamethonium, volatile anaesthetic agents	Enhanced effect in myasthenia gravis. Effects antagonized by anticholinesterases, e.g. neostigmine. Monitor response with peripheral nerve stimulator	Intubation: 0.08 mg/kg. Maintenance: 0.01–0.04 mg/kg	Intubation: 0.08 mg/kg. Maintenance: 0.01–0.04 mg/kg

IV = intravenous. IM = intramuscular. SC = subcutaneous. PO = per os (oral). SL = sublingual. ET = endotracheal. od = once daily. bd = twice daily. tds = three

Drug	Description and perioperative indications	Cautions and contraindications	Side-effects	IV dose (paediatric)	IV dose (adult)
Piroxicam	NSAID analgesic for moderate pain. High incidence of side-effects	Hypersensitivity to aspirin, asthma, severe renal impairment, peptic ulceration. Avoid in porphyria	Gastrointestinal upset or bleeding, bronchospasm, tinnitus, fluid retention, platelet inhibition		PO/PR: 10–30 mg od
Potassium chloride	Electrolyte replacement	Dilute solution before administration	Rapid infusion can cause cardiac arrest. High concentration causes phlebitis	0.5 mmol/kg over 1 h. Maintenance: 2–4 mmol/kg/day	10–20 mmol/h (max. concentration 40 mmol/litre peripherally). With ECG monitoring: up to 20–40 mmol/h via central line (max 200 mmol/day)
Prednisolone	Orally active corticosteroid. Less mineralocorticoid action than hydrocortisone	Adrenal suppression, severe systemic infections	Dyspepsia and ulceration, osteoporosis, myopathy, psychosis, impaired healing, diabetes mellitus	PO: 1–2 mg/kg od. Asthma: 0.5–1 mg/ kg qds day 1, bd day 2, then 1 mg/kg/day. Croup: 4 mg/kg then 1 mg/kg tds	PO: 10–60 mg od, reduced to 2.5– 15 mg od.

IV = intravenous. IM = intramuscular. SC = subcutaneous. PO = per os (oral). SL = sublingual. ET = endotracheal. od = once daily. bd = twice daily. tds = three times daily. qds = four times daily. NR = not recommended. Doses are intravenous and dilutions in 0.9% saline unless otherwise stated.

Drug	Description and perioperative indications	Cautions and contraindications	Side-effects	IV dose (paediatric)	IV dose (adult)
Prilocaine	Amide type local anaesthetic. Less toxic than lidocaine (lignocaine). Used for infiltration and IVRA. Rapid onset. Duration 30–90 min (prolonged by adrenaline)	Adrenaline-containing solutions contain preservative. Significant methaemoglobinaemia if dose >600 mg	Toxicity: tongue/circumoral numbness, restlessness, tinnitus, seizures, cardiac arrest	NR <6 months. 0.5–2% solution. Maximum dose dependent upon injection site— 6 mg/kg/4 h (9 mg/kg with adrenaline)	Local anaesthesia: 0.5–2% solution. Maximum dose dependent upon injection site— 6 mg/kg/4 h (8 mg/kg with adrenaline)
Prochlorperazine	Phenothiazine anti-emetic	Hypotension on rapid IV administration. Neuroleptic malignant syndrome	Tardive dyskinesia and extrapyramidal symptoms	>10 kg. PO: 0.1–0.4 mg/kg tds. IM: 0.1–0.2 mg/kg tds	IM: 12.5 mg tds. PO: 20 mg then 5–10 mg tds
Procyclidine	Antimuscarinic used in acute treatment of drug-induced dystonic reactions (except tardive dyskinesia)	Glaucoma, gastrointestinal obstruction	Urinary retention, dry mouth, blurred vision	<2 years: 0.5–2 mg. 2–10 years: 2–5 mg	IV: 5 mg. IM: 5–10 mg repeat after 20 min if needed
Promethazine (Phenergan®)	Phenothiazine, antihistamine, anticholinergic, antiemetic sedative. Paediatric sedation		Extrapyramidal reactions	>2 years. Sedation/premed PO: 1–2 mg/kg. Anti-emetic: 0.2–0.5 mg/kg	PO/IM: 25–50 mg

IV = intravenous. IM = intramuscular. SC = subcutaneous. PO = per os (oral). SL = sublingual. ET = endotracheal. od = once daily. bd = twice daily. tds = three times daily. qds = four times daily. NR = not recommended. Doses are intravenous and dilutions in 0.9% saline unless otherwise stated.

Drug	Description and perioperative indications	Cautions and contraindications	Side-effects	IV dose (paediatric)	IV dose (adult)
Propofol	Di-isopropylphenol intravenous induction agent. Rapid recovery and little nausea. Agent of choice for day stay surgery, sedation or laryngeal mask insertion	Reduce dose in elderly or haemodynamically unstable. Not recommended for caesarean section. Allergy to eggs or soybean oil. Caution in epilepsy	Apnoea, hypotension, pain on injection. Myoclonic spasms, rarely convulsions	Induction: 2–5 mg/kg. Infusion: 4–15 mg/kg/h. NR induction <1 month. NR maintenance <3 years	Induction: 2–3 mg/kg. Infusion: 6–10 mg/kg/h. TCI: initially 4–8 µg/ml then 3–6 µg/ml (reduce in elderly)
Propranolol	Non-selective β adrenergic antagonist. Controlled hypotension	Asthma, heart failure, AV block, verapamil treatment	Bradycardia, hypotension, AV block, bronchospasm	0.1 mg/kg over 5 min	1 mg increments up to 5–10 mg
Protamine	Basic protein produced from salmon sperm. Heparin antagonist	Weakly anticoagulant and marked histamine release. Risk of allergy	Severe hypotension, pulmonary hypertension, bronchospasm, flushing	Slow IV: 1 mg per 1 mg heparin (100 units) to be reversed	Slow IV: 1 mg per 1 mg heparin (100 units) to be reversed
Pyridostigmine	Long-acting anticholinesterase used in treatment of myasthenia gravis	See neostigmine	See neostigmine	PO: 1–3 mg/kg at intervals (4–12-hourly)	PO: 30–120 mg at intervals through day (maximum 1.2 g/day)

IV = intravenous. IM = intramuscular. SC = subcutaneous. PO = per os (oral). SL = sublingual. ET = endotracheal. od = once daily. bd = twice daily. tds = three times daily. qds = four times daily. NR = not recommended. Doses are intravenous and dilutions in 0.9% saline unless otherwise stated.

Drug	Description and perioperative indications	Cautions and contraindications	Side-effects	IV dose (paediatric)	IV dose (adult)
Ranitidine	Histamine (H$_2$) receptor antagonist. Reduction in gastric acid secretion	Porphyria	Tachycardia	IV: 1 mg/kg slowly tds. PO: 2–4 mg/kg bd	IV: 50 mg (diluted in 20 ml saline, given over 2 min) qds. IM: 50 mg qds. PO: 150 mg bd or 300 mg od
Remifentanil	Ultra short-acting opioid used to supplement general anaesthesia. Metabolized by non-specific esterases not plasma cholinesterase. Duration 5–10 min. Start at 0.1 µg/kg/min and adjust dose as necessary		Muscle rigidity, respiratory depression, hypotension, bradycardia	0.1–0.4 µg/kg/min	Slow bolus: up to 1 µg/kg. Infusion (IPPV): 0.1–0.5 µg/kg/min. Infusion (SV): 0.025–0.1 mg/kg/min

IV = intravenous. IM = intramuscular. SC = subcutaneous. PO = per os (oral). SL = sublingual. ET = endotracheal. od = once daily. bd = twice daily. tds = three times daily. qds = four times daily. NR = not recommended. Doses are intravenous and dilutions in 0.9% saline unless otherwise stated.

Drug	Description and perioperative indications	Cautions and contraindications	Side-effects	IV dose (paediatric)	IV dose (adult)
Rocuronium	Rapidly acting aminosteroid non-depolarizing muscle relaxant. Rapid sequence induction (avoiding suxamethonium). Duration 10–60 min (variable)	Neuromuscular block potentiated by aminoglycosides, loop diuretics, magnesium, lithium, hypothermia, acidosis, prior use of suxamethonium, volatile anaesthetic agents	Mild tachycardia. Enhanced effect in myasthenia gravis, effects antagonized by anticholinesterases, e.g. neostigmine. Monitor response with peripheral nerve stimulator	Intubation: 0.6–1 mg/kg. Maintenance: 0.1–0.15 mg/kg. Infusion: 0.3–0.6 mg/kg/h	Intubation: 0.6–1 mg/kg. Maintenance: 0.1–0.15 mg/kg. Infusion: 0.3–0.6 mg/kg/h
Rofecoxib (Vioxx®)	NSAID with selective inhibition of cyclo-oxygenase II (Cox II) enzyme. May therefore have reduced gastrointestinal side-effects	Hypersensitivity to aspirin, asthma, severe renal impairment, peptic ulceration			PO: 12.5–25 mg od
Ropivacaine	Amide type local anaesthetic agent. Possibly less motor block than other agents. Duration similar to bupivacaine, but lower toxicity			0.2–1% solution. Maximum dose dependent upon injection site – 3–4 mg/kg/4 h	0.2–1% solution. Infiltration/epidural: maximum dose dependent upon injection site – 3–4 mg/kg/4 h

IV = intravenous. IM = intramuscular. SC = subcutaneous. PO = per os (oral). SL = sublingual. ET = endotracheal. od = once daily. bd = twice daily. tds = three times daily. qds = four times daily. NR = not recommended. Doses are intravenous and dilutions in 0.9% saline unless otherwise stated.

Drug	Description and perioperative indications	Cautions and contraindications	Side-effects	IV dose (paediatric)	IV dose (adult)
Salbutamol	β_2 receptor agonist. Treatment of bronchospasm	Hypokalaemia possible	Tremor, vasodilatation, tachycardia	4 μg/kg slow IV then 0.1–1 μg/kg/min. Nebulizer: <5 years 2.5 mg, >5 years 2.5–5 mg	250 μg slow IV then 5 μg/min (up to 20 μg/min). Nebulizer: 2.5–5 mg prn
Suxamethonium	Depolarizing muscle relaxant. Rapid short-acting muscle paralysis. Phase II block develops with repeated doses (>8 mg/kg). Store at 2–8 °C	Prolonged block in plasma cholinesterase deficiency, hypokalaemia, hypocalcaemia. Malignant hyperthermia, myopathies	Increased intraocular pressure. Increased serum potassium (normally 0.5 mmol/litre — greater in burns, trauma, upper motor neuron injury). Bradycardia with second dose	1–2 mg/kg	1–1.5 mg/kg. Infusion: 0.5–10 mg/min
Sufentanil	More potent thiamyl analogue of fentanyl (five times potency). Analgesia. Duration 20–45 min	See fentanyl	See fentanyl		Analgesia: 10–30 μg (0.2–0.6 μg/kg). Anaesthesia: 0.6–4 μg/kg

IV = intravenous. IM = intramuscular. SC = subcutaneous. PO = per os (oral). SL = sublingual. ET = endotracheal. od = once daily. bd = twice daily. tds = three times daily. qds = four times daily. NR = not recommended. Doses are intravenous and dilutions in 0.9% saline unless otherwise stated.

Drug	Description and perioperative indications	Cautions and contraindications	Side-effects	IV dose (paediatric)	IV dose (adult)
Teicoplanin	Glycopeptide antibiotic with activity against aerobic and anaerobic Gram-positive bacteria		Ototoxicity, nephrotoxicity	10 mg/kg for 3 doses 12 hourly then 6 mg/kg od	IV/IM: 400 mg for 3 doses 12 hourly then 200 mg od
Temazepam	Benzodiazepine. Sedation or premedication. Duration 1–2 h	Decreased requirement for anaesthetic agents	Respiratory depression in combination with opioids. Amnesia	PO: 0.5–1 mg/kg preop.	PO: 10–40 mg 1 h preop. (elderly 10–20 mg)
Tenoxicam	NSAID analgesic for mild to moderate pain	Hypersensitivity to aspirin, asthma, severe renal impairment, peptic ulceration	Gastrointestinal upset or bleeding, bronchospasm, tinnitus, fluid retention, platelet inhibition		PO: 20 mg od. IV/IM: 20 mg od
Tetracaine (amethocaine) (Ametop®)	Ester type local anaesthetic. Topical analgesia prior to venepuncture. Ametop® gel contains 4% amethocaine. (Also available as eye drops, but has temporary disruptive effect on corneal epithelium). Duration 4 h	Apply only to intact skin under occlusive dressing. Remove after 45 min		As adult. <1month NR	Each tube expels 1 g (sufficient for area 6 x 5 cm)

IV = intravenous. IM = intramuscular. SC = subcutaneous. PO = per os (oral). SL = sublingual. ET = endotracheal. od = once daily. bd = twice daily. tds = three times daily. qds = four times daily. NR = not recommended. Doses are intravenous and dilutions in 0.9% saline unless otherwise stated.

Drug	Description and perioperative indications	Cautions and contraindications	Side-effects	IV dose (paediatric)	IV dose (adult)
Thiopental	Short-acting thiobarbiturate. Induction of anaesthesia, anticonvulsant, cerebral protection. Recovery due to redistribution	Accumulation with repeated doses. Caution in hypovolaemia and elderly. Porphyria	Hypotension	Induction: neonate 2–4 mg/kg, child 5–6 mg/kg.	Induction/cerebral protection: 3–5 mg/kg. Anticonvulsant: 0.5–2 mg/kg prn
Tramadol	Opioid analgesic thought to have less respiratory depression, constipation, euphoria, or abuse potential than other opioids. Has opioid and non-opioid mechanisms of action	Only 30% antagonized by naloxone. Caution in epilepsy. Previously not recommended for intra-operative use. MAOI	Nausea, dizziness, dry mouth. Increased side effects in conjunction with other opioids		PO: 50–100 mg 4-hourly. Slow IV/IM: 50–100 mg 4-hourly (100mg initially then 50 mg increments to maximum 250 mg). Maximum 600 mg/day
Tranexamic acid	Inhibits plasminogen activation reducing fibrin dissolution by plasmin. Reduced haemorrhage in prostatectomy or dental extraction	Avoid in thromboembolic disease and renal impairment	Dizziness, nausea	PO: 15–20 mg/kg tds	Slow IV: 0.5–1 g tds. PO: 15–25 mg/kg tds

IV = intravenous. IM = intramuscular. SC = subcutaneous. PO = per os (oral). SL = sublingual. ET = endotracheal. od = once daily. bd = twice daily. tds = three times daily. qds = four times daily. NR = not recommended. Doses are intravenous and dilutions in 0.9% saline unless otherwise stated.

Drug	Description and perioperative indications	Cautions and contraindications	Side-effects	IV dose (paediatric)	IV dose (adult)
Triamcinolone hexacetonide (Lederspan®)	Relatively insoluble corticosteroid for depot injection. (Epidural unlicensed use)	Dose depends upon site of injection. Strict asepsis essential. Dilute 20 mg/ml solution prior to use		Intra-articular or intrasynovial: 2.5–15 mg	Intra-articular or intrasynovial: 2–30 mg. Epidural: 40–60 mg diluted with local anaesthetic (triamcinolone 4 mg = prednisolone 5 mg)
Trimetaphan	Ganglion blocking hypotensive agent	Tachyphylaxis with prolonged use	Tachycardia, mydriasis	0.04–0.1 mg/kg/min	2–4 mg/min
D-Tubocurare	Intermediate acting non-depolarizing muscle relaxant	Neuromuscular block potentiated by aminoglycosides, loop diuretics, magnesium, lithium, hypothermia, hypokalaemia, acidosis, prior use of suxamethonium, volatile anaesthetic agents. Asthma	Enhanced effect in myasthenia gravis. Effects antagonized by anticholinesterases. Hypotension due to histamine release and ganglion blockade	Intubation: 0.6 mg/kg. Maintenance: 0.15 mg/kg	Intubation: 0.3–0.6 mg/kg. Maintenance: 0.05–0.3 mg/kg

IV = intravenous. IM = intramuscular. SC = subcutaneous. PO = per os (oral). SL = sublingual. ET = endotracheal. od = once daily. bd = twice daily. tds = three times daily. qds = four times daily. NR = not recommended. Doses are intravenous and dilutions in 0.9% saline unless otherwise stated.

Drug	Description and perioperative indications	Cautions and contraindications	Side-effects	IV dose (paediatric)	IV dose (adult)
Vancomycin	Glycopeptide antibiotic with activity against aerobic and anaerobic Gram-positive bacteria. Peak level <30 mg/litre. Trough level <10 mg/litre	Avoid rapid infusion (hypotension, wheezing, urticaria, red man syndrome). Reduce dose in renal impairment	Ototoxicity, nephrotoxicity, phlebitis	>1 month: 15 mg/kg over 2 h tds	1 g over 100 min bd (check blood levels after third dose)
Vasopressin (Pitressin®)	ADH used in treatment of diabetes insipidus	Extreme caution in coronary vascular disease	Pallor, coronary vasoconstriction, water intoxication	Diabetes insipidus SC/IM: 2–10 units 4-hourly	Diabetes insipidus SC/IM: 5–20 units 4-hourly
Vecuronium	Aminosteroid non-depolarizing muscle relaxant. Cardiostable and no histamine release. Duration 30–45 min	Neuromuscular block potentiated by aminoglycosides, loop diuretics, magnesium, lithium, hypothermia, hypokalaemia, acidosis, prior use of suxamethonium, volatile anaesthetic agents	Enhanced effect in myasthenia gravis. Effects antagonized by anticholin-esterases, e.g. neostigmine. Monitor response with peripheral nerve stimulator	Intubation: <4 months 10–20 μg/kg, plus increments as required >5 months 100 μg/kg	Intubation: 80–100 μg/kg. Maintenance: 20–30 μg/kg. Infusion: 0.8–1.4 μg/kg/min

IV = intravenous. IM = intramuscular. SC = subcutaneous. PO = per os (oral). SL = sublingual. ET = endotracheal. od = once daily. bd = twice daily. tds = three times daily. qds = four times daily. NR = not recommended. Doses are intravenous and dilutions in 0.9% saline unless otherwise stated.

Drug	Description and perioperative indications	Cautions and contraindications	Side-effects	IV dose (paediatric)	IV dose (adult)
Warfarin	Coumarin derivative oral anticoagulant. DVT prophylaxis: INR 2.0–2.5. DVT/PE treatment, AF, mitral valve disease: INR 2.5–3.0. Recurrent DVT/PE, prosthetic heart valve: INR 3.0–4.5	Pregnancy, peptic ulcer disease	Haemorrhage	PO: 0.2 mg/kg up to 10 mg od for 2 days, then 0.05–0.2 mg/kg od	PO: 10 mg od for 2 days then 3–9 mg od dependent on INR
Zolpidem	Short-acting imidazopyridine hypnotic with little hangover effect	Obstructive sleep apnoea, myasthenia gravis			PO: 10 mg nocte (elderly 5 mg)
Zopiclone	Short-acting cyclopyrrolone hypnotic with little hangover effect	Obstructive sleep apnoea, myasthenia gravis			PO: 7.5 mg nocte (elderly 3.75 mg)

IV = intravenous. IM = intramuscular. SC = subcutaneous. PO = per os (oral). SL = sublingual. ET = endotracheal. od = once daily. bd = twice daily. tds = three times daily. qds = four times daily. NR = not recommended. Doses are intravenous and dilutions in 0.9% saline unless otherwise stated.

Infusion regimes

Appendix 2

Drug	Indication	Diluent	Dose	Suggested regime (60 kg adult)	Infusion range	Initial rate (adult)	Comments
Adrenaline	Treatment of hypotension	0.9% saline, 5% dextrose	2–20 μg/min (0.04–0.4 μg/kg/min)	5 mg/50 ml (100 μg/ml)	1.2–12+ ml/h	5 ml/h	Via central catheter. Suggest 1 mg/50ml for initial intra-operative use (or 1 mg/500ml if no central access)
Alfentanil	Analgesia	0.9% saline, 5% dextrose	0.5–1 μg/kg/min	Undiluted (500 μg/ml)	0–8 ml/h	4 ml/h	1–2 mg can also be added to 50 ml propofol for infusion
Aminophylline	Bronchodilation	0.9% saline, 5% dextrose	0.5 mg/kg/h	250 mg/50 ml (5 mg/ml)	0–6 ml/h	6 ml/h	After 5 mg/kg slow IV bolus over 30 min
Amiodarone	Treatment of arrhythmias	5% dextrose only	Loading infusion 5 mg/kg over 1–2 h, then 900 mg over 24 h	300 mg/50 ml (6 mg/ml)	25–50 ml/h then 6 ml/h	25 ml/h	Via central line. Maximum 1.2 g in 24 h
Atracurium	Muscle relaxant	0.9% saline, 5% dextrose	0.3–0.6 mg/kg/h	undiluted (10 mg/ml)	1.5–4 ml/h	3 ml/h	Assess rate with nerve stimulator
Cis-atracurium	Muscle relaxant	0.9% saline, 5% dextrose	0.06–0.18 mg/kg/h	undiluted (2 mg/ml)	2–5 ml/h	5 ml/h	Assess rate with nerve stimulator

Alternative regimes for any infusion: 3 mg/kg/50 ml then 1 ml/hr = 1 μg/kg/min
3 mg/50 ml then 1 ml/hr = 1 μg/min

Drug	Indication	Diluent	Dose	Suggested regime (60 kg adult)	Infusion range	Initial rate (adult)	Comments
Digoxin	Rapid control of ventricular rate	0.9% saline, 5% dextrose	250–500 µg over 30–60 min	250–500 µg/ 50 ml	0–100 ml/h	50 ml/h	ECG monitoring suggested
Dobutamine	Cardiac failure/ inotrope	0.9% saline, 5% dextrose	2.5–10 µg/kg/min	250 mg/50 ml (5 mg/ml)	2–7 ml/h	2 ml/h	
Dopamine	Inotrope	0.9% saline, 5% dextrose	2–10 µg/kg/min	200 mg/50 ml (4 mg/ml)	2–9 ml/h	2 ml/h	Via central line
Dopexamine	Inotrope	0.9% saline, 5% dextrose	0.5–6 µg/kg/min	50 mg/50 ml (1 mg/ml)	2–22 ml/h	2 ml/h	May be given via large peripheral vein
Doxapram	Respiratory stimulant	0.9% saline, 5% dextrose	2–4 mg/min	200 mg/50 ml (4 mg/ml)	30–60 ml/h	30 ml/h	Maximum dose 4 mg/kg
Enoximone	Inodilator	0.9% saline only	90 µg/kg/min for 10–30 min, then 5–20 µg/kg/min	100 mg/50 ml (2 mg/ml)	9–36 ml/h	162 ml/h for 10–30 min	Maximum 24 mg/kg/day
Esmolol	Beta-blocker	0.9% saline, 5% dextrose	50–200 µg/ kg/min	2.5 g/50 ml (50 mg/ml)	3–15 ml/h	3 ml/h	
Glyceryl trinitrate	Controlled hypotension	0.9% saline, 5% dextrose	0.5–12 mg/h	50 mg/50 ml (1 mg/ml)	0.5–12 ml/h	5 ml/h	
Heparin	Anticoagulation	0.9% saline, 5% dextrose	24 000–48 000 units per 24 h	50 000 units/50 ml (1000 units/ml)	1–2 ml/h	2 ml/hr	Check APTT after 12 h
Insulin (soluble)	Diabetes mellitus	0.9% saline, haemaccel	Sliding scale	50 units/50 ml (1 unit/ml)	Sliding scale	Sliding scale	See p. 74

Alternative regimes for any infusion: 3 mg/kg/50 ml then 1 ml/hr = 1 µg/kg/min
3 mg/50 ml then 1 ml/hr = 1 µg/min

Drug	Indication	Diluent	Dose	Suggested regime (60 kg adult)	Infusion range	Initial rate (adult)	Comments
Isoprenaline	Treatment of heart block or bradycardia	5% dextrose D. saline	0.5–10 μg/min	1 mg/50 ml (20 μg/ml)	1.5–30 ml/hr	7 ml/h	
Ketamine	General anaesthesia	0.9% saline, 5% dextrose	1–3 mg/kg/h	500 mg/50 ml (10 mg/ml)	6–18 ml/h	10 ml/h	Induction 0.5–2 mg/kg
Ketamine	Analgesia	0.9% saline, 5% dextrose	0.2 mg/kg/h	200 mg/50 ml (4 mg/ml)	0–6 ml/h	3 ml/h	
Ketamine	'Trauma' mixture	0.9% saline	0.5 ml/kg/h	50 ml mixture (4 mg/ml ketamine)	15–45 ml/h	30 ml/h	200 mg ketamine + 10 mg midazolam + 10 mg vecuronium in 50 ml
Lidocaine (lignocaine)	Ventricular arrhythmias	0.9% saline	4 mg/min for 30 min, 2 mg/min for 2 h, then 1 mg/min for 24 h	500 mg/50 ml (10 mg/ml = 1%)	6–24 ml/h	24 ml/h	After 50–100 mg slow IV bolus. ECG monitoring
Milrinone	Inodilator	0.9% saline, 5% dextrose	50 μg/kg over 10 min, then 0.375–0.75 μg/kg/min	10 mg/50 ml (0.2 mg/ml)	7–14 ml/h	90 ml/h for 10 min	Maximum 1.13 mg/kg/day
Mivacurium	Muscle relaxant	0.9% saline, 5% dextrose	0.3–0.6 mg/kg/min	Undiluted (2 mg/ml)	9–18ml/h	18 ml/h	Assess rate with nerve stimulator

Alternative regimes for any infusion: 3 mg/kg/50 ml then 1 ml/hr = 1 μg/kg/min
3 mg/50 ml then 1 ml/hr = 1 μg/min

Drug	Indication	Diluent	Dose	Suggested regime (60 kg adult)	Infusion range	Initial rate (adult)	Comments
Morphine	Analgesia	0.9% saline	0–3.5 mg/h	50 mg/50 ml (1 mg/ml)	0–3.5 ml/h	2 ml/h	Monitor respiration and sedation hourly. Administer oxygen
Naloxone	Opioid antagonist	0.9% saline, 5% dextrose	>1μg/kg/h	2 mg/500 ml (4 μg/ml)			Rate adjusted according to response
Nimodipine	Prevention of vasospasm after subarachnoid	0.9% saline, 5% dextrose	0.5–1 mg/h increasing to 2 mg/h over 2 h	Undiluted (0.2 mg/ml)	2.5–10 ml/h	2.5–5 ml/h	Via central line. Incompatible with polyvinyl chloride
Nitroprusside (sodium)	Controlled hypotension	5% dextrose	0.3–1.5 μg/kg/min	25 mg/50 ml (500 μg/ml)	2–10 ml/h	5 ml/h	Maximum dose 3.5 mg/kg. Protect from light
Noradrenaline	Treatment of hypotension	5% dextrose	2–20 μg/min (0.04–0.4 μg/kg/min)	4 mg/40 ml (100 μg/ml)	1.2–12+ ml/h	5 ml/h	Via central line
Octreotide	Somatostatin analogue	0.9% saline	25–50 μg/h	500 μg/50 ml (10 μg/ml)	2–5 ml/h	5 ml/h	Use in variceal bleeding unlicensed
Oxytocin	Prevention of uterine atony	5% dextrose	0.02–0.04 units/min	20 units in 500 ml (0.04 units/ml)	30–60 ml/h	60 ml/h	
Phenytoin	Anticonvulsant prophylaxis	0.9% saline	15 mg/kg	900 mg/90 ml (administer through 0.22–0.5 μm filter)	Up to 50 mg/min	180 ml/h	ECG and BP monitoring. Complete within 1 h of preparation

Alternative regimes for any infusion: 3 mg/kg/50 ml then 1 ml/hr = 1 μg/kg/min
3 mg/50 ml then 1 ml/hr = 1 μg/min

Drug	Indication	Diluent	Dose	Suggested regime (60 kg adult)	Infusion range	Initial rate (adult)	Comments
Propofol	Anaesthesia		6–10 mg/kg/h	Undiluted (10 mg/ml)	36–60 ml/h		TCI: initially 4–8 μg/ml then 3–6 μg/ml
Propofol	Sedation		0–3 mg/kg/hr	Undiluted (10 mg/ml)	0–20 ml/h		TCI: 0–2.5 μg/ml
Remifentanil	Analgesia during general anaesthesia	0.9% saline, 5% dextrose	0.1–0.5 μg/kg/min	2 mg/40ml (50 μg/ml)	5–40 ml/h IPPV. 2–7 ml/ h SV	8 ml/h IPPV. 2 ml/ h SV	Suggest starting at 0.1 μg/kg/min (8 ml/h) then adjust up to 0.25 μg/kg/min (20 ml/h) as required
Rocuronium	Muscle relaxant	0.9% saline, 5% dextrose	0.3–0.6 mg/kg/h	undiluted (10 mg/ml)	1.5–4 ml/h	3 ml/h	Assess rate with nerve stimulator
Salbutamol	Bronchospasm	5% dextrose	5–20 μg/min	1 mg/50 ml (20 μg/ml)	15–60 ml/h	30 ml/h	After 250 μg slow IV bolus
Sodium bicarbonate	Acidosis		[weight (kg) x base deficit x 0.3] mmol	Undiluted (8.4% solution)			8.4% = 1000 mmol/ litre. Via a central line if possible
Vancomycin	Antibiotic	0.9% saline, 5% dextrose	1 g	1 g/500 ml	500 ml/ 100 min	500 ml/ 100 min	
Vecuronium	Muscle relaxant	0.9% saline, 5% dextrose	0.05–0.08 mg/ kg/h	undiluted (2 mg/ml)	1.5–3 ml/h	2.5 ml/h	Assess rate with nerve stimulator

Alternative regimes for any infusion: 3 mg/kg/50 ml then 1 ml/hr = 1 μg/kg/min
3 mg/50 ml then 1 ml/hr = 1 μg/min

Volatile agents

Appendix 3

	MAC in oxygen (%)	MAC in 66% N$_2$O (%)	Boiling point (°C)	Saturated vapour pressure at 20°C (kPa)	Oil/gas partition coefficient 37°C	Blood/gas partition coefficient 37°C	Molecular weight	Biotransformation %
Desflurane	6	2.8	23.5	88.5	18.7	0.42	168	minimal
Enflurane	1.7	0.65	56.5	22.9	96	1.91	184.5	3
Halothane	0.77	0.29	50.2	32.5	224	2.3	197.4	25
Isoflurane	1.15	0.5	48.5	31.9	91	1.4	184.5	0.2
Sevoflurane	1.71	0.66	58.5	21.3	53	0.59	200	2.5
Nitrous oxide	104	NA	-88	5200	1.4	0.47	44	0

$$CF_3 \quad\quad H$$
$$|\quad\quad\quad\quad |$$
$$H-C-O-C-F$$
$$|\quad\quad\quad\quad |$$
$$CF_3 \quad\quad H$$

sevoflurane

$$F \quad H \quad\quad F$$
$$|\quad\;\; | \quad\quad\;\; |$$
$$F-C-C-O-C-H$$
$$|\quad\;\; | \quad\quad\;\; |$$
$$F \quad Cl \quad\quad F$$

isoflurane

$$F \quad H \quad\quad F$$
$$|\quad\;\; | \quad\quad\;\; |$$
$$F-C-C-O-C-H$$
$$|\quad\;\; | \quad\quad\;\; |$$
$$F \quad F \quad\quad F$$

desflurane

$$F \quad Br$$
$$|\quad\;\; |$$
$$F-C-C-H$$
$$|\quad\;\; |$$
$$F \quad Cl$$

halothane

$$F \quad F \quad\quad F$$
$$|\quad\;\; | \quad\quad\;\; |$$
$$H-C-C-O-C-H$$
$$|\quad\;\; | \quad\quad\;\; |$$
$$Cl \quad F \quad\quad F$$

enflurane

Chemical structure of inhaled anaesthetic agents

Normal values

Vijaya Nathan

ASA classification of physical state

Grade	Description
1	A healthy patient with no systemic disease
2	Mild to moderate systemic disease treated and not limiting patient's activities
3	Severe systemic disturbance imposing definite functional limitation on patient
4	Severe systemic disease which is a constant threat to life
5	Moribund patient unlikely to survive 24 h, with or without surgery

CEPOD classification

Grade	Description of surgery	
1	Elective	Operation at a time to suit both patient and surgeon (e.g. cholecystectomy, joint replacement)
2	Scheduled	An early operation but not immediately life-saving (e.g. malignancy). Operation usually within 3 weeks
3	Urgent	Operation as soon as possible after resuscitation (e.g. irreducible hernia, intestinal obstruction, major fracture). Operation within 24 h
4	Emergency	Immediately life-saving operation, resuscitation simultaneous with surgical treatment (e.g. trauma, ruptured AAA). Operation usually within 1 h

Cardiovascular pressures (mmHg)

	Range	Mean
Central venous pressure (CVP)	0–8	4
Right atrial (RA)	0–8	4
Right ventricular (RV):		
Systolic	14–30	25
End–diastolic (RVEDP)	0–8	4
Pulmonary arterial (PA):		
Systolic	15–30	23
Diastolic	5–15	10
Mean (PAP)	10–20	15
Mean pulmonary artery wedge (PAWP)	5–15	10
Left atrial (LA)	4–12	7
Left ventricular (LV):		
Systolic	90–140	120
End–diastolic (LVEDP)	4–12	7

Arterial/Mixed venous blood gases

	Mixed venous blood gases		Arterial blood gases	
	mmHg	kPa	mmHg	kPa
O_2	37–42	4.93–5.60	90–110	12.00–14.67
CO_2	40–52	5.33–6.93	34–46	4.53–6.13
N_2	573	76.39	573	76.39
pH	7.32–7.42		7.36–7.44	

Lung volumes

	Adult (65 kg)
Dead space (V_D)	2.2 ml/kg
Tidal volume (V_T)	7–10 ml/kg
Alveolar ventilation (V_A)	70 ml/kg/min
Minute ventilation (V_E)	85–100 ml/kg/min
Vital capacity (VC)	50–55 ml/kg
Respiratory rate (RR)	12–18 breaths/min
Total lung capacity (TLC)	5000–6500 ml
Inspiratory reserve volume (IRV)	3300–3750 ml
Expiratory reserve volume (ERV)	950–1200 ml
Functional residual capacity (FRC)	2300–2800 ml
Residual volume (RV)	1200–1700 ml

Derived haemodynamic variables

Variable value	Formula	Normal values
Cardiac output (CO)	SV x HR	4.5–8 litre/min
Cardiac index (CI)	CO/BSA	2.7–4 litre/min/m^2
Stroke volume (SV)	(CO/HR) x 1000	60–130 ml/beat
Stroke volume index (SI)	SV/BSA	38–60 ml/beat/m^2
Systemic vascular resistance (SVR)	80 x (MAP − CVP)/CO	770–1500 dyn s/cm^5
Systemic vascular resistance index (SVRI)	80 x (MAP − CVP)/CI	1860–2500 dyn s/cm^5/m^2
Pulmonary vascular resistance (PVR)	80 x (PAP − PCWP)/CO	100–250 dyn s/cm^5
Pulmonary vascular resistance index (PVRI)	80 x (PAP − PCWP)/CI	225–315 dyn.sec/cm^5/m^2
Left ventricular stroke work index (LVSWI)	SI x MAP x 0.0144	50–62 g.m/m^2/beat
Rate–pressure product (RPP)	SAP x HR	9600
Ejection fraction (EF)	(ESV − EDV)/EDV	>0.6

BSA = body surface area; HR = heart rate; MAP = mean arterial pressure; CVP = central venous pressure; PAP = mean pulmonary arterial pressure; PCWP = pulmonary capillary wedge pressure; SAP = systolic arterial pressure; ESV = end-systolic volume; EDV = end-diastolic volume.

Gas flows in anaesthetic breathing systems

	Spontaneous ventilation	Intermittent positive pressure ventilation
Mapleson A (Lack or Magill)	MV (theoretically V_A) 80 ml/kg/min	2.5 x MV (200 ml/kg /min)
Mapleson D (Bain or coaxial Mapleson D)	(2–3) × MV (150–250 ml/kg/min)	70 ml/kg/min for $PaCO_2$ of 5.3 kPa. 100 ml/kg/ min for PaCO2 of 4.3 kPa
Mapleson E (Ayre's T-piece)	2 × MV	As Mapleson D. Minimum of 3 litre/min fresh gas flow
Mapleson F (Jackson Rees modification of Ayre's T-piece)	As Mapleson E	As Mapleson E

MV = minute ventilation; V_A = alveolar ventilation

Ayre's T-piece system (spontaneous ventilation)

Patient age	Fresh gas flow (litres/min)	Reservoir limb (ml)
0–3 months	3–4	6–12
3–6 months	4–5	12–18
6–12 months	5–6	18–24
1–2 years	6–7	24–42
2–4 years	7–8	42–60

Pulmonary function tests (females)

Age (years)	Height (cm)	FEV$_1$ (litres)	FVC (litres)	FEV$_1$/FVC (%)	PEFR (litre/min)
20	145	2.60	3.13	81.0	377
	152	2.83	3.45	81.0	403
	160	3.09	3.83	81.0	433
	168	3.36	4.20	81.0	459
	175	3.59	4.53	81.0	489
30	145	2.45	2.98	79.9	366
	152	2.68	3.30	79.9	392
	160	2.94	3.68	79.9	422
	168	3.21	4.05	79.9	448
	175	3.44	4.38	79.9	478
40	145	2.15	2.68	77.7	345
	152	2.38	3.00	77.7	371
	160	2.64	3.38	77.7	401
	168	2.91	3.75	77.7	427
	175	3.14	4.08	77.7	457
50	145	1.85	2.38	75.5	324
	152	2.08	2.70	75.5	350
	160	2.34	3.08	75.5	380
	168	2.61	3.45	75.5	406
	175	2.84	3.78	75.5	436
60	145	1.55	2.08	73.2	303
	152	1.78	2.40	73.2	329
	160	2.04	2.78	73.2	359
	168	2.31	3.15	73.2	385
	175	2.54	3.48	73.2	415
70	145	1.25	1.78	71.0	282
	152	1.48	2.10	71.0	308
	160	1.74	2.48	71.0	338
	168	2.01	2.85	71.0	364
	175	2.24	3.18	71.0	394

FEV$_1$ = forced expiratory volume in 1s; FVC = forced vital capacity;
PEFR = peak expiratory flow rate.

Pulmonary function tests (males)

Age (years)	Height (cm)	FEV$_1$ (litres)	FVC (litres)	FEV$_1$/FVC (%)	PEFR (litre/min)
20	160	3.61	4.17	82.5	572
	168	3.86	4.53	82.5	597
	175	4.15	4.95	82.5	625
	183	4.44	5.37	82.5	654
	191	4.69	5.73	82.5	679
30	160	3.45	4.06	80.6	560
	168	3.71	4.42	80.6	584
	175	4.00	4.84	80.6	612
	183	4.28	5.26	80.6	640
	191	4.54	5.62	80.6	665
40	160	3.14	3.84	76.9	536
	168	3.40	4.20	76.9	559
	175	3.69	4.62	76.9	586
	183	3.97	5.04	76.9	613
	191	4.23	5.40	76.9	636
50	160	2.83	3.62	73.1	512
	168	3.09	3.98	73.1	534
	175	3.38	4.40	73.1	560
	183	3.66	4.82	73.1	585
	191	3.92	5.18	73.1	608
60	160	2.52	3.40	69.4	488
	168	2.78	3.76	69.4	509
	175	3.06	4.18	69.4	533
	183	3.35	4.60	69.4	558
	191	3.61	4.96	69.4	579
70	160	2.21	3.18	65.7	464
	168	2.47	3.54	65.7	484
	175	2.75	3.96	65.7	507
	183	3.04	4.38	65.7	530
	191	3.30	4.74	65.7	551

FEV$_1$ = forced expiratory volume in 1 s; FVC = forced vital capacity;
PEFR = peak expiratory flow rate.

Haematology

Measurement	Reference interval	Your hospital
White cell count (WCC)	$4.0-11.0 \times 10^9$/L	
Red cell count	♂$4.5-6.5 \times 10^{12}$/L	
	♀$3.9-5.6 \times 10^{12}$/L	
Haemoglobin	♂$13.5-18.0$ g/dL	
	♀$11.5-16.0$ g/dL	
Packed red cell volume (PCV)	♂$0.4-0.54$ L/L	
or haematocrit	♀$0.37-0.47$ L/L	
Mean cell volume (MCV)	$76-96$ fL	
Mean cell haemoglobin (MCH)	$27-32$ pg	
Mean cell haemoglobin concentration (MCHC)	$30-36$ g/dL	
Neutrophils	$2.0-7.5 \times 10^9$/L	
	$40-75\%$ WCC	
Lymphocytes	$1.3-3.5 \times 10^9$/L	
	$20-45\%$ WCC	
Eosinophils	$0.04-0.44 \times 10^9$/L	
	$1-6\%$ WCC	
Basophils	$0.0-0.10 \times 10^9$/L)	
	0.1% WCC	
Monocytes	$0.2-0.8 \times 10^9$/L	
	$2-10\%$ WCC	
Platelet count	$150-400 \times 10^9$/L	
Reticulocyte count	$0.8-2.0\%$* $25-100 \times 10^9$/L	
Erythrocyte sedimentation rate	depends on age	
Prothrombin time (factors I, II, VII, X)	$10-14$ seconds	
Activated partial thromboplastin time (VIII, IX, XI, XII)	$35-45$ seconds	

* Only use percentages as reference intervals if red cell count is normal; otherwise use the absolute value. Express as a ratio versus control.

For INR values see p. 1088.

Biochemistry

Drugs (and other substances) may interfere with any chemical method; as these effects may be method-dependent, it is difficult for the clinician to be aware of all the possibilities. If in doubt, discuss with the lab.

Substance	Spec-imen	Reference interval	Your hospital
Adrenocorticotrophic hormone	P	<80ng/L	
Alanine aminotransferase (ALT)	P	5–35 iu/L	
Albumin	P¶	35–50 g/L	
Aldosterone	P‡	100–500 pmol/L	
Alkaline phosphatase	P	30–300 iu/L (adults)	
α-amylase	P	0–180 Somogyi u/dL	
α-fetoprotein	S	<10 ku/L	
Angiotensin II	P‡	5–35 pmol/L	
Antidiuretic hormone (ADH)	P	0.9–4.6 pmol/L	
Aspartate transaminase	P	5–35 iu/L	
Bicarbonate	P¶	24–30 mmol/L	
Bilirubin	P	3–17 μmol/L	
Calcitonin	P	<0.1 μg/L	
Calcium (ionized)	P	1.0–1.25 mmol/L	
Calcium (total)	P¶	2.12–2.65 mmol/L	
Chloride	P	95–105 mmol/L	
*Cholesterol	P	3.9–7.8 mmol/L	
VLDL	P	0.128–0.645 mmol/L	
LDL	P	1.55–4.4 mmol/L	
HDL	P	0.9–1.93 mmol/L	
Cortisol	P	a.m. 450–700 nmol/L	
		midnight 80–280 nmol/L	
Creatine kinase (CK)	P	♂ 25–195 iu/L	
		♀ 25–170 iu/L	
Creatinine (∝ to lean body mass)	P¶	70–≤150 mmol/L	
Ferritin	P	12–200 μg/L	
Folate	S	2.1 μg/L	
Follicle-stimulating hormone (FSH)	P/S	2–8 u/L in ♀ (luteal); >25 u/L in menopause	
Gamma-glutamyl transpeptidase	P	♂ 11–51 iu/L	
		♀ 7–33 iu/L	
Glucose (fasting)	P	3.5–5.5 mmol/L	
Glycated (glycosylated) Hb	B	2.3–6.5%	
Growth hormone	P	<20 mu/L	
HbA$_{1c}$ (= glycosylated Hb)	B	2.3–6.5%	
Iron	S	♂ 14–31 μmol/L	
		♀ 11–30 μmol/L	

Lactate dehydrogenase (LDH)	P	70–250 iu/L
Lead	B	<1.8 mmol/L
Luteinizing hormone (LH) (pre-menopausal)	P	3–16 u/L (luteal)
Magnesium	P	0.75–1.05 mmol/L
Osmolality	P	278–305 mosmol/kg
Parathyroid hormone (PTH)	P	<0.8–8.5 pmol/L
Phosphate (inorganic)	P	0.8–1.45 mmol/L
Potassium	P	3.5–5.0 mmol/L
Prolactin	P	♂ <450 u/L; ♀ <600 u/L
Prostate specific antigen	P	0–4 nanograms/mL, p. 653
Protein (total)	P	60–80 g/L
Red cell folate	B	0.36–1.44 μmol/L
		(160–640 μg/L)
Renin (erect/recumbent)	P‡	2.8–4.5/1.1–2.7 pmol/mL/h
Sodium	P	135–145 mmol/L
Thyroid-binding globulin (TBG)	P	7–17 mg/L
Thyroid-stimulating hormone (TSH) NR widens with age	P	0.5–5.7 mu/L
Thyroxine (T₄)	P	70–140 mmol/L
Thyroxine (free)	P	9–22 pmol/L
Total iron binding capacity	S	54–75 μmol/L
Triglyceride	P	0.55–1.90 mmol/L
Tri-iodothyroinine (T₃)	P	1.2–3.0 nmol/L
Urate	P	♂ 210–480 μmol/L
		♀ 150–390 μmol/L
Urea	P	2.5–6.7 mmol/L
Vitamin B₁₂	S	0.13–0.68 nmol/L (>150 ng/L)

* Desired upper limit of cholesterol would be ~ 6 mmol/L.

‡ The sample requires special handling: contact the laboratory.

P = plasma (eg heparin bottle); S = serum (clotted; no anticoagulant);
B = whole blood (edetic acid EDTA bottle)

Checklist for Anaesthetic Apparatus

The following checks should be made prior to each operating session.

1. **Check that the anaesthetic machine is connected to the electricity supply (if appropriate) and switched on.**
   - Take note of any information or labelling on the anaesthetic machine referring to the current status of the machine. Particular attention should be paid to recent servicing. servicing labels should be fixed in the service logbook.

2. **Check that an oxygen analyser is present on the anaesthetic machine.**
   - Ensure that the analyser is switched on, checked and calibrated.
   - The oxygen sensor should be placed where it can monitor the composition of the gases leaving the common gas outlet.

3. **Identify and take note of the gases which are being supplied by pipeline, confirming with a "tug-test" that each pipeline is correctly inserted into the appropriate gas supply terminal.**

   Note: Carbon dioxide cylinders should not be present on the anaesthetic machine unless requested by the anaesthetist. A blanking plug should be fitted to any empty cylinder yoke.
   - Check that the anaesthetic machine is connected to a supply of oxygen and that an adequate supply of oxygen is available from a reserve oxygen cylinder.
   - Check that adequate supplies of other gases (nitrous oxide, air) are available and connected as appropriate.
   - Check that all pipeline pressure gauges in use on the anaesthetic machine indicate 400 kPa.

4. **Check the operation of flowmeters.**
   - Ensure that each flow control valve operates smoothly and that the bobbin moves freely throughout its range.
   - Check the operation of the emergency oxygen bypass control.

5. **Check the vaporiser(s).**
   - Ensure that each vaporiser is adequately but not over filled.
   - Ensure that each vaporiser is correctly seated on the back bar and not tilted.
   - Check the vaporiser for leaks (with vaporiser on and off) by temporarily occluding the common gas outlet.
   - When checks have been completed turn the vaporiser(s) off.
   - A leak test should be performed immediately after changing any vaporiser.

6. **Check the breathing system to be employed.**
   - The system should be visually inspected for correct configuration. All connections should be secured by "push and twist".
   - A pressure leak test should be performed on the breathing system by occluding the patient port and compressing the reservoir bag.
   - The correct operation of unidirectional valves should be carefully checked.

7. **Check that the ventilator is configured appropriately for its intended use.**
   - Ensure that the ventilator tubing is correctly configured and securely attached.
   - Set the controls for use and ensure that an adequate pressure is generated during the inspiratory phase.
   - Check that the pressure relief valve functions.
   - Check that the disconnect alarm functions correctly.
   - Ensure that an alternative means to ventilate the patient's lungs is available.

8. **Check that the anaesthetic gas scavenging system is switched on and is functioning correctly.**
   - Ensure that the tubing is attached to the appropriate expiratory port(s) of the breathing system or ventilator.

9. **Check that all ancillary equipment which may be needed is present and working.**
   - This includes laryngoscopes, intubation aids, intubation forceps, bougies etc. and appropriately sized facemasks, airways, tracheal tubes and connectors.
   - Check that the suction apparatus is functioning and that all connections are secure.
   - Check that the patient can be tilted head-down on the trolley, operating table or bed.

10. **Ensure that the appropriate monitoring equipment is present, switched on and calibrated ready for use.**
    - Set all default alarm limits as appropriate.

      (It may be necessary to place the monitors in the stand-by mode to avoid unnecessary alarms before being connected to the patient.)

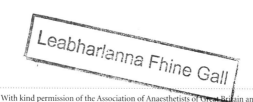

With kind permission of the Association of Anaesthetists of Great Britain and Ireland

Useful web sites

http://www.rcoa.ac.uk/	Royal College of Anaesthetists
http://www.aagbi.org/	Association of Anaesthetists of Great Britain and Ireland
http://www.anzca.edu.au/	Australian and New Zealand College of Anaesthetists
http://www.asahq.org/ homepageie.html	American Society of Anesthesiologists
http://www.bja.oupjournals.org/	British Journal of Anaesthesia
http://www.anesthesiology.org/	Anesthesiology
http://www.anesthesia-analgesia.org/	Anesthesia and Analgesia
http://www.bmj.com/	British Medical Journal
http://www.thelancet.com/	The Lancet
http://www.aaic.net.au/	Anaesthesia & Intensive Care
http://www.esraeurope.org/	European Society of Regional Anaesthesia
http://www.scata.org.uk/	Society of Computing and Technology in Anaesthesia
http://www.pedsanesthesia.org/	Society for Pediatric Anesthesia
http://www.histansoc.org.uk/	History of Anaesthesia Society
http://www.vasgbi.com/	Vascular Anaesthesia Society of Great Britain and Ireland
http://www.oaa-anaes.ac.uk/	Obstetric Anaesthetists Association
http://www.nda.ox.ac.uk/wfsa	World Anaesthesia
http://www.cochrane.org/	Cochrane Collaboration
http://www.virtual-anaesthesia-textbook.com/	Virtual Anaesthesia Textbook
http://www.eguidelines.co.uk/	eGuidelines
http://www.ncbi.nlm.nih.gov/ PubMed/	PubMed
http://www.ohsu.edu/cliniweb/	Cliniweb
http://www.medexplorer.com/	MedExplorer
http://www.medimatch.com	MediMatch
http://www.bma.org.uk	British Medical Association
http://www.mps.org.uk	The Medical Protection Society
http://www.the-mdu.com/	The Medical Defence Union
http://www.mddus.com	The Medical and Dental Defence Union of Scotland

Index